Tongue Lesions

Mahmoud F. Sakr

Tongue Lesions

Diagnostic Challenges and Therapeutic Strategies

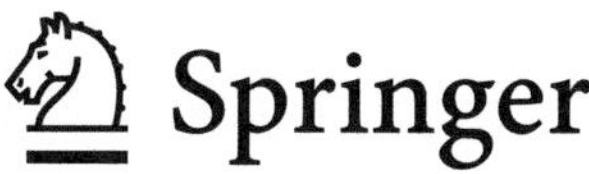

Mahmoud F. Sakr
Faculty of Medicine
Alexandria University
Alexandria, Egypt

ISBN 978-3-031-08197-2 ISBN 978-3-031-08198-9 (eBook)
https://doi.org/10.1007/978-3-031-08198-9

© The Editor(s) (if applicable) and The Author(s), under exclusive license to Springer Nature Switzerland AG 2022
This work is subject to copyright. All rights are solely and exclusively licensed by the Publisher, whether the whole or part of the material is concerned, specifically the rights of translation, reprinting, reuse of illustrations, recitation, broadcasting, reproduction on microfilms or in any other physical way, and transmission or information storage and retrieval, electronic adaptation, computer software, or by similar or dissimilar methodology now known or hereafter developed.
The use of general descriptive names, registered names, trademarks, service marks, etc. in this publication does not imply, even in the absence of a specific statement, that such names are exempt from the relevant protective laws and regulations and therefore free for general use.
The publisher, the authors, and the editors are safe to assume that the advice and information in this book are believed to be true and accurate at the date of publication. Neither the publisher nor the authors or the editors give a warranty, expressed or implied, with respect to the material contained herein or for any errors or omissions that may have been made. The publisher remains neutral with regard to jurisdictional claims in published maps and institutional affiliations.

This Springer imprint is published by the registered company Springer Nature Switzerland AG
The registered company address is: Gewerbestrasse 11, 6330 Cham, Switzerland

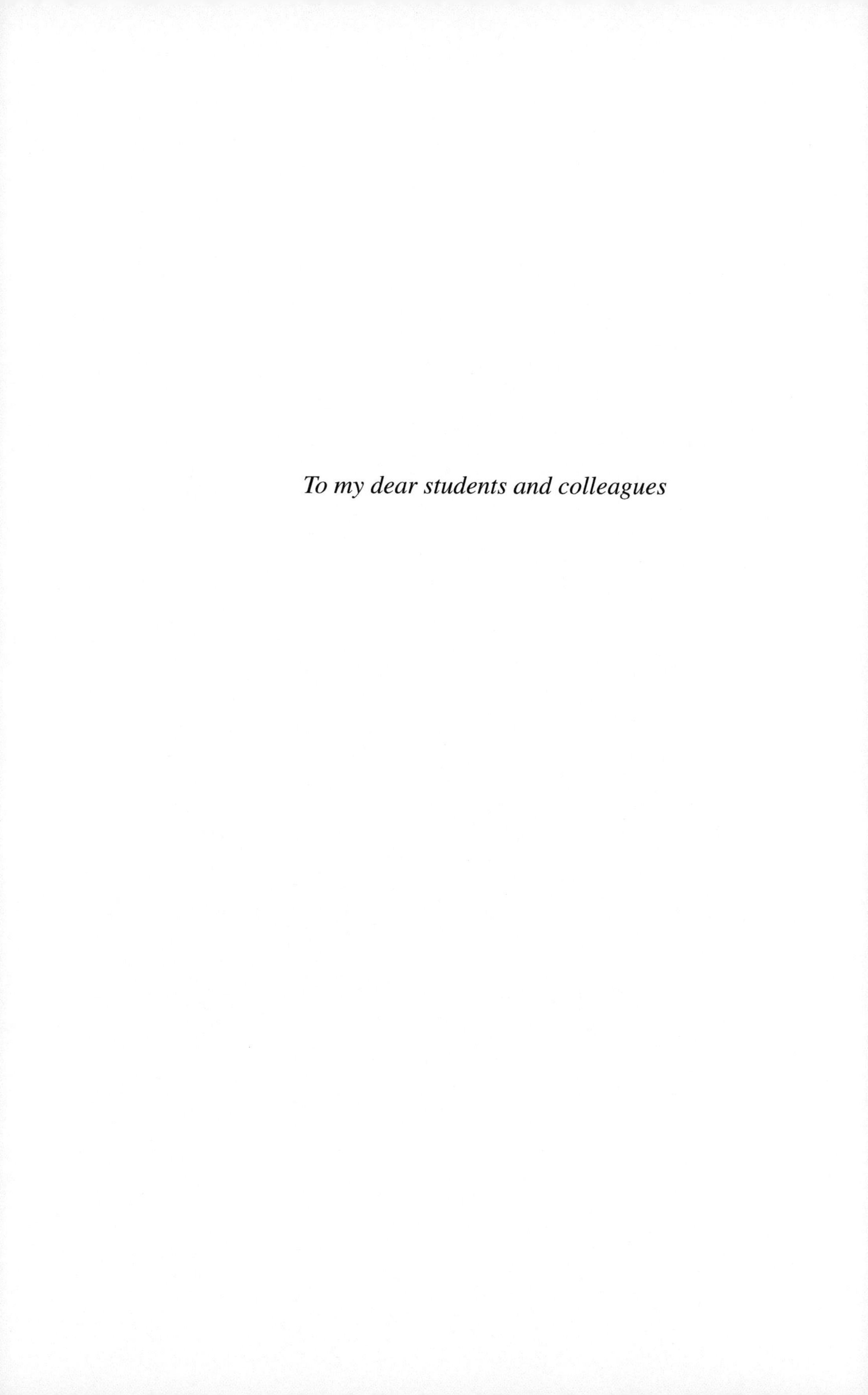

To my dear students and colleagues

Preface

In this authored book, we aim at emphasizing established concepts, displaying the ongoing arguments, controversies, challenges, and debates on diagnosis and treatment of different tongue lesions with a view of clarifying some uncertainties, making suggestions to resolve others, and establishing strategies to reach therapeutic success.

This book, with 1229 references, will provide a valuable source of knowledge and reference for all specialists and trainees entrusted with the care of patients suffering from tongue lesions. It includes 19 chapters, namely, embryology of the tongue, surgical anatomy of the tongue, histology of the tongue, physiology of the tongue, congenital anomalies, tongue trauma, tongue piercing, inflammation (glossitis), swellings of the tongue, neoplastic lesions of the tongue, tongue manifestations of systemic disease, tongue discoloration, tongue fissures, ulcers of the tongue, glossectomy, surgical management of the neck, reconstruction after glossectomy, tongue replantation after trauma, and tongue allo-transplantation.

It is my collective hope that head and neck surgeons, dentists, maxillofacial surgeons, dermatologists, oncologists, pediatricians, and clinicians of other specialties will find this book to be a useful and indispensable resource as they face the most challenging of tongue lesions to help provide individual patients with the best possible functional and esthetic outcome.

Alexandria, Egypt — Mahmoud F. Sakr

Acknowledgments

I would like to thank all those who helped and encouraged me during the writing, editing, and revision of this book. I would like to express my appreciation and gratitude to my wife and children for their continuous support and unconditioned love.

Contents

Embryology of the Tongue

1

1.1 Development of the Tongue

The *pharyngeal apparatus* is the main embryological structure that gives rise to numerous components of the *head and neck region*. It is divided into *arches, pouches, and clefts*, which fuse and reshape throughout early development to give the adult structures of the head and neck. The pharyngeal apparatus begins to form around day 23 of embryonic development and is fully formed by day 28. Subsequently, it begins to transform into the definitive head and neck structures. This is preceded by the formation of the *stomodeum* (primitive mouth) and rupture of the oropharyngeal membrane which separates the stomodeum from the primitive pharynx; thereby allowing communication of the foregut with the amniotic cavity (around day 26 of embryonic development). Within the pouches of the pharyngeal apparatus are neurovascular bundles and mesenchymal tissue that develop into the nerves and blood vessels, and bones and muscles, respectively within the region [1].

1.1.1 Anterior Two-Thirds: From First Arch

Towards the end of the fourth gestational week, the mesenchyme of the ventromedial aspect of the first pharyngeal arches begins to proliferate in the floor of the primitive pharynx to form the median lingual swelling (*tuberculum impar*). This triangular protuberance is located cranial to the *foramen cecum* (opening of the thyroglossal duct) and is later joined by the two distal tongue buds (lateral lingual swellings) that arise on either side of the median lingual swelling.

The rate of growth of the lateral lingual swellings exceeds that of the median lingual swelling. By the fifth to sixth gestational week, they outgrow the median lingual swelling and fuse in the midline to form the *oral part of the tongue*. The

© The Author(s), under exclusive license to Springer Nature Switzerland AG 2022
M. F. Sakr, *Tongue Lesions*, https://doi.org/10.1007/978-3-031-08198-9_1

fibrous lingual septum represents the point of fusion of the two lateral lingual swellings, which lies deep to the midline groove (a central groove along the longitudinal axis) of the tongue [2].

1.1.2 Posterior Third: From Third Arch

Caudal to the foramen cecum, two mesenchymal derivatives arise from the ventromedial part of the second to the fourth pharyngeal arches. The *copula linguae* are the product of the second pharyngeal arches, while the hypopharyngeal eminence, which develops below the copula, arises from the third and fourth pharyngeal arches. Similar to the lateral lingual swellings, the hypopharyngeal eminences grow at a faster rate than the copula. As a result, the copula regresses between the fourth and fifth week of development and the hypopharyngeal eminence becomes the *pharyngeal part* of the tongue.

The oral and pharyngeal parts of the tongue eventually fuse, forming a V-shaped junction known as the *sulcus terminalis*. While the connective tissue and vascular supply of the tongue mostly originate from the preceding pharyngeal arches, the intrinsic and extrinsic muscles are myoblast derivatives that originate from the *occipital myotomes* [2].

The tongue and the *hard palate* also develop simultaneously. It contributes to moulding the palate into the arched structure that it eventually becomes during post-natal life.

Most of the morphological changes of the tongue occur during the first trimester of pregnancy. By the second trimester and into extrauterine life, the rest of the changes are related to elongation and repositioning of the organ. Both the pre-sulcal and post-sulcal parts of the tongue are within the oral cavity proper at birth. Caudal migration of the posterior third of the tongue is *not* completed until the age of 4 years [3].

1.2 Development of Taste Buds and PapillaE

The coarse texture of the dorsal surface of the tongue can be attributed to the numerous lingual papillae that are found on its surface. Close to the end of the eighth gestational week, *foliate* and *vallate papillae* are the first of the 4 papillae to develop, followed by the appearance of *fungiform* papillae. By the 10th–11th week of gestation, the thread-like *filiform* papillae can be observed on the dorsal surface of the tongue. Each type of papillae has a particular role in tongue physiology, and as such, has a unique innervation based on the nerve endings they developed closest to [4].

The development of *taste buds* begins as the last of the papillae are formed in the 11th week of gestation. Their formation is influenced by the invading special sensory nerve fibers and inductive factors from the surrounding epithelium. Although the majority of these specialized gustatory receptors will develop on the dorsum of the tongue, they also arise on the hard and soft palates, dorsum of the epiglottis, palatoglossal arches, and the posterior oropharyngeal wall. Taste bud development is concluded around the 13th week of gestation [4].

1.3 Development of the Nerve Supply

Owing to the fact that each pharyngeal arch has its own neurovascular bundle, the derivatives of these pouches will also take their nerve supply from these sources. The *mandibular division of the trigeminal nerve* (*CN-V3*) carries sensory impulses arising from the derivatives of the first pharyngeal arch. Since this arch gives rise to the tuberculum impar and lateral lingual swellings (which forms the oral part of the tongue), the mucosa of this entire area sends afferent impulses via the lingual branch of CN-V3 [5].

Although the second pharyngeal arch does *not* contribute to a visible structure on the surface of the tongue, a part of its nerve supply—the *chorda tympani*; a branch of the *facial nerve* (*CN-VII*)—carries special afferent signals from the taste buds (excluding vallate papillae) of the pre-sulcal part of the tongue. Vallate papillae and mucosa of the post-sulcal part pass afferent stimuli to the *glossopharyngeal nerve* (*CN-IX*), which is the nerve of the third pharyngeal arch. This innervation is also supplemented by the nerve of the fourth pharyngeal arch (*vagus nerve-CN-X*), which carries the sensory stimuli from the base of the tongue that is anterior to the epiglottis [5].

Since both intrinsic and extrinsic *muscles* of the tongue arise from occipital myotomes that migrated ventrally to populate the developing tongue, the migrating myocytes take the *hypoglossal nerve* (*CN-XII*) along with it. Therefore, the hypoglossal nerve provides efferent stimuli to all the muscles of the tongue except the *palato-glossus*, which has a vagal nerve (CN-X) supply [6, 7].

1.4 Summary of Tongue Development

- Development of the tongue begins toward the end of the fourth gestational week.
- The anterior two-thirds of the organ is known as the pre-sulcal (oral) part, and the posterior third is the post-sulcal (pharyngeal) part.
- The pre-sulcal tongue originates from the first pharyngeal arch, while the post-sulcal part arises from the third and fourth pharyngeal arches.
- Neither the tuberculum impar (from the first pharyngeal arch) nor the copula (second pharyngeal arch) contributes to structures of the adult tongue.
- The pre-sulcal tongue has lingual papillae and taste buds; while the post-sulcal part has lingual tonsils and taste buds.
- Innervation of the tongue is dependent on the pharyngeal arch that the area was derived from.

References

1. Yamane A. Embryonic and postnatal development of masticatory and tongue muscles. Cell Tissue Res. 2005;322:183–9.
2. Hong SJ, Cha BG, Kim YS, Lee SK, Chi JG. Tongue growth during prenatal development in korean fetuses and embryos. J Pathol Transl Med. 2015;49:497–510.
3. Achiron R, Ben Arie A, Gabbay U, Mashiach S, Rotstein Z, Lipitz S. Development of the fetal tongue between 14 and 26 weeks of gestation: in utero ultrasonographic measurements. Ultrasound Obstet Gynecol. 1997;9:39–41.
4. Kim JY, Lee MJ, Cho KW, Lee JM, Kim YJ, Kim JY, Jung HI, Cho JY, Cho SW, Jung HS. Shh and ROCK1 modulate the dynamic epithelial morphogenesis in circumvallate papilla development. Dev Biol. 2009;325:273–80.
5. Mu L, Sanders I. Human tongue neuroanatomy: nerve supply and motor endplates. Clin Anat. 2010;23:777–91.
6. Smith JC, Goldberg SJ, Shall MS. Phenotype and contractile properties of mammalian tongue muscles innervated by the hypoglossal nerve. Respir Physiol Neurobiol. 2005;147:253–62.
7. Alves P. Imaging the hypoglossal nerve. Eur J Radiol. 2010;74:368–77.

Surgical Anatomy of the Tongue

2

2.1 Overview: Key Facts About the Tongue

The tongue (Latin, *lingua*; Greek, *glos sa*) is a unique organ located in the oral cavity. It has importance in the digestive system and is the primary organ of taste in the gustatory system. It also plays important roles in mastication and deglutition. Additionally, the tongue is an integral component of the speech pathway, as it helps with articulation. Typically, the length of a human tongue is around 3.3 in. (8.5 cm) for men and 3.1 in. (7.9 cm) for women [1].

The tongue is embryologically divided into an anterior and a posterior part. The anterior part of the tongue is also called the *oral or pre-sulcal* part of the tongue. The posterior part of the tongue is referred to as the *pharyngeal or post-sulcal* part of the tongue. The left and right sides of the tongue are separated along most of its length by a vertical section of fibrous tissue (*lingual septum*) that results in a groove, the *median sulcus*, on the tongue's surface. The *base of the tongue* refers to the post-sulcal part that forms the ventral wall of the oropharynx, while the *root of the tongue* refers to a part of the pre-sulcal tongue that is attached to the floor of the oral cavity.

There are four paired intrinsic muscles of the tongue; they are named by the direction in which they travel: the superior longitudinal, inferior longitudinal, transverse, and vertical muscles. These muscles affect the shape and size of the tongue. There are also four paired extrinsic muscles, namely genioglossus, hyoglossus, styloglossus, and palatoglossus. All of the intrinsic and extrinsic muscles are innervated by the hypoglossal nerve (CN-XII) except the palatoglossus, which has a vagal innervation (CN-X) [1].

Most of the arterial supply to the tongue is provided by the lingual artery, a branch of the external carotid artery, and drainage is by the lingual vein. Lymphatics of the anterior two-thirds of the tongue drain initially into the submental and submandibular lymph nodes (LNs), which empty into the deep cervical LNs, which also receive direct drainage from the posterior third.

In the anterior two-thirds of the tongue, *general sensation* is supplied by the trigeminal nerve (CN-V), specifically the lingual branch of the submandibular nerve

© The Author(s), under exclusive license to Springer Nature Switzerland AG 2022

M. F. Sakr, *Tongue Lesions*, https://doi.org/10.1007/978-3-031-08198-9_2

Table 2.1 Key facts about the tongue [1, 2]

Embryology	Starts with day 23 of conception
Parts	Tip (apex), body, base
Surfaces	Dorsal (superior) and ventral (inferior)
Relations	• *Anterior and lateral*—Teeth • *Superior*—hard and soft palates • *Inferior*—mucosa of the floor of the oral cavity, sublingual salivary glands, posterior wall of oropharynx • *Posterior*—epiglottis, pharyngeal inlet • *Lateral*—Palatoglossal and palatopharyngeal arches
Muscles	• *Intrinsic*—superior longitudinal, vertical, transverse, inferior longitudinal • *Extrinsic*—genioglossus, hypoglossus, styloglossus, palatoglossus
Blood supply	Lingual artery (dorsal lingual, sublingual, deep lingual arteries), ascending palatine, tonsillar, ascending pharyngeal arteries
Lymphatics	Marginal, central, dorsal, submandibular, jugulo-omohyoid, deep cervical lymph nodes.
Innervation	Hypoglossal nerve (CN-XII), pharyngeal plexus, lingual nerve, glossopharyngeal nerve (CN-IX), facial nerve (CN-VII), vagus nerve (CN-X), chorda tympani
Mucosa	Stratified squamous keratinized (dorsal surface) and nonkeratinized (ventral surface) epithelia
Lingual papillae	Filiform, fungiform, foliate, and circumvallate
Taste buds	• *Epithelium*—stratified squamous • *Structure—gustatory cells, supportive cells, basal stem cells, taste pore*

CN Cranial nerve

(CN-V3), while *taste sensation* is supplied by the facial nerve (CN-VII) via the chorda tympani, which arises from the facial nerve in the petrous part of the temporal bone, travels through the middle ear, and continues on to the tongue. In the posterior third of the tongue, both general and taste sensations are supplied by the glossopharyngeal nerve (CN-IX) [2].

The anatomical key facts about the tongue are summarized in Table 2.1.

2.2 Structure of the Tongue

The tongue is a pink, muscular organ located within the oral cavity proper. It is kept moist by the products of the major and minor salivary glands, which aid the tongue as it facilitates deglutition, speech, and gustatory perception. While there is significant variability in the length of the tongue among individuals, on average, the organ is roughly 10-cm long. The tongue has three main parts as follows [3–5].

- *The tip or apex* of the tongue is the most anterior and most mobile aspect of the organ.
- *The body* of the tongue follows the tip and has a rough dorsal (superior) surface that abuts the palate and is populated with taste buds and lingual papillae, and a

smooth ventral (inferior) surface that is attached to the floor of the oral cavity by the lingual frenulum.
- *The base* of the tongue is the most posterior part. It is populated by numerous lymphoid aggregates (*the lingual tonsils*) along with foliate papillae along the posterolateral surface.

2.2.1 Important Relations

There are many important structures surrounding the tongue, which is limited *anteriorly* and *laterally* by the upper and lower rows of teeth. *Superiorly*, it is bordered by the hard (anterior part) and soft (posterior part) palates. *Inferiorly*, the root of the tongue is continuous with the mucosa of the floor of the oral cavity; with the sublingual salivary glands and vascular bundles being located below the mucosa of the floor of the oral cavity.

The palatoglossal and palatopharyngeal arches (and palatine tonsils) have *lateral* relations to the posterior third of the tongue. Posterior to the base of the tongue is the dorsal surface of the epiglottis and laryngeal inlet, and the posterior wall of the oropharynx. As mentioned earlier, the pre-sulcal and post-sulcal parts of the tongue differ based on not only anatomical location but also embryological origin, innervation, and the type of mucosa found on its surface [3–5].

2.2.2 Anterior Two-Thirds

The pre-sulcal tongue includes the apex and body of the organ. It terminates at the sulcus terminalis; which can be seen extending laterally in an oblique direction from the foramen cecum towards the palatoglossal arch. The mucosa of the dorsal surface of the oral tongue is made up of circumvallate, filiform, and fungiform papillae (Fig. 2.1). There is a longitudinal midline groove running in an anteroposterior direction from the tip of the tongue to the foramen cecum. This marks the embryological point of fusion of the lateral lingual swellings that formed the oral tongue. It also represents the location of the median lingual (fibrous) septum of the tongue that inserts in the body of the hyoid bone [3–5].

2.2.3 Terminal Sulcus (Sulcus Terminalis Linguae)

On the lateral surface of the oral tongue are foliate papillae arranged as a series of vertical folds. The ventral mucosa of the oral tongue is comparatively unremarkable. It is smooth and continuous with the mucosa of the floor of the mouth and the inferior gingiva. The lingual veins are relatively superficial and can be appreciated on either side of the lingual frenulum. Lateral to the lingual veins are pleated folds of mucosa known as the *plica fimbriata*. They are angled anteromedially toward the apex of the tongue [3–5].

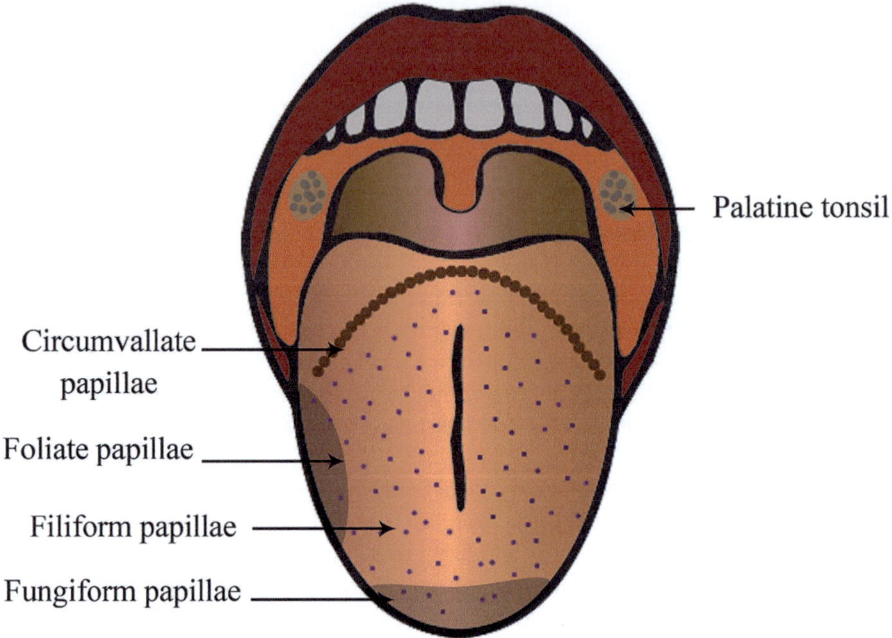

Fig. 2.1 Tongue papillae on the dorsal surface of the anterior two-thirds of the tongue. Note also the palatine tonsils

2.2.4 Posterior Third

The remainder of the tongue that lies posterior to the sulcus terminalis is made up by the base of the organ. It lies behind the palatoglossal folds and functions as the anterior wall of the oropharynx. Unlike the oral tongue, the pharyngeal tongue does *not* have lingual papillae. Instead, its mucosa is populated by aggregates of lymphatic tissue known as the *lingual tonsils*. The mucosa is also continuous with that of the laterally located palatine tonsils, the lateral oropharyngeal walls, and the posterior epiglottis and glosso-epiglottic folds [3–5].

2.2.5 Lingual Frenulum

Frenulum is a general term for a small fold of integument (skin) or mucous membrane that limits the movements of an organ or part. There are several anatomical frenula associated with the genital system, while the lingual frenulum is associated with the inferior side of the tongue.

The short length of the lingual frenulum and its anterior position of insertion can lead to speech disorders and may affect postnatal feeding [6]. It is the prevalence of pain in mothers breastfeeding infants with ankyloglossia that presents many problems in breastfeeding [7].

Children with a frenulum length of more than 2 cm do not show speech problems. Ankyloglossia (tongue-tie) is the general clinical term for the short frenulum, which limits the range of movement of the tongue. There is still no accurate classification for this condition (ankyloglossia) [8]. Frenotomy, frenectomy, and frenuloplasty are the main surgical treatment options to release or remove an ankyloglossia.

2.2.6 Muscles of the Tongue

The tongue is chiefly a muscular organ with some amount of fatty and fibrous tissue distributed throughout its substance. All the muscles of the tongue are paired structures, with each copy being found on either side of the median fibrous septum. There are muscles that extend outside of the organ to anchor it to the surrounding bony structures known as *extrinsic muscles*. The other set of muscles are confined to each half of the organ and contribute to altering the shape of the organ; these are the *intrinsic muscles*.

2.2.6.1 Intrinsic Tongue Muscles

The intrinsic tongue muscles are responsible for adjusting the shape and orientation of the organ. There are *four paired intrinsic muscles*, which are discussed below in a dorsoventral manner and summarized in Table 2.2.

Table 2.2 Intrinsic Muscles of the Tongue

Summary of intrinsic muscles of the tongue	
Superior longitudinal	• *Origin*: Submucosa of posterior tongue, lingual septum • *Insertion*: Apex/anterolateral margins of tongue • *Innervation*: Hypoglossal nerve (CN-XII) • *Blood supply*: Lingual branch of external carotid artery (ECA) • *Action:* Retracts and broadens tongue, elevates apex of tongue
Inferior longitudinal	• *Origin*: Root of tongue, body of hyoid bone • *Insertion*: Apex of tongue • *Innervation*: Hypoglossal nerve • *Blood supply*: Lingual branch of ECA • *Action*: Retracts and broadens tongue, lowers apex of tongue
Transverse muscle	• Origin: Lingual septum • *Insertion*: Lateral margin of tongue • *Innervation*: Hypoglossal nerve • *Blood supply*: Lingual branch ECA • *Action*: Narrows and elongates tongue
Vertical muscle	• Origin: Root of tongue, genioglossus muscle • Insertion: Lingual aponeurosis • Innervation: Hypoglossal nerve • Blood supply: Lingual branch of ECA • *Action*—broadens and elongates tongue

The intrinsic tongue muscles can operate independently or in combination with each other to give rise to numerous shapes. This is an important feature of the tongue as it facilitates molding of the food particles into a bolus in preparation for deglutition and speech.

1. *Superior longitudinal muscles* (musculus longitudinalis superior linguae): These are made up of a thin layer of muscle fibers that travel in a mixture of oblique and longitudinal axes just deep to the superior mucosal surface of the tongue. They arise from the median fibrous septum and the fibrous layer of submucosa from the level of the epiglottis. They insert along the lateral and apical margins of the organ. These muscles are responsible for retracting and broadening the tongue, as well as elevating the tip of the tongue. The net effect of these muscles results in shortening of the organ.
2. *Vertical muscles*: These are a set of muscles that occupy the dorsoventral plane of the tongue deep to the superior longitudinal muscles. They arise from the root of the tongue and genioglossus muscle and insert into the median fibrous septum, along the entire length of the organ. These muscles facilitate flattening and widening of the tongue.
3. *Transverse muscles*: These muscles are deep to the ventral muscles of the tongue. They take a lateral route, extending from either side of the medial lingual septum (origin) to the fibrous submucosa along the lateral margins of the tongue (insertion). As these muscles contract, they cause the tongue to narrow and elongate.
4. *Inferior longitudinal muscles*: These muscles travel above the ventral submucosa of the tongue. These fibers travel between the hyoglossus and genioglossus muscles as they arise from the base of the tongue and body of the hyoid bone. The fibers end in the apex of the tongue; allowing the muscle to pull the tip of the tongue inferiorly and also shortening the organ.

2.2.6.2 Extrinsic Tongue Muscles

While the *shape* of the tongue is determined by the intrinsic muscles, *movement* of the tongue within and out of the oral cavity is dependent on the extrinsic tongue muscles. There are four pairs of extrinsic muscles that originate outside the tongue and insert into the body of the tongue. They can be viewed as those arising from *above* the tongue (styloglossus and palatoglossus muscles), and those that originate from *below* the tongue (hyoglossus and genioglossus muscles) [9].

The extrinsic muscles play an important role in pressing and molding the food bolus in preparation for the initial phase of swallowing. Additionally, they are used to move the bolus posteriorly into the oropharyngeal inlet. Furthermore, the action of palatoglossus closes off the oropharyngeal isthmus in order to prevent food from moving cranially during swallowing. Although some of these muscles are able to act in isolation, it is the combined effect of all the intrinsic and extrinsic muscles that allows the tongue to have significant flexibility. Extrinsic muscles of the tongue are summarized in Table 2.3 [9].

Table 2.3 Extrinsic muscles of the tongue

Summary of extrinsic muscles of the tongue	
Palatoglossus	• *Origin*: Palatine aponeurosis of soft palate • *Insertion*: Lateral margins of tongue, blends with intrinsic muscles of tongue • *Innervation*: Vagus nerve (CN-X) (via branches of pharyngeal plexus) • *Blood supply*: Ascending palatine branch of facial artery, ascending pharyngeal artery • *Action*: Elevates root of tongue, constricts isthmus of fauces
Styloglossus	• *Origin*: Anterolateral aspect of styloid process (of temporal bone), stylomandibular ligament • *Insertion:* Blends with inferior longitudinal muscle (longitudinal part); blends with hyoglossus muscle (oblique part) • *Innervation*: Hypoglossal nerve (CN-XII) • *Blood supply*: Sublingual branch of lingual artery • *Action*: Retracts and elevates lateral aspects of tongue
Genioglossus	• *Origin*: Superior mental spine of mandible • *Insertion*: Entire length of dorsum of tongue, lingual aponeurosis, body of hyoid bone • *Innervation*: Hypoglossal nerve (CN-XII) • *Blood supply*: Sublingual branch of lingual artery, submental branch of facial artery • *Action*: Depresses and protrudes tongue (bilateral contraction), deviates tongue contralaterally (unilateral contraction)
Hyoglossus	• *Origin*: Body and greater horn of hyoid bone • *Insertion*: Inferior/ventral parts of lateral tongue • *Innervation*: Hypoglossal nerve (CN-XII) • *Blood supply*: Sublingual branch of lingual artery, submental branch of facial artery • *Action*: Depresses and retracts tongue

1. *Palatoglossus muscle:* It is anatomically a part of the pharyngeal group of muscles. However, its attachments to the tongue mean that it is also an extrinsic tongue muscle. It originates from the oral part of the aponeurosis of the soft palate. Here, and also at its insertion in the lateral margins of tongue, the muscle is wider than along its middle section. Its role as an extrinsic tongue muscle is to elevate the dorsal surface of the tongue, and to act as a sphincter at the oropharyngeal isthmus (by working synergistically with the contralateral palatoglossus).
2. *Styloglossus muscle:* It originates from the anterolateral surface of the styloid process. It contributes to the stylomandibular ligament and assists in retraction of the tongue (moving it posterosuperiorly). It is the smallest and shortest of the three styloid muscles. At the lateral margin of the tongue, the muscle bifurcates into longitudinal and oblique components. The former pierces the tongue on the dorsolateral aspect and integrates with the inferior longitudinal muscle; while the latter crosses over and decussates with hyoglossus.
3. *Genioglossus muscle:* It originates from a slender tendon that is attached to the superior genial tubercle found on the inner surface of the symphysis menti. This attachment prevents the tongue from falling backward and obstructing the air-

way when an individual is in the supine position. The lower fibers of the muscle also have indirect attachments to the anterior part of the body of the hyoid bone via its slender aponeurosis. It is a triangular, midline structure that travels posterosuperiorly at which point the upper fibers of the muscle interdigitate with the intrinsic muscles, before attaching along the length of the inferior surface of the tongue (extending from the root to the tip).

4. *Hyoglossus* muscle: It originates from the entire greater cornu of the hyoid bone as a slender, quadrilateral muscle. It is often accompanied by the chondroglossus muscle (may be considered as part of the hyoglossus), which arises from the base of the lesser cornu of the hyoid bone. The hyoglossus muscle takes a vertical course cranially, where it pierces the inferolateral margins of the tongue and subsequently blends between the inferior longitudinal muscles and the styloglossus.

A particular pharyngeal arch defect (known as *Pierre Robin Syndrome*) causes *glossoptosis* among other symptoms. This defect causes the tongue to be displaced posteriorly and may cause airway obstruction or apnea.

2.3 Blood Supply and Lymphatic Drainage

2.3.1 Arterial Supply

The vascular supply to the tongue muscles is provided by derivatives of the *lingual artery*, a branch of the external carotid artery (ECA) that arises at the tip of the greater cornu of the hyoid bone. It traverses the region between the middle pharyngeal constrictor and hyoglossus in order to access the floor of the mouth. It takes a sharp superior turn at the anterior border of hyoglossus as it travels alongside the glossopharyngeal nerve (CN-IX). The tongue has a good collateral supply as the lingual artery also anastomosis with the contralateral vessel [10].

The course of the lingual artery is divided into three parts by the hyoglossus muscle; (1) the first part lies in the carotid triangle, (2) the second part lies deep to the hyoglossus along the upper border of the hyoid bone, and (3) the third part is called the *deep lingual artery* or arteria profunda, where the lingual artery terminates near the lingual frenulum on the ventral surface of the tongue. The lingual artery is supported by other branches of the ECA. The *facial artery* gives off the ascending *palatine and tonsillar arteries* that also supply the tongue. The *ascending pharyngeal branch* of the ECA also supplies the organ [10].

The named branches of the lingual artery are the dorsal lingual artery and the sublingual artery [10].

1. *Dorsal Lingual Artery*

   It is a relatively small branch that originates medial to the hyoglossus muscle. It supplies the dorsal mucosa of the tongue, and gives branches to the palatoglossus, soft palate, palatine tonsils, and epiglottis.

2. *Sublingual Artery*

   It emerges at the anterior limit of the hyoglossus and courses between the mylohyoid and genioglossus as it travels towards the sublingual glands in the floor of the oral cavity. As it arborizes, one of its branches anastomoses with the submental branches of the facial artery, while another traverses the gingiva of the mandible to anastomose with the analogous contralateral vessel.

2.3.2 Venous Drainage

The veins of the tongue are named similarly to the arteries that they accompany. They are formed from numerous venous tributaries that eventually coalesce. As the *deep lingual vein* forms adjacent to the apex of the tongue, it courses along the ventral surface of the tongue (deep to the mucosa). As the deep lingual vein anastomosis with the *sublingual vein*, they become the *vena commitants of CN-XII*. This venous network eventually drains to the *lingual vein* that later joins the *facial* or the *anterior division of the retromandibular* veins. Here, they form the *common facial vein*, which is a tributary to the *internal jugular vein* (IJV). Alternatively, the venae comitantes may drain directly to the IJV [10].

The *dorsal lingual veins* are responsible for draining the lateral margins and dorsal surface of the tongue. They travel alongside the similarly named artery as they drain into the IJV [8].

2.3.3 Lymphatic Drainage

When discussing the lymphatic drainage of the tongue, it helps to group them according to the region of the tongue that they drain. The marginal and central groups drain the anterior parts of the tongue, while the dorsal group drains lymph from the posterior third of the organ. It is not uncommon to see the central area of the tongue draining to both marginal and dorsal groups of lymph vessels.

The marginal lymph vessels will carry lymph to the submandibular lymph nodes (LNs) or to the jugulo-omohyoid LNs. It is not uncommon to see lymph vessels decussating to drain to contralateral LNs. The vessels from the central region may go to the deep cervical nodes, with a particular preference for the jugulo-omohyoid or jugulo-digastric nodes. The dorsal group of vessels also passes laterally on either side to eventually join the marginal vessels in their course to the jugulo-omohyoid and jugulo-digastric vessels (Fig. 2.2).

Thus, lymphatic drainage from the oral tongue is primarily to levels I through III of the neck. This includes the submental (level Ia) and submandibular (level Ib) LN basins, as well as the upper and middle jugular chain neck lymphatics (levels II and III, respectively). Lymphatic drainage from the *tongue base* is primarily to levels II through IV (lower jugular chain) [11, 12]. Understanding lymphatics is important in locoregional control of tongue cancers.

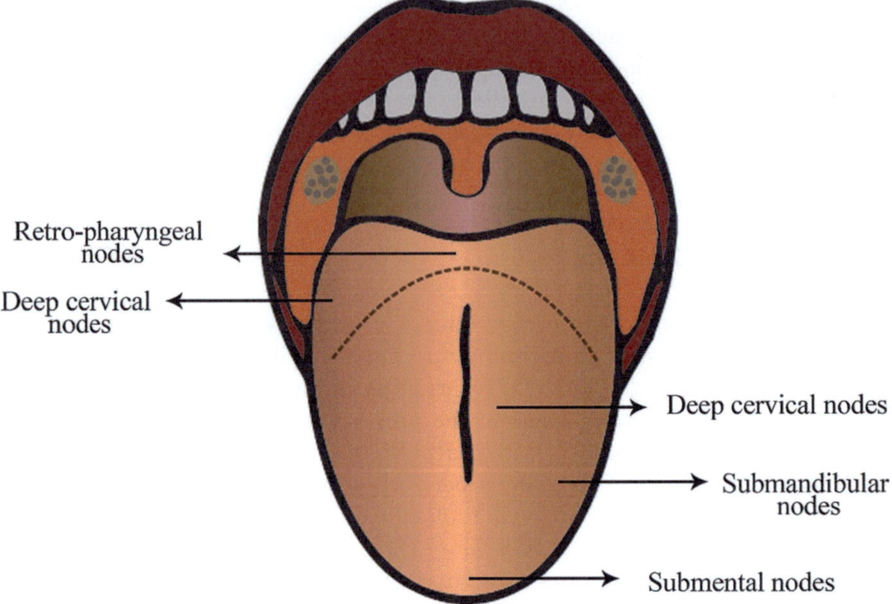

Fig. 2.2 Lymphatic drainage of the tongue. Note that the mid-dorsum and tip of the tongue can drain into lymph nodes on both sides of the neck

2.4 Innervation of the Tongue

The tongue has multiple sources of innervation based on its embryological origins. The nerve supply to the tongue can be grouped based on *efferent fibers* that carry motor impulses, general sensory that conveys touch and proprioception, and special *afferent* that conveys gustatory (taste) impulses.

The human tongue innervation has recently been analyzed histologically and has been described as being extremely dense and complex [13]. Clinically, the nerve pathway of the tongue can be divided into the following regions: intra-axial, cisternal, skull base, and extracranial segments [14].

2.4.1 Motor Innervation: The Hypoglossal Nerve (CN-XII)

The muscles of the tongue arise from occipital myotomes that migrated to the floor of the pharyngeal apparatus during development. These primitive myocytes took the fibers of the hypoglossal nerve (Nervus Hypoglossus) (CN-XII) along with them during their journey. As a result, the hypoglossal nerve provides motor innervation to all muscles of the tongue, except the palatoglossus. Motor units within the hypoglossal motor system can be categorized as predominantly "fast fatigue-resistant" [15].

The hypoglossal nerve originates from the hypoglossal nucleus and exits the skull base through the hypoglossal canal. Once in the neck, it crosses anterior to the internal and external carotid arteries and can be seen deep to the posterior belly of the digastric muscle. It can often be found inferior to the digastric muscle as it proceeds anteriorly, putting it at risk for injury during dissection of cervical levels IB and IIA. The nerve proceeds superomedially deep to the mylohyoid muscle to innervate the intrinsic and extrinsic tongue muscles. As the hypoglossal nerve pierces the ventrolateral part of the pharyngeal tongue, it gives a branch to the *geniohyoid* muscle. Subsequently, it bifurcates into medial and lateral branches. The medial branch innervates the posterior part of the transverse and vertical muscles, as well as the medial part of the inferior longitudinal muscle, and the entire genioglossus. The lateral branch innervates the lateral part of the inferior longitudinal, superior longitudinal, hyoglossus, and styloglossus muscles.

While there is an agreement regarding the fact that the pharyngeal plexus brings motor fibers to the muscle, there is still some discrepancy regarding which component of the pharyngeal plexus (i.e. cranial part of accessory nerve [CN-XI] or the vagus nerve [CN-X]) that the fibers arise from. Some sources state that CN-XI piggybacks on CN-X to supply palatoglossus. However, others consider absence of hitchhiking, and that CN-X is the nerve that supplies the palatoglossus. The nucleus ambiguus provides efferent fibers that innervate the skeletal muscles of the soft palate. Whether or not these fibers travel via CN-X or CN-XI is still uncertain.

2.4.2 Tactile Sensory Innervation: The Lingual Nerve (CN-V3)

The lingual nerve (*nervus lingualis*) is a branch of the *trigeminal verve* (CN-V3). It lies at first beneath the lateral pterygoid muscle, medial to, and in front of the inferior alveolar nerve, and is occasionally joined to this nerve by a branch which may cross the artery. The chorda tympani (a branch of the facial nerve, CN VII) joins it at an acute angle here, carrying taste fibers from the anterior two-thirds of the tongue and parasympathetic fibers to the submandibular ganglion.

The lingual nerve then passes between the medial pterygoid muscle and the ramus of the mandible, and crosses obliquely to the side of the tongue beneath the constrictor pharyngis superior and styloglossus, and then between the hyoglossus and deep part of the submandibular gland; it finally runs from laterally to medially inferiorly crossing the duct of the submandibular gland, and along the tongue to its tip becoming the sublingual nerve, lying immediately beneath the mucous membrane.

The lingual nerve is responsible for conveying general somatic afferent impulses from the anterior two-thirds of the tongue. Additionally, it also carries sensory information from the oral mucosa beneath the ventral surface of the tongue and the gingival mucosa of the lingual side of the mandible. General afferent impulses from the circumvallate papillae, along with the posterior third of the tongue, are carried by fibers of the glossopharyngeal nerve (CN-IX).

The lingual nerve is best considered as a "*two-way nerve*":

1. *General sensory:* anterior two-thirds of the tongue.
2. *Taste (Gustatory)* (via the chorda tympani): anterior two-thirds of the tongue.
3. *Secretory motor* (via the chorda tympani): submandibular and sublingual glands.

2.4.3 Taste Innervation

There are three cranial nerves responsible for conveying taste sensation from the tongue to the brain: the facial nerve (CN-VII), glossopharyngeal nerve (CN-IX), and (to a lesser extent) the vagus nerve (CN-X). The region of the tongue covered by each nerve is dependent on the proximity of the developing taste bud (and lingual papilla) to the free nerve ending.

Taste from the anterior two-thirds of the tongue travels along the chorda tympani, which travels early in its course with the lingual nerve (V3) and later in its course with the facial nerve (CN-VII) [16]. Taste in the posterior one-third of the tongue is from the glossopharyngeal nerve (CN-IX) [17].

The post-sulcal tongue, circumvallate papillae, palatoglossal arches, and oropharynx are governed by the glossopharyngeal nerve [18]. The vagus nerve provides supply to only the taste buds in the extreme areas of the pharyngeal tongue. These impulses are conveyed by the internal laryngeal branch of the vagus nerve.

2.4.4 Lingual Nerve Injuries

Any injury to sensory nerves can result in pain, altered sensation, and/or numbness, or more usually, a combination of all three. This can have a significant negative effect on the patient's quality of life affecting their daily function and psychological health.

The most common cause of lingual nerve injuries is third molar (wisdom tooth) surgery, less commonly the lingual nerve can be injured by local anesthetic dental injections (particularly inferior dental block injections) and sublingual or submandibular surgery. Patients should be routinely warned about lingual nerve injuries prior to wisdom tooth and floor of mouth surgery. The risk associated with wisdom tooth surgery is commonly accepted to be 2% temporary and 0.2% permanent [19]. Infiltration dentistry is a technique that may reduce the possibility of lingual nerve injuries by avoiding deep injections [20].

Common causes of injuries of the lingual nerve are summarized below as follows [21]:

- Administration of local anesthetics
- Removal of mandibular third molars
- Surgical insertion of dental implants
- Inadverent instrumentation during mandibular osteotomy
- Primary soft tissue suture closure

- Flap manipulation and handling
- Manipulation of the soft tissues of the floor of the mouth
- Blunt instrumentation (e.g. periosteal elevators)
- Crush injuries (e.g. rongeurs and hemostats)
- Cutting instruments (e.g. scalpel blades, drills, and needles)
- Stretch injury (e.g. inappropriate tension or tearing of the lingual mucosa)
- Chemical injury (e.g. local anesthetic, hemostatic, and endodontic materials)
- Thermal injury (e.g. cautery, laser, and rotary burns)

References

1. Kato H, Shimizo T. Tongue anatomy, kinametics and diseases (human anatomy and physiology). Nova Biomedical, UK Ed, Edition; 2012.
2. Singh H. Anatomy of tongue and its clinical relevance in orthodontics. Saarbrucken: Lap Lambert Academic Publishing; 2014.
3. Netter FH. Atlas of human anatomy (neeter basic science). 7th ed. Philadelphia, PA: Elsevier; 2019.
4. Drake R, Vogle AW, Mitchell AWM, Tibbittis R, Richardson P. Gray's atlas of anatomy. 3rd ed. Philadelphia, PA: Elsevier; 2017.
5. Iwasaki S. Evolution of the structure and function of the vertebrate tongue. J Anat. 2002;201(1):1–13.
6. Queiroz Marchesan I. Lingual frenulum: classification and speech interference. Int J Orofacial Myology. 2004;30:31–8.
7. Segal LM, Stephenson R, Dawes M, Feldman P. Prevalence, diagnosis, and treatment of ankyloglossia: methodologic review. Can Fam Physician. 2007;53:1027–33.
8. Suter VG, Bornstein MM. Ankyloglossia: facts and myths in diagnosis and treatment. J Periodontol. 2009;80:1204–19.
9. Sakamoto Y. Configuration of the extrinsic muscles of the tongue and their spatial interrelationships. Surg Radiol Anat. 2017;39(5):497–506.
10. Ferreira JR, Nogueira DJ, Rodrigues BF, Alvarenga BF. Blood supply in the tongue of Nellore Bos indicus (Linnaeus, 1758). Anat Histol Embryol. 2009;38(2):103–7.
11. Shah JP. Patterns of cervical lymph node metastasis from squamous carcinomas of the upper aerodigestive tract. Am J Surg. 1990;160(4):405–9.
12. Farmer RW, McCall L, Civantos FJ, Myers JN, Yarbrough WG, Murphy B, O'Leary M, Zitsch R, Siegel BA. Lymphatic drainage patterns in oral squamous cell carcinoma: findings of the ACOSOG Z0360 (Alliance) study. Otolaryngol Head Neck Surg. 2015;152(4):673–7.
13. Mu L, Sanders I. Human tongue neuroanatomy: nerve supply and motor endplates. Clin Anat. 2010;23:777–91.
14. Alves P. Imaging the hypoglossal nerve. Eur J Radiol. 2010;74:368–77.
15. Smith JC, Goldberg SJ, Shall MS. Phenotype and contractile properties of mammalian tongue muscles innervated by the hypoglossal nerve. Respir Physiol Neurobiol. 2005;147:253–62.
16. Weiss MH, Harrison LB, Isaacs RS. Use of decision analysis in planning a management strategy for the stage N0 neck. Arch Otolaryngol Head Neck Surg. 1994;120(7):699–702.
17. Jerjes W, Upile T, Petrie A, Riskalla A, Hamdoon Z, Vourvachis M, Karavidas K, Jay A, Sandison A, Thomas GJ, Kalavrezos N, Hopper C. Clinicopathological parameters, recurrence, locoregional and distant metastasis in 115 T1-T2 oral squamous cell carcinoma patients. Head Neck Oncol. 2010;20:2–9.
18. Ho AS, Kim S, Tighiouart M, Gudino C, Mita A, Scher KS, Laury A, Prasad R, Shiao SL, Van Eyk JE, Zumsteg ZS. Metastatic lymph node burden and survival in oral cavity cancer. J Clin Oncol. 2017;35(31):3601–9.

19. Renton T, Yilmaz Z. Profiling of patients presenting withpostraumatic neuropathy of the trigeminal nerve. J Orofacial Pain. 2011;25(4):333–44.
20. Meechan JG. The use of the mandibular infiltration anesthetic technique in adults. J Am Dent Assoc. 2011;142(3):19S–24S.
21. Nizam SA, Ziccardi VB. Trigeminal nerve injuries: avoidance and management of iatrogenic injury. Oral Maxillofac Surg Clin North Am. 2015;27(3):411–24.

Histology of the Tongue

3

Layers of the tongue are formed of mucosa, submucosa, and musculosa (muscle layer). There is a fibrous raphe in the midline of the tongue that marks the point of fusion of the embryonic lateral lingual swellings. Posteriorly, there is a variable amount of adipose tissue within the pharyngeal tongue [1].

Mucosa

The *lingual mucosa* is covered by stratified squamous epithelium with varying degrees of keratinization. Since the dorsal surface of the oral tongue is more at risk of desiccation and abrasions from contact with food boluses of varying temperatures and textures, it is covered by keratinized epithelium. On the other hand, the ventral surface of the oral part of the tongue and the pharyngeal part are relatively well protected from the harsh environment. Thus, the epithelia in these areas are characteristically nonkeratinized [2].

The mucosa of the dorsal surface of the oral part of the tongue is characterized by the presence of "lingual papillae" giving it a characteristic rough surface. On the other hand, the pharyngeal part has lymphatic aggregates throughout its mucosa known as "lingual tonsils."

Submucosa

The epithelium is adherent to the underlying striated muscle fibers of the tongue. The submucosa contains minor salivary glands that secrete both mucous and serous secretions.

Musculosa

The intrinsic muscles of the tongue are arranged in four layers; superior longitudinal muscles, vertical muscles, transverse muscles, and lastly inferior longitudinal muscles.

© The Author(s), under exclusive license to Springer Nature Switzerland AG 2022

M. F. Sakr, *Tongue Lesions*, https://doi.org/10.1007/978-3-031-08198-9_3

3.1 Lingual Papillae

The dorsal mucosa of the oral tongue is characterized by numerous raised structures known as *lingual papillae*. They give the characteristic rough appearance of the dorsal surface that is not appreciated on the ventral surface of the tongue. The pharyngeal tongue also has raised dome-like structures throughout the mucosa. However, these are lymphatic aggregates (i.e. *lingual tonsils*) and should *not* be confused with papillae [3].

There are four types of lingual papillae found on the surface of the human tongue, namely, filiform papillae, fungiform papillae, foliate papillae, and circumvallate (vallate) papillae as shown in Fig. 3.1.

The "lingual papillae" contain taste buds and taste cells with the exception of the filiform papillae, which are the most abundant and scattered on the whole dorsal surface of the oral tongue. The other three types of lingual papillae, circumvallate, foliate, and fungiform, have certain characteristic distributions on the tongue surface as shown in Fig. 3.2.

The four types of lingual papillae found on the surface of the human tongue can be described as follows:

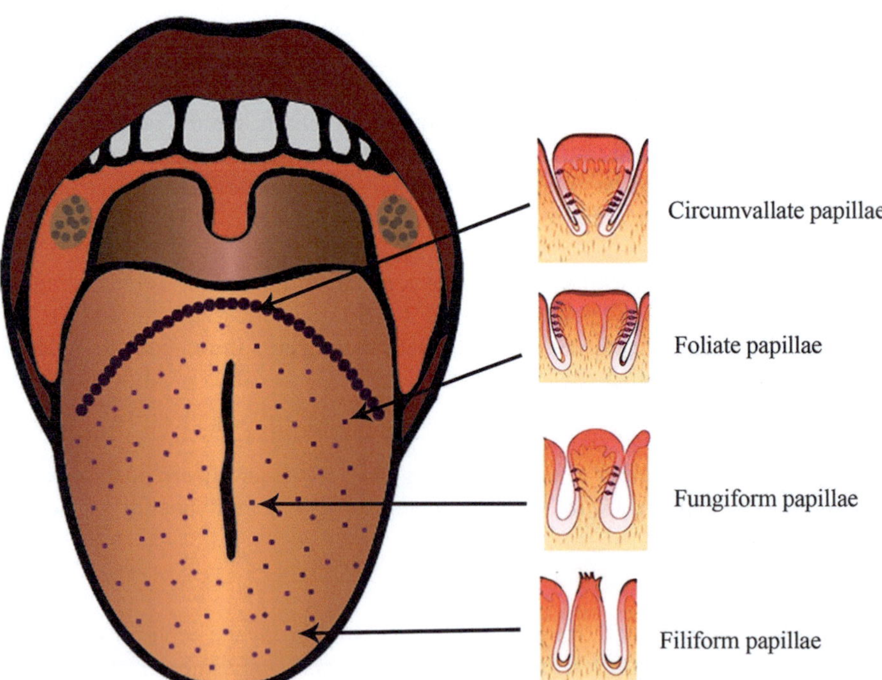

Fig. 3.1 The four types of lingual papillae present on the dorsal surface of the oral tongue: filiform, fungiform, foliate, and circumvallate (vallate) papillae

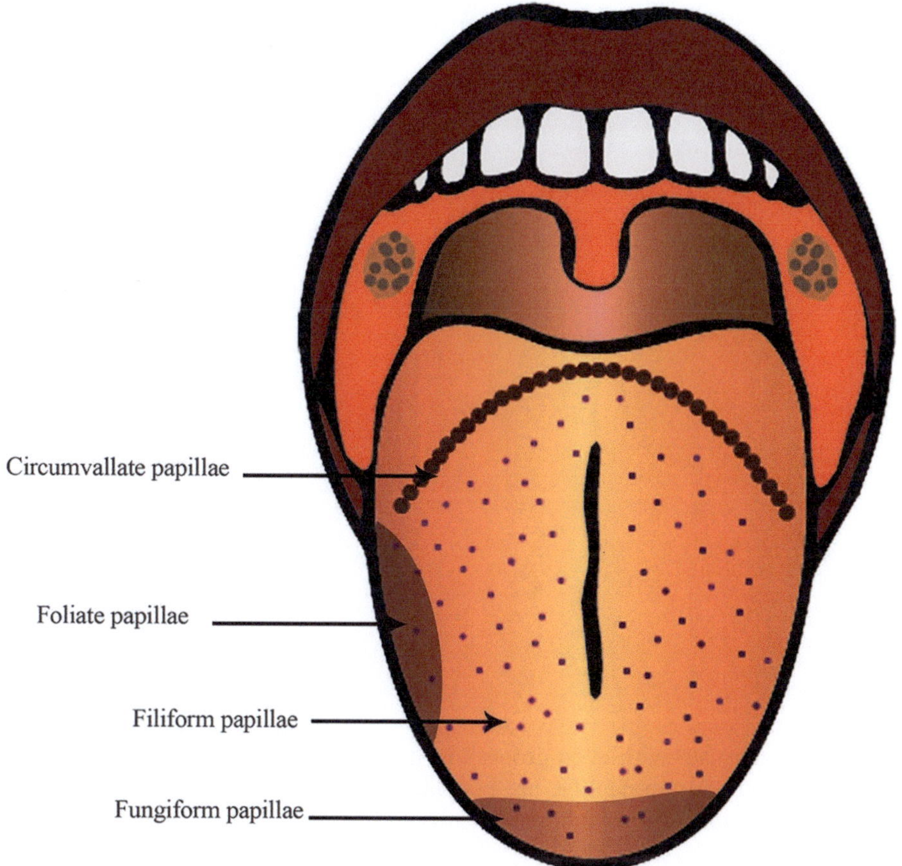

Fig. 3.2 Papillae of the tongue. Note the location of the circumvallate, foliate, and fungiform papillae. Filiform papillae occupy the dorsum of the tongue

Filiform Papillae (Papillae Filiformes)
Filiform papillae are the most abundant of the four types of papillae. They are stretched, conical, gray-white papillae that are covered in a heavy coat of keratinized squamous epithelium. By making the dorsal surface of the tongue rough, these papillae provide friction to allow movement of the food bolus during chewing. It should be noted that these papillae do *not* possess taste buds.

Fungiform Papillae
Fungiform papillae are weakly keratinized, less abundant than the filiform papillae, but scattered across the entire dorsal surface of the tongue. These highly vascular, mushroom-shaped papillae contain a few taste buds on the apical aspect.

Foliate Papillae (Leaf-Like)
Foliate papillae appear as bilaterally paired, parallel, longitudinal slits on the posterolateral margin of the tongue, near the sulcus terminalis. They consist of 4–11

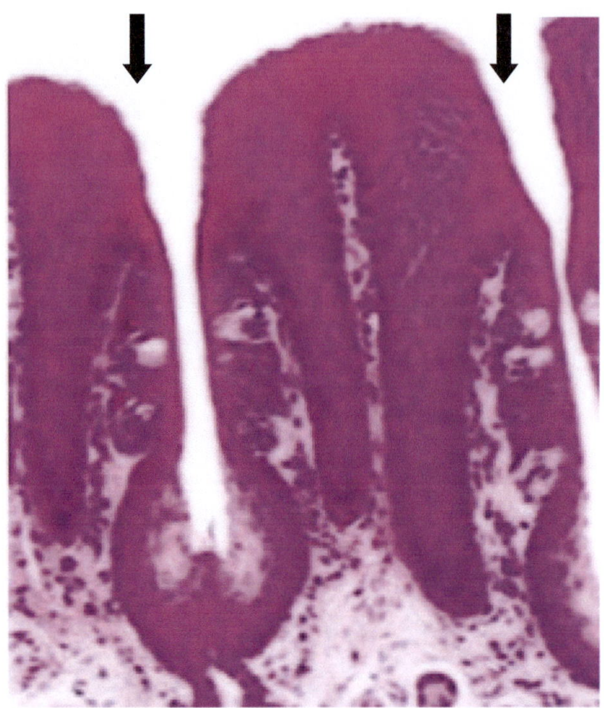

Fig. 3.3 Foliate papillae. They appear as bilaterally paired, parallel, longitudinal slits (black arrows) on the posterolateral margin of the tongue

ridges that alternate with deep grooves in the mucosa (Fig. 3.3). The mucosa is nonkeratinized and the papillae are populated with numerous taste buds. Foliate papillae also contain serous glands underlying the taste buds, which cleanse the grooves.

Circumvallate (Vallate) Papillae

Circumvallate papillae (also known as vallate papillae) are organized linearly, as a set of four to six large papillae anterior to each limb of the sulcus terminalis (total = 8–12 papillae). The characteristic furrow found within the papillae can be appreciated. These moats facilitate drainage of serous salivary *von Ebner glands* that empty into the structure. The persistent lubrication creates a favorable environment for gustatory particles to dissolve so that they can be detected by the taste buds [4].

3.2 Taste Buds (Caliculi Gustatererius)

While taste buds are distributed throughout the entire oral cavity, they are at higher concentrations on the tongue. Each taste bud is clear, oval in shape, and covered by stratified squamous epithelium. A combination of elongated taste (gustatory) cells, supportive cells, and basal stem cells can be found within each taste bud.

The *gustatory* cells have an apical taste pore surrounded by numerous microvilli that bind dissolved molecules and bring them closer to the receptors responsible for taste. However, these cells have a relatively high turnover rate, as their shelf life is roughly seven to ten days only.

There are five *gustatory sensations* that are perceived by individuals: *sweet*, *salty*, *sour*, *bitter*, and *umami*. The microvilli found on the apical surface of the taste cells are equipped with various receptors that bind to varying molecules. The reaction generated from this compound–receptor interaction gives rise to varying action potentials that are subsequently perceived as taste [5].

Saltiness is often associated with the cationic component of a compound (i.e. sodium ions), while sourness is related to the acidity (concentration of hydrogen ions) in the compound. Organic compounds such as carbohydrates or amino acids give rise to *sweet taste*, while *bitterness* is associated with long-chain organic compounds. The final taste, *umami*, also known as *savory*, is related to compounds with the left-handed chiral isomer of glutamic acid [6].

References

1. Young B, O'Dowd G, Woodford P. Wheater's functional histology: a text and color atlas. 6th ed. Amsterdam: Elsevier; 2014.
2. Iwasaki S. Evolution of the structure and function of the vertebrate tongue. J Anat. 2002;201(1):1–13.
3. Ross MH, Pawlina W. Histology: a text and atlas with correlated cell and molecular biology. 8th ed. Amsterdam: Wolters Kluwer Health; 2017.
4. Kim JY, Lee MJ, Cho KW, Lee JM, Kim YJ, Kim JY, Jung HI, Cho JY, Cho SW, Jung HS. Shh and ROCK1 modulate the dynamic epithelial morphogenesis in circumvallate papilla development. Dev Biol. 2009;325:273–80.
5. Lumerman HS, Bowe RB. Atlas of oral and maxillo-facial histopathology. 1st ed. Philadelphia: Lippincott, Williams & Wilkins; 2012.
6. Bhaskar SN. Synopsis of oral pathology. 6th ed. St. Louis: Mosby; 1981.

Physiology of the Tongue

4

The tongue is a mobile muscular organ that lies within the mouth and partly extends into the upper throat. The tongue is covered by a mucous membrane that is important for taste sensation. Beyond its obvious role in eating—manipulating food into a bolus that can be safely passed into the throat with swallowing—it also, among other functions, has a vital contribution to speech and may even affect breathing, especially in sleep.

4.1 Functions of the Tongue

4.1.1 Tongue: Tool to Taste Food

The ability of tongue to taste food is because of the presence of taste buds on its surface. According to traditional belief, different parts of the tongue sense only a specific taste. Modern research, however, rejects this belief. It suggests that different parts of tongue detect a specific taste more easily (and strongly), but they can detect other tastes as well. However, each receptor cell is sensitive to a particular taste only. The *taste receptors* are of five main types—sweet taste receptors, bitter taste receptors, salty taste receptors, sour taste receptors, and umami (savory) taste receptors. The latter helps detecting the taste of amino acids in food (characteristic of broths and cooked meats).

The dorsum (upper surface) of the tongue contains lots of lingual papillae. The papillae house the taste buds and the taste receptors. These receptors assist in the sensation of taste of different types of dietary components, which come into contact with them. On the tip of the tongue there are taste buds for sensing sweet. Behind the apex of the tongue and along its sides, there are receptors for tasting bitter, sour, and salty substances as demonstrated in Fig. 4.1 [1].

© The Author(s), under exclusive license to Springer Nature Switzerland AG 2022
M. F. Sakr, *Tongue Lesions*, https://doi.org/10.1007/978-3-031-08198-9_4

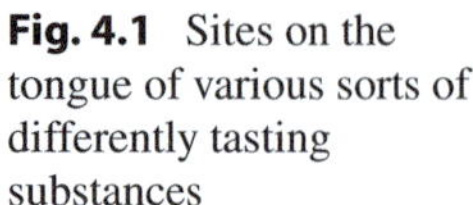

Fig. 4.1 Sites on the tongue of various sorts of differently tasting substances

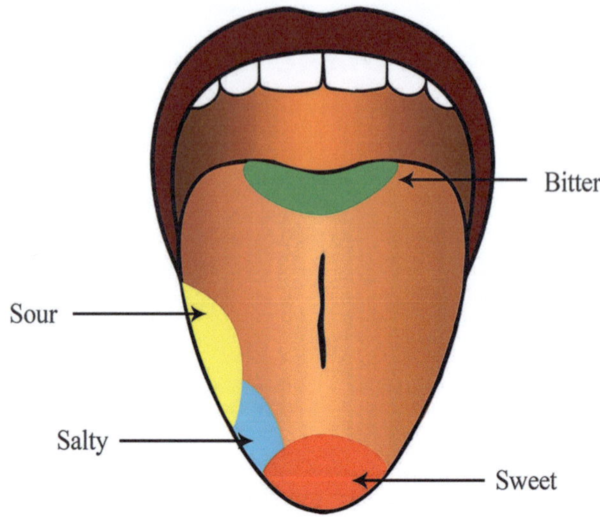

4.1.2 Tongue's Role in Mastication

After the food enters the mouth cavity, two processes start and go side by side, *grinding* and *mastication*. During grinding, the teeth break down the large food particles into smaller ones.

Thus, there is easy mixing of these particles with saliva to form the "bolus". Mastication (chewing) involves the mixing of finely ground food with saliva. This is facilitated by the tongue, which particularly helps in the positioning of food between the teeth. Secondly, as the food turns around, it is mixed with saliva.

The masticatory muscles provide the enormous strength of jaw closure. It is in large part due to the pinnate arrangement of fibers in the masseter (the masticatory muscle of the posterior cheek) [2].

4.1.3 Removal of Hard and Ill-Tasting Substances

The tongue has also a role in separating, sorting out, and removing unsuitable particles that may accidently come with the food, such as bones and the ill-tasting soft or hard substances.

4.1.4 Swallowing Food

The masticated food forms a rounded mass, the *bolus*, with the help of tongue, which then expels the bolus at the back of the mouth cavity into esophagus. The food bolus then moves through the esophagus with the help of peristaltic contractions and enters the stomach.

4.1.5 The Tongue: An Organ for Sucking

Almost all mammals suck milk from the breasts of their mothers in infancy. They do so with the help of their tongue by creating negative pressure within their oral cavity.

4.1.6 Tongue as an Organ of Speech

Individuals produce different speech sounds as a stream of air coming from the lungs leaves the body through the mouth. The mouth cavity is the home to various organs of speech. Different speech organs include the tongue, teeth, lips, palate, and uvula. Here, the tongue is of incredible importance. The tip of the tongue, the body, and the back significantly contribute to the production of vowel and other sounds.

Different parts of tongue play their own part in producing and modifying sounds. For example, labiodental sounds are produced while the tip of tongue touches the upper teeth. To produce the/k/and/g/sounds, the back of the tongue raises against the roof top. Composed of a set of extremely movable tongue muscles, it can quickly assume various shapes for the efficient performance of all the assigned tasks.

4.1.7 Intimacy

The tongue plays a role in physical intimacy and sexuality. The tongue is part of the erogenous zone of the mouth and can be used in intimate contact for pleasure and conception.

4.1.8 Medication Delivery

The sublingual region underneath the front of the tongue is an ideal location for the administration of certain medications into the body. The oral mucosa is very thin underneath the tongue, and is underlain by a plexus of veins. The sublingual route takes advantage of the highly vascular quality of the oral cavity, and allows for the speedy application of medication into the cardiovascular system, bypassing the gastrointestinal tract. This is the only convenient and efficacious route of administration (apart from intravenous therapy) of nitroglycerin to a patient suffering chest pain from angina pectoris.

4.1.9 The Tongue: An Indicator of Health

The appearance of the tongue serves as an indicator of health. It takes time for the tongue to change its appearance. Therefore, the color of tongue at a particular time reflects the health of the individual. When the tongue color is pale-red, it means there is good circulation of blood in the body reflecting a good health. In case of anemia, the color changes to nearly white or extremely pale.

The appearance of a thicker *white coat* is the sign of predominance of common cold. It represents a weakness in some physiological function or a viral infection. The individuals with thick, *yellow coating* on the tongue are likely to have some bacterial infection or inflammation.

Different tongue problems are likely to cause changes in taste. In addition, changes in the color and texture of the tongue may occur. Sometimes, the variations in the color and texture are also indicative of different diseases in other parts of the human body [3].

The tongue is susceptible to various tongue conditions, including glossitis, pain, tongue swelling, and tongue ulcers. Severe tongue diseases include cancer, ulcer, tongue blisters, and hemangioma.

4.2 Taste (Gustatory) Pathway

Taste buds house the chemoreceptors responsible for taste. They are stimulated by chemicals termed *testants* that are dissolved in saliva. Each grape-like taste bud contains 50–125 chemorecptors termed *gustatory cells*, which are surrounded by supportive capsules [4–8]. Tiny cilia-like structures extend from each gustatory cell and project into an opening called *taste pores*, which are bathed in saliva.

All taste cells can respond at least to most taste-producing chemicals. Functionally, however, there are five "*primary taste sensations*", namely, *sour* [9], *sweet* [10, 11], *bitter* [12–15], salty [16], and umami (from glutamate) [17] (Fig. 4.2). *Primary sensation* plus sense of *smell* results in the ability to detect many different *flavors*.

Areas of sensitivity on the tongue include the tip of the tongue (sweetness), back of the tongue (bitterness), and sides of the tongue (saltiness and sourness). The five

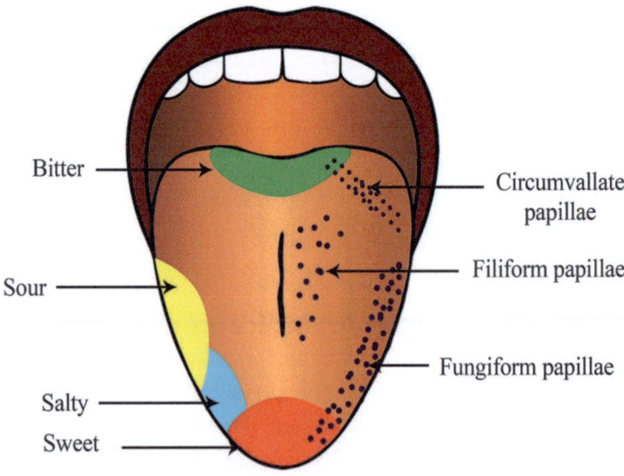

Fig. 4.2 The tongue with circumvallate, filiform, and foliate papillae. Note the sites of primary taste sensations

taste qualities combine with other oral sensations, such as texture, spiciness, temperature, and aroma to produce what is commonly referred to as "flavor."

Flavor is recognized largely through the sense of smell. Taste and smell are closely linked senses. It is therefore common for people who lose their sense of smell to say that food has lost its taste. This is incorrect; the food has lost its aroma, but taste remains.

4.2.1 Neuronal Pathway for Taste

The neuronal pathway for taste begins with the creation of a receptor potential in the gustatory cells of a taste bud. It is then transmitted via sensory input to the brain. The anterior two-thirds of the tongue cells are conducted via the facial nerve (CN-VII), while the posterior third tongue cells are conducted by the fibers of the glossopharyngeal nerve (CN-IX). The vagus nerve (CN-X) transmits taste sensation from the taste buds located on the walls of the pharynx and epiglottis only. The three cranial nerves carry impulses into the medulla, into the thalamus, and then into the taste area of the cerebral cortex in the *parietal lobe*.

Key Points [18]

- Taste buds are composed of two excitable cell types and a glia-like cell; each type of cell has distinct functions.
- Basic taste qualities are detected by G protein-coupled type 1 and type 2 taste receptors, by other receptors and ion channels, and possibly by transporters.
- ATP is an afferent taste transmitter and is secreted by taste bud cells through an unconventional, nonvesicular release mechanism.
- ATP, serotonin, and GABA mediate cell–cell interactions in the taste bud that may shape transmission to sensory afferent fibers.
- Controversy remains regarding whether peripheral taste coding follows a labeled line or combinatorial pattern.
- Taste preferences and appetites seem to have a genetic component that is being revealed by molecular and population studies.

4.3 Taste Disorders

4.3.1 Types of Taste Disorders

4.3.1.1 Dysgeusia

Dysgeusia means "an altered sense of taste." The gustatory system may misread and/or distort an odor, a taste, or a flavor. A person may also detect a foul taste from a substance that is normally pleasant tasting.

4.3.1.2 Hypogeusia

Hypogeusia means a reduced ability to taste sweet, sour, bitter, salty, and umami

4.3.1.3 Ageusia

In ageusia, the patient cannot detect taste at all. True taste loss is rare; perceived loss usually reflects a smell loss, which is often confused with a taste loss.

4.3.2 Etiology of Taste Disorders

Problems with taste are caused by anything that interrupts the transfer of taste sensations to the brain, or by conditions that affect the way the brain interprets the sensation of taste.

The most common causes of taste disorders are

- Certain medications (e.g. anti-thyroid drugs [ATDs], zinc preparations, antibiotics, and neurologic drugs)
- Chemotherapy or radiotherapy
- Aging (decreased ability to taste and smell)
- Medical conditions (e.g. Bells' Palsy, Parkinsons' disease, diabetes mellitus [DM], and gastroesophageal reflux disease [GERD])
- Injuries to the mouth, nose, or head
- Poor oral hygiene
- Fungal infections on the tongue or in the oral cavity
- Head and neck cancers

4.3.3 Symptoms

People who have taste disorders usually lose their ability to taste or can no longer perceive taste in the same way. The most common taste complaint is "phantom taste perception" i.e. tasting something when nothing is in the mouth. There may be a specific ageusia of one or more of the five taste categories: sweet, sour, bitter, salty, and umami or savory.

4.3.4 Diagnosis

4.3.4.1 History-Taking

- How long has the taste problem been going on?
- What kind of taste change has occurred?
- What medication is she/he currently, or was recently, taking?
- Does she/he smoke, use recreational drugs, or drink alcohol?
- When was her/his last dental visit?
- How is her/his appetite?
- Are there any foods that taste normal?

- Has there been any recent change in smell?
- Any recent injury or illness?
- Did she/he recently change her/his brand of mouthwash or toothpaste?

4.3.4.2 Investigations

Tests can be used to evaluate senses of taste and smell. Certain chemicals made to produce the four major tastes—sour, sweet, bitter, salty—can be applied to areas of the tongue; or the patient may be asked to take a taste test. In this test, the patient will sip certain liquids and try to identify their tastes. The chemicals or liquids used to test taste have no odor.

A "*scratch and sniff*" test can be used to check out the sense of smell. The test uses *special cards*. Each one contains an odor that is released when scratched. The patient is asked to identify the odor on each card.

Other tests that may be performed include imaging such as computed tomography (CT) scan and magnetic resonance imaging (MRI), blood tests, and saliva flow.

4.3.5 Prevention

Taste disorders may be prevented by practicing good oral hygiene, keeping-up to date with dental appointments, consulting the doctor on noticing any problems with the sense of taste, avoiding contact with insecticides and solvents, and quitting smoking

4.3.6 Treatment

Dysgeusia is treated by treating the cause. If no cause can be found, this is called "*idiopathic dysgeusia*." It is hard to say what the outlook for this condition will be. In some cases, idiopathic dysgeusia may resolve on its own. In others, it will not. It is important to thoroughly evaluate the patient so that the known causes of dysgeusia can be ruled out.

A distorted sense of taste can be a serious risk factor for heart disease, diabetes, stroke, and other illnesses that require sticking to a specific diet. When taste is impaired, a person may change his or her eating habits. Some people may eat too little and lose weight, while others may eat too much and gain weight. This can be a problem for people with certain medical conditions, such as diabetes or hypertension. In severe cases, loss of taste can lead to depression.

4.3.7 Prognosis

How long dysgeusia lasts depends on the cause. Sometimes the problem disappears once the cause is removed. This can occur if the cause is gum disease, plaque, a medication received for a short time or a short-term condition such as a common cold.

If the cause is a fungal infection, dysgeusia should disappear after the fungal infection is properly treated. In some cases, as in "nerve damage," dysgeusia may be permanent.

References

1. Iwasaki S. Evolution of the structure and function of the vertebrate tongue. J Anat. 2002;201(1):1–13.
2. Yamane A. Embryonic and postnatal development of masticatory and tongue muscles. Cell Tissue Res. 2005;322:183–9.
3. Du Toit DF. The tongue: structure and function relevant to disease and oral health. SADT. 2003;58(9):375–6.
4. Zhang Y, Hoon MA, Chandrashekar J, Mueller KL, Cook B, Wu D, et al. Coding of sweet, bitter, and umami tastes: different receptor cells sharing similar signaling pathways. Cell. 2003;112:293–301.
5. Calvo SS, Egan JM. The endocrinology of taste receptors. Nat Rev Endocrinol. 2015;11:213–27.
6. Larson ED, Vandenbeuch A, Voigt A, Meyerhof W, Kinnamon SC, Finger TE. The role of 5-HT3 receptors in signaling from taste buds to nerves. J Neurosci. 2015;35:15984–95.
7. Roper SD, Chaudhari N. Handbook of brain microcircuits. 2nd ed. Oxford: Oxford University Press; 2017. p. 277–83.
8. Dando R, Holland VF, Zampighi GA, Simon SA. A permeability barrier surrounds taste buds in lingual epithelia. Am J Physiol Cell Physiol. 2015;308:21–32.
9. Ye W, Chang RB, Bushman JD, Tu YH, Mulhall EM, Wilson CE, et al. The K^+ channel KIR2.1 functions in tandem with proton influx to mediate sour taste transduction. Proc Natl Acad Sci U S A. 2016;113:229–38.
10. Sukumaran SK, Yee KK, Iwata S, Kotha R, Quezada-Calvillo R, Nichols BL, et al. Taste cell-expressed α-glucosidase enzymes contribute to gustatory responses to disaccharides. Proc Natl Acad Sci U S A. 2016;113:6035–40.
11. Lapis TJ, Penner MH, Lim J. Humans can taste glucose oligomers independent of the hT1R2/hT1R3 sweet taste receptor. Chem Senses. 2016;41:755–62.
12. Meyerhof W, Batram C, Kuhn C, Brockhoff A, Chudoba E, Bufe B, et al. The molecular receptive ranges of human TAS2R bitter taste receptors. Chem Senses. 2010;35:157–70.
13. Kuhn C, Bufe B, Winnig M, Hofmann T, Frank O, Behrens M, et al. Bitter taste receptors for saccharin and acesulfame K. J Neurosci. 2004;24:10260–5.
14. Sainz E, Cavenagh MM, Gutierrez J, Battey JF, Northup JK, Sulivan SL. Functional characterization of human bitter taste receptors. Biochem J. 2007;403:537–43.
15. Nolden AA, McGeary JE, Hayes JE. Differential bitterness in capsaicin, piperine, and ethanol associates with polymorphisms in multiple bitter taste receptor genes. Physiol Behav. 2016;156:117–27.
16. Lewandowski BC, Sukumaran SK, Margolskee RF, Bachmanov AA. Amiloride-insensitive salt taste is mediated by two populations of type III taste cells with distinct transduction mechanisms. J Neurosci. 2016;36:1942–53.
17. Yamaguchi S. Basic properties of umami and effects on humans. Physiol Behav. 1991;49:833–41.
18. Roper SD, Chaudhari N. Taste buds: cells, signals and synapses. Naute Rev Neurosci. 2017;18:485–97.

5 Congenital Anomalies

Developmental Anomalies

Congenital (developmental) anomalies (malformations) of the tongue reported in the literature include the following:

- Aglossia
- Hemiglossia (Half tongue)
- Microglossia
- Macro-glossia
- Congenital bifid-tongue (Cleft tongue)
- Double tongue/Accessory Tongue
- Ankyloglossia (tongue tie)
- Black hairy tongue
- Fissured tongue
- Lingual varices
- Lingual thyroid nodule

5.1 Aglossia

Aglossia (also known as "aglossia congenita") means "absence of the tongue" resulting from complete agenesis of the tongue primordia (Fig. 5.1). It is believed to be caused by heat-induced vascular disruption near the fourth week of embryonic development.

Aglossia is commonly associated with craniofacial and limb defects (*Adactylia syndrome*) and is thought to belong to a family of oromandibular limb hypogenesis syndrome (OLHS). The incidence of OLHS is very low (1/175,000 live births), and most cases are actually hypoglossia rather than true aglossia. Isolated aglossia without limb defects is even rarer.

© The Author(s), under exclusive license to Springer Nature Switzerland AG 2022
M. F. Sakr, *Tongue Lesions*, https://doi.org/10.1007/978-3-031-08198-9_5

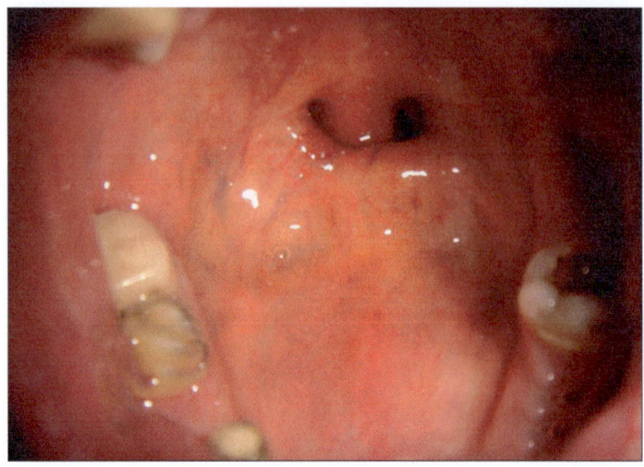

Fig. 5.1 Aglossia congenita. A rare congenital anomaly of the oromandibular limb hypogenesis syndrome (OLHS). Isolated aglossia may occur, though very rarely

The first known case of aglossia was reported in the early eighteenth century by a member of the prominent De Jussieu family in France and cases remain rare to date [1].

5.2 Hemiglossia (Half-Tongue)

Hemiglossia is a very rare anomaly and refers to "congenital absence of half of the anterior two-thirds of the tongue." It occurs if one of the tongue swellings fails to develop.

5.3 Microglossia

5.3.1 Definition

Microglossia is another rare congenital anomaly in which only a tiny or rudimentary tongue has developed from the cupola resulting in an "abnormally small tongue" (Fig. 5.2).

5.3.2 Epidemiology

Since the first case reported by Antoine De Jussieu in 1718, there have been less than 50 cases reported so far [2, 3]. This anomaly shows no predilection for gender and has no genetic implications. No teratogen has been detected in patients with microglossia [4].

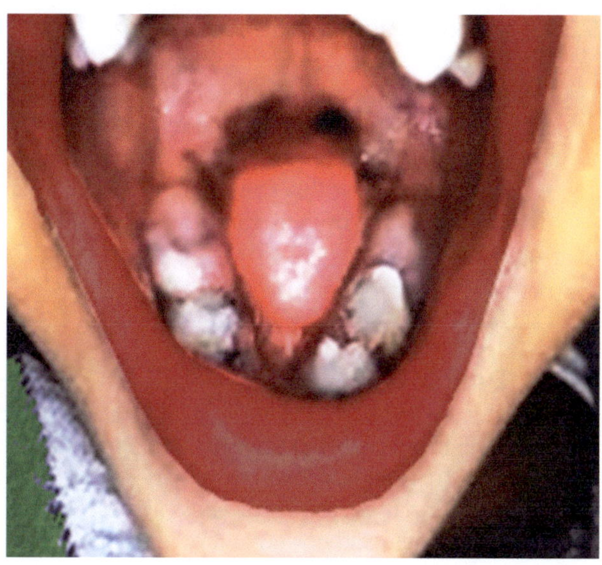

Fig. 5.2 Microglossia. Rudimentary or abnormally small tongue in the oral cavity

Table 5.1 Types of Oromandibular Limb Hypogenesis Syndrome (OLHS) proposed by Chicarilli in 1985 [7]

Type I	• *Micrognathia (mandibular)* • Pierre Robin syndrome • Hanhart's syndrome
Type II	• *Microglossia* • Hypoglossia • Hypoglossia hypodactyly
Type III	• *Dysgnathia (maxillomandibular)* • Glosso-palatine ankylosis • Glosso-palatine ankylosis hypodactyly
Type IV	• Mobius syndrome • Charlie M syndrome • Amniotic band syndrome

5.3.3 Etiology

The cause of microglossia is poorly understood. Although microglossias may develop as *isolated* cases [5], in most of the cases they occur in association with *other anomalies* [6], such as oromandibular limb hypogenesis syndrome (OLHS) (Table 5.1) [7] or hypoglossia-hypodactylia syndrome. Microglossias without limb deformity can occur, but they are also associated with some other birth defects such as partial anodontia, sublingual gland hypertrophy, and dextrocadia.

Iwata et al. reported that cranial neural crest fibroblasts noncanonical transforming growth factor beta (TGF-β) regulation of fibroblast growth factor (FGF) and bone morphogenic protein signaling can cause similar tongue muscle developmental defects [8].

5.3.4 Clinical Picture and Treatment

Clinically, there is difficulty in speech and swallowing. As size of the tongue often determines the growth and size of the mandibular arch, in case of microglossia the length of the mandibular arch will be smaller due to the smaller size of tongue. There is no treatment for this condition, and the affected persons will have to train their tongue to the best of their abilities.

5.4 Macroglossia

5.4.1 Definitions

Macroglossia means an "abnormally large tongue" in proportion to other structures in the mouth. It usually occurs secondary to an underlying disorder that may be present from birth (*congenital*) or *acquired.* It can be *localized* or *generalized*, and it leads to functional and cosmetic problems.

True macroglossia refers to macroglossia caused by histological abnormalities within the tongue, such as muscular hypertrophy and vascular malformation (Fig. 5.3).

Pseudo-macroglossia (also called "relative macroglossia") refers to a condition in an individual who has a normal-sized tongue that, as a result of oral or skeletal abnormalities such as a narrow mandible, maxillary retraction, or restricted naso-pharynx (as found in many head and neck syndromes), seems unusually large.

Apparent macroglossia is a condition where the tongue appears abnormally large due to poor muscular control of tongue, although there is no real increase in the bulk

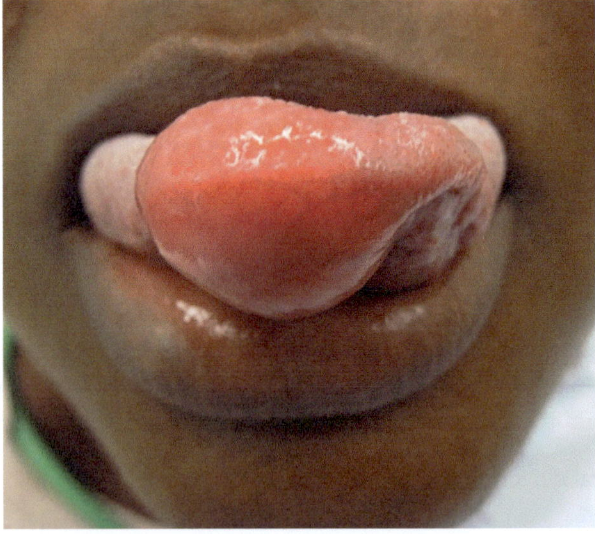

Fig. 5.3 Clinical appearance of "true macroglossia"

of the tongue tissue. Apparent macroglossia is seen in cases of cretinism and happy puppet syndrome (also known as "*Angelman syndrome*"). It is a genetic disorder, which causes severe learning difficulties along with walking and talking trouble, but the affected child never stops smiling because the disorder puts a permanent smile on the face [9].

5.4.2 Epidemiology

5.4.2.1 Frequency

Although the exact incidence of macroglossia in the general population is unknown (because the etiologies are too numerous to quantify), the condition is found in some congenital syndromes, such as Down syndrome (1/700 live-births) and Beckwith-Wiedemann syndrome (0.07/1000 live-births). In Beckwith-Wiedemann syndrome, 97.5% of patients have macroglossia. The literature also documents two families with autosomal dominant inheritance of isolated macroglossia. Using the Kids' Inpatient Database, a study by Simmonds et al. reported congenital macroglossia to be present in 4.63/100,000 births, with 48.1% of cases being isolated and 51.9% being syndromic [10].

5.4.2.2 Gender

Simmonds et al. reported that the incidence of isolated congenital macroglossia is greater in females than males, with a ratio of 1.93:1 [10].

5.4.2.3 Race

The aforementioned recent study by Simmonds et al. found the incidence of isolated congenital macroglossia to be greater in African Americans, with a 2.02 odds ratio [10].

5.4.3 Etiology

Macroglossia is more common than microglossia. It can be associated with a wide range of congenital and acquired conditions, or it can occur as an isolated feature (with no other abnormalities). In most cases, macroglossia results from vascular malformations and muscular hypertrophy [11].

5.4.3.1 Causes of Pseudo-Macroglossia

Causes of pseudo-macroglossia, i.e. conditions that force the tongue to sit in an abnormal position, include the following:

1. Allergic reactions to medications that cause the tongue to swell.
2. Enlarged tonsils and/or adenoids that displace the tongue.
3. Low palate and decreased oral cavity volume.
4. Severe maxillary deficiency with narrow palatal arch.

5. Severe mandibular deficiency (retrognathism).
6. Local oral tumor that displaces the tongue.

5.4.3.2 Causes of True Macroglossia

Congenital or inherited causes of true macroglossia may include the following [12].

1. Idiopathic tongue muscle hypertrophy (over-development of tongue musculature).
2. Various syndromes such as trisomy 21 (Down syndrome), Beckwith-Seidermann hypoglycemic syndrome, multiple endocrine neoplasia syndrome, Behmel syndrome, Laband syndrome, and lysosomal storage disease (mucopolysaccharoidosis) such as Hurler syndrome, Hunters syndrome, and Marteaux-Lamy syndrome (Table 5.2).
3. Hemangioma.
4. Lymphangioma [13].
5. Hamartomas.
6. Salivary gland tumors.
7. Congenital hypothyroidism.
8. Primary amyloidosis.

Table 5.2 Hereditary syndromes associated with macroglossia

Behmel syndrome (also known as *Simpson-Golabi-Behmel syndrome*) is a condition that affects many parts of the body and occurs primarily in males. It is classified as an overgrowth syndrome, which means that affected infants are considerably larger than normal at birth (macrosomia) and continue to grow and gain weight at an unusual rate
Laband syndrome (also known as *Zimmerman-Laband syndrome*), is an extremely rare genetic disorder characterized by abnormalities of the head and facial (craniofacial) area and the hands and feet. Most children with this disorder have abnormally large gums (gingival fibromatosis)
Hurler syndrome (also known as *muco-polysaccharidosis type IH (MPS-IH), Hurler's disease,* and formerly *gargoylism*), is a genetic disorder that results in the build-up of large sugar molecules called glycosaminoglycans (AKA GAGs or mucopolysaccharides) in lysosomes
Hunter syndrome, also called *mucopolysaccharidosis II* or *MPS II*, is a rare disease that is passed on in families. It mainly affects boys. Their bodies cannot break down a kind of sugar that builds bones, skin, tendons, and other tissue. Those sugars build up in their cells and damage many parts of the body, including the brain. Exactly what happens is different for every person
Maroteaux-Lamy syndrome, also known as *arylsulfatase-B deficiency, and deficiency mucopolysaccharidosis type VI (MPS IV),* is an error of MPS metabolism characterized by excretion of the "dermatan sulfate" in urine, growth retardation, lumbar kyphosis, sternal protrusion, genu valgum, usually hepatosplenomegaly, and no mental retardation; onset occurs after 2 years of age; autosomal recessive inheritance, caused by mutation in the arylsulfatase B gene (ARSB) on chromosome 5q. It takes its name from two French doctors, Dr. Maroteaux and Dr. Lamy, who first described the condition in 1963

In some cases, macroglossia occurs as an *isolated hereditary* trait that is inherited an autosomal dominant manner [14].

Acquired causes of true macroglossia may be:

1. *Metabolic/endocrine* such as hypothyroidism, acromegaly, and myxedema [15].
2. *Inflammatory/infectious* such as Ludwig angina, pemphigus vulgaris, diphtheria, tuberculosis (TB), actinomycosis, candidiasis, and sarcoidosis
3. *Systemic/medical* such as neurofibromatosis
4. *Traumatic* such as hemorrhage and hematoma, direct trauma (tongue biting), and intubation injury
5. *Neoplastic* such as lymphangioma [13], hemangioma, plasmacytoma, and various malignancies (e.g. carcinoma and lymphoma) [11].

5.4.4 Clinical Presentation

Normal *speech* and *swallowing* requires normal tongue anatomy and function. Swallowing begins as a tongue mixes food with saliva to form food bolus which is then propelled into the pharynx. Articulation also depends on the tongue ability to alter the impedance of air and change the resonant characteristics of the upper airway. In macroglossia, increase in tongue bulk impairs these functions.

In macroglossia the tongue is always protruded, which makes it prone to trauma and drying due to which the upper respiratory tract infections are common. There is speech impairment along with drooling of saliva. Patient has difficulty in swallowing, chances of air way obstruction are there, and the patient fails to thrive.

5.4.5 Clinical Evaluation

Macroglossia due to an *allergic reaction* may require life-saving measures and emergency intervention to maintain a patent airway. The cause of the allergy must be determined and eliminated or treated. An association between macroglossia and a syndrome or congenital disorder can be determined by assessing family history and through genetic counseling. Severe congenital cases may require surgical intervention in infancy.

Should the cause of macroglossia go undetermined on initial presentation, further investigation is indicated to narrow the list of differential diagnoses. Direct questions regarding the etiological factors (e.g. inflammatory, neoplastic) will lead to the exact diagnosis and ultimate treatment.

Physical examination and diagnostic testing can significantly aid in the diagnosis. Physical examination of the *tongue* alone should reveal signs of the cause or at least help to rule out the etiologic classes that are not involved. For example, hemangiomas can often be observed on the surface of the tongue in a variety of positions, bearing a characteristic blue coloration. Infectious processes often present with characteristic findings, such as painful swelling or white plaques (pathognomonic for candidiasis).

Physical examinations of the head and neck, the oral cavity, maxilla, and mandible are helpful in differentiating true macroglossia from pseudo-macroglossia. Severe retrognathia and unusually small maxillary or mandibular size may indicate the latter.

General physical examination may indicate congenital or systemic syndromes. Certain vitamin deficiencies may manifest with angular stomatitis, non-pitting edema of the lower extremities may indicate hypothyroidism, and unusual body morphologies may indicate the early signs of diseases such as acromegaly [15].

5.4.6 Complications

The pathophysiology of the enlarged tongue is related to the specific etiological factors. The locoregional complications of macroglossia are generally the same relative to the magnitude of the enlargement and the size of the tongue. Macroglossia may cause obstruction of the oral airway, which is usually worsened when the patient lies supine, allowing an enlarged tongue base to more directly block the oropharynx and hypopharynx. Speech and swallowing are also affected by macroglossia.

The size of the tongue affects the shape and structures of the oral cavity, including the teeth, palate, and alveolar ridges. Macroglossia may lead to open bite deformities, prognathism, malocclusion, anterior or posterior cross bite, buccal tipping of posterior teeth, accentuated curve of Spee in the maxillary arch, reverse curve of Spee in the mandibular arch, and increased transverse width of mandibular or maxillary arches. Furthermore, difficulty with mastication may lead to temporomandibular joint pain. If the tongue protrudes beyond the lips, exposing it to the air, it can become dry, with resultant glossitis and stomatitis.

5.4.7 Treatment

5.4.7.1 Medical Therapy

Large tongue has been treated medically and surgically in the last century. To avoid surgical intervention, sclerosing agents, leeches, and physical muscular entrapment of the tongue within the oral cavity have all been tried, but with limited success.

Medical therapy for macroglossia is useful when the underlying cause is identified, and the cause is medically treatable such as hypothyroidism, infection, or amyloidosis. No medical treatments have been proven useful when the cause is unclear.

5.4.7.2 Sclerotherapy/Embolisation

The use of sclerotherapy to cause scarring of the tongue and vascular strangulation, or embolization of the blood vessels supplying the tongue were tried in the past, with many complications and limited success [11].

5.4.7.3 Mechanical Therapy

Mechanical therapy may be useful in macroglossia with hypotonicity due to hypoglossal nerve deficit. Such treatment can be carried out using complex electrical stimulation and construction of a palatal prosthesis, which can be connected to the stimulation device. When the prosthesis is placed in the mouth, the tongue reflexively seeks this foreign body, moving backward and upward to meet it. When the tongue touches the prosthesis, it activates a lingual electrode, which further stimulates the tongue into the backward and upward position.

5.4.7.4 Surgical Treatment

Surgical procedures to reduce tongue size and, more recently, orthognathic surgical intervention have become the treatment modalities of choice. Resection of part of the tongue (partial glossectomy) with anterior wedge technique is indicated when there is airway obstruction, difficulty in speech or swallowing, and because of cosmetic reasons. In some cases, an elective tracheostomy is performed prior to surgical correction. The goal of nearly all surgical procedures in macroglossia is to return the patient to an anatomically and physiologically normal condition that includes articulation, mastication, deglutition, protection of the airway, and gestation. Most studies have shown that surgical procedures for macroglossia lead to improved physical appearance, speech, chewing, and feeding [11].

5.5 Bifid (Cleft) Tongue

Congenital bifid-tongue (also known as "*cleft tongue*") (Fig. 5.4) is a rare congenital anomaly and results from failure of fusion of the two lingual swellings.

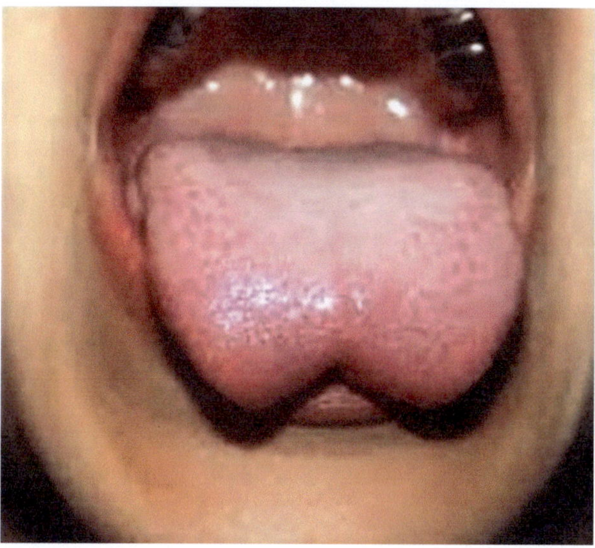

Fig. 5.4 Bifid-tongue (cleft tongue). The tip of the tongue is divided longitudinally for a certain distance

5.5.1 Etiology

The tongue develops during the fourth week of intrauterine life, originating from a median swelling, the tuberculum impar on the floor of the pharynx and two lateral lingual swellings joining this central structure. These lateral lingual structures grow rapidly to cover the tuberculum impar to form the anterior two-thirds of the tongue. When this process is disturbed, the tip of the tongue is divided longitudinally for a certain distance giving rise to cleft tongue/bifid tongue. The occurrence of bifid tongue in the absence of other orofacial abnormalities is a rare entity by itself and usually receives attention much later compared to those seen in association with certain syndromes.

Bifid tongue has been reported in syndromic cases such as Opitz G/BBB syndrome, oral–facial–digital syndrome type I, Klippel–Feil anomaly, and Larsen syndrome. It has also been reported as a rare feature associated with infants of diabetic mother syndrome and as a complication of tongue piercing. Associations have also been postulated with cleft palate, mandibular cleft, midline palatomandibular bony fusion, and cervical vertebrae.

5.5.2 Treatment

Surgical correction of the defect can be undertaken under local anesthesia or general anesthesia. The median parts of the defect are freshened and the tongue is reconstructed by suturing the tongue muscles in layers. Postsurgical healing is usually uneventful with no speech therapy sessions required.

5.6 Double Tongue/Accssory Tongue

5.6.1 Double Tongue

Double tongue means the presence of two tongues in the oral cavity (Fig. 5.5). It results from formation of a double pair of lingual swellings.

5.6.2 Accessory Tongue

Accessory tongue is an extremely uncommon anomaly and difficult to estimate in terms of incidence. It is characterized by a tongue-like neoformation that can be found in the oral cavity, pharynx, or dorsal portion of the tongue (Fig. 5.6). This extremely rare deformity is normally asymptomatic and can be identified at the initial neonatal examination. It is important to distinguish it from a duplication of the tongue [1], lingual ectopic thyroid, and hamartomatous lingual neoformations.

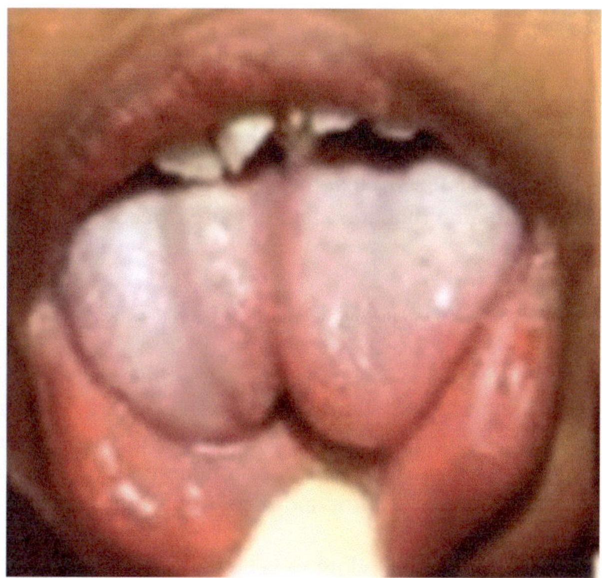

Fig. 5.5 Double tongue in the oral cavity. A very rare congenital anomaly

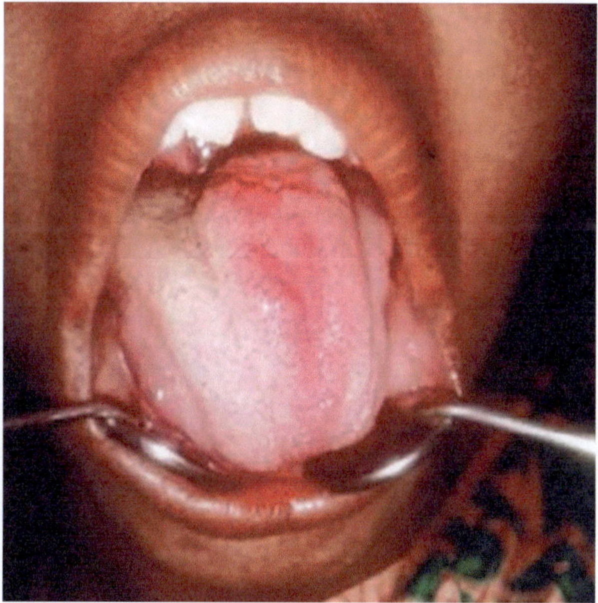

Fig. 5.6 Accessory tongue in the oral cavity on the dorsal portion of the tongue

5.7 Ankyloglossia

5.7.1 Definition

Ankyloglossia (*tongue-tie*) is the general clinical term for the "short lingual frenulum" (less than 2 cm) that limits the range of movement of the tongue (Fig. 5.7) and impacts lingual function including breastfeeding.

5.7.2 Prevalence

Ankyloglossia has been reported to range between 2% and 16% of neonates (depending on the definition of authors), with a male predominance (male: female ratio equals approximately, 3:1). This significant wide range can be attributable to the lack of diagnostic criteria for tongue-tie [16–19]. However, because the tongue normally is short at birth and then grows longer at the tip, the prevalence is much lower in adults.

Most cases of Ankyloglossia are believed to be sporadic rather than genetic, and commonly it is an isolated anomaly; although, associations with other genetic disorders have been reported.

5.7.3 Etiology

The exact etiopathogenesis of tongue-tie is unknown. It is claimed to result from failure of deepening of the alveolo-lingual sulcus.

A short lingual frenulum is also associated with a number of *genetic syndromes* such as ROR2-Related Robinow syndrome, dystrophic epidermolysis bullosa,

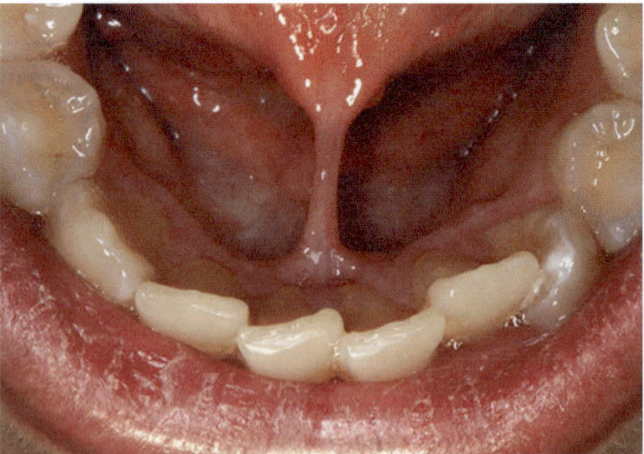

Fig. 5.7 Ankyloglossia (*tongue tie*). Note the thick lingual frenulum attached to the tongue limiting the range of its free movement

Table 5.3 Genetic syndromes associated with ankyloglossia

Robinow syndrome is an extremely rare genetic disorder characterized by short-limbed dwarfism, abnormalities in the head, face, and external genitalia, as well as vertebral segmentation. The disorder was first described in 1969 by human geneticist Meinhard Robinow, along with physicians Frederic N. Silverman and Hugo D. Smith. By 2002, over 100 cases had been documented
Epidermolysis bullosa (DEB) is a group of genetic conditions that cause the skin to be very fragile and to blister easily. Blisters and skin erosions form in response to minor injury or friction, such as rubbing or scratching. DEB is one of the major forms of epidermolysis bullosa
Oral-facial-digital syndrome, type 1 (OFDSI) is a multiple anomaly syndrome inherited as an X-linked dominant trait. It is caused by defects in the OFD1 gene, which maps to Xp22.2
Opitz syndrome, also known as *oculo-genito-laryngeal syndrome and BBB/G compound syndrome*, is a genetic condition characterized by widely spaced eyes and, in males, hypospadias
Van der Woude syndrome (VDWS) is a genetic disorder characterized by the combination of lower lip pits, cleft lip with or without cleft palate, and cleft palate only

oral-facial-digital syndrome type I, Opitz syndrome (X-Linked Opitz G/BBB Syndrome) and Van der Woude syndrome (Table 5.3) [5]. Nevertheless, ankyloglossia occurs mostly as an isolated congenital anomaly.

Studies of *nonsyndromic ankyloglossia* have suggested both autosomal-dominant and X-linked inheritance, although in one of the studies 47% of those affected had no family history of ankyloglossia. Familial cleft palate with or without ankyloglossia is caused by mutation in the *TBX22* gene.

5.7.4 Classification

Ankyloglossia can be observed at different ages with specific indications for treatment for each group. Still, however, there is no accurate classification for this condition [20].

5.7.4.1 Anterior/Posterior [21–23]

The term *anterior ankyloglossia* is used for examples in which the attachment of the frenum extends toward the tip of the tongue (Fig. 5.8).

Posterior ankyloglossia is often more difficult to appreciate, being caused by short submucosal collagen fibers in the posterior midline floor of the mouth that prevent full tongue motion (Fig. 5.9).

5.7.4.2 Complete/Partial [21–23]

Complete Ankyloglossia: The tongue is unable to protrude past the alveolar ridge or to move laterally (it is uncommon but, when present, requires frenuloplasty).

Partial Ankyloglossia: In this case, there is variability in the lingual range of motion. It has been reported in up to 5% of newborns.

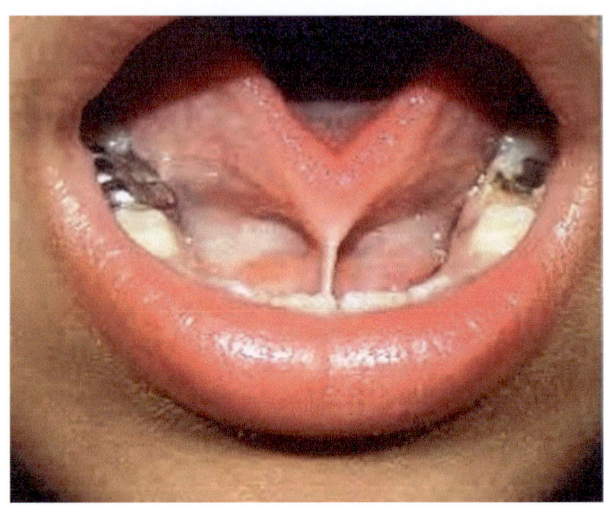

Fig. 5.8 Anterior ankyloglossia. Note the thin lingual frenulum attached to the tip of the tongue

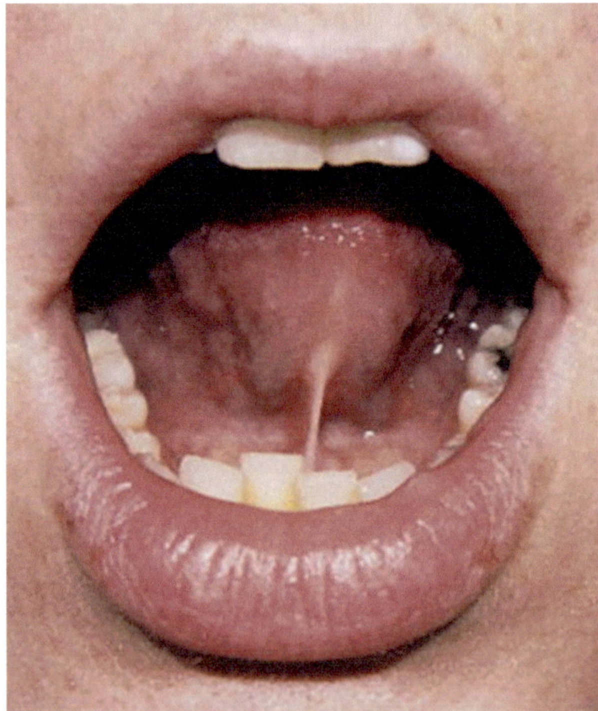

Fig. 5.9 Posterior ankyloglossia in a 16-year-old lady with inability to protrude the tongue i.e. (tongue-tie)

5.7.4.3 Hazelbaker Assessment Tool for Lingual Frenulum Function (HATLFF) [24, 25]

This tool was developed to evaluate the severity of tongue-ties in newborns. It is based on the tongue's anatomy and its functional aspects as follows:

- *Anatomy*: appearance of tongue when lifted, elasticity of frenulum, length of lingual frenulum when tongue lifted, attachment of lingual frenulum to tongue, and attachment of lingual frenulum to inferior alveolar ridge.
- *Function*: lateralization, lift of tongue, extension of the tongue, spread, cupping of tongue, peristalsis, snap-back.

This tool consists of 10 points for frenulum anatomy and 14 points for tongue function. It uses a scoring system to classify babies' tongues into one of three categories:

1. Functionally impaired
2. Acceptable
3. Perfect.

However, it is complex, lengthy, and has not been validated in a controlled manner [26].

5.7.4.4 Coryllos Classifications of Tongue-Tie [27]

This classification divided ankyloglossia into four types, according to how close to the tip of the tongue the leading edge of the frenulum is attached as shown in Table 5.4:

Coryllos types 1 and 2, considered as "classical" tongue-tie, are the most common and obvious tongue-ties and probably account for 75%. Types 3 and 4 are less common and, because they are more difficult to visualize, are the most likely to go untreated. Type 4 is most likely to cause symptoms that are more significant for mother and infant.

5.7.4.5 Kotlow Classification of Tongue-Tie

It is the most commonly used classification tool. Kotlow described upper lip-tie classification for infants. Four classes were described as seen in Table 5.5.

Table 5.4 Coryllos classifications of tongue-tie

Type 1	Attachment of the frenulum to tip of tongue
Type 2	Attachment is 2–4 mm behind tip of tongue/on or behind alveolar ridge
Type 3	Attachment to mid-tongue and the middle of the floor of the mouth, usually tighter and less elastic
Type 4	Attachment against base of tongue, thick, shiny, and inelastic

Table 5.5 Kotlow classification of ankyloglossia [28, 29]

Type	Frenular attachment	Free tongue length
Clinically acceptable	Normal	Normal free tongue movement >16 mm
Class I (mild)	No significant attachment	12–16 mm
Class II (moderate)	Attachment mostly into the gingival tissue	8–11 mm
Class III (severe)	Attachment in front of the anterior papilla	3–7 mm
Class IV (complete)	Attachment into the papilla or extending into hard palate	<3 mm

5.7.5 Clinical Presentation

Tongue tie may occur with varying degrees of severity, which does not always correlate with severity of functional impairment. Some children have no problems with eating/drinking or speech and others do.

Some derangements that may result from ankyloglossia include the following:

5.7.5.1 Feeding and Swallowing Difficulties

Feeding difficulties may be encountered such as (1) breastfeeding difficulties (prolonged feeding, difficulty latching, and irritability while feeding), (2) poor tongue movement and chewing due to restricted tongue movement laterally, and (3) persistent messy eating (due to the child being unable to clear food from the buccal cavities and the lips).

Ngerncham et al. (2013), reported that poor latch with maternal nipple pain and insufficient milk transfer may result, although less than half of infants with even moderate to severe tongue tie appear to be affected [30].

As described in ABM Clinical Protocol 11, neonatal ankyloglossia, standardized clinical tools to assess the degree of tongue tie and its impact on breastfeeding include the *Hazelbaker assessment tool for lingual frenulum function* [31]. In 2008, Geddes and colleagues reported that one-week pre-frenotomy and post-frenotomy changes in sucking pattern and milk transfer were demonstrated on submental ultrasonography [32]. However, whether or not frenulotomy (division of the frenulum), frenulectomy (removal of the frenulum), or frenuloplasty (frenulotomy with stitches) clearly improves breastfeeding has been controversial. Systematic reviews including five randomized controlled studies, of which four used validated measures of latch as a primary outcome, concluded that frenotomy in selected infants appears to provide objective improvements in breastfeeding measures, with subjective improvement in maternal pain [33].

5.7.5.2 Speech Impairment/Development Disorders [34]

In ankyloglossia, a short lingual frenulum extending from the tip of the tongue to the floor of the mouth and onto the lingual gingival tissue limits movements of the tongue and causes speech difficulties. Stripping of the lingual tissues may occur if the tongue-tie is not corrected.

Substitution and distortion of tongue tip (alveolar) sounds /l/, /t/, /d/, /n/, /s/, /z/ caused by restricted elevation of the tongue tip may occur. Slower-than-normal speech rate or reduced speech intelligibility in conversational speech has been reported. Reduced speech precision during shouting (shouting requires the mouth to open more widely and thereby may result in the tongue tie having a more negative effect on speech precision) is also encountered.

If a child's speech or feeding appears to be affected by tongue tie, an assessment by a speech pathologist and a pediatric dentist is useful to determine whether lingual frenectomy is required.

5.7.5.3 Gingival Recession/Dental Caries

It also has been theorized that ankyloglossia might contribute to gingival recession if the frenulum attaches high on the lingual alveolar mucosa. Ankyloglossia (tongue tie) can lead to dental caries in older children because it may be difficult to clean the lower teeth.

5.7.5.4 Other Reported Problems

Other reported problems include difficulty eating certain foods that include licking (ice cream), playing certain wind instruments (e.g. flutes, clarinets, tubas, trumpets), and orthodontic problems (open bite and malocclusion).

5.7.5.5 Social Concerns

Possible social concerns related to the reduction of tongue mobility may include speech, oral hygiene, excessive salivation, kissing, spitting while talking, and self-esteem and psychological issues. With only one poor-quality comparative study, the evidence related to the ability of ankyloglossia treatment to alleviate social concerns is currently insufficient [35, 36].

5.7.6 Identification of Ankyloglossia (Tongue-Tie) [37]

- When the tongue protrudes, the tip is anchored behind the alveolar ridge.
- When the infant cries, the tongue remains anchored.
- The tongue is notched or heart-shaped when protruded.
- The tongue cannot be manually extended by the examiner.
- The frenulum is short (less than 1 cm or ½ in.) and inelastic.
- The tongue is attached close to alveolar ridge.

5.7.7 Treatment

The biggest question for physicians dealing with patients with ankyloglossia remains whether to treat or not to treat. There is clear evidence that supports treatment in symptomatic patients [38–42].

Frenotomy (division of the frenulum by clipping and freeing the frenulum), *frenectomy* (removal of the frenulum), and *frenuloplasty* (frenulotomy with stitches) are the main surgical treatment options to release or remove an ankyloglossia, though there is still debate about surgical intervention.

Because most cases of ankyloglossia do not result in significant clinical problems, treatment is often unnecessary. For infants with breastfeeding difficulty, *frenotomy* may improve the ability to nurse. However, there is insufficient evidence to support prophylactic surgical correction of tongue-tie in an effort to improve speech development. A reduction of the frenulum should be recommended only if local conditions or speech problems warrant the treatment.

Because the frenulum is thin and relatively avascular in neonates and young infants, it can often be incised as an office procedure; anesthesia is usually not required, nor is suturing. The timing of frenotomy varies from 6 to 18 days of age. In a study of 200 infants undergoing frenotomy without analgesia, researchers found that 18% cried during the procedure and 60% after the procedure. Rarely the frenulum grows back.

In older children, surgical treatment may require a short general anesthetic because the frenulum is thicker and more vascular, requiring surgical correction that includes *frenulectomy* in which the frenulum is released in a similar manner as in frenotomy although occasionally limited division of the genioglossus may be required for adequate release. The wound is sutured with or without a z-plasty flap closure (*frenuluplasty*). However, the latter procedure is rarely required. Some complications have been reported after frenulectomy [43]. Observation for bleeding is brief. In the rare case of bleeding for more than 3 min, a strip of gelatin foam can be applied to achieve rapid hemostasis and removed before feeding.

5.7.8 Prognosis

Prognosis of a patient with ankyloglossia is good, and overall, patients develop normally. Some complications could include low self-esteem and psychological issues, but that can be easily addressed.

5.7.9 Pearls for Clinical Practice [44]

- Ankyloglossia occurs most commonly in *males*.
- The most commonly feared *complication* is difficulty with breastfeeding that leads to failure to gain weight.
- In most patients in whom ankyloglossia is an incidental finding, the best management is *observation and reassurance*.
- In cases where management is necessary, *frenotomy* is the treatment of choice; it is simple with few side effects and can be done in an outpatient setting.

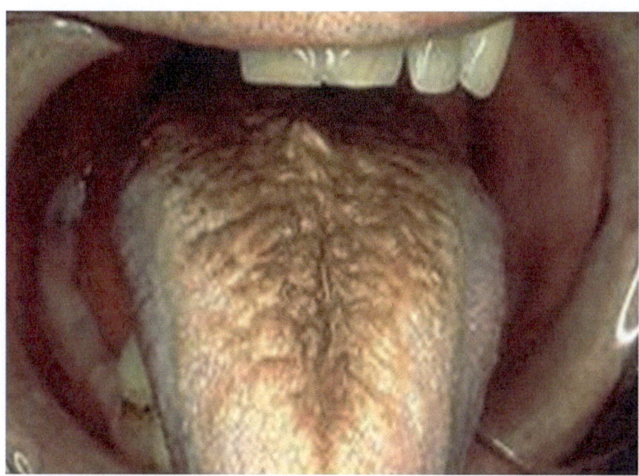

Fig. 5.10 Black hairy tongue. Note the discoloration of the dorsal surface of the tongue

5.8 Black Hairy Tongue

It is a disorder characterized by changes in the appearance of tongue color. It results from elongation of filiform papillae and their failure to desquamate or fall-off. It may also result from some antibiotics, heavy smoking, and antiseptic mouth washes. However, there is no known cause in the majority of cases [45].

Clinically, it produces brownish or black areas of discoloration of the tongue appearing as if there is hair on the tongue. It is more common in middle of the tongue (Fig. 5.10) [46].

Treatment of black hairy tongue consists of good oral hygiene and the use of a toothbrush or tongue scraper to aid with the desquamation of the tongue. Antifungal drugs may be warranted if there is a suspicion of Candida infection [46].

Details of black hairy tongue are mentioned in Chap. 8 (Tongue Discoloration).

5.9 Fissured Tongue

5.9.1 Definition

It means "presence of multiple fissures (deep grooves) on the dorsum of the tongue." The mucosa looks normal. It is also known as *plicated or scrotal tongue* (Fig. 5.11). Although these grooves may look unsettling (Fig. 5.12), the condition is usually painless. Some individuals may complain of an associated burning sensation [47].

5.9.2 Epidemiology

Fissured tongue is relatively common with a prevalence ranging between 6.8% [48] and 11% [49]. Often hereditary in children, may also be part of degenerative process. Prevalence increases significantly with age, occurring in approximately 40% of the population after the age of 40 years [50].

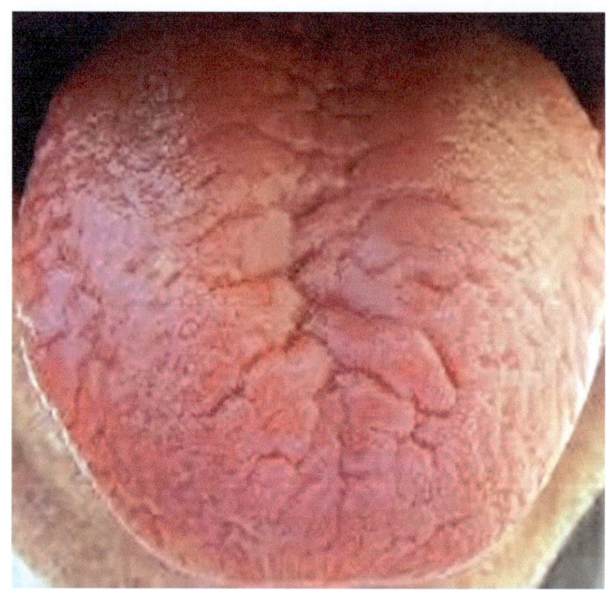

Fig. 5.11 Fissure tongue (plicated or scrotal tongue)

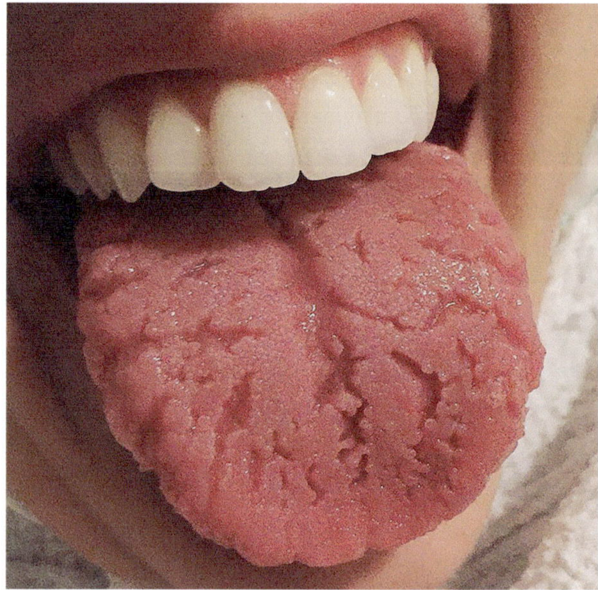

Fig. 5.12 Fissure tongue (deep fissures that look unsettling)

Table 5.6 Genetic syndromes associated with fissured tongue

Melkersson-Rosenthal syndrome is a rare neurological disorder characterized by recurring facial paralysis, swelling of the face and lips (usually the upper lip—cheilitis granulomatosis) and the development of folds and furrows in the tongue (fissured tongue)
Down syndrome (also known as ***trisomy 21***), is a genetic disorder caused by the presence of all or part of a third copy of chromosome 21. It is usually associated with physical growth delays, mild to moderate intellectual disability, and features. The average IQ of a young adult with down syndrome is 50, equivalent to the mental ability of an 8- or 9-year-old child, but this can vary widely
Cowden's syndrome (also known as multiple hamartoma syndrome) is an autosomal dominant inherited condition characterized by benign hamartomas as well as an increased lifetime risk of breast, thyroid, uterine, and other cancers

5.9.3 Etiology

The cause of fissured tongue is exactly unknown, but it may be partly a *genetic* trait. *Aging and environmental* factors may also contribute to the appearance.

Fissured tongue is seen in *Melkersson-Rosenthal syndrome* (along with facial nerve paralysis and granulomatous cheilitis). It is also seen in the majority of patients with *Down syndrome*, in association with geographic tongue, in patients with oral manifestations of psoriasis, and in healthy individuals. Fissured tongue is also sometimes a feature of *Cowden's syndrome* (Table 5.6).

5.9.4 Treatment

A fissured tongue does not typically require treatment. Often, it does not have any symptoms, and a person may not know they have the condition until a dentist discovers it during a routine checkup. Complications of fissured tongue typically occur if food or other debris gets caught in the grooves. If this happens, it can cause irritation or allow bacteria to grow. The bacteria trapped in the fissures can cause *bad breath* or promote *tooth decay*.

In extreme cases, *Candida albicans* may infect very deep grooves and require treatment with a topical antifungal medication. The best prevention against fissured tongue is to practice proper oral hygiene, including cleaning of the mouth at least twice a day and regular visits to the dentist.

5.10 Lingual (Sublingual) Varices

Everyone has veins in and around the tongue that may vary in size, shape, or color. *Lingual varicosities* are "veins under and on the sides of the tongue." They can be red, blue, or purple in color (Fig. 5.13) and generally occur in clusters.

Sublingual varices are not unusual. They are a common clinical finding [51]. Their prevalence increases with age, with surveys indicating that they are present in up to 60% of elderly patients, in both sexes, and in different population groups [51–53].

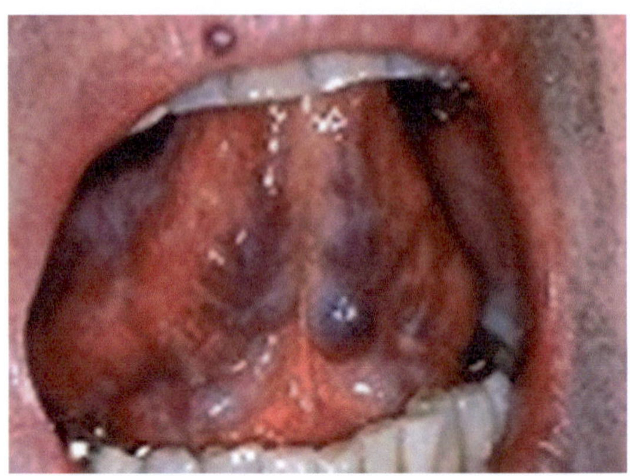

Fig. 5.13 Sublingual varicosities, bluish in color

Hemoptysis has once been reported due to bleeding from varices at the base of the tongue, associated with portal hypertension, but review of literature for spontaneous hemorrhage from sublingual varices does not show any similar reported cases to that described [54]. The advice given that sublingual varices can cause subtle and potentially dangerous bleeding is based on negligible evidence. It would be unfortunate if it induced unnecessary cauterization and misled clinicians from searching for the true cause of a patient's hemoptysis [55].

5.11 Lingual Thyroid Nodule

Hickman in 1869 was the first person to report the presence of lingual ectopia of the thyroid gland. The reported incidence of this condition has been 1 in 100,000 cases, which shows the rarity of this ectopic lesion [56, 57].

5.11.1 Definition

Lingual thyroid is a rare clinical entity of the oropharyngeal region caused by failure of the thyroid gland to descend to its normal position during embryogenesis. Although "*lingual thyroid*" is an accepted terminology, the term "*ectopia*" may be used better to describe those general conditions where thyroid tissues are seen in places other than tongue [56].

5.11.2 Pathogenesis

The exact pathogenesis of this accessory thyroid tissue is not clearly understood, it generally arises from failure of migration of the median thyroid rudiment or unobliterated thyroglossal duct epithelium [57].

The thyroid gland normally descends along the midline with growth of the neck but at times all or part of the gland may fail to migrate along the path from ventral floor of the pharynx to its normal location in front of trachea over thyroid cartilage and it sequestrates within the tongue substance giving rise to an embryological defect with location at the base of the tongue, in a zone posterior to the circumvallate papillae [58–60].

5.11.3 Epidemiology

There is no age predilection for lingual thyroid nodules, although Thomas et al. found that the peak incidence of occurrence is seen in the third decade of life. Male to female ratio of occurrence is has been reported to be 1:7 [56, 61]. Lingual thyroid is mostly seen in females particularly during puberty, pregnancy, or menopause when the plasma TSH level increases in the body leading to hypertrophy of ectopic tissue [62].

5.11.3.1 Other Rare Sites

Other rare sites of occurrence such as submandibular, prelaryngeal, tracheal, laterocervical, esophageal, and substernal have also been reported. The most frequent sites of ectopic thyroid tissue are lingual, sublingual, thyroglossal, laryngotracheal, and lateral cervical. Thyroid tissue can also be found, though very rarely, in remote structures that were associated with the thyroid anlage during development, including the esophagus, mediastinum, heart, aorta, adrenal, pancreas, gall bladder, and skin. Ectopic thyroid tissue usually occurs in a single site, although presence of dual ectopic tissue in lingual and subhyoid region has been reported [63].

5.11.3.2 Clinical Presentation

Female predominance of occurrence is seen seven times higher than male counterpart. It may also occur in more than one ectopic site in the human body. It usually presents as a reddish lobulated mass behind the foramen cecum. It lies at the *foramen cecum* at the back of the tongue. It may be *lingual,* projecting from the tongue (Fig. 5.14) or *sublingual*, between the tongue and the mylohyoid muscle.

Clinically, a rounded reddish brown swelling is seen at the back of the tongue as shown in Fig. 5.15 [60, 64]. It may cause dysphagia, speech problems, respiratory obstruction, hemorrhage, hypothyroidism (about 70% of patients with ectopic thyroid are hypothyroid [61], and less commonly, hyperthyroidism [65, 66], though most of them remain asymptomatic until late adolescence. Rare cases of sleep apnea syndrome due to lingual thyroid have also been reported in the literature [67].

Conditions such as thyroid adenoma, hyperplasia, inflammation, and carcinoma which may affect the thyroid gland in normal position are also seen in ectopic tissues [61]. Malignant transformation of lingual thyroid is rather a rare entity [67].

Technetium (Tc-99) scintigraphy is the most important diagnostic technique employed in the identification of this ectopic thyroid [68].

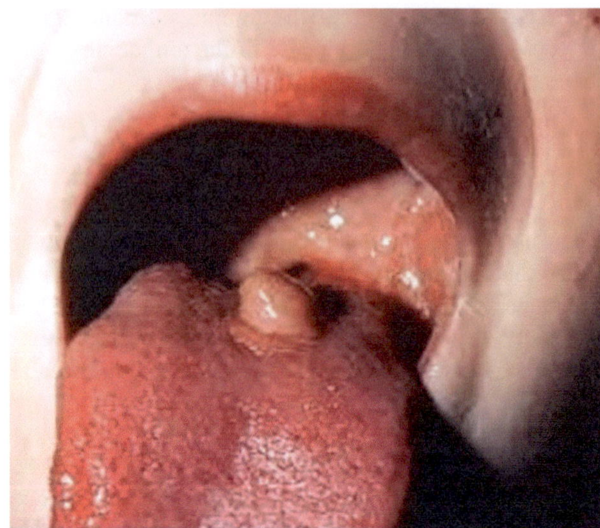

Fig. 5.14 Lingual thyroid nodule at the foramen cecum at the back of the tongue

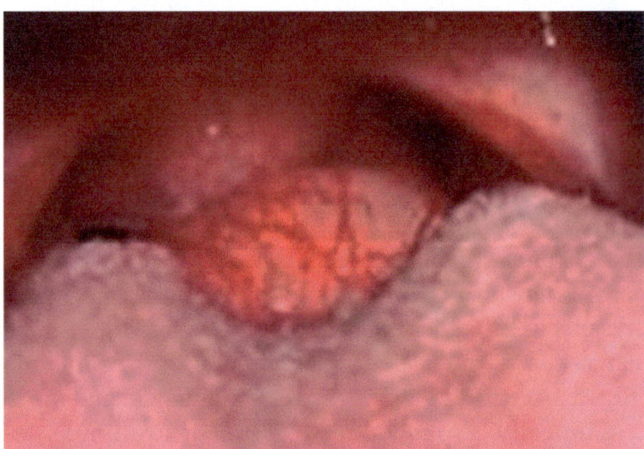

Fig. 5.15 Lingual thyroid tissue seen as a round reddish mass seen at the back of the tongue

5.11.4 Differential Diagnosis

The differential diagnosis of lingual thyroid should include vascular tumors, telangiectatic granuloma, teratomas, and benign or malignant processes in the posterior region of the tongue [69, 70]. Lingual thyroid should be investigated based on thyroid function tests and scintigraphy. Increased TSH value with decreased T3 and T4 level are usually seen in thyroid function test denoting hypothyroidism [71]. Very few studies have found labeled thyroglobulin as a powerful immunohistological marker to confirm the thyroid origin of the tissue [67].

5.11.5 Treatment

Treatment modalities employed in lingual thyroid depends on factors such as a general condition of patient, size, and degree of discomfort.

A lingual thyroid nodule may be the only thyroid tissue, or an accessory thyroid tissue (proved by scanning). If *asymptomatic*, there is no need for removal and patients are followed-up regularly *without any treatmen*t and supplemental thyroxine should be given in hypothyroid patients. El-troxin tablets should be given to reduce the size of the gland. *Thyroxine* suppresses TSH stimulation and minimizes goitrous enlargement [60].

Failure of medical therapy, obstructive symptoms, and complications such as ulceration, bleeding, cystic degeneration, or malignancy are indications for *surgery*. Excision should be done, but if it is the only thyroid tissue in the body, it must be implanted in the infrahyoid muscle otherwise, El-troxin is given as a replacement for life.

Despite providing limited accessibility, the trans-oral approach with cold instruments with monopolar coagulation and laser CO_2 is the most widely employed technique for smaller lesions as they avoid injury to deep neck structures such as lingual nerve. Other methods usually used include lateral pharyngotomy, suprahyoid, and transhyoid techniques. Occasionally, midline mandibular split osteotomy is employed for larger lesions [49, 62, 72].

Ablative *radioiodine therapy* is an alternative approach recommended in older patients or patients who are unfit for surgery. This treatment should be avoided in children and young adults because of slow response to medication, fibrosis, and dependence on life-long thyroid hormone replacement and often the systemic doses required have potentially damaging effects on the gonads or other organs [73].

References

1. Gupta SR. Isolated aglossia congenita: a rare case of oromandibular limb hypogenesis syndrome type I B. J Oral Maxillofac Pathol. 2012;16:414–9.
2. Weingarten RT, Walner DL, Holinger LD. Tongue hypoplasia in a newborn. Int J Pediatr Otorhinolaryngol. 1993;25:235–41.
3. Thorp MA, de Waal PJ, Prescott CA. Extreme microglossia. Int J Pediatr Otorhinolaryngol. 2003;67:473–7.
4. Jang GY, Lee KC, Choung JT, Son CS, Tockgo YC. Congenital aglossia with situs inversus totalis - a case report. J Korean Med Sci. 1997;12:55–7.
5. Nepram SS, Jain P, Devi R, Huidrom RD. Isolated microglossia. A case report. J Med Soc. 2015;29:180–1.
6. Emmanouil-Nikoloussi EN, Kerameos-Foroglou C. Developmental malformations of human tongue and associated syndromes (review). Bull Group Int Rech Sci Stomatol Odontol. 1992;35:5–12.
7. Chicarilli ZN, Polayes IM. Oromandibular limb hypogenesis syndromes. Plast Reconstr Surg. 1985;76:13–24.
8. Iwata J, Suzuki A, Pelikan RC, Ho TV, Chai Y. Noncanonical transforming growth factor β (TGFβ) signaling in cranial neural crest cells causes tongue muscle developmental defects. J Biol Chem. 2013;288:60–70.

9. Boyd SG, Harden A, Patton MA. The EEG in early diagnosis of Angelman's (happy puppet) syndrome. Eur J Pediatr. 1988;147:503–13.
10. Simmonds JC, Patel AK, Mildenhall NR, Mader NS, Scott AR. Neonatal macroglossia: demographics, cost of care, and associated comorbidities. Cleft Palate Craniofac J. 2018;55(8):1122–9.
11. Najjar T. Macroglossia. Medscape reference. March 25, 2015. http://emedicine.medscape.com/article/873658-overview.
12. Prada CE, Zarate YA, Hopkin RJ. Genetic causes of macroglossia: diagnostic approach. Pediatrics. 2012;129(2):431–7.
13. Sivasankari T, Jeelani S, et al. Lymphangioma of the tongue - a case report and review of literature. J Clin Diagn Res. 2014;8(9):12–4.
14. Isaacson GC. Congenital anomalies of the jaw, mouth, oral cavity, and pharynx. UpToDate. Waltham; 2015.
15. Dudhia SB, Dudhia BB. Undetected hypothyroidism: a rare dental diagnosis. J Oral MaxillofacPathol. 2014;18(2):315–9.
16. Campanha SMA, Martinelli RLC, Palhares DB. Association between ankyloglossia and breastfeeding. Codas. 2019;31(1):e20170264.
17. Hill R. Implications of ankyloglossia on breastfeeding. MCN Am J Matern Child Nurs. 2019;44(2):73–9.
18. Wood NK. Home-based interventions in a case of first latch at 27 days. NursWomens Health. 2019;23(2):135–40.
19. Mills N, Pransky SM, Geddes DT, Mirjalili SA. What is a tongue tie? Defining the anatomy of the in-situ lingual frenulum. Clin Anat. 2019;32(6):749–61.
20. Suter VG, Bornstein MM. Ankyloglossia: facts and myths in diagnosis and treatment. J Periodontol. 2009;80:1204–19.
21. Martin MS, Schwartz RH. Tackling ankyloglossia in the office. Contemp Pediatr. 2008;25:59–64.
22. Krol DM, Keels MA. Oral conditions. Pediatr Rev. 2007;28:17–8.
23. Lalakea ML, Messner AH. Ankyloglssia: does it matter? Pediatr Clin N Am. 2003;50:381–97.
24. Hazelbaker AK. The assessment tool for lingual frenulum function: use in a lactation consultant private practice (Master's thesis). Pasadena, CA: Pacific Oaks College; 1993.
25. Hazelbaker AK. Tongue-tie: morphogenesis, impact, assessment and treatment. Columbus, OH: Aidan and Eva Press; 2010.
26. Ingram J, Johnson D, Copeland M, et al. The development of a tongue assessment tool to assist with tongue-tie identification. Arch Dis Child Fetal Neonatal Ed. 2015;100:F344–8.
27. Watson Genna C, editor. Supporting sucking skills in breastfeeding infants. Burlington, MA: Jones & Bartlett Learning; 2016.
28. Kotlow LA. Ankyloglossia (tongue-tie): a diagnostic and treatment quandary. Quintess Int. 1999;30:259–62.
29. Kotlow L. Diagnosing and understanding the maxillary lip-tie (superior labial, the maxillary labial frenum) as it relates to breastfeeding. J Hum Lact. 2013;29:458–64.
30. Amir L, James J, Beatty J. Review of tongue tie release at a tertiary maternity hospital. J Paediatr Child Health. 2005;41:243–5.
31. Geddes DT, Kent JC, Mitoulas LR, Hartmann PE. Tongue movement and intra-oral vacuum in breastfeeding infants. Early Hum Dev. 2008;84(7):471–7.
32. Francis DO, Krishnaswami S, McPheeters M. Treatment of ankyloglossia and breastfeeding outcomes: a systematic review. Pediatrics. 2015;135(6):e1458–66.
33. Marchesan QI. Lingual frenulum: classification and speech interference. Int J Orofacial Myology. 2004;30:31–8.
34. Daggumati S, Cohn JE, Brennan MJ, Evarts M, McKinnon BJ, Terk AR. Caregiver perception of speech quality in patients with ankyloglossia: comparison between surgery and non-treatment. Int J Pediatr Otorhinolaryngol. 2019;119:70–4.
35. Srinivasan A, Al Khoury A, Puzhko S, Dobrich C, Stern M, Mitnick H, Goldfarb L. Frenotomy in infants with tongue-tie and breastfeeding problems. J Hum Lact. 2019;35(4):706–12.

36. Adewumi AO, Wallen J. In: Nowak AJ, Christensen JR, Wells MH, editors. Pediatric dentistry. 6th ed. WB Saunders; 2019.
37. Kapoor P. The tongue tie: untied. Indian Pediatr. 2018;55(10):917.
38. Perez-Aguirre B, Soto-Barreras U, Loyola-Rodriguez JP, Reyes-Macias JF, Santos-Diaz MA, Loyola-Leyva A, Garcia-Cortes O. Oral findings and its association with prenatal and perinatal factors in newborns. Korean J Pediatr. 2018;61(9):279–84.
39. Dixon B, Gray J, Elliot N, Shand B, Lynn A. A multifaceted programme to reduce the rate of tongue-tie release surgery in newborn infants: observational study. Int J Pediatr Otorhinolaryngol. 2018;113:156–63.
40. Belmehdi A, Harti KE, Wady WE. Ankyloglossia as an oral functional problem and its surgical management. Dent Med Probl. 2018;55(2):213–6.
41. Patel J, Anthonappa RP, King NM. All tied up! Influences of oral frenulae on breastfeeding and their recommended management strategies. J Clin Pediatr Dent. 2018;42(6):407–13.
42. Maciag M, Sediva I, Alexander-Scott N. Submandibular swelling and fever following frenulectomy in a 13-day-old infant. Clin Pediatr (Phila). 2016;55(10):990–2.
43. Segal LM, Stephenson R, Dawes M, Feldman P. Prevalence, diagnosis, and treatment of ankyloglossia: methodologic review. Can Fam Physician. 2007;53:1027–33.
44. Garg A, Wadhera R, Gulati SP, Goyal R. Hairy tongue. J Assoc Physic India. 2008;56:816.
45. Gurvits GE, Tan A. Black hairy tongue syndrome. World J Gastroenterol. 2014;20(31):10845–50.
46. Crispian S. Oral and maxillofacial medicine: the basis of diagnosis and treatment. 2nd ed. Edinburgh: Churchill Livingstone; 2008.
47. Aljawfi K. Frequency of tongue anomalies among Yemeni children in dental clinics. Yemeni. J Med Sci. 2013;7:27–32.
48. Rabiei M, Mohtashame Amiri Z, Masoodi Rad H, Niazi M, Niazi H. Frequency of tongue anomalies in primary school of Lahidjan. Journal of Guilan University of Medical Sciences. 2003;12(45):36–42.
49. Chernoff R. Geriatric nutrition: the health professional's handbook. Burlington, MA: Jones & Bartlett Learning; 2006. p. 176.
50. Ettinger RL, Manderson RD. A clinical study of sublingual varices. Oral Surg Oral Med Oral Path. 1974;38:540–5.
51. Kleinman HZ. Lingual varicosities. Oral Surg Oral Med Oral Path. 1967;23:546–8.
52. Kovac-Kavcic M, Skaleric U. The prevalence of oral mucosal lesions in a population in Ljubljana,Slovenia. J Oral Pathol Med. 2000;29:331–5.
53. Jassar P, Jaramillo M, Nunez DA. Base of tongue varices associated with portal hypertension. Postgrad Med J. 2000;76:576–7.
54. Pemberton MN. Sublingual varices are not unusual. BMJ. 2006;22:333.
55. Douglas PS, Baker AW. Lingual thyroid. Br J Oral MaxillofacSurg. 1994;32:123–4.
56. Hickman W. Congenital tumour of the base of the tongue passing down the epiglottis on the larynx and causing death by suffocation sixteen hours after death (sic.). Trans Path Soc Lond. 1869;20:160.
57. Prasad KC, Bhat V. Surgical management of lingual thyroid: a report of four cases. J Oral Maxillofac Surg. 2000;58:223–7.
58. Batsakis JG, El-Naggar AK, Luna MA. Thyroid gland ectopias. Ann Otol Rhinol Laryngol. 1996;105:996–1000.
59. Ueda D, Yoto Y, Sato T. Ultrasonic assessment of the lingual thyroid gland in children. Pediatr Radiol. 1998;28:126–8.
60. Thomas G, Hoilat R, Daniels JS, Kalagie W. Ectopic lingual thyroid: a case report. Int J Oral Maxillofac Surg. 2003;32:219–21.
61. Farrell ML, Forer M. Lingual thyroid. Aust NZ J Surg. 1994;64:135–8.
62. Klubo-Gwiezdzinska J, Manes RP, Chia SH, Burman KD, Stathatos NA, Deeb ZE, et al. Clinical review: ectopic cervical thyroid carcinoma – review of the literature with illustrative case series. J Clin Endocrinol Metab. 2011;96:2684–91.

63. Polo Tomás I, AlemánLópez O, López Rico JJ, Talavera Sánchez J, Córdoba C. Follicular carcinoma originating in the lingual thyroid: a case report. Acta Otorrinolaringol Esp. 1996;47:407–10.
64. Gallo A, Leonetti F, Torri E, Manciocco V, Simonelli M, DeVincentiis M. Ectopic lingual thyroid as unusual cause of severe dysphagia. Dysphagia. 2001;16:220–3.
65. Hafidh MA, Sheahan P, Khan NA, Colreavy M, Timon C. Role of CO2 laser in the management of obstructive ectopic lingual thyroids. J Laryngol Otol. 2004;118:807–9.
66. Rashid M, Majeed S, Tariq KM, Inam-ul-Haq, Niwaz A, Saeed A. Lingual thyroid as a cause of snoring and sleep apnea. J Coll Physicians Surg Pak. 2004;14:681–2.
67. Kumar LKS, Kurien NM, Jacob MM, Menon PV, Khalam SA. Lingual thyroid. Ann Maxillofac Surg. 2015;5(1):104–7.
68. Akyol MU, Ozcan M. Lingual thyroid. Otolaryngol Head Neck Surg. 1996;115:483–4.
69. Koch CA, Picken C, Clement SC, Azumi N, Sarlis NJ. Ectopic lingual thyroid: an otolaryngologic emergency beyond childhood. Thyroid. 2000;10:511–4.
70. Anand SS, Sood V, Kumar PG, Suryanayna KM, Kotwal N. Case report – lingual thyroid. Med J Armed Forces India. 2006;62:2.
71. Wapshaw H. Lingual thyroid; a report of a case with unusual histology. Br J Surg. 1942;30:160.
72. Giovagnorio F, Cordier A, Romeo R. Lingual thyroid: value of integrated imaging. Eur Radiol. 1996;6:105–7.
73. Collins P. Embryology and development. In: Williams PL, Bannister LH, Berry MM, editors. Gray's anatomy – the anatomical basis of medicine and surgery. 38th ed. New York, NY: Churchill Livingston; 1995. p. 174–99.

6 Tongue Trauma

6.1 Common Tongue Injuries

6.1.1 Etiology

A *fall at home* is the most common situation that causes accidental tongue injury. Lateral *tongue biting* is 100% specific for epileptic seizures and may be helpful in differentiating seizures from syncope and pseudo-seizure [1].

The most common *location* of a tongue injury is the anterior dorsum of the tongue (Fig. 6.1) followed by the mid-dorsal and anterior ventral surfaces. Other causes of tongue injury include tongue piercing, tongue burn, intoxication, road traffic accidents, iatrogenic causes or self-mutilation. The frequency of injury reduces from anterior to posterior on both surfaces [2].

6.1.2 Sequelae

Hemorrhage and disfigurement are the two most common concerns in lacerated tongue injuries, although loss of function, infection, and swelling that compromises the airway are also mentioned as sequelae. The tongue has a rich blood supply, and the airway may be compromised sometime after trauma to the tongue or lacerations of the floor of the mouth if veins are injured, resulting in swelling of the tongue into the oropharynx and the possibility of suffocation.

6.1.3 Management

6.1.3.1 To Suture or Not?

The largely anecdotal literature on tongue lacerations can confuse clinicians. Andreasen and Andreasen [3] suggested suturing both dorsum and lateral border injuries. Powers et al. [4] suggested loosely suturing tongue wounds and placing

© The Author(s), under exclusive license to Springer Nature Switzerland AG 2022

M. F. Sakr, *Tongue Lesions*, https://doi.org/10.1007/978-3-031-08198-9_6

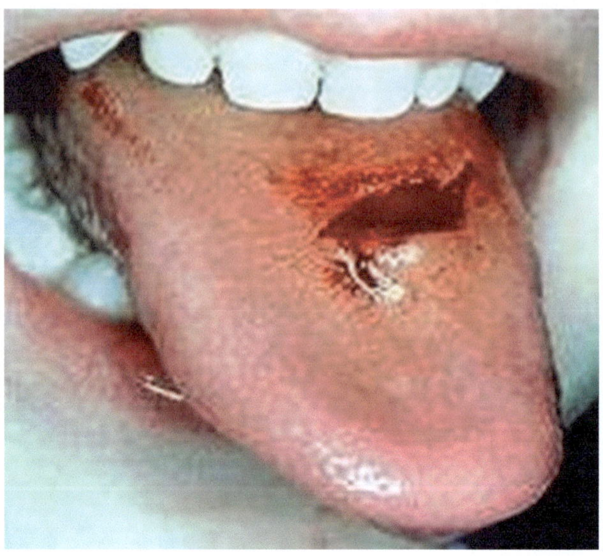

Fig. 6.1 Tongue injury involving the dorsum of the tongue caused by tongue biting

deep sutures in layers. Donat et al. [5], however, recommended suturing only wounds larger than 2 cm or when hemorrhage is a concern. English [6] agrees that small lacerations need not be sutured when wound margins are in good approximation. Furthermore, Touloukian [7] warned that suturing may predispose the tongue to invasive, closed space infection.

6.1.3.2 Principles of Management

Management principles of soft tissue injuries are similar except that treatment should be initiated within hours because healing occurs sooner. Although immature collagen in the soft tissue provides very cosmetic results, hypertrophic scars and keloids may form [8].

6.1.3.3 Injuries of the Dorsal Surface

A wound located on the dorsal surface of the tongue should always be examined for a ventral counterpart. If there are concomitant crown fractures, pieces of teeth or restoration fragments may be located within the wound. These fragments can be revealed by a radiographic examination with an exposure time 25% of normal exposure time.

6.1.3.4 Penetrating Injuries

Treatment of penetrating tongue wounds include (1) administration of anesthesia (local, regional, or general), (2) cleansing of the wound, (3) removal of foreign bodies to prevent infection and/or scar formation, (4) tight suturing of the dorsal and ventral aspects of the lesion, and (5) administration of antibiotics as indicated.

Sutures are removed after 4–5 days for lateral border wounds; buried resorbable sutures are sometimes indicated in order to approximate the wound edges and relieve tension on the mucosal sutures. Deep lacerations should be closed in layers, with chromic catgut sutures in the muscle layers to prevent formation of a hematoma [9].

6.1.3.5 Lateral or Tip Injuries

Loss of lateral tongue or tongue tip from extensive injury usually produces no permanent deficit, since the tongue hypertrophies to restore its bulk in a period of 6 months.

6.1.3.6 Large Lacerations or Avulsion

Reconstruction of laceration or avulsion tongue injuries is *not* usually required; primary wound healing often occurs rapidly because of the rich vascular supply. Only with lacerations larger than 2 cm or with difficulties in obtaining hemostasis it is necessary to effect closure [9].

6.1.3.7 Injuries of the Tongue Base

Injuries involving the *tongue base* are more likely to affect function in the event of hypoglossal nerve injury or late fibrosis from large transecting lacerations. Mostly, a laceration in which a flap of muscle is elevated may be ignored [9].

6.1.3.8 Tongue Injuries in Children with Coagulopathy

A special group of injuries to the tongue are those that occur in children with coagulopathy. These tend to heal slowly, and although they may heal primarily, the process may take weeks in a child who has hemophilia. Suture repair of relatively small injuries in these cases may expedite healing and is advisable since it is necessary to maintain these children with replacement coagulation factors. Dental fabrication of a smooth splint for the prevention of wound irritation by the maxillary teeth is additionally warranted [9].

6.1.3.9 Postoperative Care

Early motion is advisable for effective function after the proper lip and tongue repair. Within several days after suture removal, the patient should perform stretching exercises, which should be continued until the tissues soften and the period of wound contracture has passed [9].

6.2 Complex Tongue Lacerations

6.2.1 Introduction

The tongue is a muscular organ that sits on the floor of the oropharynx. It is enveloped by mucosa and contains glands, sensory organs, and four pairs of extrinsic muscles. The tongue is essential for several important functions, including jaw articulation, taste, food manipulation, and swallowing, as well as the production of speech.

6.2.2 Etiology

A tongue laceration is often the result of a fall, seizure, psychogenic non-epileptic seizure, or other blunt or penetrating force mechanism [10–12]. Piercings, intoxication, and iatrogenic cause are also commonly associated with tongue injury [13–21]. Case studies have also implicated dystonia, self-mutilation, anesthesia, and exploding electronic cigarettes [22–25]. Lacerations secondary to seizures are most often found to the side of the tongue [9, 26, 27].

Though uncommon, practitioners should keep in mind that such injuries can be the result of physical abuse [28–30]. Oral and facial trauma occurs in 50% of abused children [28].

6.2.3 Operative Management - Repair

6.2.3.1 Goals of Repair

The goals of laceration repair of the tongue are to attain adequate closure, stop bleeding, minimize complications, preserve mobility, and optimize articulation and deglutition.

6.2.3.2 Indications of Repair

Because of the tongue's generous blood supply, most tongue lacerations do not become infected and many heal well without repair. The tongue itself hypertrophies to regain its bulk in a period of 6 months, so even loss of lateral tongue and tip often produces no permanent deficit [9]. However, repair is required when the injury has certain characteristics, which include the following [31–34]:

- Bisecting wounds
- Large flaps
- Persistent bleeding
- Wounds larger than 1–2 cm
- Wounds to tip of tongue
- Gaping wounds
- U-shaped lacerations
- Avulsion or amputation injuries. (The tongue may be primarily closed if the defect is less than 30% of the tongue.)

6.2.3.3 Contraindications

Most tongue lacerations do not require sutures. Small flaps may be simply excised. Tongue lacerations in children are known to heal well without intervention [35]. Simple linear lacerations, especially if centrally located, heal with minimal risk of infection. Mouth protectors and tooth guards are also noninvasive modalities to assist tongue healing [36].

Amputations or avulsions of more than 30% require a flap procedure, which should be performed by a specialist [37–39]. Case reports have demonstrated the efficacy of using 2-octyl cyanoacrylate (Dermabond) for a pediatric tongue laceration [9, 40, 41].

6.2.3.4 Anesthesia

The following anesthesia techniques may be used:

- Topical anesthesia with Lidocaine 4% on gauze for 5 min
- Local infiltration with Lidocaine 1%. The pain associated with local anesthesia injections can be diminished with the use of a smaller-gauge needle and administration of the anesthetic slowly [42].
- Lingual nerve block for the anterior two-thirds of the tongue
- Procedural sedation, especially in children
- General anesthesia

6.2.3.5 Positioning

The supine position is preferable for most repairs. The patient may sit in an ENT (ear, nose, and throat) chair, if available.

6.2.3.6 Preparation

Once the patient is anesthetized, the wound should be inspected carefully. Some through-and-through lacerations may not be obvious without gentle probing. Chipped, missing, or mobile teeth in mouth injuries should always be checked for. Tooth fragments may be lodged inside the wound and, if not removed, may serve as a nidus for infection. Obtaining a radiographic imaging to locate missing tooth fragments may be considered.

Intraoral wounds are prone to considerable contamination, and therefore, thorough irrigation is necessary.

The major difficulty in closing a tongue laceration is maintaining control of the area being sutured. To stabilize and hold in protrusion for repair, the tip of the tongue is grasped with gauze or a towel clip or punctured and withdrawn with a large suture. A bite block may be used to protect both the patient and physician, as necessary.

6.2.3.7 Technique

Recommendations on technique for repair are based on anecdotal literature [9]. Through-and-through lacerations can be closed in one, two, or three layers, as described below. If the muscular layer is closed, bleeding is sufficiently controlled, and motor function is returned, then the superficial mucosal layers will heal rapidly.

The frequent movements of the tongue often untie the sutures. This can be avoided by burying the stitches or tying many knots. Nylon sutures in the mouth and tongue should be avoided.

6.2.3.7.1 Three-Layer Technique

Using 4–0 absorbable sutures, the muscular mucosa is close first. The inferior mucosa is then sutured. The repair is then extended up and around the lateral aspect of the tongue to close the superior mucosa.

6.2.3.7.2 Two-Layer Technique

One stitch is used to approximate half the thickness of the tongue superiorly. Another stitch is used to approximate half the thickness inferiorly. The edges of the tongue are then closed. Sutures do not have to be buried.

6.2.3.7.3 One-Layer Technique

Some authors suggest using a deep absorbable suture to close only the muscular layer leaving the other layers open to heal without sutures. This technique is successful because of the rapidly healing superficial mucosa.

6.2.4 Aftercare

After repair, the patient should be on a soft diet for 2–3 days. Daily dilute peroxide or Chlorohexidine mouth rinses may be used. The patient's tetanus vaccination should be updated, if necessary. Broken teeth and embedded foreign bodies should be evaluated.

The use of prophylactic antibiotics for tongue injury is controversial, but they should be considered in any contaminated wound [43]. A 2008 review on this topic concluded that, "treatment decisions must be guided by clinical and scientific rationale rather than evidence-based medicine" [44]. It is recommended that patients use a mouth-guard to prevent future lacerations if they are at high risk of recurrence or engaged in high-risk activities like contact sports [20, 36, 45, 46].

6.2.5 Complications

Complications of tongue injuries include infection, hemorrhage (in patients with coagulopathy or severe arterial bleeding, specialty consultation and interventional assistance for arterial ligature may be necessary), disfigurement, impaired articulation, impaired deglutition, swelling, and airway compromise [47].

6.3 Tongue Bites

6.3.1 Introduction

Injuries caused by tongue biting are common and often minor, especially in children. They are usually more severe in adults. Healing time for a tongue bite depends on the severity of injury. Minor injuries usually heal spontaneously within a week. More severe injuries require treatment and may take several weeks or months to fully heal. With tongue biting, it is also possible to bite the lips or the inside of the cheeks, the treatment of which is similar to that of the tongue.

6.3.2 Etiology

Tongue biting is relatively common and usually occurs accidentally. It may occur in the following conditions: during eating, after dental anesthesia, using illicit (illegal) drugs [48], during a seizure [49], during sleep [50], due to stress, and in the course of a traumatic event such as a bike or car accident or during a fall, or while playing sports.

6.3.3 Treatment

6.3.3.1 Indications

In adults, a good rule of thumb is to get medical attention when the edges of a tongue injury do not come together when the tongue is still. Immediate medical attention should be sought if the tongue bleeds excessively (or bleeding recurs), appears inflamed or swollen, feels warm, has red streaks or pus, is very painful, accompanied by a fever, or visibly deformed.

Immediate medical care for a child is indicated in presence of (1) a gaping cut on the tongue, lips, or inside of the mouth, (2) intense pain that does not improve within 2 hours of taking analgesics, (3) difficulty in swallowing liquids or spitting, (4) inability to fully open or close the mouth, and (5) signs of infection and fever.

6.3.3.2 Procedure

Depending on the severity of injury, treatment may include (1) stitches to close a wound, (2) antibiotics to treat or prevent infection, and (3) reattachment to connect part of the tongue that was bitten off (very uncommon).

6.3.4 Prognosis

A small laceration on the tongue, lips, or inside of the mouth is expected to heal in 3–4 days. A more severe laceration that required stitching or reattachment may take several weeks to a few months to heal. Infections of the mouth are rare, but can occur. They usually clear-up completely after a few weeks. Using an oral device may prevent recurrent biting of the tongue [51].

6.4 Tongue Biting During Sleep

6.4.1 Introduction

While there are no statistics on how many people bite their tongues, it happens to everyone from time to time, most commonly accidentally while eating. However, tongue biting is also common during sleep. Seizures and any condition causing facial muscle spasms may result in tongue biting at night. People who bite their tongues are at risk of developing ulcers, infections, and scalloping on their tongues.

6.4.2 Etiology

Underlying medical conditions leading to tongue biting during sleep include the following:

6.4.2.1 Bruxism

Bruxism, or "teeth grinding and clenching," is a common movement problem that most often affects the teeth and jaws, causing soreness, pain, and injury. However, it can also cause a person to bite their tongue and cheeks. The exact cause is exactly unknown [52].

6.4.2.2 Facial Muscle Spasms

Facial and jaw muscle spasms, also known as "*facio-mandibular myoclonus*," can cause tongue biting during sleep. This condition is most commonly seen in children, and often causes uncontrollable trembling of the chin during sleep. People who experience these spasms are unable to control their facial and jaw muscles during sleep, and thus often bite their tongues [53].

6.4.2.3 Illicit Drug Use

Methylene-dioxy-meth-amphetamine (MDMA), also known as "molly" and "ecstasy," is an amphetamine-derived psychostimulant and is considered an illicit drug that causes extreme euphoria. It also appears to cause bruxism (probably by intensifying the desire to bite or chew), which can cause severe injury to the teeth, cheeks, and tongue. Research on rats suggests that MDMA may lead to a reduced ability to keep the jaws open [48].

6.4.2.4 Lyme Disease

Lyme disease is not a very well understood illness. It appears to affect the central nervous system and bodily reflexes resulting in accidentally biting the tongue or cheeks. Other signs of Lyme disease include abnormal sensitivities to heat and cold, fatigue, slurred speech, frequent diarrhea, vision changes, and generalized pain and tingling [54].

6.4.2.5 Nighttime Seizures

Nighttime seizures are a common cause of tongue biting during sleep since about 50 million people worldwide have epilepsy. Such patients lose control of their bodies during a seizure causing them to unconsciously bite down on the tip and sides of their tongue [49, 55].

6.4.2.6 Rhythmic Movement Disorder

Rhythmic movement disorder strikes while a person, mostly a child, is drowsy or asleep. It causes a person to repeat body movements over and over again. It may cause the child to produce humming sounds, body motions like rocking and head banging, or rolling. These movements may be rapid and cause tongue biting [56].

6.4.2.7 Sleep Apnea

Sleep apnea does *not* cause tongue biting, but tongue biting is common in many people with sleep apnea. This is because people with sleep apnea often have tongues that are especially large or muscles in the mouth that relax abnormally during sleep, which can lead to tongue biting. Other signs of sleep apnea include loud snoring, gasping for air during sleep, morning headache, and excessive daytime sleepiness [50].

6.4.3 Symptoms

There are some signs and symptoms that can make nighttime tongue biting easier to identify. These include tongue bleeding, inflammation (redness) or swelling of the tongue, pain, cuts or marks on the tongue, ulcer on the tongue, and raw, scalloped edges on the tongue.

6.4.4 Treatment

Tongue injuries usually heal quickly without any medical intervention. However, if an ulcer, redness, excessive bleeding, pus, or lacerations are noticed, medical attention should be sought. Treatment of tongue biting usually involves treating the underlying condition.

- Those suffering from sleep bruxism or sleep apnea may benefit from wearing a mouth-guard at night. Sleep apnea can also be treated with weight loss, quitting smoking, continuous positive airway pressure (CPAP) machine, or surgery [50, 52].
- If illicit drug use is causing tongue biting during sleep, stopping use of the drug is usually enough to stop symptoms [48].
- Nighttime seizures caused by epilepsy are best treated with anti-seizure medication. According to researchers, those experiencing muscle spasms in their face and jaw at night may also benefit from anti-seizure medication [50, 52].

- Most children grow out of rhythmic movement disorder [56].
- Those patients with Lyme disease should receive a combination of an antibiotic and supportive therapy to help reduce symptoms [54].

6.4.5 Prevention

6.4.5.1 Sleep Study

In a sleep facility, the recordings of brainwave activity, eye movement, muscle tone, heart rhythm, and breathing rate may help determine the cause of tongue biting during sleep, and consequently prevention and treatment [55].

6.4.5.2 Mouth-Guard

For many people who bite their tongue, wearing a mouth-guard can prevent future injuries. The mouth-guard should be customized to perfectly fit the patient's teeth [51].

6.4.5.3 Reduction of Stress

One major cause of nighttime bruxism that leads to tongue biting is stress during the day. Some relaxation techniques such as deep breathing, meditation, or yoga may be of help.

6.4.5.4 Avoidance of Illegal Drugs

Avoiding illicit drugs (including MDMA), which increase the risk of bruxism, may prevent tongue biting during sleep [48].

6.4.5.5 Medications

Anti-seizure medications can help prevent seizures and tongue biting [50, 52].

6.5 Tongue Burn: Burning Mouth Syndrome

6.5.1 Introduction

A "*tongue burn*" typically occurs after eating or drinking something that is too hot. Standard first-aid treatment for burns can also work for a tongue burn. In some cases, a burning sensation on the tongue is felt without an actual burn. This condition may be due to ***"burning mouth syndrome"*** **(*BMS*)**, which is also known as "*idiopathic glossopyrosis*."

The International Association for the Study of Pain (IASP) has described burning mouth syndrome as a "chronic condition characterized by a burning sensation of the oral mucosa for which no cause can be found" [57]. The anterior part of the tongue is most commonly affected, followed by the labial mucosa, and occasionally the palate. The burning pain is often accompanied by tingling or numbness and the sensation of dryness of the mouth [58–60]. Reduced taste intensity and a bitter or a metallic taste are experienced by about two-thirds of those with BMS. Despite all these symptoms, the oral mucosa and the salivary flow rate are normal [61, 62].

6.5.2 Prevalence

The worldwide prevalence of BMS is unknown because nearly all studies have been of European or North American populations and different diagnostic criteria have been used in different studies [58]. The frequency of BMS increases with age in both women and men and is highest in women aged 60–69 years [63]. The higher frequency of BMS in women (F:M = 5:1) [64] may very well be owing to biological, sociocultural, and psychological factors [65].

6.5.3 Etiology of Tongue Burn

6.5.3.1 Tongue Burn (from Food or Liquid)

Underestimating the temperature of steam, hot food, or liquids can cause a burn on the tongue, mouth, or lips. Frequently eating and drinking extremely hot food and beverages without testing the temperature puts the person at a higher risk for tongue burn.

6.5.3.2 Burning Mouth Syndrome (BMS)

There is no known cause for BMS (i.e. idiopathic). It has been linked to abnormal function in the nerves of the mouth. Genetic and environmental factors are believed to play a role as well. In BMS, the saliva and anatomy of the mouth are otherwise normal. Extreme stress, anxiety, and depression can affect how pain is managed by the body. These conditions can make the symptoms of BMS worse [66]. There are other conditions that can lead to similar symptoms. These must *not* be present in order for BMS to be diagnosed. They are known as secondary causes of burning mouth pain as summarized in Table 6.1.

6.5.4 Pathogenesis of BMS

6.5.4.1 Peripheral and Central Neuropathies

Apart from psychogenic factors, both peripheral and central neuropathies appear to play a role in the pathogenesis of BMS [72]· Genetic and environmental factors seem to play an important role in determining individual differences in the experience of pain [66]. In patients with BMS who suffer from anxiety or depression and those who do not have immediate relief after local anesthetic regional nerve block, or after topical treatment with capsaicin or with clonazepam, central neuropathy is probably the dominant mechanism of the pain [60, 72, 73].

Table 6.1 Causes of a burning sensation in the mouth, which, by definition is *not* burning mouth syndrome [60, 67–71]

Causes	Examples
Oral mucosal conditions	• Erythema/erosion of whatever cause • Atrophic tongue • Candidiasis (oral thrush) • Geographic tongue • Oral lichen planus • Pemphigoid, pemphigus
Para-functional habits	• Teeth grinding • Cheek-sucking • Tongue-thrusting • Bad oral habits (e.g. using mouth wash too often).
Trauma (injury)	• Mechanical (e.g. dentures) • Chemical (e.g. acid from gastroesophageal reflux disease - GERD). • Thermal
Xerostomia and altered salivary quality	• Radiotherapy • Chemotherapy • Other drugs • Sjogren's syndrome
Systemic factors	• Diabetes mellitus (DM) • Decreased levels of vitamins B_1, B_2, B_{12}, folate, iron, zinc • Abnormal thyroid function and other endocrine disorders • Hormonal imbalance (e.g. menopause) • Allergic reaction to food or dental materials • Lichenoid tissue reactions • Autoimmune conditions • Parkinson disease
Drugs	• Paroxetine • Angiotensin-converting enzyme inhibitors
Local nerve damage	• Chemotherapy-associated neuropathy • Local physical irritation
Neuropathy	• Various peripheral or central neuropathies

Several neuronal dysfunctions are linked to BMS pain. The lingual mucosa exhibits a decreased number of small diameter nerve fibers; and these show upregulation of the transient receptor potential subfamily member V1 (TRPV1) ion channel, and upregulation of the P2X3 receptors and of nerve growth factor (NGF). This explains the role of trigeminal small-fiber sensory neuropathy in the pathogenesis of BMS [60, 63, 67, 72, 74].

TRPV1 channels are mostly found in nociceptive terminals of peripheral Aδ and C fibers but also centrally in the dorsal root and trigeminal ganglia. They respond to chemical irritants including the chili pepper ingredient capsaicin [75]. P2X3 ion channel receptors are expressed by a subpopulation of small-diameter primary nociceptors in the trigeminal nervous system, and when activated by adenosine trisphosphate they can evoke a sensation of burning pain [76, 77].

It has been further proposed that downregulation of central dopaminergic pain-inhibitory pathways also plays a role in the pathogenesis of BMS [58, 60, 72], particularly in persons with anxiety or depression, which are both associated with dysregulation of central mood-mediating dopaminergic pathways.

In case of persistent peripheral neuropathy, the central afferent nociceptor terminals in the dorsal horn of the spinal cord release excitatory biological mediators, which can activate postsynaptic NMDA receptors which under physiological conditions are silent, thus resulting in central sensitization with increased excitability [78]. There may also be a decrease in the functional activity of the GABA-mediated pain-inhibitory interneuron circuits in the dorsal horn of the spinal cord which under physiological circumstances inhibit the glutamate/NMDA-mediated central sensitization [78], possibly contributing to the neuropathic pain of BMS [61].

Thus, central sensitization characterized by structural and functional neural plasticity results in increased excitability and increased tonic activity of central nociceptive neurons, playing an important role in the pathogenesis of BMS [58, 79]. However, surprisingly, despite the possible roles of central sensitization and of psychogenic factors such as anxiety or depression in burning mouth syndrome neuropathic pain, it appears that, in persons with burning mouth syndrome, the co-occurrence of other chronic neuropathic pain disorders (central sensitivity syndromes) including fibromyalgia, atypical facial pain, trigeminal neuralgia, temporomandibular joint pain, back pain, and vulvodynia is rare [66, 80]. This suggests that the neural pathogenic mechanisms of burning mouth syndrome are distinct, probably localized somewhere in the trigeminal nerve pathway [80].

6.5.4.2 Psychological Factors

The chronic burning sensation of BMS has the characteristics of neuropathic pain and is debilitating with a negative impact on quality of life [65]. As attempts of treatment are often unsuccessful, owing to the chronicity of the burning sensation, some patients become cancero-phobic, believing that either they have or are developing cancer, and this exaggerates their anxiety [61, 70, 71].

6.5.5 Symptoms

6.5.5.1 Tongue Burn

A burn of the tongue looks and feels different, depending on the degree of the burn:

- *A first-degree burn* involves the outermost layer of the tongue. The patient experiences pain and the tongue may become red and swollen.
- *A second-degree burn* is more painful because both the outermost layer and the under layer of the tongue are injured. Blisters may form, and the tongue appears red and swollen.
- *A third-degree burn* affects the deepest tissue of the tongue. The effect is white or blackened, burnt skin. The patient may also experience numbness or severe pain.

When the tongue becomes red or swollen, the tongue papillae may disappear giving the tongue a smooth, rather than bumpy, appearance. A burn may reduce the sense of taste as well. But this is most often a temporary side effect unless the burn is severe [81].

6.5.5.2 Burning Mouth Syndrome

The burning sensation of BMS is moderate to severe in intensity, is usually bilaterally symmetrical, and is present every day for most of the day. It is minimal or even absent early in the morning and during mealtimes and it seldom interferes with sleep. In most cases, BMS starts spontaneously [58, 60–62, 82] and continues for several years. Only about 3% of cases resolve over a 5-year observation period, and even with treatment, only about 30% of affected persons report any improvement [58, 59, 61, 67].

In addition to feeling a burning sensation on the tongue, symptoms of BMS may include (1) a feeling of little discomfort of the tongue in the morning that steadily increases throughout the day, (2) a daily repetition of burning symptoms, (3) numbness and tingling of the tongue and mouth, (4) a metallic or bitter taste that accompanies the burning sensation, and (5) a feeling of having a dry mouth despite normal saliva production.

6.5.6 Complications

6.5.6.1 Tongue Burn

If it is not identified and treated properly, a severe burn of the tongue can become *infected.* Medical advice should be sought for second-degree and third-degree burns.

A burn of the tongue can also destroy taste buds, creating loss of sensation where the burn occurred. This is typically a short-term complication because taste buds typically regenerate about every 2 weeks.

6.5.6.2 Burning Mouth Syndrome

Persistent pain, which does not respond significantly to treatment as in the case of burning mouth syndrome, is debilitating in that it negatively affects the psyche, evoking feelings of vulnerability, helplessness, and desperation partly because of the fear that the pain will never let up or might even become worse. Such negative emotions can overwhelm the BMS sufferer causing anxiety and depression, interfering with everyday activities, and significantly reducing the quality of life [83].

6.5.7 Diagnosis

6.5.7.1 Tongue Burn

Redness, swelling, and blistering are signs of a tongue burn. Simple tongue examination will reveal the degree of burn.

6.5.7.2 Burning Mouth Syndrome

A diagnosis of burning mouth syndrome can be made only if the oral mucosa is clinically normal and all systemic and local causes for a burning sensation have been excluded (Table 6.1), bearing in mind that BMS may be superimposed upon a burning sensation of known systemic or local origin [61, 67, 82]. It is essential for treatment purposes thus to differentiate between BMS which is an *idiopathic condition* and oral mucosal burning sensations secondary to a known cause (Table 6.1) [68, 69]. Treating these secondary causes is the key to managing symptoms in such cases, for example, changing a medication that is causing dry mouth or management of GERD.

In addition to history-taking and physical examination, the following tests may be performed to rule out other conditions than BMS:

- *Blood tests* to exclude nutritional deficiencies, hormone imbalances, and endocrine disorders.
- *Oral samples* to rule out oral conditions, such as thrush and lichen planus.
- *Allergy tests* to rule out burning of tongue caused by allergies to certain foods or additives.
- *Saliva analysis* to rule out xerostomia.
- *Gastric reflux tests* for GERD, if suspected.
- *Imaging* studies as indicated. One functional magnetic resonance imaging (fMRI) study suggested that in patients with BMS, painful thermal trigeminal stimuli generate different patterns of brain activation in terms of their location and amplitude when compared to healthy control subjects without BMS [84]. Another fMRI study investigating the functional connectivity of brain neural circuits associated with pain and emotions in subjects with BMS suggested that these subjects show different patterns of functional brain connectivity in relation to different reported intensities of burning/pain: high intensity burning/pain is associated with increased functional activity of those affective-motivational neural circuits regulating symptoms of depression and anxiety [85].

Burning mouth syndrome is frequently associated with stressful life events, anxiety, and depressive disorders [64, 79], and as these psychogenic factors can either enhance or reduce perception of pain, BMS can be managed by pharmacological or by psychological means or by a combination of the two [66, 79]. As with other chronic neuropathic pain conditions, BMS can induce or promote psychic symptoms or can itself be a somatic feature of a psychic disorder [65], but it is unclear, however, whether psychogenic factors are primary or secondary in any particular case of BMS.

6.5.8 Treatment

6.5.8.1 Tongue Burn

Initial treatment for a burn of the tongue should include basic first-aid. To avoid infection and reduce pain the following is advised:

- Drinking and rinsing the area well with cool water for a few minutes or rinsing with cool salt water (1/8 teaspoon of salt dissolved in 8 ounces of water).
- Sucking on ice chips to soothe the pain.
- Avoiding warm or hot liquids, which could irritate the burn.
- Taking acetaminophen or ibuprofen for pain and inflammation.
- Considering honey on the tongue to relieve pain.

6.5.8.2 Burning Mouth Syndrome

Patients should be told that BMS is a complex disorder for which there is no cure and treatment is purely symptomatic, and therefore expectations of the outcome of treatment should not be unrealistic [73]. As the etio-pathogenesis of BMS is poorly understood, there is no standard treatment for the condition, and treatment is empirical and largely based on personal and expert opinion [79].

Some pain modulating neural pathways descending from the cortex, hypothalamus, midbrain, and medulla to the spinal cord, influenced by emotional states such as excitement, stress, anxiety, or depression, can either potentiate or suppress spinal nociceptive pathways and may also have the capacity to spontaneously induce nociceptive signals without the peripheral input [78, 86]. This mechanism may be the link between psychogenic factors and BMS pain. The descending inhibitory pathways of this conditioned pain modulatory system are mediated by serotonin, noradrenalin, gamma aminobutyric acid (GABA), and enkephalins. Thus, both *nonpharmacological approach* such as cognitive-behavioral therapy and *pharmacological agents* targeting neuronal central sensitization pathways such as anticonvulsants, and N-methyl-D-aspartate [NMDA] receptor antagonists, alone or in combination, are beneficial in the treatment of neuropathic pain conditions, including BMS [66].

Pain in BMS is associated with irritability, fatigue, anorexia, diminished social activity, and depression. Psychological/psychiatric intervention might therefore be beneficial [60, 67]. Furthermore, the strong association between anxiety and depression on the one hand and BMS pain on the other hand provides the biological rationale for the use of anxiolytics and antidepressants in the treatment of BMS [65].

Various *systemic and topical medications* (Table 6.2) have been used in the treatment of BMS with varying degrees of success [67]. Psychological/psychiatric intervention should be considered only when BMS does *not* respond favorably to medication. In particular, cognitive-behavioral therapy which helps the patient to develop pain-coping strategies was found to be beneficial in reducing suffering [61, 67].

6.5.8.2.1 Topical and Systemic Medications

Capsaicin is the "hot" component of chili pepper and has been used both topically and systemically in the treatment of BMS, reportedly to bring about symptomatic relief. Topical capsaicin has the capacity to bind to the TRPV1 ion channels of small-diameter peripheral sensory nerve fibers, mediating desensitization of afferent nociceptors, and causing reversible degeneration of peripheral sensory nerve endings, with consequent reduction in the syndromal burning pain sensation [73,

Table 6.2 Pharmacological and nonpharmacological management of burning mouth syndrome (BMS) [58]

Pharmacological agents	
Topical	*Systemic*
• Clonazepam • Capsaicin • Doxepin • Lidocaine	• Tricyclic antidepressants • Selective serotonin reuptake inhibitors • Serotonin-adrenalin reuptake inhibitors • Anticonvulsants (e.g., gabapentin) • Opioids • Benzodiazepines • Alpha-lipoic acid
Nonpharmacological therapy	
• Cognitive-behavioral therapy • Mindfulness meditation • Other relaxation techniques	

75]. It has also been reported that capsaicin can downregulate the biosynthesis of neurotransmitters and their axonal transport by primary nociceptors, thus inhibiting central sensitization in response to peripheral nociceptive stimuli [87, 88]. Systemic capsaicin is not well tolerated because of its side effects and therefore is seldom used.

Clonazepam, a benzodiazepine, is a GABAnergic agonist, which activates pain-inhibitory pathways in the spinal cord and in peripheral nociceptors. When applied topically to the oral mucosa, clonazepam is thought to decrease excitability of peripheral sensory nerve fibers, and when given systemically, it has central sedative, anxiolytic, and analgesic effects. The use of both topical and systemic clonazepam has been reported to reduce the intensity of the pain of burning mouth syndrome [60, 61, 67, 71, 89, 90].

Antidepressants are often used to treat BMS most probably because of their documented effects in reducing the intensity of neuropathic pain and because of the close association between BMS and generalized anxiety and depressive disorders [59]. Several studies have shown that tricyclic antidepressants (e.g. amitriptyline) bring relief to a significant number of sufferers of BMS [60, 71].

Alpha lipoic acid, a potent antioxidant, has been shown to be beneficial in the treatment of BMS, either alone or particularly in combination with anticonvulsants or with *psychotherapy* (cognitive behavior therapy) [73]. The *anticonvulsant* gabapentin, which is often used for the treatment of neuropathic pain disorders, has been shown also to reduce BMS pain [67].

6.5.8.2.2 Psychological/Psychiatric Intervention

Cognitive-behavioral therapy (CBT) has been shown to reduce the intensity of the pain of BMS in a significant number of patients, either alone or with medications [60, 91]. The CBT is a "directed, structured, short-term psychological treatment aimed at correcting dysfunctional emotional responses such as pain, fear, helplessness, vulnerability, or exhaustion, by changing thoughts and behaviors" [92]. The rationale for this therapy is based on the concept that cognition, emotion, and behavior are interrelated, forming a "complex adaptive system." Accordingly, modifications in dysfunctional cognition and/or behavior may be beneficial in correcting irrational emotional responses, and modifying cognition may correct dysfunctional behavior [92].

With CBT, harmful thoughts and problematic behaviors are identified, and the dysfunctional relationship between cause and disordered emotional response is explained to the patient. An understanding of the mechanisms that drive dysregulated relationships between thought, behavior, and emotion may decrease the level of anxiety. Undoubtedly, CBT can be an effective part of the management of BMS [58, 91, 92].

6.5.9 Prevention

6.5.9.1 Tongue Burn

A primary tongue burn can be prevented by testing the temperature of hot liquids and food before eating or drinking. Extra caution should be taken with beverages or food heated in a microwave as they may not be heated evenly.

6.5.9.2 Burning Mouth Syndrome

There is no known way to prevent BMS. The patient may be able to lower the burning sensation by reducing stress and avoiding tobacco and certain types of foods and drinks. These include carbonated beverages, acidic foods, and spicy foods.

6.5.10 Prognosis

6.5.10.1 Tongue Burn

A primary tongue burn can heal in about 2 weeks or less without specific treatment. However, some burns can last up to 6 weeks depending on the cause and severity.

6.5.10.2 Burning Mouth Syndrome

Burning mouth syndrome can persist for months or even years. It can be difficult to manage. Some studies suggest only 3 out of 10 people find improvement with treatment. Additional research is necessary into the roles of genetic factors, familial patterns, and the nature of the complex interactions between stressful life events, personality, comorbid psychic factors, and the lack of social support in the pathogenesis of BMS as it may allow for the identification of predictors of successful treatment [64, 92].

6.6 Conclusion

A primary tongue burn can be prevented by testing the temperature of hot liquids and food before eating or drinking. It usually heals in 2 weeks or less without a specific treatment.

The pathogenesis of burning mouth syndrome is complex involving psychogenic factors and dysregulated peripheral and central pain pathways. Genetic factors determining the function of neural pain pathways may play an important role in individual susceptibility to BMS, and while there is no standard treatment protocol for its management, both drugs and psychological services may be required.

References

1. Benbadis SR. Tongue biting as a lateralizing sign in partial epilepsy. Seizure. 1996;5(3):175–6.
2. Lamell CW, Fraone G, Casamassimo PS, Wilson S. Presenting characteristics and treatment outcomes for tongue lacerations in children. Pediatr Dent. 1999;21(1):34–8.
3. Andreasen JO, Andreasen FM. Textbook and color atlas of traumatic injuries to the teeth. St. Louis, MI: Mosby-Year Book; 1994. p. 511–4.
4. Powers MP, Bertz J, Fonseca RJ. Management of soft tissue injuries. In: Fonseca RJ, Walker RV, editors. Oral and maxillofacial trauma. Philadelphia, PA: WB Saunders; 1991. p. 618–48.
5. Donat TL, Maisel RH, Mathog RH. Injuries to the mouth, pharynx and esophagus. In: Bluestone CD, Stool SE, Kenna MA, editors. Pediatric otolaryngology. Philadelphia, PA: WB Saunders; 1996. p. 1183–4.
6. English GM. Otolaryngology. New York, NY: Harper and Row; 1976. p. 463.
7. Touloukian RJ. Pediatric trauma. St Louis, MI: CV Mosby; 1990. p. 204.
8. Das UM, Nagarathna C, Viswanath D, Keerthi R, Gadicherla P. Management of facial trauma in children: a case report. J Indian Soc Pedod Prev Dent. 2006;24(3):161–3.
9. Das UM, Gadicherla P. Lacerated tongue injury in children. Int J Clin Pediatr Dent. 2008;1(1):39–41.
10. Bringhurst C, Herr RD, Aldous JA. Oral trauma in the emergency department. Am J Emerg Med. 1993;11(5):486–90.
11. Asadi-Pooya AA, Emami M, Emami Y. Ictal injury in psychogenic non-epileptic seizures. Seizure. 2014;23(5):363–6.
12. Colgan L, Shannon D. Dento-alveolar and facial injury caused by air gun pellets. Dent Update. 2010;37(5):323–5.
13. Hua M, Brady J, Li G. The epidemiology of upper airway injury in patients undergoing major surgical procedures. Anesth Analg. 2012;114(1):148–51.
14. Sanaei-Zadeh H. Medical image. Tramadol intoxication and tongue laceration. N Z Med J. 2013;126(1370):113–4.
15. Aren G, Sepet E, Pınar Erdem A, Tolgay CG, Kuru S, Ertekin C, et al. Predominant causes and types of orofacial injury in children seen in the emergency department. Ulus Travma Acil Cerrahi Derg. 2013;19(3):246–50.
16. Lent GS, Schraga ED, Windle ML. Complex tongue laceration. Drugs Dis. Updated: Jan 25, 2019.
17. Woo SW, Do SH. Tongue laceration during electroconvulsive therapy. Korean J Anesthesiol. 2012;62(1):101–2.
18. Vieira EP, Ribeiro AL, PinheiroJde J, AlvesSde M Jr. Oral piercings: immediate and late complications. J Oral Maxillofac Surg. 2011;69(12):3032–7.
19. Davis SF, Kalarickal P, Strickland T. A report of two cases of lip and tongue bite injury associated with transcranial motor evoked potentials. Am J Electroneurodiagnostic Technol. 2010;50(4):313–20.
20. Mahmoud M, Spaeth J, Sadhasivam S. Protection of tongue from injuries during transcranial motor-evoked potential monitoring. Paediatr Anaesth. 2008;18(9):902–3.
21. Vézina MC, Trépanier CA, Nicole PC, Lessard MR. Complications associated with the esophageal-tracheal Combitube in the pre-hospital setting. Can J Anaesth. 2007;54(2):124–8.
22. Beena JP. Management of tongue and lip laceration due to dystonia in a 1-year-old infant. J Indian Soc Pedod Prev Dent. 2017;35(1):90–3.

23. Brooks JK, Kleinman JW, Brooks JB, Reynolds MA. Electronic cigarette explosion associated with extensive intraoral injuries. Dent Traumatol. 2017;33(2):149–52.
24. Shapira J, Birenboim R, Shoshani M, Abdel-Kader A, Behar O, Moskovitz M, et al. Overcoming the oral aspects of -self-mutilation: description of a method. Spec Care Dentist. 2016;36(5):282–7.
25. Hao TJ, Liu G, Ang P. A rare complication of tongue laceration following posterior spinal surgery using spinal cord monitoring: a case report. Indian J Anaesth. 2014;58(6):773–5.
26. Oliva M, Pattison C, Carino J, Roten A, Matkovic Z, O'Brien TJ. The diagnostic value of oral lacerations and incontinence during convulsive "seizures". Epilepsia. 2008 Jun;49(6):962–7.
27. Lagunju IA, Oyinlade AO, Babatunde OD. Seizure-related injuries in children and adolescents with epilepsy. Epilepsy Behav. 2016;54:131–4.
28. Maguire S, Hunter B, Hunter L, Sibert JR, Mann M, Kemp AM. Diagnosing abuse: a systematic review of torn frenum and other intra-oral injuries. Arch Dis Child. 2007;92(12):1113–7.
29. Costacurta M, Benavoli D, Arcudi G, Docimo R. Oral and dental signs of child abuse and neglect. Oral Implantol (Rome). 2015;8(2–3):68–73.
30. George CLS, Theesfeld SSN, Wang Q, Hudson MJ, Harper NS. Identification and characterization of oral injury in suspected child abuse cases: one health system's experience. Pediatr Emerg Care. 2018; https://doi.org/10.1097/PEC.0000000000001715.
31. Brown DJ, Jaffe JE, Henson JK. Advanced laceration management. Emerg Med Clin North Am. 2007;25(1):83–99.
32. Steinig JP, DeLoach ED, Boyd CR. Transection of the base of the tongue caused by penetrating injury. Am Surg. 1999;65(2):133–4.
33. Patel A. Tongue lacerations. Br Dent J. 2008;204(7):355.
34. Seiler M, Massaro SL, Staubli G, Schiestl C. Tongue lacerations in children: to suture or not? Swiss Med Wkly. 2018;22:148.
35. Ud-din Z, Aslam M, Gull S. Towards evidence based emergency medicine: best BETs from the Manchester Royal Infirmary. Should minor mucosal tongue lacerations be sutured in children? Emerg Med J. 2007;24(2):123–4.
36. Yamanaka R, Soga Y, Moriya Y, Okui A, Takeuchi T, Sato K, et al. Management of lacerated and swollen tongue after convulsive seizure with a mouth protector: interprofessional collaboration including dentists in intensive care. Acta Med Okayama. 2014;68(6):375–8.
37. Egozi E, Faulkner B, Lin KY. Successful revascularization following near-complete amputation of the tongue. Ann Plast Surg. 2006;56(2):190–3.
38. Kim JS, Choi TH, Kim NG, Lee KS, Han KH, Son DG, et al. The replantation of an amputated tongue by supermicrosurgery. J Plast Reconstr Aesthet Surg. 2007;60(10):1152–5.
39. Vyloppilli S, Prathap A. Lingual frenectomy using multiple series Z-plasty. J Maxillofac Oral Surg. 2010;9(2):195–7.
40. Kazzi MG, Silverberg M. Pediatric tongue laceration repair using 2-octyl cyanoacrylate (dermabond (®)). J Emerg Med. 2013;45(6):846–8.
41. Perera AGN, Tavarez MM. 2-octyl cyanoacrylate. Treasure Island, FL: StatPearls Publishing; 2020.
42. Forsch RT. Essentials of skin laceration repair. Am Fam Physician. 2008;78(8):945–51.
43. Armstrong BD. Lacerations of the mouth. Emerg Med Clin North Am. 2000;18(3):471–80.
44. Mark DG, Granquist EJ. Are prophylactic oral antibiotics indicated for the treatment of intraoral wounds? Ann Emerg Med. 2008;52(4):368–72.
45. Hino S, Takeda A, Kaneko T, Horie N, Shimoyama T. Oral lacerations during motocross: a case report. Dent Traumatol. 2017;33(6):482–4.
46. Badel T, Jerolimov V, Pandurić J, Carek V. Custom-made mouthguards and prevention of orofacial injuries in sports. Acta Med Croatica. 2007;1:9–14.
47. Faverani LP, Gaetti-Jardim EC, Ramalho-Ferreira G, Gulinelli JL, Queiroz TP, Garcia Júnior IR. Ligature of external carotid artery as an optional technique in a patient with von Willebrand disease. Braz Dent. 2011;2(5):435–8.
48. Arrue A, Gomez FM, Giralt MT. Effects of 3,4-methylenedioxymethamphetamine ('Ecstasy') on the jaw-opening reflex and on the alpha-adrenoceptors which regulate this reflex in the anesthetized rat. Eur J Oral Sci. 2004;112:127–33.

49. Brigo F, Starti M, Lochner P, Tezzon F, Fiaschi A, Bongiovanni LG, et al. Tongue biting in epileptic seizures and psychogenic events: an evidence-based perspective. Epilepsy Behavior (E&B). 2012;25(2):251–5.
50. Dylgjeri S, Dylgjeri S, Pincherle A, Ciano C, Binelli S, Villani F. Sleep-related tongue biting may not be a sign of epilepsy: a case of sleep-related facio-mandibular myoclonus. Epilepsia. 2009;50(1):157–9.
51. Pigno MA, Funk JJ. Prevention of tongue biting with a removable oral device: a clinical report. J Prosthet Dent. 2000;83(5):508–10.
52. Mayo Clinic Staff. Bruxism (teeth grinding). 2017. http://mayoclinic.org/diseases-conditions/bruxism/symptoms-causes/syc-20356095.
53. Mahmoudi M, Kothare SV. Tongue biting: a case of sporadic genio-spasm during sleep. J Clin Sleep Med. 2014;10(12):1339–40.
54. Kaplan M. Master Lyme symptoms list. 2014. http://anapsid.org/lyme/symptoms.
55. Goraya JS, Virdi V, Parmar V. Recurrent nocturnal tongue biting in a child with hereditary chin trembling. J Child Neurol. 2006;21(11):985–7.
56. Hoban T. Rhythmic movement disorder in children. CNS Spectr. 2003;8(2):135–8.
57. IASP orofacial pain fact sheet. Burning mouth syndome. 2016. Available: https://www.iasp-pain.
58. Patton LL, Siegel MA, Benoliel R, de Laat A. Management of burning mouth syndrome: systematic review and management recommendations. Oral Surg Oral Med Oral Pathol Oral Radiol Endod. 2007;103(39):1–39.
59. Buchanan JAG, Zakrzewska JM. Burning mouth syndrome. BMJ Clin Evid. 2010;2010:1301.
60. Gurvits GE, Tan A. Burning mouth syndrome. World J Gastroenterol. 2013;19(5):665–72.
61. Grushka M, Epstein J, Mott A. An open-label, dose escalation pilot study of the effect of clonazepam in burning mouth syndrome. Oral Surg Oral Med Oral Pathol Oral Radiol Endod. 1998;86(5):557–61.
62. Forssell H, Jääskeläinen S, List T, Svensson P, Baad-Hansen L. An update on pathophysiological mechanisms related to idiopathic oro-facial pain conditions with implications for management. J Oral Rehab. 2015;42(4):300–22.
63. Puhakka A, Forssell H, Soinila S, Virtanen A, Röyttä M, Laine M, et al. Peripheral nervous system involvement in primary burning mouth syndromeresults of a pilot study. Oral Dis. 2016;22(4):338–44.
64. Bogetto F, Maina G, Ferro G, Carbone M, Gandolfo S. Psychiatric comorbidity in patients with burning mouth syndrome. Psychosom Med. 1998;60(3):378–85.
65. Schiavone V, Adamo D, Ventrella G, Morlenio M, DeNotaris EB, Ravel MG, et al. Anxiety, depression, and pain in burning mouth syndrome: first chicken or egg? Headache. 2012;52(6):1019–25.
66. Yunus MB. Editorial review: an update on central sensitivity syndromes and the issues of nosology and psychobiology. Curr Rheumatol Rev. 2015;11(2):70–85.
67. Speciali JG, Stuginski-Barbosa J. Burning mouth syndrome. Curr Pain Headache Rep. 2008;12(4):279–84.
68. Balasubramaniam R, Klasser GD, Delcanho R. Seperating oral burning from burning mouth syndrome: unravelling a diagnostic enigma. Aust Dent J. 2009;54(4):293–9.
69. Renton T. Burning mouth syndrome. Rev Pain. 2011;5(4):12–7.
70. Lamey PJ, Lamb AB. Prospective study of aetiological factors in burning mouth syndrome. BMJ (Clin Res ed). 1988;296(6631):1243–6.
71. Grushka M, Epstein JB, Gorsky M. Burning mouth syndrome. Am Fam Phys. 2002;65(4):615–22.
72. Jääskeläinen SK. Pathophysiology of primary burningmouth syndrome. Clin Neurophysiol. 2012;123(1):71–7.
73. De Moraes M, Do Amaral Bezerra BA, Da Rocha Neto PC, De Oliveira Soares ACA, Pinto LP, De Lisboa Lopes Costa A. Randomized trials for the treatment of burning mouth syndrome: an evidence-based review of the literature. J Oral Pathol Med. 2012;41(4):281–7.

74. Yilmaz Z, Renton T, Yiangou Y, Zakrzewska J, Chessell IP, Bountra C, et al. Burning mouth syndrome as a trigeminal small fibre neuropathy: increased heat and capsaicin receptor TRPV1 in nerve fibres correlates with pain score. J Clin Neurosci. 2007;14(9):864–71.
75. Laklouk M, Baranidharan G. Profile of the capsaicin 8% patch for the management of neurolp-pathic pain associated 6 Pain Research and Management with postherpetic neuralgia: safety, efficacy, and patient acceptability. Patient Prefer Adherence. 2016;10:1913–8.
76. Shinoda M, Kawashima K, Ozaki N, Asai H, Nagamine K, Sugiura Y. P2X3 receptor mediates heat hyperalgesia in a rat model of trigeminal neuropathic pain. J Pain. 2007;8(7):588–97.
77. Baccei ML, Fitzgerald M. Development of pain pathways andmechanisms. In: McMahon MB, Tracey I, Koltzenburg M, Turk DC, editors. Wall and Melzack's textbook of pain. Philadelphia, PA: Elsevier; 2013. p. 143–54.
78. Basbaum AI, Bautista DM, Scherrer G, Julius D. Cellular and molecular mechanisms of pain. Cell. 2009;139(2):267–84.
79. Savage NW, Abetz LM. Burning mouth syndrome and psychological disorders. Aust Dent J. 2009;54(2):84–93.
80. Moisset X, Calbacho V, Torres P, Gremeau-Richard C, Dallel R. Co-occurrence of pain symptoms and somatosensory sensitivity in burning mouth syndrome: a systematic review. PLoS One. 2016;11(9):e0163449.
81. van Heerden WFP, van Zyl AW. Burning mouth syndrome. S Afr Fam Pract. 2011;53(1):8–10.
82. Scala A, Checchi L, Montevecchi M, Marini I, Giamberardino MA. Update on burning mouth syndrome: overview and patient management. Crit Rev Oral Biol Med. 2003;14(4):275–91.
83. Brailo V, Firić M, Vučićević Boras V, Andabak Rogulj A, Krstevski I, Alajbeg I. Impact of reassurance on pain perception in patients with primary burning mouth syndrome. Oral Dis. 2016;22(6):512–6.
84. Albuquerque RJC, de Leeuw R, Carlson CR, Okeson JP, Miller CS, Andersen AH. Cerebral activation during thermal stimulation of patients who have burning mouth disorder: an fMRI study. Pain. 2006;122(3):223–34.
85. Khan SA, Keaser ML, Meiller TF, Seminowicz DA. Altered structure and function in the hippocampus andmedial prefrontal cortex in patients with burning mouth syndrome. Pain. 2014;155(8):1472–80.
86. Rathmell JP, Fields HL. Pain: pathophysiology and management. In: Kasper DL, Hauser J, Jameson JL, editors. Harrison's principles of internal medicine, vol. 1. New York, NY: Mc-Graw Hill; 2015. p. 87–95.
87. Takenoshita M, Sato T, Kato Y, et al. Psychiatric diagnoses in patients with burningmouth syndrome and atypical odontalgia referred from psychiatric to dental facilities. Neuropsych Dis Treat. 2010;6:699–705.
88. Silvestre FJ, Silvestre-Rangil J, Tamarit-Santafé C, Bautista D. Application of a capsaicin rinse in the treatment of burning mouth syndrome. Med Oral Patol Oral Cir Bucal. 2012;17(1):e1–4.
89. Tan SN, Song E, Dong XD, Somvanshi RK, Cairns BE. Peripheral GABAA receptor activation modulates rat tongue afferent mechanical sensitivity. Arch Oral Biol. 2014;59(3):251–7.
90. Cui Y, Xu H, Chen MF, et al. Efficacy evaluation of clonazepam for symptom remission in burning mouth syndrome: a meta-analysis. Oral Dis. 2016;22(6):503–11.
91. Komiyama O, Nishimura H, Makiyama Y, et al. Group cognitive-behavioral intervention for patients with burning mouth syndrome. J Oral Sci. 2013;55(1):17–22.
92. Kaczkurkin AN, Foa EB. Cognitive-behavioral therapy for anxiety disorders: an update on the empirical evidence. Dial Clin Neurosci. 2015;17(3):337–46.

7 Tongue Piercing

7.1 Introduction

Oral and perioral piercing, which involve the insertion of jewellery into the *tongue*, lip, cheek, frenulum, uvula, or other part of the mouth, has long been practiced in the world for religious, tribal, cultural, sexual, or identity reasons [1].

Tongue piercing (Fig. 7.1a, b) is one of those things that a lot of people do on an impulse and then end up regretting for a very long time because of its complications, which may be severe. Unlike piercings in other parts of the body where the skin is pierced, the tongue is *all muscle*. It has a lot of important structures running through it, as well as communications with other parts of the body.

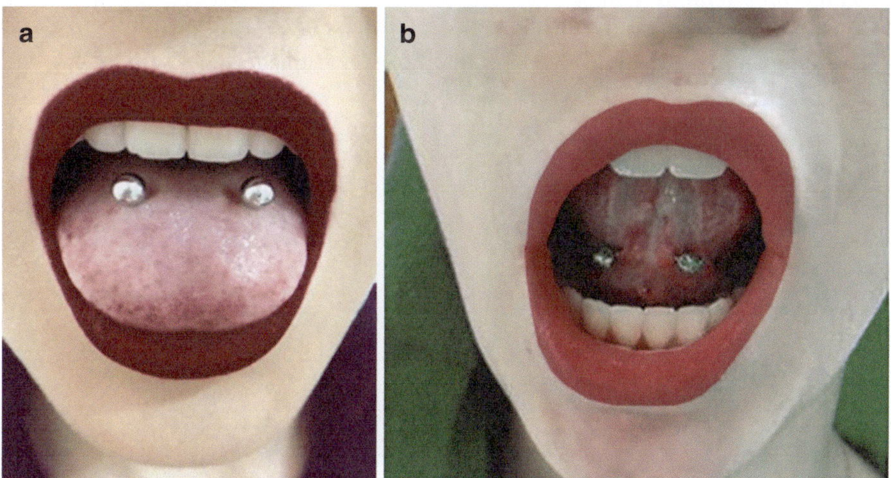

Fig. 7.1 Tongue piecing seen on the dorsum of the tongue (**a**) and in the tongue frenulum (**b**)

© The Author(s), under exclusive license to Springer Nature Switzerland AG 2022
M. F. Sakr, *Tongue Lesions*, https://doi.org/10.1007/978-3-031-08198-9_7

7.2 Historical Review

The earliest known representation of this piercing was in the figure of a dog created in *Egypt* in around 1500 BC, when it was considered a symbol of royalty. For *ancient Mayans*, piercing was a symbol of spirituality, virility, and courage. *Eskimos* inserted a "labret" into the lower lip as a symbol of passage to adulthood in boys and as an act of purification in girls. The piercing of lips, cheek, or tongue was also a traditional practice in *Hindu*, *Chinese*, and *American Indian* cultures [2]. In *Southern India*, a vow of silence was accompanied by tongue piercing [3].

In *developed countries*, piercing became fashionable with the punk movement and then as part of a wider "body art," i.e. the voluntary modification of physical appearance by tattoos, branding, scars, or piercing [4, 5]. Hypoallergenic and non-toxic materials are used for piercing jewellery, e.g. 14 or 18K gold, titanium, stainless steel, niobium, tygon, acrylic, stone, wood, bone, or ivory [2, 3, 5, 6].

7.3 Types of Piercing Jewellery

Four types of piercing jewellery are applied in the oral/perioral area, namely:

1. *Labret*, which is a bar with ball, disc, or point at one end and flat closing disc at the other (Fig. 7.2).
2. *Barbell*, which is a straight or curved bar with balls at each end
3. *Unclosed ring* with a ball at one or both ends [4, 6].
4. *Magnet*, which consists of two components of the stud held together by a *magnetic force* tenfold greater than that of conventional magnet ends [5]. Various authors have reported the adverse effects that can be produced during the act of piercing and as a result of the constant presence of this jewellery [6].

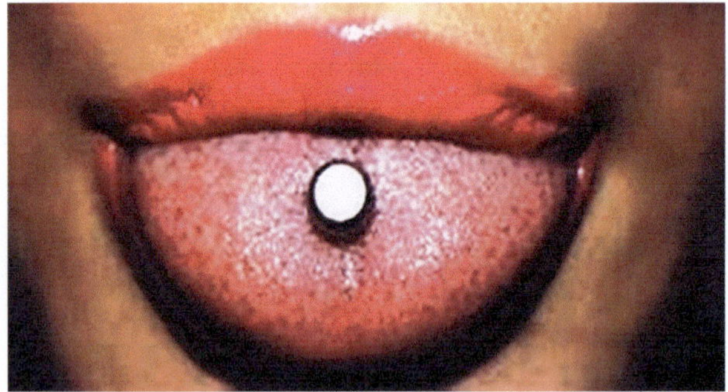

Fig. 7.2 *Labret* is a bar with ball, disc, or point at one end and flat closing disc at the other

7.4 Complications of Tongue Piercing

7.4.1 Hemorrhage

The tongue is highly vascularized and innervated, and controlled bleeding can be expected during the piercing of this organ (Fig. 7.3). However, there is evidence that a major hemorrhage can be produced [5, 7].

7.4.2 Nerve Injury

Piercing sites in the tongue are innervated with sensory or motor fibers. These are easily and commonly injured during tongue piercings resulting in lost or altered taste sensation, severe pain or parasthesia, or even partial loss of tongue movement. Nerve damage is slow to heal and recovery may never be complete [4, 5].

7.4.3 Painful Ulceration and Inflammation

The most frequent complication of tongue piercing, besides bleeding, is painful ulceration, being reported in almost half of recipients [3, 4, 8]. In the tongue, the primary lesions disappear after 3–5 weeks [9]. The onset of local inflammation is

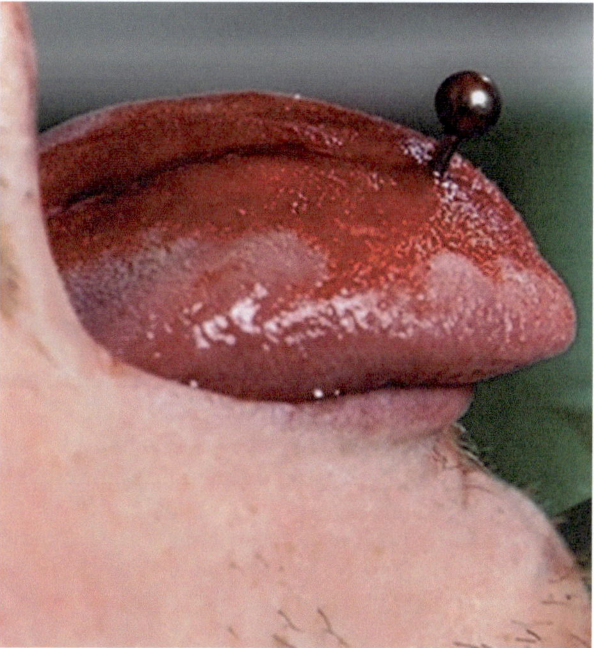

Fig. 7.3 Hemorrhage may be encountered during tongue piercing. It may be severe

at 6–8 h after the piercing, reaching a peak on Day 3 or 4. Inflammation can persist for weeks and, although usually temporary, may produce a granulomatous inflammation in response to the foreign body, interfering with mastication and swallowing and sometimes even responsible for asphyxia or respiratory difficulties [5].

7.4.4 Infection

Many authors have described infections as a common complication of oral/perioral piercing, observed in 10–20% of cases. Tongue piercings appear especially prone to infection, by *Staphylococcus aureus*, Streptococcus group A, *Pseudomonas aeruginosa*, Erysipelas, and β-hemolytic Streptococcus, among other microorganisms.

The proximity of cervical lymph node chains to this initially local focus of infection may favor its spread, leading to speech impairment, airway obstruction, or even damage to vital organs, e.g., endocarditis [5, 7, 10–12]. The spread of these microorganisms to the bloodstream can cause bacteremia [2, 4, 6], which is normally asymptomatic but can produce fever, shivers, tremors, and inflammation or redness around the jewellery. Ludwig's angina can also be induced by the presence of anaerobic microorganisms related to perioral or tongue piercing. In isolated cases, sepsis can lead to a life-threatening septic shock [5, 6, 8, 13].

7.4.5 Bacterial Endocarditis

Any subject who has had a valvular replacement is extremely susceptible to bacterial endocarditis. Technically speaking, anything from eating to brushing the teeth can cause an increase in the bacterial levels in the bloodstream, ultimately allowing them to colonize the artificial valve. The oral cavity is a rich source of infection as there are a number of bacteria colonizing it on a daily basis. Procedures like tongue piercing increase this release of bacteria into the bloodstream and can cause bacterial endocarditis.

7.4.6 Transmission of Communicable Diseases

During tongue piercing, a hygiene protocol must be strictly followed to avoid transmission of disease by the use of common or unsterile needles. Commonly transmitted diseases include human immunodeficiency virus (HIV), hepatitis B and C, herpes simplex virus, Epstein-Barr virus (EBV), Candida albicans, tetanus, syphilis, and tuberculosis (TB) [4, 5].

7.4.7 Allergic Reactions

Allergic reactions can be produced by some of the materials inserted [5] such as *nickel*, which is the metal that causes most contact allergies. The most widely reported allergic reaction in piercing is *contact dermatitis* produced by nickel, chromium, or nickel-cobalt [4, 5, 7, 14]. In the mid-1990s, the European Union issued a directive to limit the amount of nickel in all products in direct contact with human tissue, with a limit of 0.05 g for the nickel used in oral/perioral piercing jewellery. It also recommended that gold used for this purpose should be at least 14–18K [4, 5].

7.4.8 Dental and Gum Alterations

The constant friction that the gums are subjected to from tongue piercing will result in recession leading to poor esthetics, sensitivity, and loss of support for the teeth.

A study by Botchway and Kuc (1998), found some type of dental structure loss like enamel and dentine in 80% of patients with tongue piercings [15]. This type of alteration is more frequent with the use of tongue barbells, especially in the molar and premolar area (with a higher prevalence on lingual cusps) and in lower incisors [4, 6]. It is also extremely easy to damage the teeth during everyday functions like mastication or even during sleep, causing a very painful cracked or fractured tooth (Fig. 7.4). Dental fracture can also result from nerve block due to the local anesthetic administered for the insertion [2]. Bearers of porcelain crowns have an increased risk of fractures or erosions if they also have oral piercing [15, 16] and patients with large restorations or caries have an increased risk of cusp fractures [5].

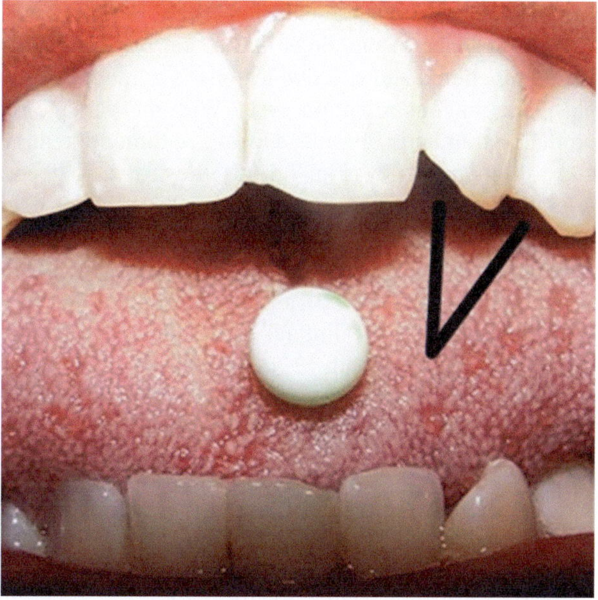

Fig. 7.4 Fracture of the left incisors due to a tongue piercing (black lines)

7.4.9 Formation of Bacterial Plaque

A greater incidence of plaque can be produced at the site of oral/perioral piercings due to the difficulty of maintaining hygiene and the retention of food remains, creating an ideal environment for a large accumulation of plaque and calculus [3]. Moreover, constant contact with a barbell in the tongue, for example, increases the probability of supra- and subgingival plaque accumulation at the lower front teeth [10]. These accumulations can produce halitosis and possible infection [8]. Thus, oral piercings have been associated with *gingivitis* [8], which requires the presence of bacteria in plaque for its onset although factors related to microorganisms and host predisposition also affect this pathogenesis [17].

7.4.10 Tissue Alteration

Mucosal trauma produced by oral/perioral piercings can cause localized erythema and edema. Piercing can be followed by hyperplastic scarring [4], which may be accompanied by pain and edema [5, 6]. Hypertrophic or keloid scarring can also occur, possibly influenced by the presence of systematic disease, medication, or smoking, although tobacco was reported not to be a statistically significant factor [18]. Tissue overgrowth can be caused by continuous movement of the jewellery in the inserted tissue [9] and surgery may even be required, with a high risk of recurrence if the piercing is repeated [5]. In some cases, the insertion wound can become covered with epithelium, complicating removal of the jewellery [4]. Continuous contact with the jewellery can also cause alterations to the lingual papillae, which results in a reduced taste sensation [5].

The presence of piercings in the oral/perioral cavity can cause various lesions, including edema and reactive lesions, e.g. mucoceles, inflammatory fibrous hyperplasia, or mucous retention cysts. With the passage of time, tongue piercings can produce a traumatic fibroma, a localized tumor that has the same color as the mucosa and a soft consistency (Fig. 7.5) [5]; they can also generate fibrous repair tissue with re-epithelization of the perforated area [10].

Oral mucosa lesions can also be produced by repeated trauma of the jewellery on adjacent tissue, which can sometimes cause gingival recessions, abrasions, or ulcerations [19, 20]. In 2003, Brooks et al. reported that tongue piercings produced gingival recession on the lingual aspect of lower front incisors and an increase in periodontal pocket depth [21]. Because of the inflammation produced by tongue piercing, longer bars (> 20 mm) are initially inserted, which are then reduced in size after 2 weeks when the inflammation has abated [2, 4, 6].

7.4.11 Sialorrhea

Several studies have confirmed that piercings in the oral/perioral cavity can stimulate salivary flow (sialorrhea) [1, 4, 5, 8]. Venta et al. (2005) reported increased salivary flow in 63% of their tongue piercing series [22].

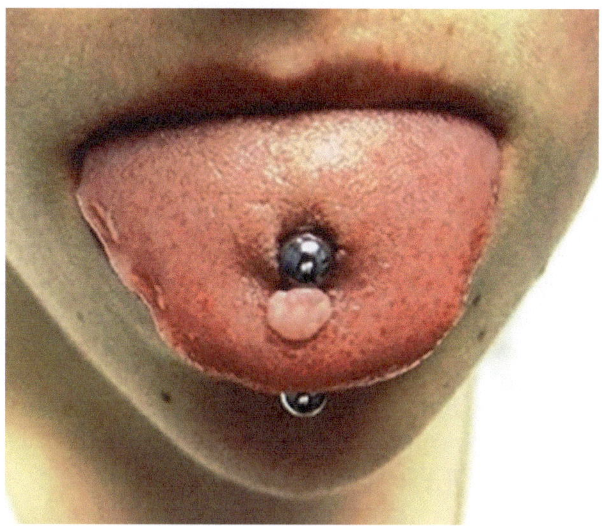

Fig. 7.5 Traumatic fibroma; a localized tumor that has a soft consistency and almost the same color as the mucosa

7.4.12 Panoramic X-ray Alteration

Oral and perioral piercings produce radiopaque areas and must be not be worn during X-ray examinations. For panoramic *X-rays*, any metal object above the neck must be removed [4–6].

7.4.13 Aspiration

Accidentally swallowing a piece of jewellery on the tongue is rather common. Often, the body tries to reject it. This is seen as delayed healing, pain, and eventually loss of the pierced object. As it becomes looser with time, it can easily be ingested leading to other problems because of its length and pointed end. In piercings with barbells, labrets or rings, the jewellery can be ingested or aspirated, producing digestive or respiratory disorders, respectively, due to an incorrect fixing, poor placement, or exertion of high pressure [4, 5]. The risk of ingestion is higher with magnet piercing [5]. Considerable controversy has arisen over the need to remove oral piercing during surgery under general anesthesia to avoid the risk of ingestion/aspiration or of trauma to tissue and the possible obstruction of intubation.

7.4.14 Other Complications

The presence of piercing jewellery on the *tongue* may hamper *chewing, phonation,* and *distorts the pronunciation of certain sounds*, e.g., "s," "sh," "th," "ph," "t," or "v" [4–6, 8].

7.5 Conclusions and Recommendations

The most hazardous oral sites for piercing are the uvula, due to the high risk of airway obstruction [4, 6], and the side of the tongue because of the higher vascularity. The type of piercing jewellery most associated with buccal alterations is a long barbell in the tongue [6, 18, 21]. Jewellery should be exclusively composed of soft, hypoallergenic, nontoxic materials to minimize anaphylactic reactions and trauma to adjacent oral structures. The most affected oral site is at the lower incisors because of the loss of gingival tissue [4, 5], largely due to tongue and lip piercings, with a high incidence of gingival recessions in this sector [8, 21]. The most frequent oral lesions produced by piercings are inflammation, erythema, and trauma to dental tissue and bone [4, 6, 16, 23], and the most frequent traumas are tissue tears. The disease most commonly transmitted by piercing is hepatitis [1, 4, 6]. There is a need for greater awareness by dentists of these possible adverse effects and for a closer follow-up of patients with oral and perioral piercing [24].

References

1. Huber MA, Terezhalmy GT, Moore WS. Oral/perioral piercing. Quintessence Int. 2003;34(9):722–3.
2. Brennan M, O'Connell B, O'Sullivan M. Multiple dental fractures following tongue barbell placement: a case report. Dent Traumatol. 2006;22(1):41–3.
3. Berenguer G, Forrest A, Horning GM, Towle HJ, Karpinia K. Localized periodontitis as a long-term effect of oral piercing: a case report. Compend Contin Educ Dent. 2006;27(1):24–7.
4. De Urbiola AI, Viñals IH. Some considerations about oral piercings. Av Odontoestomatol. 2005;21(5):259–69.
5. Barbería Leache E, García Naranjo AM, González Couso R, Gutiérrez GD. Are the oral piercing important in the clinic? Dent Pract. 2006;1:45–9.
6. Peticolas T, Tilliss TS, Cross-Poline GN. Oral and perioral piercing: a unique form of self-expression. J Contemp Dent Pract. 2000;1(3):30–46.
7. Sardella A, Pedrinazzi M, Bez C, Lodi G, Carrassi A. Labial piercing resulting in gingival recession. A case series. J Clin Periodontol. 2002;29(10):961–3.
8. Levin L, Zadik Y, Becker T. Oral and dental complications of intra-oral piercing. Dent Traumatol. 2005;21(6):341–3.
9. Boardman R, Smith RA. Dental implications of oral piercing. J Calif Dent Assoc. 1997;25(3):200–7.
10. Dubose J, Pratt JW. Victim of fashion: endocarditis after oral piercing. Curr Surg. 2004;61(5):474–7.
11. Guidard-Schmid JB, Picard H, Slama L, Masloc C, Amiel C, Pialox G. Piercing and its infectious complications. A public health issue in France. Presse Med. 2000;29:1948–56.
12. Friedel JM, Stehlik J, Desai M, Granato JE. Infective endocarditis after oral body piercing. Cardiol Rev. 2003;11(5):252–5.
13. Perkins CS, Meisner J, Harrison JM. A complication of tongue piercing. Br Dent J. 1997;182(4):47–8.
14. Lhotka CG, Szekeres T, Fritzer-Szekeres M, et al. Are allergic reactions to skin clips associated with delayed wound healing? Am J Surg. 1998;176(4):320–3.
15. Botchway C, Kuc I. Tongue piercing and associated tooth fracture. J Can Dent Assoc. 1998;64(11):803–5.
16. De Moor RJ, De Witte AM, De Bruyne MA. Tongue piercing and associated oral and dental complications. Endod Dent Traumatol. 2000;16(5):232–7.

17. Elena BMF. Periodontal diseases as bacterial infection. Av Periodontol Implantol. 2005;17(3):111–8.
18. Leichter JW, Monteith BD. Prevalence and risk of traumatic gingival recession following elective lip piercing. Dent Traumatol. 2006;22(1):7–13.
19. Lopez Jornet P, Vicente Ortega V, Yanez Gascon J, et al. Clinicopathological characteristics of tongue piercing: an experimental study. J Oral Pathol Med. 2004;33(6):340–5.
20. Bascones Martínez A, Figuero E, Esparza G. Oral ulcers. Med Clin. 2005;125(15):590–7.
21. Brooks JK, Hooper KA, Reynolds MA. Formation of mucogingival defects associated with intraoral and perioral piercing: case reports. J Am Dent Assoc. 2003;134(7):837–43.
22. Venta I, Lakoma A, Haahtela S, Peltola J, Ylipaavalniemi P, Turtola L. Oral piercings among first-year university students. Oral Surg Oral Med Oral Pathol Oral Radiol Endod. 2005;99(5):546–9.
23. Palacios-Sanchez B, Cerero-Lapiedra R, Campo-Trapero J, Esparza-Gomez G. Oral piercing: dental considerations and the legal situation in Spain. Int Dent J. 2007;57(2):60–4.
24. Escudero-Castaño N, Perea-García MA, Campo-Trapero J, Cano-Sánchez A, Bascones-Martínez A. Oral and perioral piercing complications. Open Dent J. 2008;2:133–6.

Inflammation (Glossitis)

8

8.1 Overview

8.1.1 Introduction

Glossitis, also known as "burning tongue syndrome" or "smooth tongue" means soreness of the tongue, or more usually inflammation [1] with loss of the lingual papillae (depapillation) of the dorsal surface of the tongue, leaving a smooth, shiny, and erythematous surface [2, 3] (sometimes specifically termed *atrophic glossitis*). Glossitis is often caused by nutritional deficiencies and may be painless or cause discomfort. Severe cases of glossitis can be painful and cause tongue swelling and difficulty in speech or swallowing. Glossitis usually responds well to treatment if the cause is identified and corrected. Tongue soreness caused by glossitis is differentiated from "burning mouth syndrome," where there is no identifiable change in the appearance of the tongue, and there are no identifiable causes [4].

8.1.2 Clinical Presentation

The symptoms of glossitis vary from one person to another. They may also differ according to the underlying cause of the condition. Common symptoms of glossitis include the following [2, 4]:

- A swollen tongue. Severe swelling may block the airway and interfere with breathing.
- Pain or itching in the tongue or burning sensation that may involve the whole mouth
- Change in the texture of the surface of the tongue due to the change in the size and shape of papillae e.g. smooth, shiny appearance of the tongue, caused by loss of lingual papillae

© The Author(s), under exclusive license to Springer Nature Switzerland AG 2022
M. F. Sakr, *Tongue Lesions*, https://doi.org/10.1007/978-3-031-08198-9_8

- Discoloration of the tongue's surface usually to a darker red color than the normal white-pink color of a healthy tongue
- Difficulty in proper speech because of tongue soreness or swelling.
- Difficulty in chewing and swallowing, also because of tongue soreness or swelling.
- Change in taste or loss of taste sensation
- Dry mouth sensation, increased thirst and sore throat
- Depending upon the underlying cause, there may be additional signs and symptoms such as pallor, oral ulceration, and angular cheilitis [2].

8.1.3 Diagnosis

Physical examination may reveal abnormalities in the tongue's surface, color, or presence of blisters or bumps on the tongue or gums. A swab of saliva may be taken for testing and blood sample to check for underlying nutritional deficiencies or diseases.

8.1.4 Etiology

There is a variety of possible causes of glossitis, including the following [5]:

8.1.4.1 Allergic Reaction

When glossitis occurs due to an allergic reaction, the patient is most likely to develop acute glossitis and have sudden tongue swelling and pain. An allergy to a particular *food* (food dyes), *drug* (e.g. diuretics), *dyes* in confectionery, *plastic* in dentures or retainers, or *specific irritant* (e.g. mouthwash, toothpaste, breath-fresheners) can cause this type of reaction.

8.1.4.2 Mechanical Irritation or Injury to the Mouth

Injuries to the mouth, such as small cuts from rough edges of teeth or dental appliances or burns from hot food, might cause the tongue to inflame and swell. When dental braces cause glossitis, the patient is more at risk for chronic glossitis due to the risk of repeated injury to the mouth and tongue. Tongue piercing [6] can cause glossitis by the constant irritation by the ornament and by colonization of *Candida albicans* in site and on the ornament [7].

8.1.4.3 Exposure to Irritants

Exposure to irritants such as tobacco, alcohol, hot foods, or spices is a known, common cause of glossitis.

8.1.4.4 Infections

Bacterial, viral, and fungal infections can all cause glossitis. However, oral herpes viral infection and fungal infections are among the most likely infections to cause glossitis. Chronic Candida infections of the tongue can cause an atrophic glossitis known as "median rhomboid glossitis."

Syphilis is now relatively rare, but the tertiary stage can cause diffuse glossitis and atrophy of lingual papillae, termed "syphilitic glossitis" [2], "luetic glossitis," or "atrophic glossitis of tertiary syphilis." It is caused by *Treponema pallidum* and is a sexually transmitted infection.

8.1.4.5 Anemias

Iron-deficiency anemia is mainly caused by blood loss, such as may occur during menses or gastrointestinal hemorrhage. This often results in a depapilled, atrophic glossitis, giving the tongue a bald and shiny appearance, along with pallor of the lips and other mucous membranes and a tendency towards recurrent oral ulceration [8], and cheilosis [9]. The appearance of the tongue in iron deficiency anemia has been described as diffuse or patchy atrophy with tenderness or burning [10]. One cause of iron deficiency anemia is sideropenic dysphagia (Plummer–Vinson or Paterson–Brown–Kelly syndrome) which is also characterized by esophageal webbing and dysphagia [8].

Pernicious anemia is usually caused by autoimmune destruction of gastric parietal cells. Parietal cells secrete intrinsic factor which is required for the absorption of vitamin B_{12}. Vitamin B_{12} deficiency results in megaloblastic anemia and may present as glossitis. In this case, the appearance of the tongue is "beefy" or "fiery red and sore" [8]. There may be linear or patchy red lesions [2].

8.1.4.6 Vitamin B Deficiencies

- *Vitamin B_1 deficiency* (thiamin deficiency) can cause glossitis [10].
- *Vitamin B_2 deficiency* (ariboflavinosis) can cause glossitis (known as *magenta*) [11], along with angular cheilitis, cheilosis, peripheral neuropathy, and other signs and symptoms [9].
- *VitaminB$_3$ deficiency* (pellagra) can cause glossitis [9].
- *Vitamin B_6 deficiency* (pyridoxine deficiency) can cause glossitis, along with angular cheilitis, cheilosis, peripheral neuropathy, and seborrheic dermatitis [9].
- *Vitamin B_9 deficiency* (folate deficiency) can cause glossitis, along with macrocytic anemia, thrombocytopenia, leukopenia, diarrhea, fatigue, and possibly neurological signs [9].
- *Vitamin B_{12} deficiency* can cause, in addition to pernicious anemia, glossitis, which tends to be painful, smooth, and shiny [9].

8.1.4.7 Other Diseases/Conditions

Certain diseases such as celiac disease, pernicious anemia, and protein-calorie malnutrition can cause glossitis through malnutrition or malabsorption [9], which creates the nutritional deficiencies described above. Other mechanisms may be involved in some of those conditions listed below such as autoimmune diseases (e.g. Sjögren's syndrome).

- Alcoholism [9].
- Sprue (celiac disease [12], or tropical sprue), secondary to nutritional deficiencies [9].
- Crohn's disease [9].
- Whipple disease [9].
- Glucagonoma syndrome [9].
- Cowden disease [9].
- Acquired immunodeficiency syndrome (AIDS) [7]
- Carcinoid syndrome [9].
- Kwashiorkor amyloidosis [9].
- Veganism and other specialized diets [2].
- Poor hydration and low saliva in the mouth, which allows bacteria to grow more readily.
- Administration of ganglion blockers (e.g. Tubocurarine, Mecamylamine) or bronchodilators (e.g. Albuterol).
- Oral lichen planus, erythema multiforme, aphthous ulcer, pemphigus vulgaris
- Heredity factors

8.1.5 Classification (Types) of Glossitis [13]

There are several clinical patterns of glossitis, which could be classified as:

- A group of tongue or *gastrointestinal* diseases [5].
- *Primary*, where there is no underlying cause, or *secondary* where it is a sign or symptom of another condition [3].
- *Acute*, which often develops suddenly and can have severe symptoms or *chronic* due an underlying chronic condition [5].

The following types of glossitis are discussed in this chapter:

1. Atrophic glossitis (Hunter's glossitis).
2. Median rhomboid glossitis (MRG)
3. Benign migratory glossitis
4. Geometric glossitis
5. Strawberry glossitis

8.1.6 Epidemiology

One review reported overall prevalence ranges of 0.1–14.3% for geographic tongue, 1.3–9.0% for atrophic glossitis, and 0.0–3.35% for median rhomboid glossitis [14].

8.1.7 Prevention

It may not always be possible to prevent glossitis. However, risk of developing the condition can be lowered by maintaining a healthful diet, practicing good oral hygiene with regular brushing, flossing, and mouth washes, and avoiding irritants, such as spicy foods, cigarettes, and acidic foods. Burning sensation can be prevented by simply drinking the correct amount of water to produce a good amount of saliva, which often prevents the growth of bacteria in the oral cavity.

8.1.8 Treatment

Treatment of glossitis depends on its cause. Generally, it responds well to treatment once the underlying cause has been determined.

Antibiotic, antifungal, or antiviral *drugs* may help clear up a bacterial, fungal, or viral infection, respectively. Dietary supplements are prescribed for patients with glossitis resulting from nutritional deficiencies. If a nutrient deficiency is due to an underlying disease, such as celiac disease, dietary changes to manage the underlying condition are recommended. In certain cases, corticosteroids such as prednisone are prescribed for reduction of inflammation and edema. Any burning sensation can be managed with a topical anesthetic. In rare cases, tongue swelling may threaten the airway; an emergency that needs immediate secure of air entry.

8.2 Atrophic Glossitis

8.2.1 Synonyms

Atrophic glossitis is also known as "bald tongue" [13], "smooth tongue," "Hunter glossitis," "Moeller glossitis," or "Möller-Hunter glossitis" [14]. Although the term Möller/Hunter glossitis was originally used to refer to specifically the glossitis that occurs in vitamin B_{12} deficiency secondary to pernicious anemia, it is now used as a synonym for atrophic glossitis [15].

8.2.2 Definition

Atrophic glossitis is a condition characterized by a smooth glossy tongue that is often tender and painful [16], caused by complete atrophy of the lingual papillae (depapillation) [3]. The dorsal tongue surface may be affected totally, or in patches, and may be associated with a burning sensation, pain, and/or erythema [17].

8.2.3 Etiology

Atrophic glossitis is a nonspecific finding [16], and has a great many causes, usually related to iron-deficiency anemia, pernicious anemia, vitamin-B complex deficiencies [17], xerostomia, and unrecognized and/or untreated celiac disease (which often presents without gastrointestinal symptoms) [18–20]. In this chapter, the term glossitis, unless otherwise specified, refers to atrophic glossitis. Candidiasis may be a concurrent finding or an alternative cause of erythema, burning, and atrophy.

8.2.4 Treatment

As mentioned before, treatment of glossitis depends on the etiological factor. Nutritional deficiencies are treated with the appropriate nutritional supplements. If the underlying cause is celiac disease, dietary changes are recommended. Concurrent candidiasis is treated with antifungal medications.

8.3 Median Rhomboid Glossitis (MRG)

Median rhomboid glossitis (MRG), or glossal central papillary atrophy, is a persistent depapillated rhomboidal area in the center line of the dorsum of the tongue, just anterior to the sulcus terminalis (i.e. anterior to the circumvallate papillae) (Fig. 8.1) [2, 16].

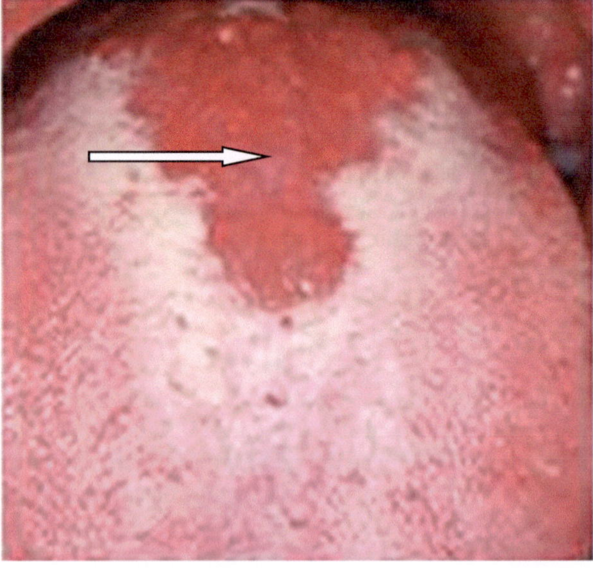

Fig. 8.1 Median rhomboid glossitis. Note the depapillated rhomboidal area on the central part of the dorsum of the tongue (arrow)

8.3.1 Incidence

- *General incidence:* It is uncommon. Incidence in adults approaches 0.2%.
- *Age*: It can occur at any age, but usually diagnosed at middle age.
- *Gender:* It can occur in either gender, but occurs among males.
- *Geographic distribution:* It has no known geographic predominance.

8.3.2 Etiology and Pathogenesis

It is *not* a developmental anomaly; it is due to localized chronic fungal infection. **Candida** species colonize mainly on the posterior dorsum of the tongue, even in healthy patients. MRG is also predisposed to by smoking, dental prostheses, corticosteroid sprays/inhalers, microtrauma (e.g., from mastication and swallowing), and human immunodeficiency virus (HIV) infection (immunosuppression) [21].

Formerly thought to be caused by failure of the lateral processes of the tongue to cover the embryonic tuberculum impar, this lesion is now thought to be related to candidosis because (1) culture frequently shows **Candida**, although often in a mixed bacterial/fungal microflora, and (2) histopathologically, candidal hyphae infiltrate the superficial layers of the parakeratotic epithelium and a neutrophil infiltrate occupies the epithelium, with elongated hyperplastic rete ridges (pseudo-epitheliomatous hyperplasia) and a lymphocyte infiltration in the corium. Thus, it can be confused with carcinoma (Fig. 8.2) [21].

Furthermore, it has been suggested that the decreased microvasculature in the midline area of the tongue predisposes to central papillary atrophy with aging and secondary candidiasis.

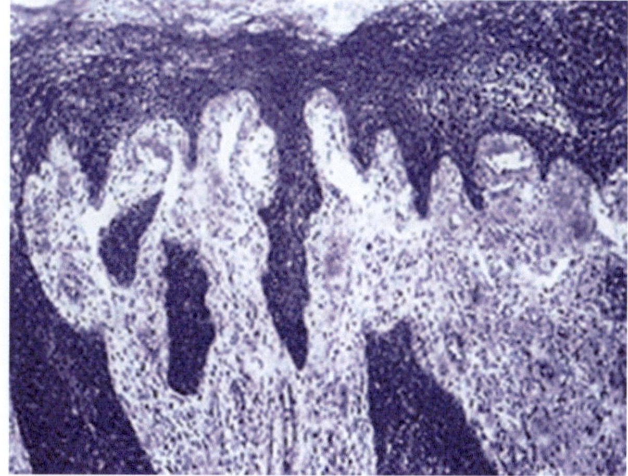

Fig. 8.2 Median rhomboid glossitis, showing histopathological appearance of pseudo-epitheliomatous hyperplasia that may lead to confusion with carcinoma

8.3.3 Clinical Features

- An ovoid, diamond-shaped atrophic area, which is usually asymptomatic, is present just anterior to circumvallate papillae (Figs. 8.3 and 8.4). Lesions are typically less than 2 cm in greatest dimension, and most demonstrate a smooth, flat surface, although it is not unusual for the surface to be lobulated.

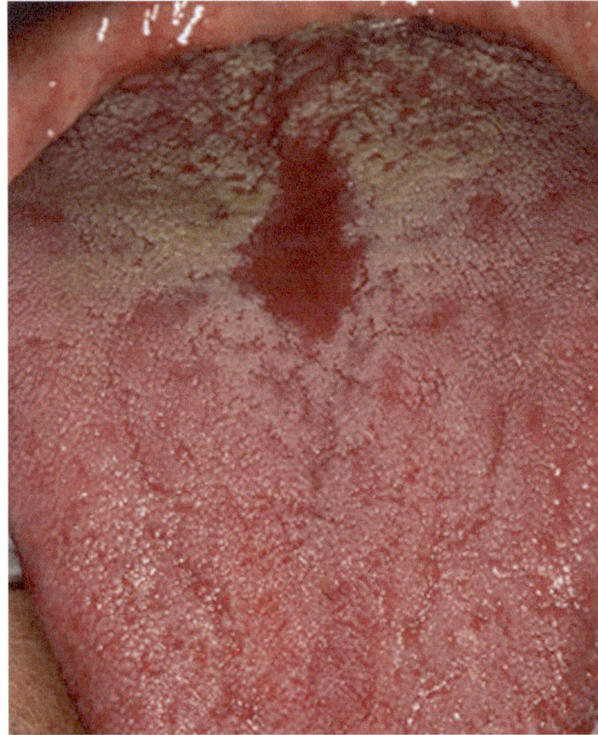

Fig. 8.3 Median Rhomboid Glossitis (MRG): Erythematous, atrophic, and roughly symmetric lesion involving the midline region of the dorsal tongue, just anterior to the circumvallate papillae

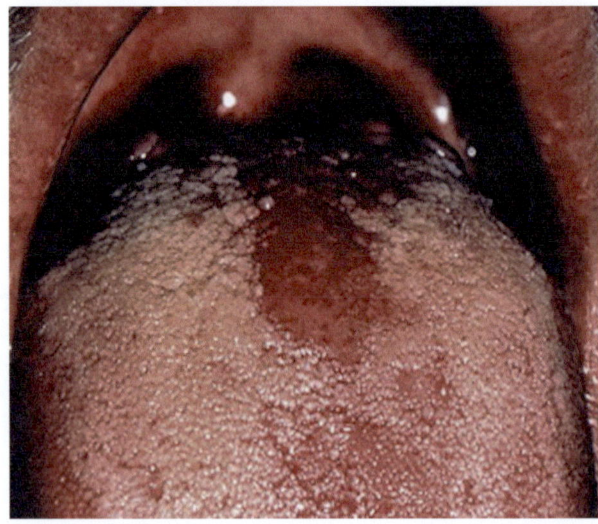

Fig. 8.4 Median rhomboid glossitis (MRG): An asymptomatic atrophic red patch on the posterior aspect of the dorsal tongue was noted on oral cavity examination

- *Age*: Most of the cases are not diagnosed until the middle age of the affected patients, but the entity is of course present in childhood.
- *Gender*: male to female ratio is 3:1
- Infected cases may also demonstrate a midline soft palate erythematic in the area of routine contact with the underlying tongue involvement; this is euphemistically referred to as a "kissing lesion" [22].

8.3.4 Diagnosis

Median rhomboid glossitis is usually a clinical diagnosis. *Biopsy* is indicated if there is any concern that it could be a neoplasm; histology shows irregular epithelial hyperplasia, which resembles, but is not, a carcinoma (because of the pseudo-epitheliomatous hyperplasia). Rarely, is there a need for blood picture, smears for fungal hyphae, or culture.

When median rhomboid glossitis presents with a thick plaque or nodule, lesions must be distinguished from a lingual thyroid, thyroglossal duct cyst, and other tumors [23].

8.3.5 Treatment

Tobacco habits should be stopped. Antifungals are indicated. However, the lesions may prove poorly responsive to topical antifungal drugs, and some cases respond only to systemic azoles [24].

8.4 Benign Migratory Glossitis (Geogrpahic Tongue)

8.4.1 Synonyms

Benign migratory glossitis is also known as "superficial migratory glossitis," "erythema migrans," "glossitis migrans," "geographic tongue," and "wandering rash of the tongue."

8.4.2 Definition

Migratory glossitis is a "psoriasis-like or psoriasis-related inflammation of the tongue resulting in the production of snaky white lines on the tops and sides, often with small parallel grooves adjacent to them" [25]. It makes the tongue look like a "map" and hence its name "geographic tongue" [26] (Fig. 8.5).

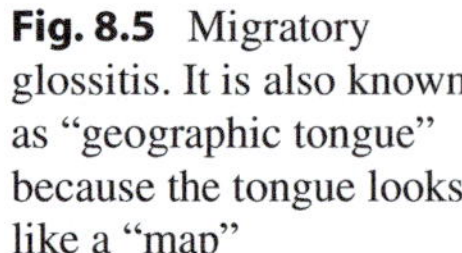

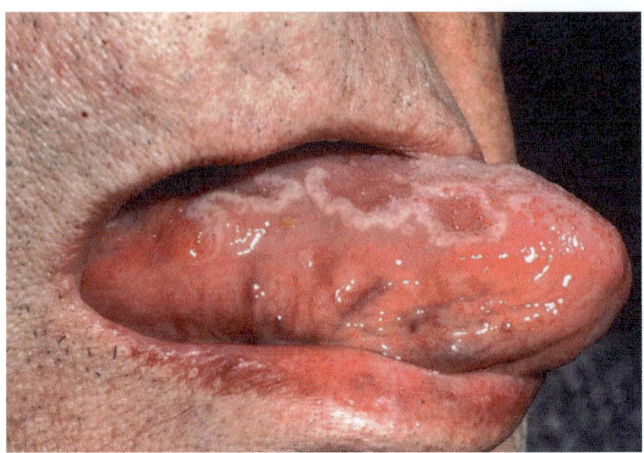

Fig. 8.5 Migratory glossitis. It is also known as "geographic tongue" because the tongue looks like a "map"

8.4.3 Prevalence

The prevalence in the general population ranges between 1.0% and 2.5% and is more prominent in adults than in children [27, 28]. Its prevalence in school children is 1% and there is no definitive gender predilection as reported by Redman [29]. The reason for its low prevalence in the pediatric age-group is because it is ignored by the parents due to its asymptomatic nature.

8.4.4 Etiology

The exact cause of erythema migrans is still unknown [13]. Since the lesions microscopically resemble those of cutaneous psoriasis, it is believed to be a psoriasis-related condition. Some studies suggested that patients with psoriasis may have an increased prevalence of oral erythema migrans [26, 30, 31].

Predisposing factors for migratory glossitis include history of psoriasis of skin [31], bronchial asthma or rhinitis [32], psychological stress [33], gastrointestinal disturbances associated with anemia [34], allergy [35], hormonal disturbances, or zinc deficiency. It has been associated with HLA-B15, suggesting the role of heredity (genetic) as one of the etiological factors [36], causing the condition to pass down from one generation to the next. Recently, it has been concluded that immunological and psychological parameters appear associated with geographic tongue and may be considered as risk factors [37–39]. Benign migratory glossitis may occur with Down's syndrome, diabetes mellitus, or fissured tongue. Some authors consider geographic tongue to be an early stage of fissured tongue, since the two conditions often occur in combination [40]. It may also present as an oral manifestation of psoriasis [41], or as a marker of severity [42].

8.4.5 Clinical Features and Diagnosis

The *diagnosis* of erythema migrans usually does *not* require biopsy because of its very characteristic *clinical features*. It presents as serpiginous white lines that may be quite pronounced and often surrounded by the erythematous areas of lost filiform papillae or edematous papillae on the dorsum of the tongue with a tendency to involve the lateral aspects of the dorsum [26]. White snaky lines with parallel grooves are characteristic (Fig. 8.6). Small grooves parallel to some lines are present. Many cases have irregular red macules without obvious white peripheral lines. Here the patient also has a mild white-coated tongue, a common comorbid feature of geographic tongue. The erythematous macules are much more obvious when combined with white-coated tongue or with a mild white hairy tongue. Occasional macules are outlined with irregular white lines, which is a pathognomonic feature (Fig. 8.7).

The lesional areas persist for a variable period, then the inflammation subsides and the papillae regenerate. Change in the location and pattern of lesion is observed after every few days, thereby giving it name "migratory" [3, 43].

In most instances, the lesions are asymptomatic, but some individuals may complain of a mild burning sensation or pain. This often happens during contact with foods or other substances. Some potential triggers include smoking, chewing tobacco, spicy or acidic foods, hot food, toothpaste or mouthwash [44].

The *differential diagnosis* of benign migratory glossitis in children should include candidiasis (oral thrush), leukoplakia, psoriasis, neutropenia, local trauma, and drug reaction [45].

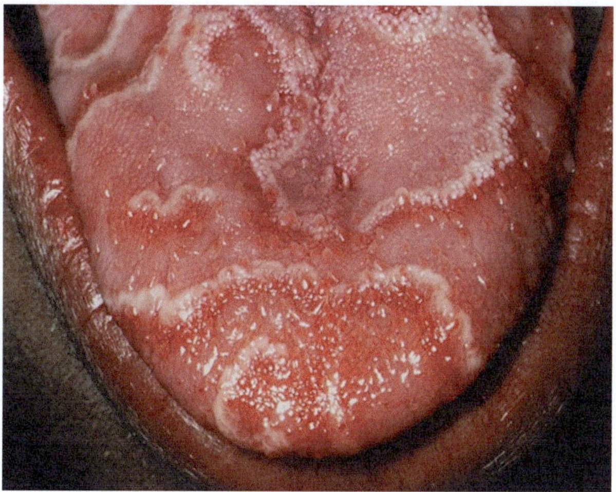

Fig. 8.6 Erythema migrans showing erythematous atrophic patches surrounded by yellow-white linear borders

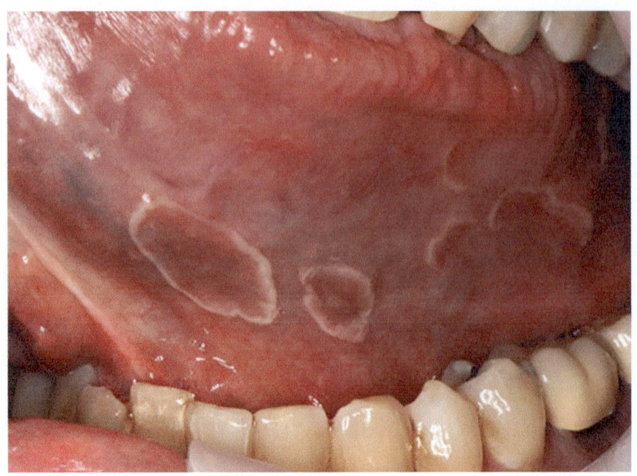

Fig. 8.7 Erythema migrans showing ovoid erythematous lesions with slightly raised yellow-white borders on the ventral tongue and floor of the mouth

Other sites of the dorsal tongue then may develop lesions. Although the dorsal tongue is the most common site of involvement, the lateral and ventral tongue mucosa also is affected rather frequently. Very uncommonly, the labial mucosa, or soft palate, and buccal mucosa may develop these lesions, which are characterized by demarcated red patches that are partially or completely surrounded by linear yellow-white borders.

8.4.6 Potential Complications

There are no major complications associated with geographic tongue. There are no illnesses or cancers that are known to stem from geographic tongue. However, due to its appearance, geographic tongue may lead some people to experience *anxiety* or other psychological complications. The anxiety may stem from the fear of negative judgment by others or the fear that there is something more seriously wrong.

8.4.7 Treatment

There are no preventive measures for migratory glossitis. In most cases, treatment is *not* necessary. Just assurance of the benign nature of the condition is all that is needed. Left untreated, most cases of geographic tongue clear up spontaneously.

The use of diphenhydramine, Lidocaine rinse, and sodium bicarbonate rinse has shown successful results in symptomatic cases of mild intensity [10]. If significant pain persists then the use of topical and systemic antihistamines [46], Vitamin A acid therapy and systemic acitretin [46], systemic cyclosporine [47], topical corticosteroids [48], and topical tacrolimus ointment [49, 50] has been reported in the literature with variable successes.

Treatment of a geographic tongue with topical or systemic antifungal drugs can be tried if secondary candidiasis is suspected.

8.4.8 Prognosis

With geographic tongue, a person will live an otherwise normal life. The appearance of the tongue and mild discomfort are often the biggest concerns a person may have. In most cases, the patches eventually clear with no intervention.

There are no lifestyle changes that the person needs to make, as nothing will help prevent the condition from appearing again in the future. However, they may need to avoid acidic or spicy foods.

8.5 Geometric Glossitis

8.5.1 Definition

Geometric glossitis, also known as "herpetic geometric glossitis" [1], is a term used by some authors to refer to a chronic lesion associated with herpes simplex virus (HSV) type I infection [51], in which there is a deep fissure in the midline of the tongue, which gives off multiple branches [10].

8.5.2 Clinical Presentation

The lesion is usually very painful, and there may be erosions present in the depths of the fissures. Similar fissured lesions which are not associated with HSV, as may occur in fissured-tongue, do not tend to be painful [51]. The name comes from the geometric pattern of the fissures which are longitudinal, crossed, or branched [52].

8.5.3 Etiology

It is described as occurring in immunocompromised patients such as those with leukemia. However, the association between herpes simplex and geometric glossitis is disputed by some authors due to a lack of gold standard techniques for diagnosis of intraoral herpetic lesions, and the high prevalence of asymptomatic viral shedding in immunocompromised individuals [10].

8.5.4 Treatment

Treatment of geometric glossitis is usually with systemic acyclovir [51].

8.6 Strawberry Glossitis

8.6.1 Definitions

- "Strawberry tongue" or "raspberry tongue" is glossitis that manifests with hyperplastic fungiform papillae, giving the appearance of a strawberry [53].
- "White strawberry tongue" is where there is a white coating on the tongue through which the hyperplastic fungiform papillae protrude.
- "Red strawberry tongue" is where the white coating is lost and a dark red, erythematous surface is revealed, interspaced with the hyperplastic fungiform papillae.

8.6.2 Etiology

White strawberry tongue is seen in early scarlet fever (a systemic infection of group A β-hemolytic streptococci) [54], and red strawberry tongue occurs later, after 4–5 days [10]. Strawberry tongue is also seen in Kawasaki disease (a vasculitic disorder primarily occurring in children under the age of 5 years) [55, 56] and toxic shock syndrome [57]. It may mimic other types of glossitis or Vitamin B_{12} deficiency [58].

8.6.3 Treatment

Treatment of strawberry glossitis is mainly treatment of the underlying cause.

References

1. Domino FJ, Baldor RA, editors. The 5-minute clinical consult. 20th ed. Philadelphia, PA: Wolters Kluwer Health/Lippincott Williams & Wilkins; 2012. p. 532–3.
2. Scully C. Oral and maxillofacial medicine, the basis of diagnosis and treatment. 2nd ed. Edinburgh: Churchill Livingstone; 2008. p. 356.
3. Rogers K, editor. The digestive system. 1st ed. New York, NY: Britannica Educational Pub., in association with Rosen Educational Services; 2010. p. 146.
4. Roddy M, Heli F, Buchanan, John Ag B, Anne-Marie G, Jo CW, Joanna MZ. Interventions for treating burning mouth syndrome. Cochrane Database Syst Rev. 2016;11:CD002779.
5. Stoopler ET, Kuperstein AS. Glossitis secondary to vitamin B12 deficiency anemia. Can Med Assoc J. 2013;185(12):E582.
6. Levin L, Zadik Y. Oral piercing: complications and side effects. Am J Dent. 2007;20(5):340–4.
7. Zadik Y, Burnstein S, Derazne E, Sandler V, Ianculovici C, Halperin T. Colonization of Candida: prevalence among tongue-pierced and non-pierced immunocompetent adults. Oral Dis. 2010;16(2):172–5.
8. Treister NS, Bruch JM. Clinical oral medicine and pathology. New York, NY: Humana Press; 2010. p. 149.
9. Yamada T, David H, Alpers DH, editors. Textbook of gastroenterology. 5th ed. Chichester, West Sussex: Blackwell Pub; 2009. p. 1717–44.
10. Neville BW, Damm DD, Allen CA, Bouquot JE. Oral and maxillofacial pathology. 2nd ed. Philadelphia, PA: WB Saunders; 2002. p. 169–70.

11. Park KK, Brodell RT, Helms SE. Angular cheilitis, part 2: nutritional, systemic, and drug-related causes and treatment. Cutis. 2011;88(1):27–32.
12. Pastore L, Carroccio A, Compilato D, Panzarella V, Serpico R, Lo Muzio L. Oral manifestations of celiac disease. J Clin Gastroenterol. 2008;42(3):224–32.
13. Reamy BV, Derby R, Bunt CW. Common tongue conditions in primary care. Am Fam Physician. 2010;81(5):627–34.
14. Dombi C, Czeglédy A. Incidence of tongue diseases based on epidemiologic studies (review of the literature). Fogorv Sz. 1992;85(11):335–41.
15. Braun-Falco O. Dermatology. 2nd ed. Berlin: Springer; 2000. p. 1173.
16. William DJ, Timothy GB. Andrews' diseases of the skin: clinical dermatology. 14th ed. Philadelphia, PA: Saunders Elsevier; 2006. p. 803.
17. Chi AC, Neville BW, Krayer JW, Gonsalves WC. Oral manifestations of systemic disease. Am Fam Physician. 2010;82(11):1381–8.
18. Rashid M, Zarkadas M, Anca A, Limeback H. Oral manifestations of celiac disease: a clinical guide for dentists. J Can Dent Assoc. 2011;77:b39.
19. National Institute of Health (NIH). Dental enamel defects and celiac disease. Bethesda, MD: NIH; n.d.. Archived from the original (PDF) on March 5, 2016.
20. Giuca MR, Cei G, Gigli F, Gandini P. Oral signs in the diagnosis of celiac disease: review of the literature. Minerva Stomatol. 2010;59(1–2):33–43.
21. Hartsfield JK Jr, Cameron AC. McDonald and Avery's dentistry for the child and adolescent. 10th ed. Amsterdam: Elsevier; 2016.
22. Cohen BA. Pediatric dermatology. 4th ed. Amsterdam: Elsevier; 2013.
23. Bouquot JE, Nikai H. Diagnostic surgical pathology of the head and neck. 2nd ed. Philadelphia, PA: WB Saunders; 2009.
24. Brad W, Neville DDS, Angela C, Chi DMD. Color atlas of oral and maxillofacial diseases. Amsterdam: Elsevier; 2019.
25. Picciani BLS, Domingos TA, Teixeira-Souza T, Batista dos Santos VC, Fernando de Sousa Gonzaga H, Cardoso-Oliveira J, et al. Geographic tongue and psoriasis: clinical, histopathological, immuno-histochemical and genetic correlation - a literature review. Anais Brasileiros de Dermatol. 2016;91(4):410–21.
26. Rajendran A, Sivapathasundharam B. Shafer's textbook of oral pathology. 7th ed. St. Louis, MO: Elsevier; 2012. p. 31–2.
27. Nandini DB, Bhavana SB, Deepak BS, Ashwini R. Paediatric geographic tongue: a case report, review and recent updates. J Clin Diagn Res. 2016;10(2):5–9.
28. Shulman JD. Prevalence of oral mucosal lesions in children and youths in the USA. Int J Pediatr Dent. 2005;15(2):89–97.
29. Redman RS. Prevalence of geographic tongue, fissured tongue, median rhomboid glossitis and hairy tongue among 3,611 Minnesota school children. Oral Surg Oral Med Oral Pathol. 1970;30(3):390–5.
30. Prinz H. Wandering rash of tongue (geographic tongue). Dent Cosmos. 1927;69:272–5.
31. Zargari O. The prevalence and significance of fissured tongue and geographical tongue in psoriatic patients. Clin Exp Dermatol. 2006;31(2):192–5.
32. Marks R, Czarny D. Geographic tongue: sensitivity to the environment. Oral Surg. 1984;58(2):156–9.
33. Redman RS, Vance FL, Gorlin RJ. Psychological component in the etiology of geographic tongue. J Dent Res. 1966;45(5):1403–8.
34. Banoczy J, Szabo L, Csiba A. Migratory glossitis. A clinical-histologic review of seventy cases. Oral Surg Oral Med Oral Pathol. 1975;39(1):113–21.
35. Barton DH, Spier SK, Crovello TJ. Benign migratory glossitis and allergy. Pediatr Dent. 1982;4(3):249–50.
36. Marks R, Tait B. HLA antigens in geographic tongue. Tissue Antigens. 1980;15(1):60–2.
37. Alikhani M, Khalighinejad N, Ghalaianj P, Khaleghi MA, Askari E, et al. Immunologic and psychologic parameters associated with geographic tongue. Oral Surg Oral Med Oral Pathol Oral Radiol. 2014;118(1):68–71.

38. Khalighinejad N, Gorsky M. Psychological parameters associated with geographic tongue: a clinical observation. Oral Surg Oral Med Oral Pathol Oral Radiol. 2015;119(1):123.
39. Stoopler ET, Thoppay JR, Sollectio TP. Psychological parameters associated with geographic tongue: a clinical observation. Oral Surg Oral Med Oral Pathol Oral Radiol. 2015;119(1):122–3.
40. Greenberg MS, Glick M, Ship JA. Burket's oral medicine. 11th ed. Hamilton, ON: BC Decker; 2008.
41. Tarakji B, Umair A, Babaker Z, Sn A, Gazal G, et al. Relation between psoriasis and geographic tongue. J Clin Diagn Res. 2014;8(11):ZE06–7.
42. Picciani BL, Souza TT, Santos Vde C, Domingos TA, Carneiro S, et al. Geographic tongue or fissured tongue in 348 patients with psoriasis: correlation with disease severity. Sci World J. 2015;2015:564326.
43. Adeyemo TA, Adeyemo WL, Adediran A, Akinbami AJ, Akanmu AS. Orofacial manifestations of hematological disorders: anemia and hemostatic disorders. Indian J Dent Res. 2011;22(3):454–61.
44. Honarmand M, Mollashahi LF, Shirzaiy M, Sehhatpour M. Geographic tongue and associated risk factors among Iranian dental patients. Iran J Public Health. 2013;42(2):215.
45. Mehta V. Benign migratory glossitis: report of a rare case with review of literature. J Dent Health Oral Disord Ther. 2017;6(4):00210.
46. Assimakopulos D, Patrikakos G, Fotika C, et al. Benign migratory glossitis or geographic tongue: an enigmatic oral lesion. Am J Med. 2002;113(9):751–5.
47. Abe M, Sogabe Y, Syuto T, Ishibuchi H, Yokoyama Y, et al. Successful treatment with cyclosporin administration for persistent benign migratory glossitis. J Dermatol. 2007;34(5):340–3.
48. Cameron AC, Widmer RP. Pediatric oral medicine and pathology. In: Handbook of pediatric dentistry. 3rd ed. St. Louis, MO: Mosby Elsevier; 2012. p. 192–3.
49. Purani JM, Purani HJ. Treatment of geographic tongue with topical tacrolimus. BMJ Case Rep. 2014;2014:bcr-2013-201268.
50. Ishibashi M, Tojo G, Watanabe M, Tamabuchi T, Masu T, Aiba S. Geographic tongue treated with topical tacrolimus. J Dermatol Case Rep. 2010;4(4):57–9.
51. Cohen PR, Kazi S, Grossman ME. Herpetic geometric glossitis: a distinctive pattern of lingual herpes simplex virus infection. South Med J. 1995;88(12):1231–5.
52. Grossman ME, Stevens AW, Cohen PR. Brief report: herpetic geometric glossitis. N Engl J Med. 1993;329(25):1859–60.
53. Stocking S, Gubili J, editors. Mosby's dental dictionary. St. Louis, MO: Mosby; 2004.
54. Yang SG, Dong HJ, Li FR, et al. Report and analysis of a scarlet fever outbreak among adults through food-borne transmission in China. J Infect. 2007;55(5):419–24.
55. Singh S, Kansra S. Kawasaki disease. Natl Med J India. 2005;18(1):20–4.
56. Park AH, Batchra N, Rowley A, Hotaling A. Patterns of Kawasaki syndrome presentation. Int J Pediatr Otorhinolaryngol. 1997;40(1):41–50.
57. Baehler EA, Dillon WP, Cumbo TJ, Lee RV. Prolonged use of a diaphragm and toxic shock syndrome. Fertil Steril. 1982;38(2):248–50.
58. Williams G, Katcher M. Skin lesions: strawberry tongue. Primary Care Dermatol Module, University of Wisconsin Madison, USA. Accessed 14 Aug 2007.

9 Swellings of the Tongue

9.1 Classification

Swellings of the tongue may be categorized as:

1. Acute tongue swellings
2. Chronic tongue swellings

Chronic tongue swellings can be further subdivided into:

1. Diffuse tongue swelling (macroglossia)
2. Localized tongue swelling (solid or cystic)

9.2 Causes of Acute Tongue Swellings

Causes of acute swellings of the tongue include the following:

1. A tongue bite or sting.
2. Injury, for instance by a fish-bone, or by tongue biting during sleep or an epileptic fit.
3. Corrosive or acute irritant applications.
4. Acute edema secondary to:
   - Inflammation (glossitis or stomatitis)
   - Certain drugs (e.g. mercury and rarely, aspirin)
   - Erythema bullosum or pemphigus
   - Angioneurotic edema of the tongue
5. Hemorrhage into the tongue substance, as in:
   - Scurvy
   - Leukemia
   - Other hemorrhagic states.

© The Author(s), under exclusive license to Springer Nature Switzerland AG 2022
M. F. Sakr, *Tongue Lesions*, https://doi.org/10.1007/978-3-031-08198-9_9

9.3 Causes of Chronic Tongue Swellings

Chronic or persistent swellings of the tongue are either "diffuse" (macroglossia) or "localized," which may be further subdivided into "solid" or "cystic." Causes are depicted in Fig. 9.1 [1–17].

9.4 Ranula

9.4.1 Definition

A ranula is a large mucous extravasation or retention cyst (a type of mucocele) found in the floor of the mouth caused by leakage of mucus from the sublingual (or rarely, submandibular) salivary gland, probably due to an unnoticed local trauma of

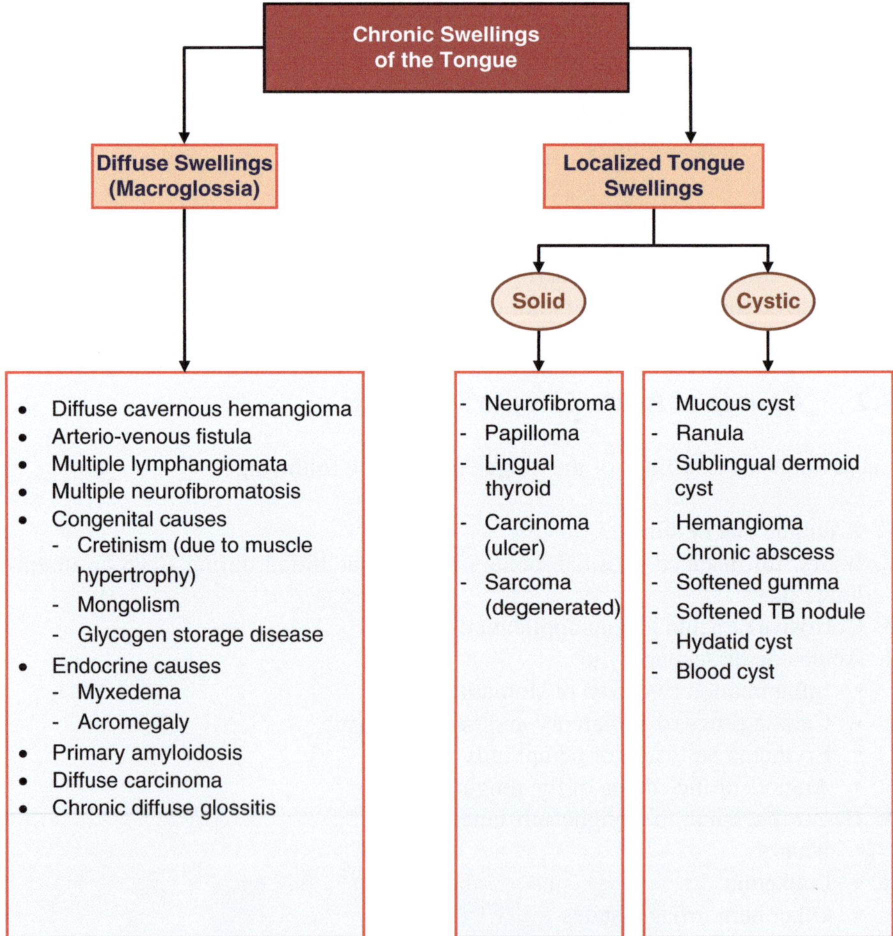

Fig. 9.1 Classification of chronic tongue swellings according to etiology

the gland. The word "ranula" means "little frog." It was coined from *rana*; a Latin word meaning "frog" because the typical swelling in the floor of mouth resembles the underbelly of a frog [18].

9.4.2 Anatomical Classification

Ranulas (ranulae) are anatomically grouped into three different types: (1) *oral ranula* (also known as simple ranula or superficial ranula), which occurs above the mylohyoid muscle and is confined to the floor of the mouth [19], (2) *plunging ranula* (also known as cervical ranula, dividing ranula, deep ranula, and oral ranula with cervical extension) [20], which is found beneath the mylohyoid muscle, lying in the neck rather than the floor of the mouth [19], and (3) *mixed type*, which has both an oral and a cervical component [21].

9.4.3 Epidemiology

The prevalence of ranula is around 0.2 cases of every 1000 individuals [22]. Ranulas are the most common pathological lesion associated with the sublingual glands accounting for approximately 6% of intraoral cysts of the salivary glands [23]. The floor of the mouth is the most common site to develop ranulas. Although sublingual glands give rise to most of the ranulas (90%), they may arise from the submandibular gland in rare cases. Age range of patients with ranula ranges from 3 years to 61 years with children and young adults in the second decade (teenagers) and third decades of life being more affected than others [18, 24]. No gender predilection has been reported for these lesions.

Plunging ranulas are rare compared to oral ranulas and only about 100 cases have been described in the English literature [20]. The ethnic variation in incidence of plunging ranula has been reported, where it was noted to be generally more prevalent in people of Asian origin, especially the Chinese, natives of New Zealand, and Eskimos.

9.4.4 Etiology

The leading cause of ranulas is minor *trauma* to the floor of the mouth, which is thought to damage the delicate ducts that drain saliva from the sublingual gland into the oral cavity [23]. The second cause is *obstruction* of the salivary duct with sialolith or mucus plug. *Other causes* leading to ranula formation include chronic inflammation (sarcoidosis and Sjogren's syndrome) or infection (human immunodeficiency virus—HIV) with periductal scarring, ductal hypoplasia, ductal stenosis, ductal agenesis, and neoplasia [25]. Anatomical variation in the ductal system of the sublingual gland may increase the risk of development of a ranula. The risk appears to be increased when the Bartholin duct is connected to and empties into the Wharton duct [26].

The most usual source of the mucin spillage is the sublingual salivary gland, but ranulas may also arise from the submandibular duct or the minor salivary glands in the floor of the mouth. A *cervical ranula* occurs when the spilled mucin dissects its way through the mylohyoid muscle [19], which separates the sublingual space from the submandibular space, and creates a swelling in the neck. It may occur following rupture of a simple ranula with subsequent formation of a non-epithelial-lined cyst [22, 27–29]. Rarely, ranulae may extend backwards into the parapharyngeal space [29]. In contrast, submandibular and parotid ducts do not usually form ranula from duct ligation because they only secrete saliva when stimulated, unlike the sublingual that constantly discharges saliva even during the interdigestive phase.

The reported ethnic variation in incidence of plunging ranula could be attributed to a *genetic alteration* in people of a certain race (Chinese, natives of New Zealand, and Eskimos), perhaps predisposing them to either develop areas of deficiencies within the mylohyoid muscle or an anatomically altered variant of the sublingual gland with easy extravasation of mucus following minor trauma [30, 31].

9.4.5 Pathophysiology

The primary pathology that lies behind the formation of ranulas is the disruption to the flow of secretions of salivary glands. Trauma is the most common cause, following which mucus extravasates and accumulates in the surrounding tissue. Another way that leads to the development of these lesions is the obstruction of the excretory duct of the salivary glands secondary to sialolith, periductal scarring or fibrosis, and tumor. The fluid within a ranula has the viscous, jelly-like consistency of egg white.

Most cervical or plunging ranulas have oral components, and four mechanisms by which they may arise have been described. These can be summarized as follows [28, 32, 33].

1. Part of the sublingual gland may move through the mylohyoid muscle, or an aberrant sublingual gland may be present below this muscle; this mechanism describes plunging ranula without an oral part.
2. The lateral part of the anterior two-thirds of the mylohyoid muscle may have a deficiency through which mucus from the sublingual gland may slip to the submandibular area. Deficiency in the anterior two-thirds of mylohyoid muscles has been reported in about 27–45% of cadavers; these sites create a path through which tissues or mucus may pass through the muscle.
3. Surgical manipulation during the removal of a ranula may mutilate and block its superior surface, and should such recur, a cervical ranula develops as this new lesion slips through the only available space which is the deficient area in the mylohyoid muscle.
4. The sublingual gland duct may join that of the submandibular gland resulting in the formation of a ranula that may form along this line between the two glands.

9.4.6 Clinical Presentation

9.4.6.1 History-Taking

A ranula is mostly seen in young children and adolescents with both sexes equally affected. Patients with *oral ranula* mostly present with a painless translucent-to-blue swelling in the floor of the mouth (Fig. 9.2). This swelling may be painful if secondarily infected, and can interfere with speech, swallowing, mastication, and even respiration, as it displaces the tongue in an upward and medial direction. In some cases, the tongue may exert pressure on the lesion, interfering with the outflow of saliva, thus leading to obstructive salivary gland signs and symptoms (pain when eating or chewing).

Patients with *cervical ranula* present with an asymptomatic mass in the neck; usually in the submandibular triangle (Fig. 9.3). There is usually a trauma to the floor of the mouth or dental surgical procedure leading to the lesion. There may

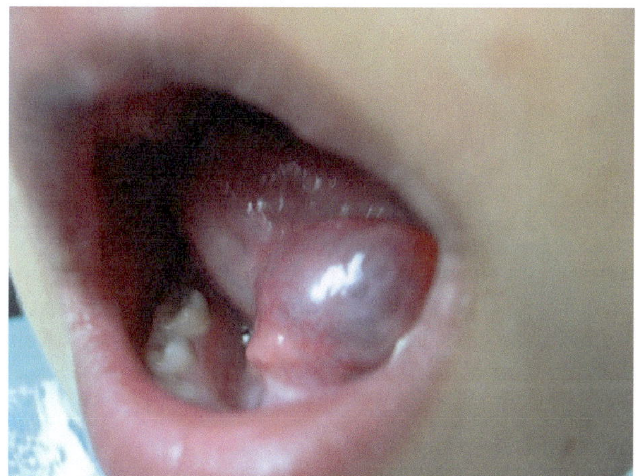

Fig. 9.2 Oral ranula: swelling in the floor of the mouth under the tongue. Note the bluish discoloration of the cyst

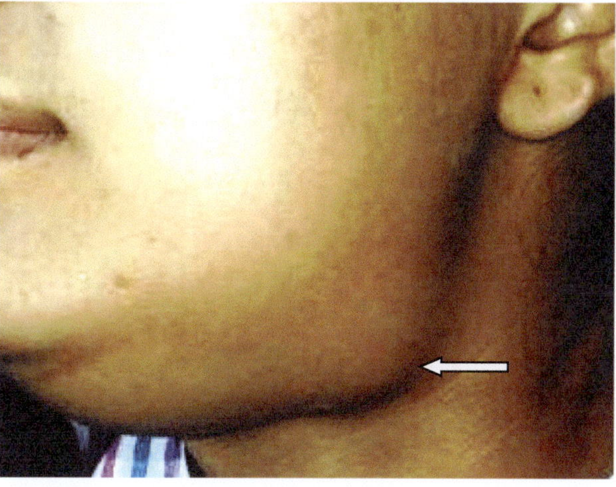

Fig. 9.3 Cervical/deep ranula presenting as a swelling in the left submandibular region of the neck (arrow)

be a history of nonsuccessful surgical treatment (incomplete removal) of a simple (oral) ranula, followed by the development of a cervical (deep or plunging ranula).

9.4.7 Clinical Examination

On physical examination, *oral ranula* appears as a cystic blue-colored swelling in the floor of mouth, between the symphysis menti and tongue, just to one side of the midline (frenulum) resembling the belly of a frog [34] (Fig. 9.4). This usual characteristic location helps to distinguish it from a midline sublingual dermoid cyst [19]. However, an oral ranula may be bilateral with a slight constriction in the middle caused by the tongue frenulum giving it a "dumbbell shape" (Fig. 9.5). If the lesion is deeper, there will be a greater thickness of tissue separating it from the oral cavity and thus the blue translucent appearance may *not* be a feature.

An *oral ranula* is characteristically spherical in shape, but only the top half is seen. It usually varies from 1–5 cm in size, but may grow so large that it almost fills the mouth. It is not tender. The surface is smooth and covered by tortuous veins, and the mucous membrane is mobile over the swelling. The submandibular duct is displaced and stretched over it. The edge is difficult to feel because it is deep, related to the arch of the mandible. It is soft in consistency, usually fluctuant and transilluminates, but cannot be compressed. It is not fixed to the overlying mucosa, tongue or jaw. Cervical lymph nodes should not be enlarged and local tissues should be normal, but an oral ranula may have extension or prolongation in the neck.

A *cervical or plunging ranula* presents as an asymptomatic, mobile, fluctuant, soft, and progressively enlarging (expanding) mass in the neck measuring about

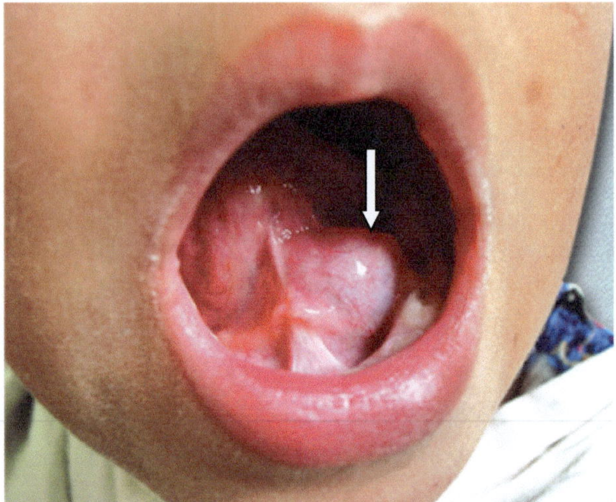

Fig. 9.4 An oral ranula appearing as a swelling in the floor of the mouth (arrow), just to one side (left) of the midline (frenulum)

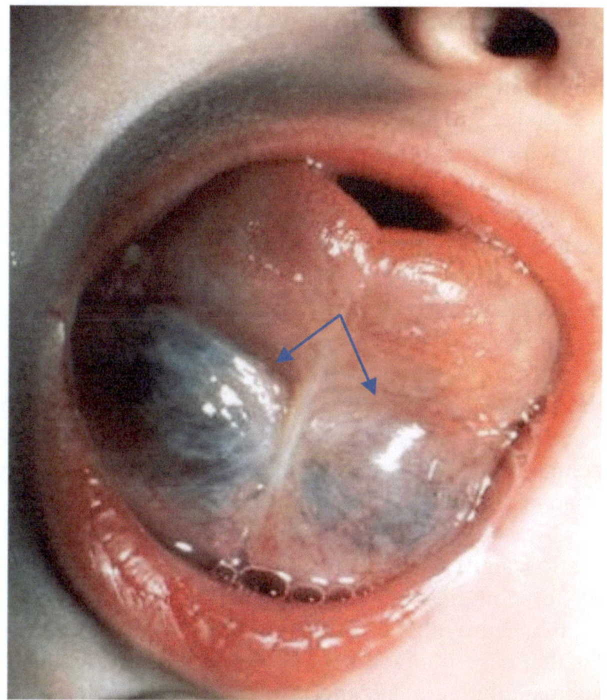

Fig. 9.5 An oral ranula appearing as a dumbbell-shaped bluish swelling in the floor of the mouth under the tongue. Note the bluish tinge (arrows)

4–10 cm in size, with or without a swelling in the mouth [35]. When an oral component is present, squeezing the neck mass may increase the size of swelling in the floor of the mouth. A plunging ranula is covered by an intact overlying skin. The submandibular space is the usual location [36]; however, plunging ranulas have been found to spread into the submental area, the contralateral side of neck, the nasopharyngeal region, including the skull of base, retropharynx, and sometimes to the upper mediastinum [20, 22].

9.4.7.1 Complications

Complications of ranulas include the following:

1. Infection
2. Repeated trauma—hematoma formation
3. Rupture and reformation
4. Dysphagia, in case of a large ranula

About half of the plunging or cervical ranulas arise as a result of the failure to excise oral ranulas completely. These plunging ranulas may enlarge and result in a respiratory compromise or acute mediastinitis, a life-threatening complication.

9.4.8 Evaluation/Investigations

The diagnosis of oral ranula is mainly based on the clinical picture. Although imaging studies are *not* generally indicated for the evaluation of oral ranulas, they can undoubtedly help in excluding other differential diagnoses, determining the cause (e.g. calculi) and the extent of the swellings, thus aiding in surgery [37]. Imaging studies include ultrasonography (US), computed tomography (CT) scan, and magnetic resonance imaging (MRI) [29].

9.4.8.1 Ultrasonography (US)

Uncomplicated ranulas appear as thin-walled cystic lesions, and can be imaged both, from the skin or trans-orally with a small probe. If infected, the walls are thicker and the fluid content is more echogenic. In expert hands, high-resolution US can detect calculi, abscesses, and cysts, and can even correctly assess up to 90% of benign *versus* malignant tumors. Vascular lesions, however, require color Doppler imaging for their evaluation.

Ultrasonography has been demonstrated to be quite successful in evaluating cystic lesions of the submandibular region in young people, with particular utility for plunging ranula [38]. The status of the mylohyoid muscle can also be established by this examination [20, 36]. It can also differentiate plunging ranulas that have plunged behind the posterior border of mylohyoid muscle into the submandibular space and the less common ranula that has herniated through a mylohyoid muscle defect (*mylohyoid boutonniere*) into submental space. The use of US suffices to investigate these lesions; it has been recommended as the preferred test (Fig. 9.6) [35].

9.4.8.2 Computed Tomography (CT) Scan

Computed tomography (CT) scan is seldom required, except if there is a large plunging or cervical ranula that has breached through a defect in the mylohyoid

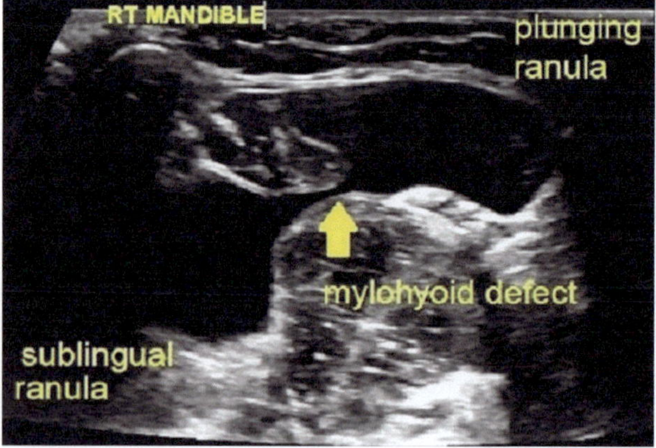

Fig. 9.6 Transverse ultrasound of the sublingual and plunging ranula through a defect in the mylohyoid muscle (arrow)

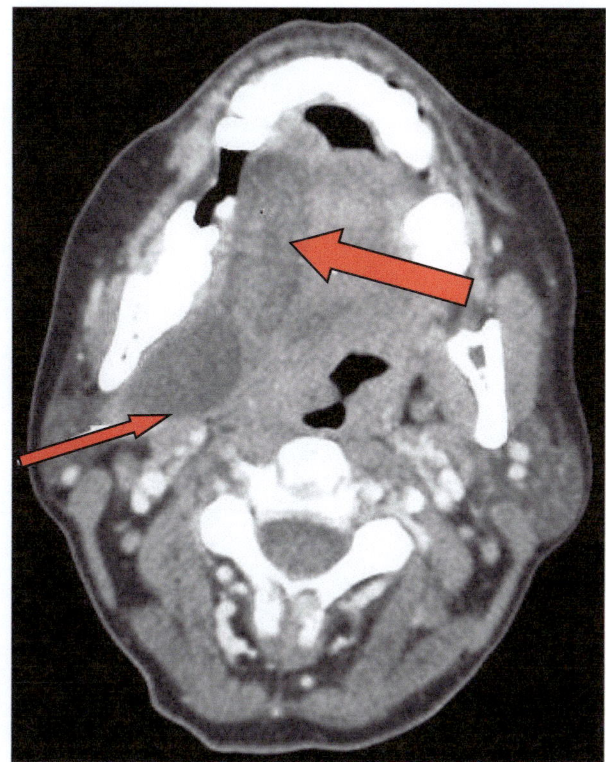

Fig. 9.7 Contrast enhanced axial CT of a plunging ranula—the superior aspect of the lesion shows a nonenhancing, water-density mass from the right sublingual space displacing the tongue to the left. A large part of the mass extends posterolaterally into the submandibular space (small arrow). Mass effect can be appreciated with displacement of the parapharyngeal space. The lesion is nonenhancing, homogenous, smoothly marginated, and without internal septations. Smooth tapering anteriorly into the sublingual space forms the "tail sign" (large arrow)

muscle (Fig. 9.7). The classical CT scan finding for plunging ranula is a lesion with a small tail that extends into the sublingual space (*tail sign*) [38]. In the absence of this sign, the diagnosis of a plunging ranula should be made if an identical cyst is seen in the submandibular or parapharyngeal space with connection to the sublingual space [20]. The CT scan also aids in determining the extent of the swelling, which is crucial to know before proceeding to the surgery [39].

On CT scan, uncomplicated ranulas appear as thin-walled cystic lesions with central fluid attenuation (10–20 HU). If the cysts have been intervened upon previously or have been infected, the content may be increased in attenuation, even occasionally resembling a nonenhancing soft tissue mass. The walls of such lesions are typically thicker. If a superimposed infection is present at the time of imaging, it will be indistinguishable from an abscess, with thicker walls and surrounding fat stranding (Fig. 9.7).

9.4.8.3 Magnetic Resonance Imaging (MRI)

Typically, MRI shows a unilocular, homogenous, well-defined, nonenhancing cystic mass with low signal on T1 and high signal on T2-weighted images (Fig. 9.8). High signal on T1 indicates high protein content.

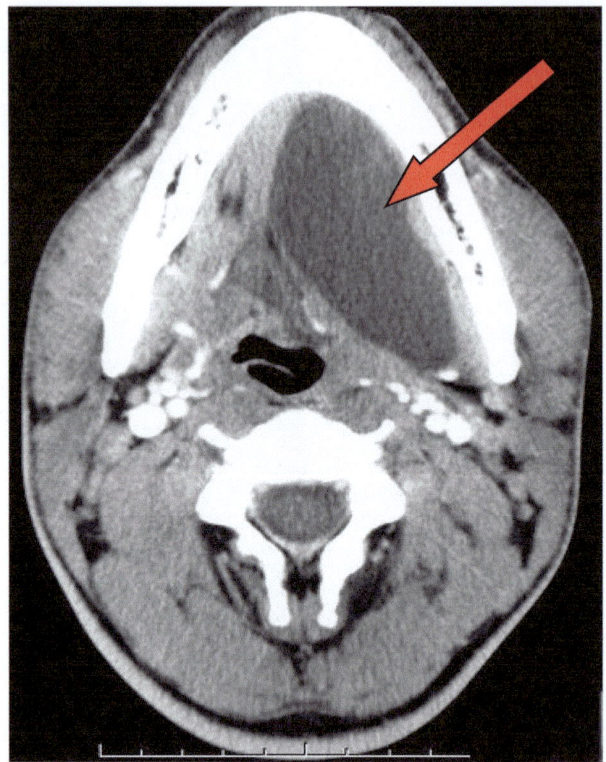

Fig. 9.8 MRI showing a ranula in the right sublingual space. It appears as a unilocular, homogenous, well-defined, nonenhancing cystic mass (arrow)

9.4.8.4 Biopsy

Histological examination is required to differentiate between benign and malignant disease. Histological appearance of a plunging ranula is typically that of a *pseudocyst* without epithelial lining; it consists of a fibrovascular stroma which contains chronic inflammatory cells including macrophages filled with mucin [36] (Fig. 9.9). Histiocytes or foamy macrophages predominate in the pseudocyst wall and mucin is also often observed. Occasionally, partial epithelial linings are seen. High amylase and protein are seen on biochemical analysis of the cystic fluid [39].

9.4.9 Differential Diagnosis

9.4.9.1 Oral (Simple) Ranula

Oral ranulas, occurring beneath the tongue, may mimic a lot of other lesions from which it must be differentiated. The broad list of differential diagnosis of these lesions includes the following:

- Hemangioma
- Lymphangioma

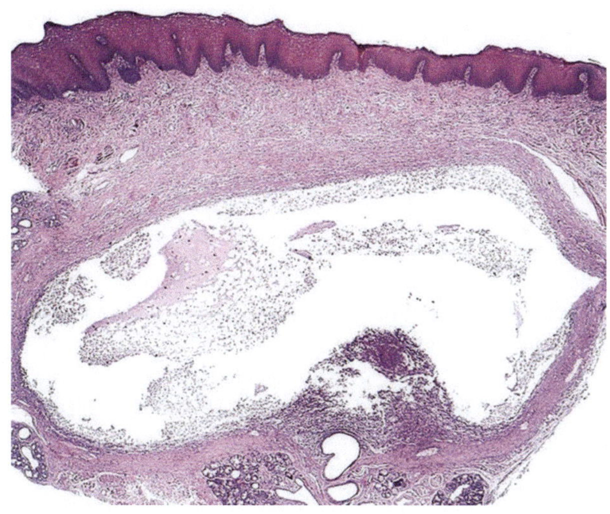

Fig. 9.9 High power micrograph (H&E, 10×) showing epithelial macrophages forming a pseudocyst around the extravasated mucin, no true capsule (epithelium) is present

- Sublingual dermoid cyst (usually in the midline)
- Benign or malignant salivary gland neoplasm
- Lipoma
- Abscess
- Venous lake
- Fibroma
- Benign mesenchymal neoplasm

9.4.9.2 Plunging (Cervical) Ranula

Plunging ranula present as a cervical swelling and thus differential diagnosis includes the following [20, 32, 36, 40, 41]:

- Cervical lymph node enlargement (necrotic/cystic)
- Abscesses (painful, with thicker walls and extensive fat strands, and usually associated with dental caries)
- Laryngocele (compressible and increases in size with straining)
- Thyroglossal duct cyst (occurs usually in the midline of the neck and characteristically moves upwards with protrusion of the tongue)
- Dermal cysts
- Cystic hygroma (usually occurs in infants)
- Second branchial cleft cyst (usually at the anterior border of the sternocleidomastoid muscle)
- Thymic cyst
- Cysts of endocrine glands of the neck
- Benign salivary gland tumors
- Some benign mesenchymal tumors

9.4.10 Treatment

9.4.10.1 Oral Ranulas: Treatment Options

Ranulas tend to resolve spontaneously. But if they are symptomatic, persistent, and are not self-resolving, multiple treatment approaches can be considered, which are discussed below.

9.4.10.1.1 Surgical Excision

Surgical resection is curative, but requires not only excision of the cystic component but of the parent sublingual gland as well. If the gland is left in situ, recurrence of the ranula is high [28].

9.4.10.1.2 Marsupialization/Micro-marsupialization

The oldest and most widely used therapy for oral ranula is marsupialization; some authors prefer marsupialization before embarking on surgical removal. Marsupialization involves the removal of the roof of the cyst (deroofing) and suturing of its borders to surrounding tissues in the floor of the mouth (Fig. 9.10). The aim is to allow the sublingual gland to reestablish connection with the oral cavity. However, this procedure recorded a very high recurrence rate of 61–89% within 6 weeks to 12 months of surgery.

Early closure of the surgery site due to compression of the tongue on the cyst has been known to increase the recurrence rate. Therefore, packing the cavity with gauze for 7–10 days is advised. This allows re-epithelialization of the cavity and also seals off the leakage site. In addition, it provokes a foreign body reaction causing fibrosis and atrophy of the offending acini, thereby reducing the recurrence rate. Thus, marsupialization and filling the cavity with gauze improves the success rate.

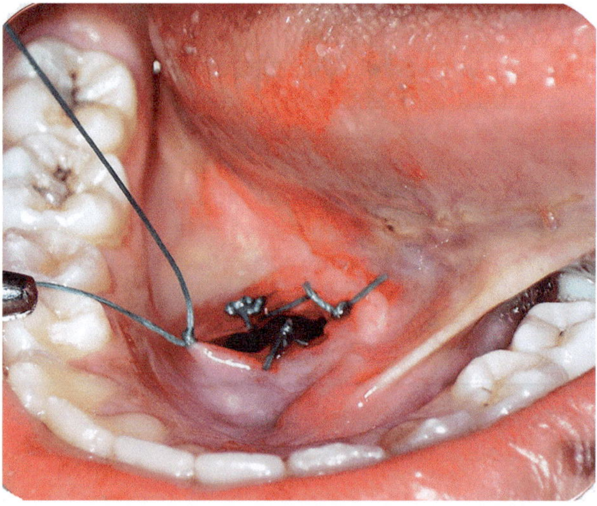

Fig. 9.10 Marsupialization: deroofing of the ranula (cyst) and suturing of its borders to surrounding tissues in the floor of the mouth

If marsupialization fails to eliminate the disease, then surgical excision is considered the next treatment of choice.

Micro-marsupialization involves the placement of a silk suture (Seton) for a minimum of 7 days during which an epithelial tract forms to allow for mucus drainage between the surface and the underlying salivary glandular tissue. Though simple, this procedure has the major disadvantage of treatment failure and the primary complication of recurrence [20].

9.4.10.1.3 Laser Ablation, Cryosurgery, and Electrocautery

These methods have also been employed for the treatment of smaller ranulas either alone or before marsupialization.

9.4.10.1.4 Intralesional Injection of a Sclerosant Agent

Although considered "experimental," intracystic injection of the streptococcal preparation, OK-432, has been reported to treat the disease with variable success rates[42, 43].

9.4.10.2 Plunging Ranulas: Treatment Options

Many methods have been used for the treatment of *cervical ranulas* and this includes (1) surgical removal of lesion, (2) use of cryosurgery, (3) marsupialization/micro-marsupialization, (4) excision of oral portion and associated sublingual gland or, rarely, submandibular gland, (5) excision of the sublingual gland via the intraoral approach, and drainage of lesion, and use of cervical approach to excise the lesion; sometimes this is combined with excision of sublingual gland, and (6) radiotherapy [22]. Recurrences have been reported to occur even after these treatments [28]. However, when the sublingual gland together with the associated lesion is excised, a low recurrence rate is recorded [44, 45].

In the management of plunging ranula, the sublingual gland could be *excised* either be via the intraoral or transcervical route. Excision of the gland through the intraoral method and drainage of the associated cervical content is enough to give cure and is presently considered as the treatment of choice [28]. With the transcervical approach, total excision of the sublingual gland is challenging because this method requires the painstaking division of the mylohyoid muscle in the floor of mouth [20]. However, this method is recommended when the plunging ranula is large in size.

Removal of the gland by a trans-oral approach after drainage of the cyst has also been advocated. Should this method fail, then the cyst should be excised via a transcervical approach. Cases restricted to the neck are also best treated by the transcervical approach [20].

Although considered experimental, *sclerosing agents* have been employed in the treatment of plunging ranula [46, 47]. Bleomycin and OK-432 have been successfully used to manage ranulas [47]. Even so, OK-432 has been shown to collapse and cause adhesion of the pseudocyst wall of a plunging ranula [46]. In a study of 32 cases of a plunging ranula, 31 (97%) achieved a marked reduction of lesion size with injection of OK-432. While about 50% of all cases experienced local pain or fever; this resolved within a few days. Rho et al., advocated that sclerotherapy is a safe and potentially curative procedure that may be used as a primary treatment before considering surgery for plunging ranula [46].

Carbon dioxide laser has also been used as a treatment option for plunging ranula; this has shown good success with a decrease in recurrence rate [48].

In very few patients who cannot endure the stress of surgery, a worthwhile substitute would be the use of *radiotherapy*, and low doses, from 20–25 grays (Gy), have been known to be effective. The attendant complications of radiotherapy, especially xerostomia, can be reduced by using low doses and protecting the contralateral parotid gland with a shield. The danger of developing malignancy due to treatment with radiation has been reported to be very low [10].

9.4.10.3 Postoperative Care

- *Diet:* A liquid or soft or bland diet is preferred postoperatively for a period ranging from a few days (in case of a minor procedure) to longer durations (in case of major salivary gland excision).
- *Activity:* Strenuous exercises are generally prohibited postoperatively for a few days to a few weeks depending on the procedure.

9.4.10.4 Intra- and Postoperative Complications

Complications common to oral ranula are also associated with plunging, with the most common being recurrence of the lesion. Possible surgical complications include the following:

9.4.10.4.1 Intraoperative Complications

1. Hemorrhage
2. Wharton duct injury leading to stenosis and obstructive sialadenitis
3. Injury to the lingual nerve causing temporary or permanent parasthesia of the tongue
4. Facial nerve marginal mandibular branch injury (it tends to occur because of the proximity of this nerve to the cyst; proper identification can prevent damage to this nerve) [49].

9.4.10.4.2 Postoperative Complications

1. Hematoma
2. Infection
3. Dehiscence of the wound
4. Recurrence

9.4.10.5 Recurrence

Parekh et al. reviewed 139 surgeries of plunging ranula in 89 patients and recorded a recurrence rate of over 50% for cases where the sublingual gland was *not* excised. Meanwhile, a recurrence rate as low as 2% or less was recorded when the sublingual gland was excised alone or in association with other treatments. They thus advocate that the sublingual gland should at all times be removed to improve the prognosis of this condition [32]. In addition, in the 15 patients treated with sublingual gland excision by Davison et al., only two cases (13%) recurred after a 2-year follow-up

Table 9.1 Recurrences after surgical treatment of ranula

Surgical procedure	Recurrence rate (%)
• Incision and drainage	70
• Marsupialization	53
• Excision of the lesion in the neck	85
• Excision of the lesion in the neck and sublingual gland	3.8
• Intraoral excision of the sublingual gland and drainage of the cyst	0

period. This further substantiates the suggestion that the sublingual gland be removed at all times [21].

Essentially, the best practice for the treatment of plunging ranula has been shown to be the excision of the sublingual gland, as its damage has been established to be the source of the condition. Thus, partial or total removal with or without the excision of the accumulated saliva would result in cure [44, 50] and although a trans-oral approach is ideal, cervical incision is recommended when the pseudocyst is of considerable size [51].

Parekh et al. [32] observed the following recurrence rates after various procedures; these are summarized in Table 9.1.

9.4.11 Prognosis

Overall, the prognosis of ranulas is quite good. Mostly, these lesions present as painless and asymptomatic swellings in the oral cavity with no associated morbidity or mortality. However, some large lesions may interfere with the speech, mastication, deglutition, or even with the respiration depending on the size and location.

With complete excision of the lesion along with the offending salivary gland (usually the sublingual), the recurrence rate is significantly low. In contrast, other procedures, including marsupialization and incision and drainage of the cyst, are associated with a higher recurrence rate as previously mentioned [52, 53].

9.5 Sublingual Dermoid Cyst

Dermoid cysts are commonly found throughout the body but are rare in the oral cavity.

9.5.1 Etiology: Classification

Dermoid cyst could be *congenital* or *acquired.*

- Congenital (developmental) dermoid cyst: It is a dysembryogenetic lesion derived from the entrapment and subsequent growth of epithelial cells, during midline fusion between the first and second brachial arches [54] that takes place during the first four weeks of development [55, 56]. Such cysts usually lie in the midline. They may lie above or below the mylohyoid muscle (*suprahyoid or infrahyoid*, respectively) [56, 57].

- Acquired dermoid cyst: They may be result from trauma [56].

9.5.2 Anatomical Classification

Dermoid cysts can be classified according to their anatomical location into three categories: (1) sublingual, (2) submental, and (3) submandibular cysts [58]. According to their relation to the mylohyoid muscle, dermoid cysts may be categorized as (1) suprahyoid or (2) infrahyoid.

9.5.3 Epidemiology

Approximately, 7% of all dermoid cysts found in the body are formed in the head or neck region, and only 1.6% may occur within the oral cavity [59]. Another study reported that out of 1007 head and neck tumors in children, 95 (9.4%) were dermoid cysts and only 3 (0.3%) occurred within the oral cavity [60]. Etarbi et al. reported that epidermoid and dermoid cysts of the oral cavity are rare, representing <0.01% of all oral cavity cysts [61]. The floor of the mouth is the second most common site for the presentation of dermoid cysts in the head and neck region, after the periorbital region [62].

9.5.4 Pathology

Histologically, midline cysts of the floor of the mouth are divided into three types: (1) *epidermoid cysts* consisting of an epithelial lined wall that may be partly keratinized, (2) *dermoid cysts* showing evidence of skin appendages such as hair follicles, hair, sweat, and sebaceous glands, and (3) *teratomas (teratoid cysts)* containing mesodermal elements such as bone, muscle, respiratory and gastrointestinal tissues, and fibrous capsules in addition to skin appendages. The latter is the rarest type [63, 64]. This type of teratoma is nearly always benign; in rare cases, squamous cell carcinoma may develop from the wall of the cyst in adults [61].

9.5.5 History-Taking

- *Age:* It usually presents between 10–25 years of age [65]. However, there are few reports of oral dermoid cysts in newborns or younger children [65]. Oluleke et al. reported 14 patients with sublingual dermoid cysts. Age range of the patients was 1 day to 25 years [66]. Table 9.2 summarizes the frequency of dermoid cysts reported in the literature from 2000 to 2020. The inclusion criteria for the selection of the reported cases were that they contain a histological report describing the characteristics of dermoid cysts (cystic lesion with stratified keratinized epithelium surrounded by a capsule of connective tissue containing skin appendages). As shown in Table 9.2, dermoid cysts appeared to most often present during the first three decades of life.

Table 9.2 Dermoid cyst frequency reported in the literature from 2000 to 2019

Authors (references)	Age (years)	Number	%
56 [66–75]	0–9	22	29.7
54, 66, 68 [76–89]	10–19	18	24.3
66, 84 [90–103]	20–29	19	25.8
[104–109]	30–39	7	9.4
[90, 110]	40–49	2	2.7
72 [111–115]	50–59	6	8.1
Total	0–59	74	100.0

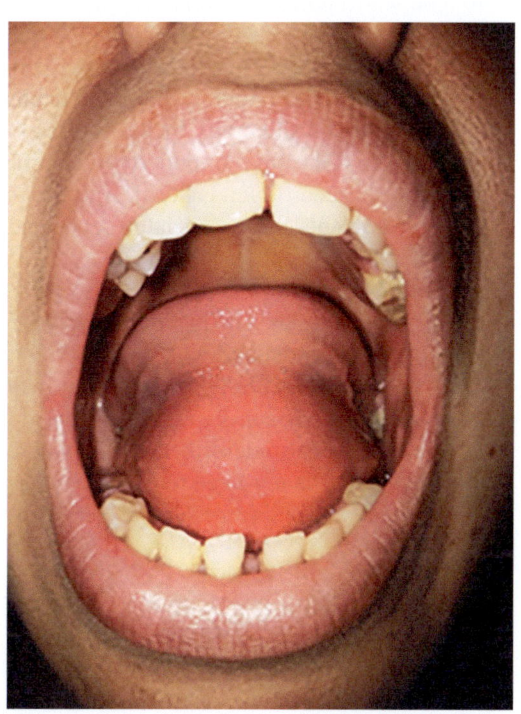

Fig. 9.11 A large sublingual dermoid cyst elevating the tongue

- *Gender:* Both sexes are affected nearly equally. Of the 14 patients with sublingual dermoid cysts reported by Olulekeand colleagues, 8 patients (57.1%) were male and 6 (42.9%) were female, with a statistically nonsignificant male-to-female ratio of 1.3: 1.0 [66].
- *Symptoms:* The patient usually complains of a painless *swelling* under the tongue, which becomes painful and tender if it gets secondarily infected. It is a slow growing mass, but when reached a large size, it may cause elevation of the tongue and interference with speech and swallowing (Fig. 9.11).

9.5.6 Physical Examination

- *Site*: The majority (52%) of dermoid cysts are found in the midline of the floor of the mouth, under the tongue, i.e. in the *sublingual space*. Approximately, 26% are found in the *submental space* below the chin (Fig. 9.12) and only 6% in the *submandibular space*. The rest involve more than one of the three possible spaces [81]. Other rare dermoid cysts in the oral cavity are those on the tongue [116]. Patients with *intralingual dermoid* cyst were described in the English literature [116, 117]. An intralingual dermoid cyst that protruded on the dorsum of the tongue was reported by Oluleke et al. [66].
- *Size:* It varies in the literature from 1.2–12 cm in size when noticed [67, 104]. When it reaches a very large size, it may involve more than one anatomical area and touch the hyoid bone when in the neck [65]. It may even fill the whole oral cavity. In certain situations, these cysts may show sudden increase in size. A possible reason is the onset of puberty with a subsequent increase in sebum secretion from the sebaceous glands [118]. Another reason may be secondary infection of the cyst contents with associated fever, pain, trismus, and cervical lymphadenopathy [54, 78].
  - *Shape*: Spherical.
  - *Surface*: Smooth. The mucous membrane appears normal.
  - *Edge*: Clearly defined.
  - *Tenderness*: It is *not* tender, unless infected.
  - *Consistency*: It can be felt bimanually. It is opaque and fluctuant. Several authors have also described it as having a doughy consistency [72, 78].
  - *Relations*: It is *not* fixed to the overlying structures.
  - *Lymph nodes and local tissues*: Cervical lymph nodes and local tissues should be normal.

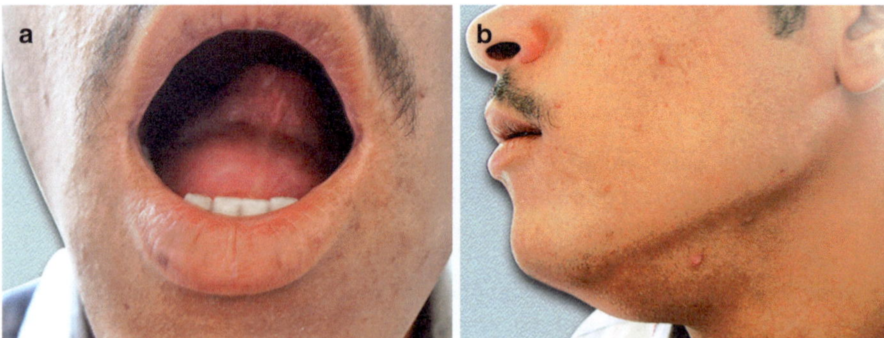

Fig. 9.12 (**a**) Central sublingual dermoid cyst in a 23-year-old patient (front view), (**b**) dermoid cyst plunging into the submental triangle in the same patient (lateral view)

9.5.7 Complications

The major complications associated with sublingual dermoid cysts include upper respiratory tract infection, anemia, respiratory obstruction, feeding difficulties, and esthetic challenges [54].

9.5.8 Evaluation/Investigations

Magnetic resonance imaging (MRI), computed tomography (CT) scan, and ultrasonography (US) are helpful in establishing the differential diagnosis. Among the available imaging modalities, CT and MRI scans are superior as they offer superior tissue characterization and more precise anatomical localization with respect to the geniohyoid and mylohyoid [90, 104]. This would be most valuable to the surgeon during the removal of the cyst [116, 117].

Recent advances in the management of sublingual dermoid cyst advocate the inclusion of *thyroid scintigraphy* in the preoperative diagnosis of the cyst of the floor of the mouth, to assess if thyroid gland is involved [119, 120].

9.5.8.1 Ultrasonography (US)

On US, a dermoid cyst would usually show up as a unilocular cystic mass, which can be heterogenous depending on the presence or absence of dermal appendages in the cyst (Fig. 9.13).

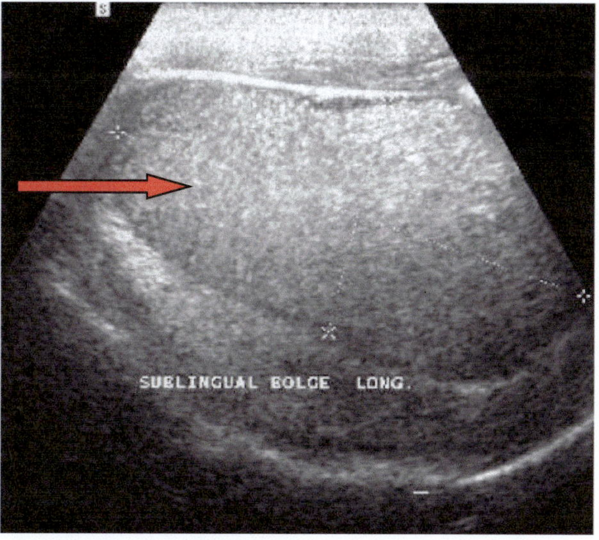

Fig. 9.13 Ultrasound picture of a sublingual dermoid cyst appearing as a unilocular cystic mass (arrow)

9.5.8.2 Computed Tomography (CT) Scan

Computed Tomography Scan (CT) of the neck would typically require contrast enhancement and show up as a central, well-encapsulated, unilocular cyst. Dermal appendages nay show up as multiple stippled calcifications [76]. Additionally, CT scan may show an encapsulated lateral mass with multiple cellular masses at the floor of the mouth (Fig. 9.14).

9.5.8.3 Magnetic Resonance Imaging (MRI)

Magnetic resonance imaging (MRI) demonstrates a sharply circumscribed cystic mass in the floor of the mouth (Fig. 9.15). A dermoid cyst would appear isointense or hypointense to muscle on T1-weighted MRI scans, and hyperintense or heterogenous on T2-weighted images [72, 121].

9.5.8.4 Cytology/Histology

Fine needle aspiration (FNA) has been described by some authors as an adjunct in diagnosing dermoid cysts of the floor of mouth. Contents of the dermoid cysts are often keratinous, caseous, sebaceous, or purulent with hair, nails, cholesterol, and even cartilage. Therefore, FNA from these cysts may yield a cheesy, keratinous-like substance, which may suggest dermoid cysts and aid the clinician to differentiate

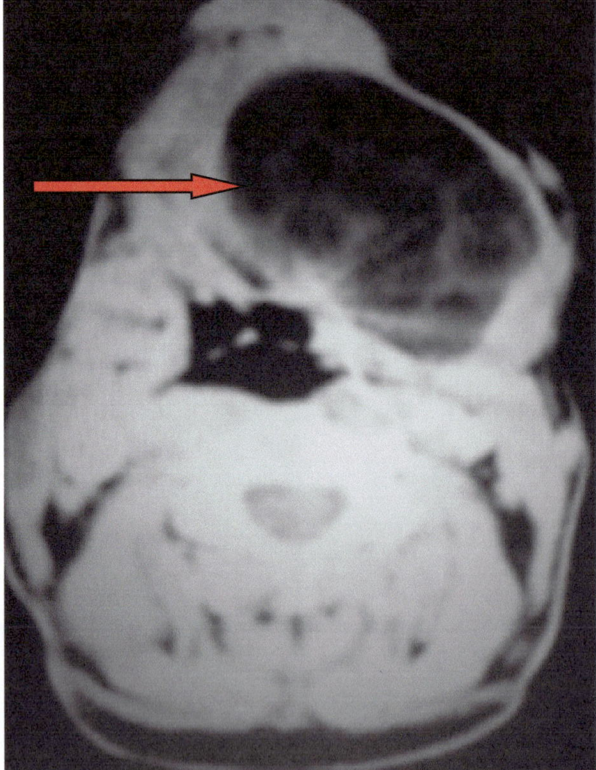

Fig. 9.14 Computed tomography (CT) scan of the neck showing an encapsulated left-sided mass with multiple cellular areas (arrow)

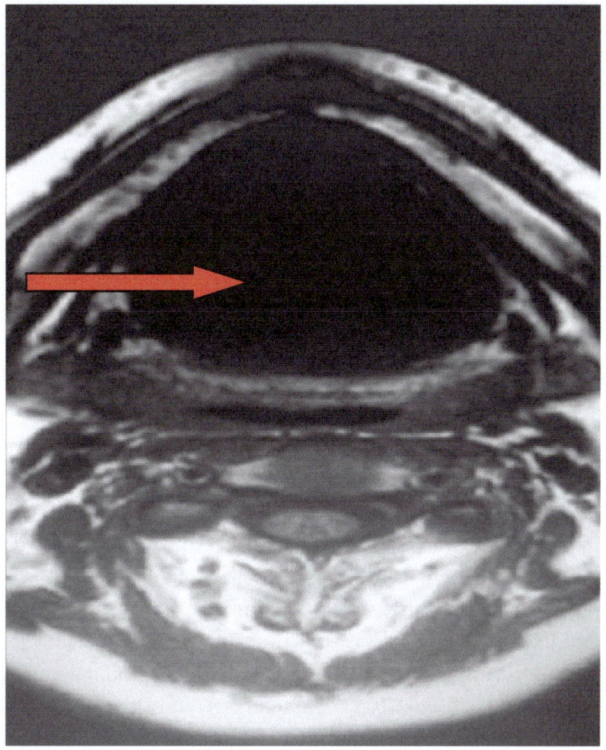

Fig. 9.15 Axial T1-weighted magnetic resonance imaging (MRI) showing sharply circumscribed, central, cystic mass (arrow)

from a salivary pathology or a vascular lesion [54, 78, 122]. However, in some cases, the high density of the cystic content prevents any meaningful aspiration and hence limits the usefulness of this technique [86].

Histopathological microscopic examination of the lesion reveals fragments of fibrous connective tissue with a central cavity lined by keratinizing stratified squamous epithelium. In some areas, there is prominent stratum granulosum with orthokeratinization. Foci of sebaceous glands and hair follicles are usually present within the cyst wall (Fig. 9.16). The microscopic features are those of a dermoid cyst and confirm diagnosis. In some cases, a foreign body giant cell reaction may result due to rupture of the cyst causing spillage of cystic contents.

9.5.9 Differential Diagnosis

Differential diagnosis of swelling of the floor of the mouth can be largely grouped into three categories: infections, neoplasms, and cystic lesions [123]. Histologically, the contents of a dermoid cyst often contain keratin, sebaceous glands, hairs, nails, fat globules, and even cartilages [117]. These features settle the diagnosis of a dermoid cyst.

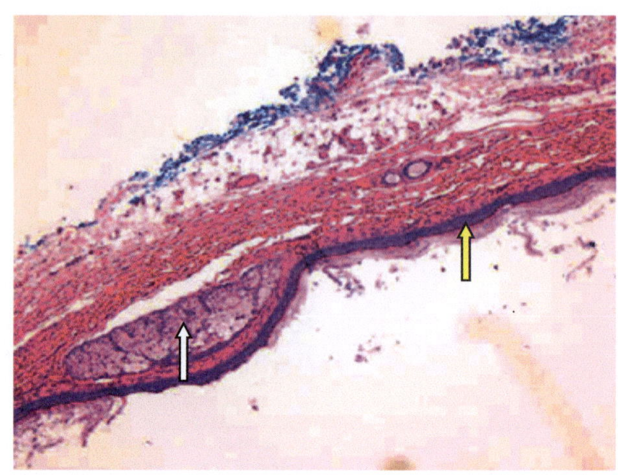

Fig. 9.16 H&E stain (×4 magnification). Dermoid cyst is lined by keratinizing stratified squamous epithelium with sebaceous glands within the cyst (white arrow) and hair follicle within the fibrous tissue wall (yellow arrow)

9.5.9.1 Infections

In an infection, there is normally pain or tenderness, erythema of the overlying mucosa, cervical lymphadenopathy, an obvious source of infection (e.g. infected pulpal necrosis or periodontal disease involving neighboring teeth), fever, and/or malaise. In a dermoid cyst without superimposed infection, these cardinal signs of infection are not present. If the lesion is nodal in nature, then the diseases to be considered, especially in teenagers or young adults, are cat scratch disease, tuberculosis, infectious mononucleosis, sarcoidosis, and actinomycosis.

9.5.9.2 Neoplasms

The neoplasms that may present as a swelling in the floor of mouth include benign and malignant salivary gland tumors, cystic hygroma, cystic lymphangioma, non-Hodgkin's lymphoma (NHL), and lipoma.

- *Mixed salivary gland tumor (minor salivary glands)*: It usually presents as a submucous, rounded, firm, mobile lobulated mass that increases in size with eating.
- *Neoplasms involving lymphatic vessels* (cystic hygroma and cystic lymphangioma): These are frequently seen in children, mostly at the posterior cervical triangle [124].
- *Lipoma*: It can present in the oral cavity, although rarely seen. It presents as a well-defined, slow growing, painless mass, with a consistency varying from soft to firm [125]. The incidence of oral lipomas is approximately 1.0–4.4% of all benign oral lesions [126, 127].
- *Lymphoma:* Hodgkin's disease is extremely rare and presents as an ulcer with cervical lymphadenopathy. On the other hand, NHL more frequently involves the head and neck region. According to Freeman et al. 28% of NHLs initially present in the head and neck region and 9.5% of such cases present in the oral cavity. Although they are usually associated with cervical lymphadenopathy, oral presentations are very rare and scarcity of cases in the literature makes interpretation of their biological behavior difficult [126].

9.5.9.3 Cystic Lesions

Cysts to be differentiated from a dermoid cyst include branchial cyst, thyroglossal cyst, ranulas, and bronchogenic cysts.

- *Branchial cysts*: These are laterally located lesions related to the anterior border of the sternocleidomastoid muscle, containing a thin, watery fluid or thick, gelatinous, mucoid material.
- *Thyroglossal cysts:* These are painless cystic lesions and expand slowly. They are normally found in the midline, are non-tender, soft, and fluctuant. Characteristically a thyroglossal cyst will move during protrusion of the tongue or swallowing since the cyst arises from a tract between the foramen caecum of the tongue and the thyroid gland.
- *Ranulas*: These are usually unilateral, to one side of the frenulum, containing thick mucus. They are blue to translucent, do not blanch on compression, and may cross the mylohyoid muscle (plunging ranula) presenting as a neck mass.
- *Detached branchogenic cysts*: These are very rare and are usually found in the mediastinum [128].

An overview of the three categories of differential diagnosis of a sublingual dermoid cyst is presented in Table 9.3 [129, 130].

Table 9.3 Overview of the three categories of differential diagnosis

Category	Salient features
Infections	• Usually rapidly growing • Associated with pain, trismus, fever, dysphagia • Swelling usually fluctuant and tender • Overlying skin at cervical area may be erythematous and warm • Source of infection usually obvious intra-orally • Leukocytosis is usually present • CT scan usually reveals a multilocular collection with surrounding inflammatory changes
Neoplasms	• Usually slow-growing • Usually firm and solid • Benign neoplasms usually have a smooth and well-defined surface while malignant neoplasms often have an ulcerated, irregular, and ragged surface • Benign neoplasms tend to displace adjacent structures, while malignant tumors tend to infiltrate underlying structures • Symptoms like restricted tongue mobility, speech impediment, and dysphagia may be present due to invasion of malignant neoplasms into the tongue musculature • Metastatic cervical lymphadenopathy may be present • CT scan reveals a dense solid mass that may or may not show invasion
Cystic lesions	• Usually slow-growing • Usually painless and fluctuant • Overlying mucosa or skin is smooth and well-defined • Tend to displace rather than invade adjacent structures • CT scan usually reveals a well-circumscribed hypodense unilocular or multilocular collection with normal surrounding structures

9.5.10 Treatment

Surgical excision is the only effective treatment of dermoid cysts [119, 120, 131, 132]. *Intraoral* sublingual dermoid cyst is treated with complete surgical excision. The approach can be either intraoral or extraoral (cervical), depending on the anatomical location and size of the mass [91]. The intraoral surgical route rather than the cervical route is preferred and seems to be ideal because it gives a good view of the cyst, an easy access as well as satisfactory esthetic results (hidden scar), even when the cyst is above the geniohyoid muscle [133]. A midline incision is created along the longitudinal ventral surface of the tongue to the floor of the mouth, and by careful dissection, the cyst is completely enucleated of the mylohyoid muscle (Fig. 9.17).

Large dermoid cysts plunging in the sublingual space have been reported to be enucleated successfully via the intraoral approach. Jain et al. [54] reported the excision of a large (9 × 9 cm) sublingual plunging dermoid cyst via the intraoral route. More recently, Aydin et al. also reported a case of a giant plunging dermoid cyst (measuring 12 × 5 × 4 cm) that was removed via intra-oral approach [107].

The *extraoral approach* is usually used for very large sublingual dermoid cysts *plunging* in the submental and/or submandibular spaces, and in cases of infection that could compromise the patient's airways [86]. Dermoid cyst is often located between the geniohyoid and mylohyoid muscles, when it bulges out in the submental or submandibular region. Careful dissection is thus needed during surgery to avoid injury of the hypoglossal nerve. In exceptionally large cysts, a combined intra-oral and extraoral approach may be necessary to provide direct visualization of important adjacent structures [72, 74].

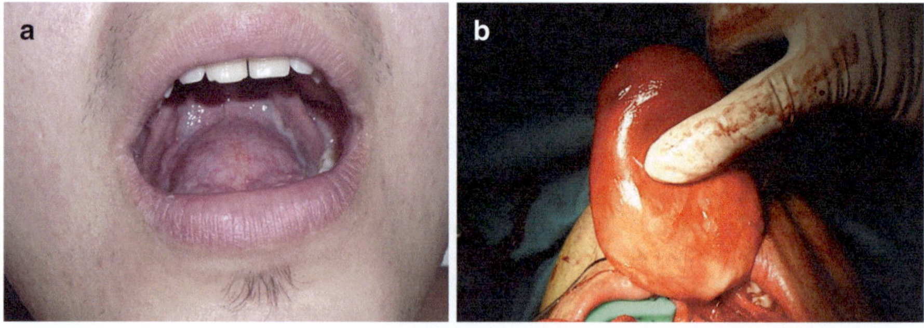

Fig. 9.17 Sublingual dermoid cyst (intraoral cystic swelling underneath the tongue) (**a**). The cyst completely excised via the intraoral route (**b**)

9.5.11 Prognosis

Prognosis of sublingual dermoid cysts is generally good. *Recurrence* is very rare with complete excision of the lesion due to the fibrous capsule around the cyst which facilitates enucleation [72, 134]. Sometimes, a recurrence may not be noticed until the child is older or becomes an adult [65]. In one study of 14 patients with sublingual dermoid cysts, 2 cases of recurrence were reported (14.3%); their first surgeries were done under local anesthesia; it was likely due to incomplete excision. A 5% rate of *malignant transformation* of the oral dermoid cysts into the teratoid type has been reported in literature [131, 132].

References

1. Wong T, Yap T, Wiesenfeld D. Common causes of 'swelling' in the oral cavity. Aust J Gen Pract. 2020;49(9):575–80.
2. Berkovitz BKB, Holland GR, Moxham BJ. Oral anatomy, embryology and histology. 3rd ed. Edinburgh: Mosby; 2002.
3. Ship II. Epidemiologic aspects of recurrent aphthous ulcerations. Oral Surg Oral Med Oral Pathol. 1972;33(3):400–6.
4. Scully C, Porter S. Oral mucosal disease: recurrent aphthous stomatitis. Br J Oral Maxillofac Surg. 2008;46(3):198–206.
5. Rhodus NL. Oral cancer: Leukoplakia and squamous cell carcinoma. Dent Clin N Am. 2005;49(1):143–65.
6. Gupta PC, Murti PR, Bhonsle RB, Mehta FS, Pindborg JJ. Effect of cessation of tobacco use on the incidence of oral mucosal lesions in a 10-yr follow-up study of 12,212 users. Oral Dis. 1995;1(1):54–8.
7. DeAngelis A, Breik O, Koo K, et al. Non-smoking, non-drinking elderly females, a 5 year follow-up of a clinically distinct cohort of oral squamous cell carcinoma patients. Oral Oncol. 2018;86:113–20.
8. Williams DW, Lewis MA. Isolation and identification of candida from the oral cavity. Oral Dis. 2000;6(1):3–11.
9. Manfredi M, Polonelli L, Aguirre-Urizar JM, Carrozzo M, McCullough MJ. Urban legends series: oral candidosis. Oral Dis. 2013;19(3):245–61.
10. Bouquot JE, Gorlin RJ. Leukoplakia, lichen planus, and other oral keratoses in 23,616 white Americans over the age of 35 years. Oral Surg Oral Med Oral Pathol. 1986;61(4):373–81.
11. Canniff JP, Harvey W. The aetiology of oral submucous fibrosis: the stimulation of collagen synthesis by extracts of areca nut. Int J Oral Surg. 1981;10(Suppl 1):163–7.
12. Hsue SS, Wang WC, Chen CH, Lin CC, Chen YK, Lin LM. Malignant transformation in 1458 patients with potentially malignant oral mucosal disorders: a follow-up study based in a Taiwanese hospital. J Oral Pathol Med. 2007;36(1):25–9.
13. van der Waal I. Oral potentially malignant disorders: is malignant transformation predictable and preventable? Med Oral Patol Oral Cir Bucal. 2014;19(4):e386–90.

14. Warnakulasuriya S, Johnson NW, van der Waal I. Nomenclature and classification of potentially malignant disorders of the oral mucosa. J Oral Pathol Med. 2007;36(10):575–80.
15. Warnakulasuriya S, Ariyawardana A. Malignant transformation of oral leukoplakia: a systematic review of observational studies. J Oral Pathol Med. 2016;45(3):155–66.
16. Holmstrup P. Oral erythroplakia – what is it? Oral Dis. 2018;24(1–2):138–43.
17. Shafer WG, Waldron CA. Erythroplakia of the oral cavity. Cancer. 1975;36(3):1021–8.
18. Suresh BV, Sk V. Huge plunging ranula. J Maxillofac Oral Surg. 2012;11:487–90.
19. Brad WB, Douglas DN, Damm ACM, Jerry E. Oral and maxillofacial pathology. 2nd ed. Philadelphia: WB Saunders; 2002. p. 391–2.
20. de Visscher JG, van der Wal KG, de Vogel PL. The plunging ranula: pathogenesis, diagnosis and management. J Craniomaxillofac Surg. 1989;17:182–5.
21. Davison MJ, Morton RP, Mclvor NP. Plunging ranula: clinical observations. Head Neck. 1998;20:63–8.
22. Gupta A, Karjodkar FR. Plunging ranula: a case report. ISRN Dent. 2011;2011:806–928.
23. Hupp JR, Ellis E, Tucker MR. Contemporary oral and maxillofacial surgery. 5th ed. St Louis: Mosby; 2008. p. 410–1.
24. Baurmash HD. Mucoceles and ranulas. J Oral Maxillofac Surg. 2003;61(3):369–78.
25. Syebele K, Bütow KW. Oral mucoceles and ranulas may be part of initial manifestations of HIV infection. AIDS Res Hum Retrovir. 2010;26(10):1075–8.
26. Mun SJ, Choi HG, Kim H, Park JH, Jung YH, Sung MW, Kim KH. Ductal variation of the sublingual gland: a predisposing factor for ranula formation. Head Neck. 2014;36(4):540–4.
27. Dietrich EM, Vasilios B, Maria L, Styliani P, Konstantinos A. Sublingual-plunging ranula as a complication of supraomohyoid neck dissection. Int J Surg Case Rep. 2011;2:90–2.
28. Ichimura K, Ohta Y, Tayama N. Surgical management of the plunging ranula: a review of seven cases. J Laryngol Otol. 2011;110:554–6.
29. La Porte SJ, Juttla JK, Lingam RK. Imaging the floor of the mouth and the sublingual space. Radiographics. 2011;31(5):1215–30.
30. Chin SJ, Zeng IS, Morton RP. The epidemiology of plunging ranula in South Auckland. Laryngoscope. 2016;2016(126):2739–43.
31. Morton RP, Ahmad Z, Jain P. Plunging ranula: congenital or acquired? Otolaryngol Head Neck Surg. 2010;142:104–7.
32. Parekh DM, Joseph SC, Lawson HH. Plunging ranula: a report of three cases and a review of the literature. Br J Surg. 1987;74:307–9.
33. Skouteris CA, Sotereanos GC. Plunging ranula: report of a case. J OralMaxillofac Surg. 1987;45:1068–72.
34. Crysdale WS, Mendelsohn JD, Conley S. Ranulas–mucoceles of the oral cavity: experience in 26 children. Laryngoscope. 1988;98(3):296–8.
35. Jain PR, Morton RP, Ahmad Z. Plunging ranulas: high-resolution ultrasound for diagnosis and surgical management. Eur Radiol. 2010;20:1442–9.
36. Langlois NE, Kolhe P. Plunging ranula: a case report and a literature review. Hum Pathol. 1992;23:1306–8.
37. Barbería E, Lucavechi T, Cárdenas D, Maroto M. An atypical lingual lesion resulting from the unhealthy habit of sucking the lower lip: clinical case study. J Clin Pediatr Dent. 2006;30(4):280–2.
38. Charnoff SK, Carter BL. Plunging ranula: CT diagnosis. Radiology. 1986;158:467–8.
39. Yamasoba T, Tayama N, Syoji M, Fukuta M. Clinicostatistical study of lower lip mucoceles. Head Neck. 1990;12(4):316–20.
40. Balakrishnan A, Ford GR, Bailey CM. Plunging ranula following bilateral submandibular duct transposition. J Laryngol Otol. 1991;105:667–9.
41. Horiguchi H, Kakuta S, Nagumo M. Bilateral plunging ranula: a case report. Int J Oral Maxillofac Surg. 1995;24:174–5.
42. Fukase S, Ohta N, Inamura K, Aoyagi M. Treatment of ranula with intracystic injection of the streptococcal preparation OK-432. Ann Otol Rhinol Laryngol. 2003;112(3):214–20.

43. Kim KH, Sung MW, Roh JL, Han MH. Sclerotherapy for congenital lesions in the head and neck. Otolaryngol Head Neck Surg. 2004;131(3):307–16.
44. Harrison JD. Modern management and pathophysiology of ranula: literature review. Head Neck. 2010;32:1310–20.
45. Yoshimura Y, Obara S, Kondoh T, Naitoh SI. A comparison of three methods used for treatment of ranula. J Oral Maxillofac Surg. 1995;52:280–3.
46. Rho MH, Kim DW, Kwon JS, Lee SW, Sung YS, Song YK, et al. OK-432 sclerotherapy of plunging ranula in 21 patients: it can be a substitute for surgery. AJNR Am J Neuroradiol. 2006;27:1090–5.
47. Woo JS, Hwang S, Lee HM. Recurrent plunging ranula treated with OK-432. Eur Arch Otorhinolaryngol. 2003;260:226–8.
48. Mintz S, Barak S, Horowitz I. Carbon dioxide laser excision and vaporization of nonplunging ranulas: a comparison of two treatment protocols. J Oral Maxillofac Surg. 1994;52:370–2.
49. Kim PD, Simental A. Management of mucocele and ranula. In: Myers EN, Ferris RL, editors. Salivary gland disorders. 1st ed. Berlin: Springer; 2007. p. 177–84.
50. Harrison JD. Sublingual gland is the origin of giant submandibular mucocele. Am J Otolaryngol. 2015;36:616–7.
51. Lesperance MM. When do ranulas require a cervical approach? Laryngoscope. 2013;123:1826–7.
52. Mínguez-Martinez I, Bonet-Coloma C, Ata-Ali-Mahmud J, Carrillo-García C, Peñarrocha-Diago M, Peñarrocha-Diago M. Clinical characteristics, treatment, and evolution of 89 mucoceles in children. J Oral Maxillofac Surg. 2010;68(10):2468–71.
53. Wu CW, Kao YH, Chen CM, Hsu HJ, Chen CM, Huang IY. Mucoceles of the oral cavity in pediatric patients. Kaohsiung J Med Sci. 2011;27(7):276–9.
54. Jain H, Singh S, Singh A. Giant sublingual dermoid cyst in floor of the mouth. J Maxillofac Oral Surg. 2012;11:235–7.
55. Woo SB. Oral pathology: a comprehensive atlas and text. 2nd ed. Philadelphia: Elsevier; 2016.
56. Hemaraju N, Nanda SK, Medikeri SB. Sub-lingual dermoid cyst. Indian J Otolaryngol Head Neck Surg. 2004;56(3):218–20.
57. Balla S, Acharya V, Ally M, Taghie A. Acute presentation of an intraoral dermoid cyst causing airway compromise in a young child. BMJ Case Rep. 2019;12(4):e228421.
58. Fomete B, Saheeb BD, Onyebuchi EP, Ogbeifun JO. Dermoid cyst of the oral cavity as seen in a Nigeria tertiary institution. Niger J Surg Res. 2013;157:3–6.
59. King RC, Smith BR, Burk JL. Dermoid cyst in the floor of the mouth. Review of the literature and case reports. Oral Surg Oral Med Oral Pathol. 1994;78(5):567–76.
60. Taylor BW, Erich JB, Dockerty MB. Dermoids of the head and neck. Minn Med. 1966;49:1535–40.
61. Etarbi MS, Aishaish H, Khalifa O. Large sublingual cyst in the floor of the mouth and submental space. Otolaryngology. 2017;7:287–91.
62. New GB, Erich JB. Dermoid cysts of the head and neck. Surg Gynecol Obstet. 1937;65:48–56.
63. Menditti D, Laino L, Ferrara N, Baldi A. Dermoid cyst of the mandibula: a case report. Cases J. 2008;1:260.
64. Park SW, Lee JJ, Chae SA, Yoo BH, Kim GJ, Lee SY. Congenital epidermoid cyst of the oral cavity: prenatal diagnosis by sonography. Clin Exp. 2013;6:191–3.
65. Di Francesco A, Chiapasco M, Biglioli F, Ancona D. Intraoral approach to large dermoid cysts of the floor of the mouth: a technical note. Int J Oral Maxillofac Surg. 1995;24:233–5.
66. Oluleke OO, Akau KS, Godwin AI, Kene AI, Sunday AO. Sublingual dermoid cyst: review of 14 cases. Ann Maxillofac Surg. 2020;10(1):279–83.
67. Ho MW, Crean SJ. Simultaneous occurrence of sublingual dermoid cyst and oral alimentary tract cyst in an infant: a case report and review of the literature. Int J Paediatr Dent. 2003;13(6):441–6.
68. Schwanke TW, Oomen KP, April MM, Ward RF, Modi VK. Floor of mouth masses in children: proposal of a new algorithm. Int J Pediatr Otorhinolaryngol. 2013;77(9):1489–94.

69. Puricelli E, Barreiro BOB, Quevedo AS, Ponzoni D. Occurrence of dermoid cyst in the floor of the mouth: the importance of differential diagnosis in pediatric patients. J Appl Oral Sci. 2017;25(3):341–5.
70. Anguita Sánchez I, Sepúlveda Rojas C, Inmaculada Isorna R, Creo Martínez T, Sánchez González FJ. Lateral dermoid cyst of the floor of the mouth. A case report. ORL Aragón. 2010;13(1):24–6.
71. Pan M, Nakamura YC, Clark M, Eisig S. Intraoral dermoid cyst in an infant: a case report. J Oral Maxillofac Surg. 2011;69(5):1398–402.
72. Gordon PE, Faquin WC, Lahey E, Kaban LB. Floor-of-mouth dermoid cysts: report of 3 variants and a suggested change in terminology. J Oral Maxillofac Surg. 2013;71(6):1034–41.
73. Tekkeşin MS, Özer N, Olgaç V. Sublingual dermoid cyst: a case report. Turk Patoloji Derg. 2016;32(2):135–8.
74. Berbel P, Ostrosky A, Tosti F. Large sublingual dermoid cyst: a case of mandibular prognathism. Craniomaxillofac Trauma Reconstr. 2016;9(4):345–8.
75. Naina P, Syed KA, Koshy L, Mathews SS. Sublingual dermoid causing stertor in an infant. BMJ Case Rep. 2016;2016:217135.
76. Dillon JR, Avillo AJ, Nelson BL. Dermoid cyst of the floor of the mouth. Head Neck Pathol. 2015;9(3):376–8.
77. Metz A, Schnorrenberg J, Daamen J, Schmeling C, Mohr C. Extensive dermoid cyst occupying almost the entire floor of the mouth in a juvenile patient. HNO. 2012;60(5):439–42.
78. Seah TE, Sufyan W, Singh B. Case report of a dermoid cyst at the floor of the mouth. Ann Acad Med Singap. 2004;33(4):77–9.
79. Lima SM Jr, Chrcanovic BR, de Paula AM, Freire-Maia B, Souza LN. Dermoid cyst of the floor of the mouth. Sci World J. 2003;3:156–62.
80. Ege G, Akman H, Fienvar A, Kuzucu K. Sublingual dermoid kist. Tanisal Giriflim Radyol. 2003;9:57–9.
81. Teszler CB, El-Naaj IA, Emodi O, Luntz M, Peled M. Dermoid cysts of the lateral floor of the mouth: a comprehensive anatomo-surgical classification of cysts of the oral floor. J Oral Maxillofac Surg. 2007;65(2):327–32.
82. Ikeda K, Koseki T, Maehara M, Ohmura N, Kurokawa H, Shimizotani K. Hourglass-shaped sublingual dermoid cyst: MRI features. Radiat Med. 2007;25(6):306–8.
83. Montoro Chavarria S, Sanz Calvo ML, Rado Peralta S, Montoya Bordón J, Alonso Torres A, Escorihuela ER. Floor of the mouth dermoid cyst. Ann Pediatr. 2010;73(3):156–8.
84. Portelles Massó AM, Torres Íñiguez AT. Dermoid cyst in the mouth floor. Rev Cuba Estomatol. 2010;47(4):455–9.
85. Makos C, Noussios G, Kim JP, et al. Endoscope-assisted intraoral resection of external dermoid cyst. Head Neck. 2012;34(6):907–10.
86. Kyriakidou E, Howe T, Veale B, Atkins S. Sublingual dermoid cysts: case report and review of the literature. J Laryngol Otol. 2015;129(10):1036–9.
87. Patel H, Mayl J, Chandra B, Pritchett C, Chandra T. Dermoid of the oral cavity: case report with histopathology correlation and review of literature. J Radiol Case Rep. 2016;10(12):19–27.
88. Derin S, Koseoglu S, Sahan L, Dere Y, Sahan M. Giant dermoid cyst causing dysphagia and dyspnea. J Craniofac Surg. 2016;27(3):e260–1.
89. Giarraputo L, Savastano S, D'Amore E, Baciliero U. Dermoid cyst of the floor of the mouth: diagnostic imaging findings. Cureus. 2018;10(4):e2403.
90. Longo F, Maremonti P, Mangone GM, De Maria G, Califano L. Midline (dermoid) cysts of the floor of the mouth: report of 16 cases and review of surgical techniques. Plast Reconstr Surg. 2003;112(6):1560–5.
91. Ohta N, Watanabe T, Ito T, et al. A case of sublingual dermoid cyst: extending the limits of the oral approach. Case Rep Otolaryngol. 2012;2012:634949.
92. Mumtaz S, Singh M. Transoral marsupialization of a large dermoid cyst. J Oral Maxillofac Surg. 2019;77(4):753–6.
93. Santos-Briz A Jr, Serrano R, del Cañizo A, Santos-Briz A, de Agustín PP. Liesegang rings in a dermoid cyst of the floor of the mouth. Report of a case with cytologic findings. Acta Cytol. 2000;44(6):1062–5.

94. Kutuya N. A case of dermoid cyst of the floor of the mouth: ultrasonography was more useful than computed tomography and magnetic resonance imaging in the preoperative diagnosis. J Med Ultrason. 2009;36(1):27–31.
95. Tuz M, Dogru H, Uygur K, Baykal B. Rapidly growing sublingual dermoid cyst throughout pregnancy. Am J Otolaryngol. 2003;24(5):334–7.
96. Licéaga Reyes R, Licéaga Escalera C, Mosqueda TA. Quiste dermoide: presentación de un caso y revisión bibliográfica. Dermatol Rev Mex. 2005;49:130–3.
97. Burger MF, Holland P, Napier B. Submental midline dermoid cyst in a 25-year-old man. Ear Nose Throat J. 2006;85(11):752–3.
98. El-Hakim IE, Alyamani A. Alternative surgical approaches for excision of dermoid cyst of the floor of mouth. Int J Oral Maxillofac Surg. 2008;37(5):497–9.
99. Jadwani S, Misra B, Kallianpur S, Bansod S. Dermoid cyst of the floor of the mouth with abundant hair: a case report. J Maxillofac Oral Surg. 2009;8(4):388–9.
100. Antunes Freitas D, Lozano Pérez J, Fang Mercado L, Díaz CA. True dermoid cyst in the floor of the mouth. Rev Cuba Estomatol. 2013;50(3):302–7.
101. Vieira EM, Borges AH, Volpato LE, et al. Unusual dermoid cyst in oral cavity. Case Rep Pathol. 2014;2014:389752.
102. Sahoo NK, Choudhary AK, Srinivas V, Tomar K. Dermoid cysts of maxillofacial region. Med J Armed Forces India. 2015;71(2):389–94.
103. Kumar NG, Arora SS, Kumar I, Pandher PK, Balwan R. Dermoid cysts of the maxillofacial region: case series. J Maxillofac Oral Surg. 2019;18(2):238–44.
104. Aydın S, Demir MG, Demir N, Şahin S, Kayıpmaz ŞS. A giant plunging sublingual dermoid cyst excised by intraoral approach. J Maxillofac Oral Surg. 2016;15(2):277–80.
105. Armstrong JE, Darling MR, Bohay RN, Cobb G, Lawen D, Daley TD. Trans-geniohyoid dermoid cyst: considerations on a combined oral and dermal surgical approach and on histogenesis. J Oral Maxillofac Surg. 2006;64(12):1825–30.
106. Fuchshuber S, Grevers G, Issing WJ. Dermoid cyst of the floor of the mouth–a case report. Eur Arch Otorhinolaryngol. 2002;259(2):60–2.
107. Santos TS, Gomes ACA, Frota R, Silva EDO, Martins Filho PRS, Andrade ESS. Iatrogenic infection in dermoid cysts of the floor of the mouth. Braz J Otorhinolaryngol. 2011;77(5):675.
108. Pirgousis P, Fernandes R. Giant submental dermoid cysts with near total obstruction of the oral cavity: report of 2 cases. J Oral Maxillofac Surg. 2011;69(2):532–5.
109. Sun Z, Sun L, Gao Y, Ma X. Lingual dermoid cyst with congenital discharging sinus: a rare entity. J Laryngol Otol. 2013;127(2):211–4.
110. Durr ML, van Zante A, Pletcher SD. An unusual presentation of a lingual dermoid cyst. Ear Nose Throat J. 2015;94(10–11):29–31.
111. Lin HW, Silver AL, Cunnane ME, Sadow PM, Kieff DA. Lateral dermoid cyst of the floor of mouth: unusual radiologic and pathologic findings. Auris Nasus Larynx. 2011;38(5):650–3.
112. Ariyoshi Y, Shimahara M. Magnetic resonance imaging of a submental dermoid cyst: report of a case. J Oral Maxillofac Surg. 2003;61(4):507–10.
113. Devine JC, Jones DC. Carcinomatous transformation of a sublingual dermoid cyst. A case report. Int J Oral Maxillofac Surg. 2000;29(2):126–7.
114. Vargas Fernández JL, Lorenzo Rojas J, Aneiros Fernández J, Sainz Quevedo M. Dermoid cyst of the floor of the mouth. Acta Otorrinolaringol Esp. 2007;58(1):31–3.
115. Otonari-Yamamoto M, Nakajima K, Sakamoto J, Imoto K, Watanabe M, Kotaki S. Atypical MRI and histopathological findings in dermoid cyst. Bull Tokyo Dent Coll. 2018;59(3):207–12.
116. Saheeb BD, Osagonona A. Submental dermoid cyst. A case report. OJM. 2005;17:24–7.
117. Chukuneke FN, Okwuowulu T. Enbloc enucleation of a large intra-oral dermoid cyst under local anaesthesia: a case report and review of the literature. J Coll Med. 2007;12:8–12.
118. Black EE, Leathers RD, Youngblood D. Dermoid cyst of the floor of the mouth. Oral Surg Oral Med Oral Pathol. 1993;75:556–8.
119. Batsaki JG. Tumours of the head and neck clinical and pathological consideration. 2nd ed. Philadelphia: Williams and Wilkins Company Publishers; 1980. p. 226–8.
120. Gleizal A, Abouchebel N, Lebreton F, Beziat JL. Dermoid cyst of the tongue: an association of dermoid cyst with bronchogenic epithelium. J Craniomaxillofac Surg. 2006;34:113–6.

121. Gol IH, Kiyici H, Yildirim E, Arda IS, Hicsonmez A. Congenital sublingual teratoid cyst: a case report and literature review. J Pediatr Surg. 2005;40:9–12.
122. Miles LP, Naidoo LC, Reddy J. Congenital dermoid cyst of the tongue. J Laryngol Otol. 1997;111:1179–82.
123. Triantafillidou E, Karakasis D, Laskin J. Swelling of the floor of the mouth. J Oral Maxillofac Surg. 1989;47:733–6.
124. Ali E, Karim N, Hicham A, Mohamed Z. Cystic lymphangioma on the floor of the oral cavity extending to the submandibular region in adult patients. Pan Afr Med J. 2016;24:202.
125. Hatziotis JC. Lipoma of the oral cavity. Oral Surg Oral Med Oral Pathol. 1971;31:511–24.
126. Fregnani ER, Pires FR, Falzoni R, Lopes MA, Vargas PA. Lipomas of the oral cavity: clinical findings, histological classification and proliferative activity of 46 cases. Int J Oral Maxillofac Surg. 2003;32:49–53.
127. Lombardi T, Odell EW. Spindle cell lipoma of the oral cavity: report of a case. J Oral Pathol Med. 1994;23:237–9.
128. Bailey BM. A detached bronchogenic cyst occurring in the tongue of a neonate. Br J Oral Surg. 1982;20:288–93.
129. Louis PJ, Hudson C, Reddi S. Lesion of floor of the mouth. J Oral Maxillofac Surg. 2002;60:804–7.
130. Lee MH, Lee CS, Sim CQ, Nagadia R. Sublingual dermoid cyst: case report and a review of the clinical, radiological and histological aspects of this rare condition. Oral Surg. 2018;11:147–52.
131. Oginni FO, Oladejo T, Braimah OP, Adenekan AT. Sulinqual epidermoid cyst. Surgery. 2014;4:96–8.
132. Mohta A, Sharma M. Congenital oral cysts in neonates: report of two cases. Oral Surg Oral Med Oral Pathol Oral Radiol Endod. 2006;102:e36–8.
133. Zeltser R, Milhem I, Azaz B, Hasson O. Dermoid cysts of floor of the mouth: report of four cases. Am J Otolaryngol. 2000;21(1):55–60.
134. Eken M, Evren C, Sanli A, Bozkurt Z. An alternative surgical approach for sublingual dermoid cysts: a case report. Kulak Burun Bogaz Ihtis Derg. 2007;17:176–8.

Neoplastic Lesions of the Tongue 10

10.1 Classification

As shown in Table 10.1, tongue neoplasms (tumors), whether benign or malignant, are classified according to tissue of origin into epithelial tumors, mesenchymal tumors, and tumors of salivary gland or thyroid gland origin.

10.2 Benign Tumors

10.2.1 Granular Cell Tumors

Granular cell tumors are small, solitary, firm, painless tumors that can occur throughout the body. More than one half of cases may occur in the oral cavity, and up to one-third involve the dorsum of the tongue [1]. In contrast to squamous cell cancers, which have a rough or ulcerated surface, granular cell tumors have a smooth

Table 10.1 Classification of tongue tumors

Origin	Benign tumors	Malignant tumors
Epithelial	1. Granular cell tumor 2. Traumatic fibroma 3. Papilloma	1. Epithelioma (SSC) 2. Lymphoepithelioma 3. Adenocarcinoma 4. Basal cell carcinoma (BCC)
Mesenchymal	1. Cavernous hemangioma 2. Lymphangioma 3. Neurofibroma 4. Fibroma 5. Lipoma (rare)	1. Fibrosarcoma 2. Hemangioendothelioma 3. Rhabdomyosarcoma 4. Lymphoma
Salivary glands	Mixed salivary gland tumor	Malignant salivary gland tumors
Thyroid Gland	Lingual thyroid nodule	Malignancy in thyroid tissue remnants

© The Author(s), under exclusive license to Springer Nature Switzerland AG 2022

M. F. Sakr, *Tongue Lesions*, https://doi.org/10.1007/978-3-031-08198-9_10

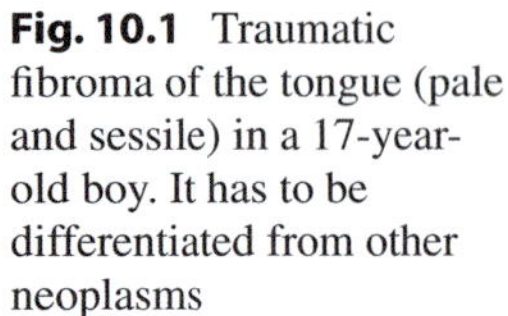
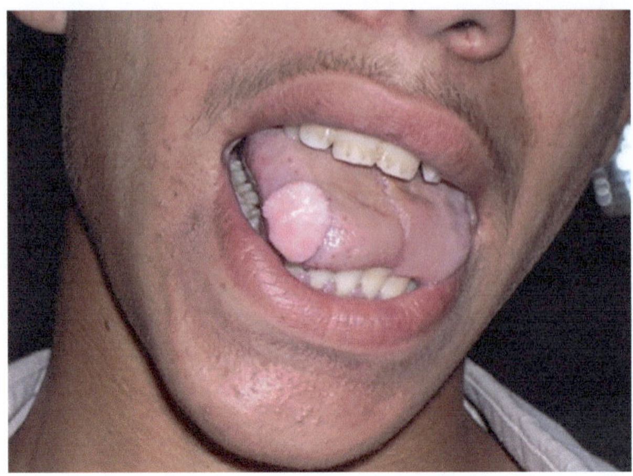

Fig. 10.1 Traumatic fibroma of the tongue (pale and sessile) in a 17-year-old boy. It has to be differentiated from other neoplasms

surface. These tumors are more common after 30 years of age and in women [1]. Biopsy is needed to confirm the diagnosis. Rarely, malignant transformation occurs requiring a wide local excision [2].

10.2.2 Fibroepithelial Polyp (Traumatic Fibroma)

Traumatic fibroma or fibroepithelial polyp (Fig. 10.1) is a common lesion of the oral cavity. It results from repeated biting or trauma and usually appears along the bite line as a focal, thickened area that is typically dome shaped, pink, and smooth. It is caused by the accumulation of dense, collagenous connective tissue at the site of chronic irritation, which can also precipitate the development of pyogenic granulomas at the site of traumatic fibromas [3]. *Excisional biopsy* is indicated.

10.2.3 Papilloma

Squamous papilloma is one of the more common oral lesions, occurring in up to 1% of adults. It may affect any age but usually between 30–50 years [4]. It is generally associated with human papilloma virus (HPV) type 6 or 11 infection [4, 5].

A papilloma usually affects the soft palate, the tongue (Fig. 10.2), lingual frenulum, lower lip [4], and uvula [6], most often presenting as a single, small lesion smaller than 1 cm, with exophytic growth and finger-like projections, and a wide basis or pedicle (Fig. 10.3). Histopathology shows epithelial proliferation and a centrally disposed fibrovascular core (Fig. 10.4-E). Koilocytosis may or may not be present.

Oral squamous papilloma may be isolated or multiple-recurring, which is more likely to affect immunosuppressed patients, such as HIV-positive patients. Multiple-recurring papilloma is also more likely to be malignant [6] and tends to relapse more often [7]. *Differential diagnoses* include exophytic carcinoma, verrucous carcinoma, and condyloma acuminatum [6]. It should be removed with an adequate margin of tissue and biopsied.

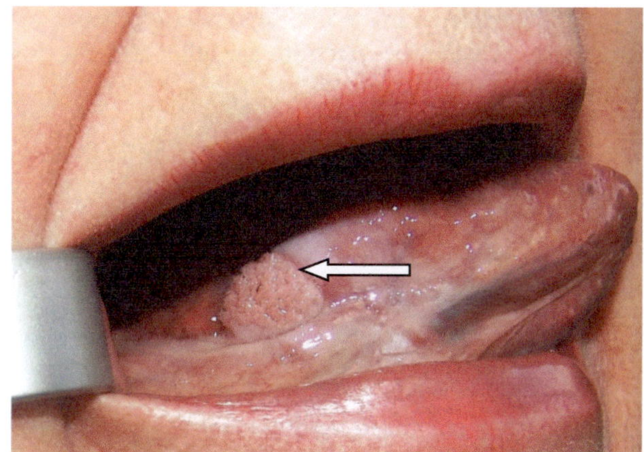

Fig. 10.2 Tongue pailloma at the lateral side of the tongue (arrow). Note the wide base and the finger-like projections

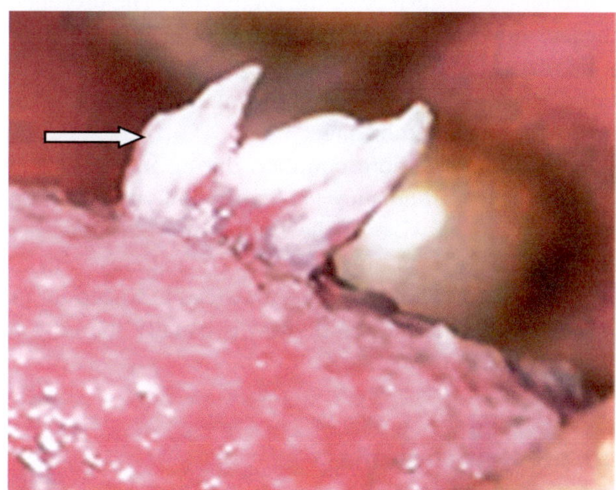

Fig. 10.3 Oral squamous papilloma. Exophytic lesion with hyperkeratotic whitish surface, forming finger-like projections on the dorsum of the tongue (arrow)

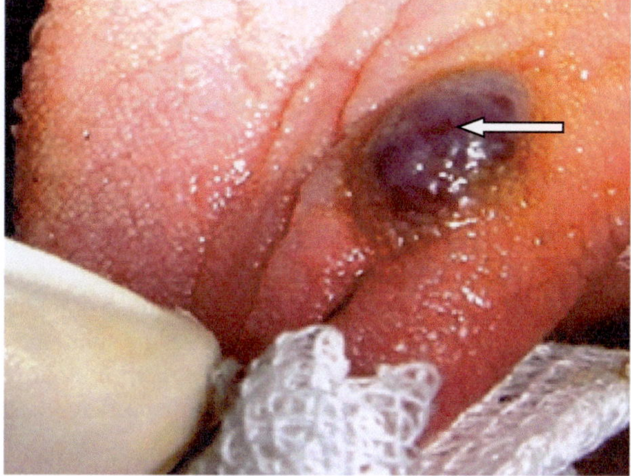

Fig. 10.4 Cavernous hemangioma of the tongue (bluish in color, small in size, and localized (arrow))

Surgical excision is the first treatment of choice, but electrocauterization, cryosurgery, and interferon injections are other effective treatment courses [8].

10.2.4 Mixed Salivary Tumor (Minor Salivary Glands)

It usually presents as a submucous, rounded, firm, mobile lobulated mass that increases in size with eating. It is treated by simple excision.

10.2.5 Lingual Thyroid Nodule

Almost 90% of ectopic thyroid tissue is associated with the dorsum of the tongue. It typically appears as a smooth nodular mass of tissue located in the midline of the posterior dorsal surface of the tongue [9]. The presence of a lingual thyroid reflects the lack of descent of thyroid tissue during development. Up to 70% of patients with a lingual thyroid have hypothyroidism [10]. Some patients have a sensation of a lump or difficulty swallowing. A lingual thyroid nodule may even cause respiratory obstruction and hemorrhage.

Symptoms are more common during increased metabolic demand, such as in adolescence or pregnancy [11]. If hypothyroidism is present, thyroid replacement can decrease the size of the lingual thyroid and improve obstructive symptoms. Surgical excision is often advised for patients with a lingual thyroid and normal thyroid function; however, this may lead to a need for postoperative thyroid replacement because the lingual thyroid is usually the only functioning thyroid tissue in these patients [10].

10.2.6 Hemangioma

Hemangioma (Greek: *Haima* blood; *angeion* vessel, *oma* tumor) by definition can be defined as "a benign tumor of dilated blood vessels." Vasoformative tumors are broadly classified into two groups: *Hemangioma* and *vascular malformation*. Hemangioma is histologically further classified into *capillary* and *cavernous* forms. Capillary hemangioma is composed of many small capillaries lined by a single layer of endothelial cells supported in a connective tissue stroma of varying density, while cavernous hemangioma is formed by large, thin-walled vessels, or sinusoids lined by epithelial cells separated by a thin layer of connective tissue septa [12].

Unlike vascular malformations, hemangiomas are real tumors arising from the rapidly dividing endothelial cells. The two main types are "infantile" and "congenital" types. An infantile hemangioma is the most common tumor in infancy and presents shortly after birth as a well-demarcated, flat, and erythematous red patch. At this stage, hemangiomas may be confused with other red lesions of birth, but rapid proliferation and vertical growth trigger the diagnosis. Hemangiomas classically grow in three developmental phases: (1) *proliferation* (endothelial proliferative growth phase), (2) *quiescence*, and (3) *involution* (involutive phase with very slow inevitable regression). In most hemangiomas, 80% of proliferation occurs by 3 months of life. Relative ischemia of the tumor due to rapid growth at this phase causes necrosis, ulceration, and eventual bleeding. Involution of 50%, 70%, and 90% of the hemangioma occurs by 5, 7, and 9 years of age, respectively.

The pathophysiology of hemangiomas is attributed to genetic and cellular factors, mainly to monocytes, which are considered the potential ancestors of hemangioma endothelial cells. Imbalance in the angiogenesis, which causes an uncontrolled proliferation of vascular elements, associated with substances such as vascular endothelial growth factor (VEGF), basic fibroblast growth factor (BFGF), and indole-amine 2,3-dioxygenase (IDO), which are found in large amount during proliferative stages, are believed to be the cause [13].

Approximately 60–70% of hemangiomas occur in the head and neck region, with the lips, *tongue*, buccal mucosa, and palate most commonly involved [14]. *Diagnosis* depends on clinical examination that shows the characteristic bluish lesion, which may be localized, whether small (Fig. 10.4) or large on the dorsal surface (Fig. 10.5) or the ventral surface (Fig. 10.6), or may be diffuse (Fig. 10.7). When in doubt, a Doppler ultrasound (US) and/or magnetic resonance imaging (MRI), will define diagnosis.

Factors such as patient's age, size, and site of lesion and the proximity of lesion to vital structure are paramount in the determination of the therapeutic approach and surgical excision. Even though radiotherapy, cryotherapy, laser therapy, medical treatment (systemic propranolol administration), injection of sclerosing substances, and the selective embolization of the lingual artery seem to have some efficacy, surgery is considered the therapy of choice in the isolated vascular lesions of the body of the tongue. Various combination protocols have also been proposed for treatment of tongue hemangiomas.

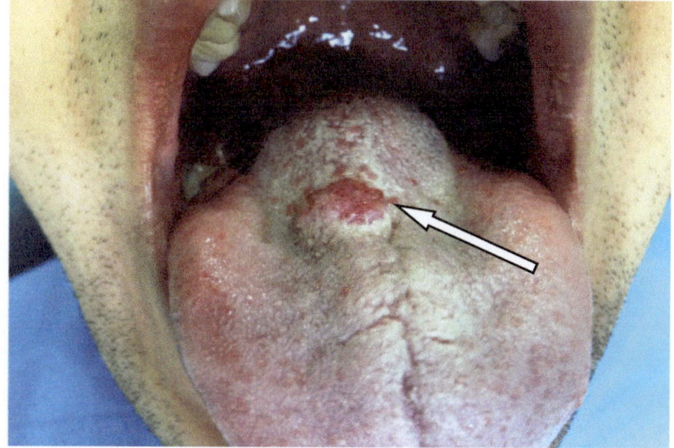

Fig. 10.5 Cavernous hemangioma on the dorsal surface of the tongue (large in size and localized (arrow))

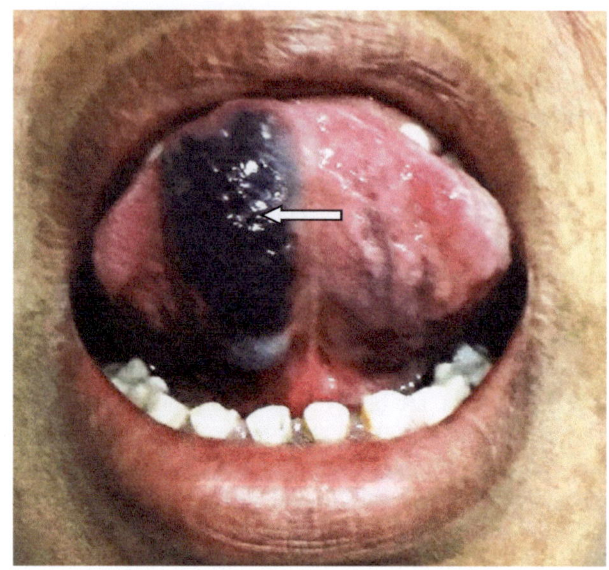

Fig. 10.6 Cavernous hemangioma on the ventral surface of the tongue (dark blue in color, large in size, and localized (arrow))

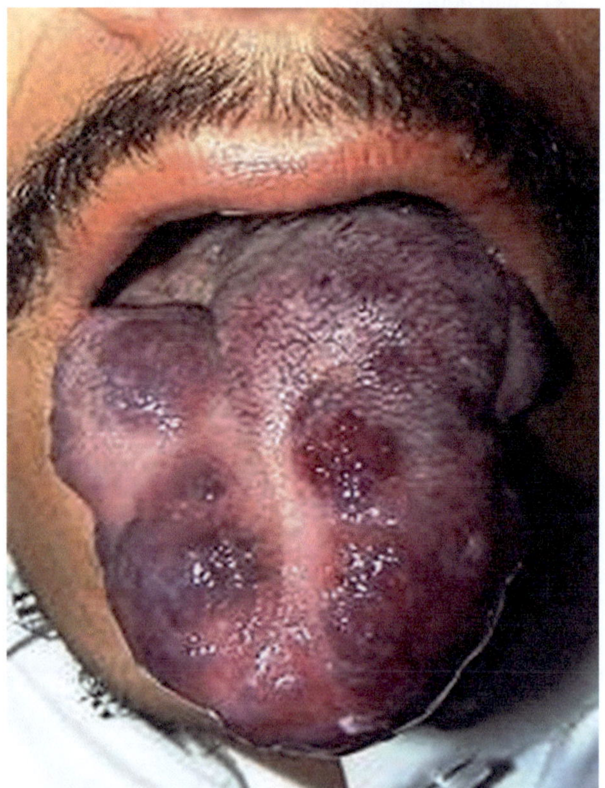

Fig. 10.7 Cavernous hemangioma of the tongue (bluish in color, large in size, and diffuse)

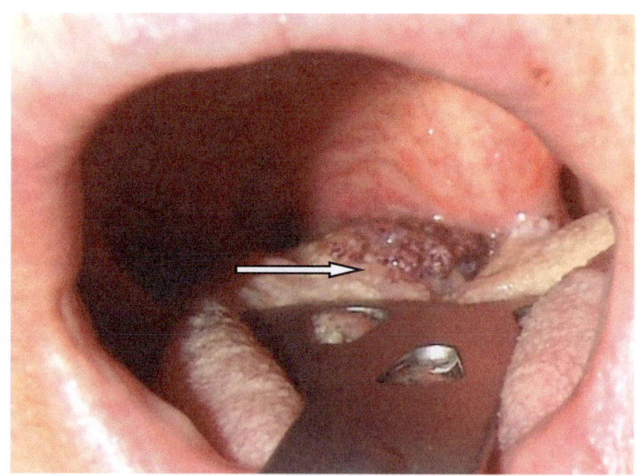

Fig. 10.8 Lymphangioma at the base of the tongue (arrow). It was partially removed and diagnosed by histology

10.2.7 Lymphoepithelial Cysts

Lymphoepithelial cysts are yellowish nodules located on the ventral surface of the tongue, tonsillar region, or floor of the mouth (Fig. 10.8). They are benign lesions and are thought to arise from the entrapment of salivary epithelium in lymphoid aggregates during embryogenesis [15]. Biopsy is required to confirm the diagnosis.

10.3 Malignant Tumors

Malignant tumors of the tongue are mainly *epithelial* in origin, most commonly squamous cell carcinoma (SCC). Mesenchymal tumors, malignant mixed salivary tumors, and malignancy in remnants of the thyroid gland may also occur.

10.3.1 Squamous Cell Carcinoma (SCC)

Risk factors of SCC include older age, tobacco use, and alcohol use [16]. It commonly involves the lateral surface of the tongue (Fig. 10.9). Patients younger than 40 years who develop intra-oral SCC often do not have risk factors [16, 17]. Initially, lesions appear as a slight thickening over a red or white base. This may lead to nodularity or ulceration, causing pain and discomfort.

Biopsy is critical to confirm diagnosis of SCC and start prompt treatment before extensive local invasion occurs. Typically, treatment of SCC of the tongue includes surgery and radiation therapy [18].

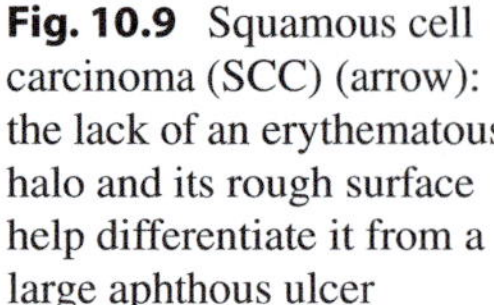
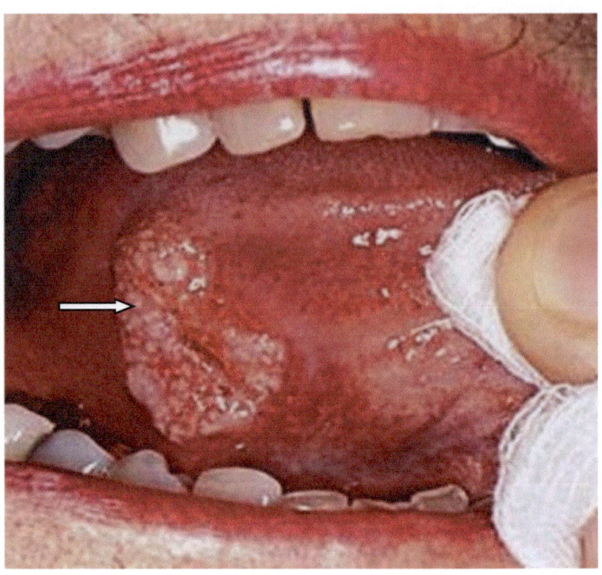

Fig. 10.9 Squamous cell carcinoma (SCC) (arrow): the lack of an erythematous halo and its rough surface help differentiate it from a large aphthous ulcer

10.3.2 Alveolar Soft Part Sarcoma (ASPS)

10.3.2.1 Pathogenesis

Alveolar soft part sarcoma (ASPS) derives its name from its histological appearance and suspected origin. As a result of formalin fixation, granular cells that are normally arranged in well-defined nests separated by a rich vascular network lose cohesion and create a pseudo-alveolar pattern. Although the histogenesis remains controversial, immunohistochemical (IHC) stains indicate a myogenic origin. The tumor's common occurrence in skeletal muscle and desmin reactivity support a myogenic origin. Although recent studies have been unable to confirm myoD1 expression or myogenin reactivity (5), this may be attributed to its derivation from a myoid precursor with lack of differentiation.

10.3.2.2 Incidence

Alveolar soft part sarcoma accounts for <1% of soft tissue sarcomas. This extremely vascular tumor is most commonly found in the lower extremities (44%) and arises in the head and neck in 27% of cases, with 25% of head and neck cases occurring in the tongue [19].

10.3.2.3 Clinical Presentation

Alveolar soft part sarcoma typically presents in young women between 15–35 years of age as a slowly enlarging, well-circumscribed, and often encapsulated mass. Vascular invasion is frequent, and metastatic disease is frequently present at diagnosis. Lung metastases are seen in 42–65% of patients at presentation [20]. Brain and bone are the next most common sites of metastasis, with lymph node (LN) involvement seen in only 10% of patients [20].

Alveolar soft part sarcoma has a close clinical and imaging resemblance to common benign vascular tumors such as hemangioma or venous malformations, the two categories of benign vascular soft tissue vascular lesions according to the system of Mulliken and Glowaski [21]. This may lead to misdiagnosis and inadequate or delayed treatment. The term "hemangioma" is restricted to the classic involuting vascular lesion of infancy. Vascular malformations are divided into low-flow and high-flow subtypes, characterized by the predominant vessel involved; namely, capillary, venous, or lymphatic involvement. Vascular malformations are present at birth, grow in proportion to patient growth, and do not involute. Rarely, they may spontaneously enlarge through the development of arteriovenous fistulas, thrombosis, or ectasia.

In contrast, ASPS is *not* present at birth, grows rapidly, and occurs in an older age group (Fig. 10.10). Patients with ASPS of the tongue experience dysphagia, dysphonia, or mild discomfort. Clinical examination often reveals pulsation with a thrill. Although there usually is no overlying ulceration or bleeding, our patient had significant hemorrhage as the tumor grossly extended through the overlying mucosa [22]. Bone erosion is also rare [22].

10.3.2.4 Imaging

Several imaging features help distinguish ASPS from benign hemangiomas and venous malformations (cavernous hemangioma).

10.3.2.4.1 Computed Tomography (CT) Scan

Unenhanced CT imaging shows a low-attenuation lesion similar to muscle with peripheral enhancement and central areas of low attenuation on enhanced images

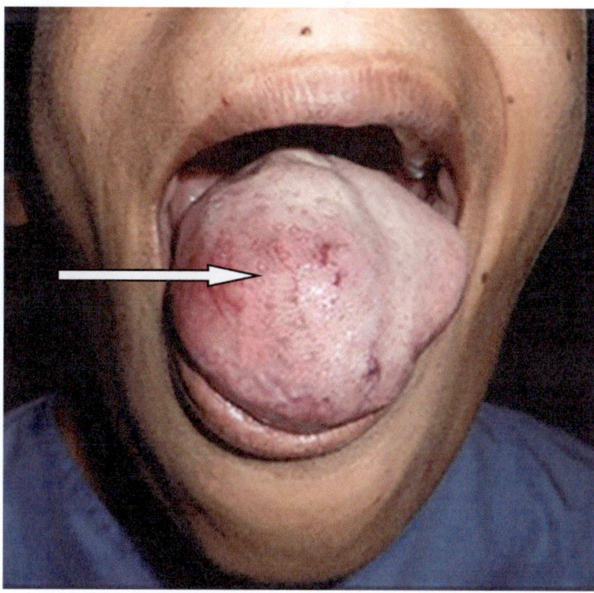

Fig. 10.10 Alveolar soft part sarcoma (ASPS) of the tongue occupying most of the tongue (arrow)

consistent with necrosis In contrast, CT imaging of hemangioma typically shows a slightly hyperattenuated lesion on unenhanced images, with intense homogeneous enhancement after contrast material administration. Hemangiomas and venous malformations may also contain phleboliths seen as punctate calcifications on unenhanced CT images.

10.3.2.4.2 Magnetic Resonance Imaging (MRI)

T1-weighted MR images typically show hyperintense signal as compared with muscle that is not as intense as that seen with hemangiomas but more intense than that of other soft tissue sarcomas that are typically isointense relative to muscle [23]. Similar to hemangioma, ASPS has very high signal intensity on T2-weighted images, but flow voids are also seen, suggesting the correct diagnosis [20, 23]. Contrast-enhanced MR images show intense, heterogeneous enhancement and central necrosis as seen on CT images.

10.3.2.4.3 Angiography

Angiography shows a hypervascular mass with multiple, enlarged tortuous vessels, arteriovenous shunts, and an intense prolonged tumor blush (Fig. 10.11) [23]. This is in contrast to a high-flow vascular malformation such as an arteriovenous malformation that has an arteriovenous shunt but no persistent tumor blush and a low-flow vascular malformation that has prolonged contrast blush but no arteriovenous shunt.

10.3.2.5 Differential Diagnosis

In addition to hemangioma and vascular malformation, other less likely differential diagnoses *include hyperplastic lingual thyroid, dermoid, and squamous cell*

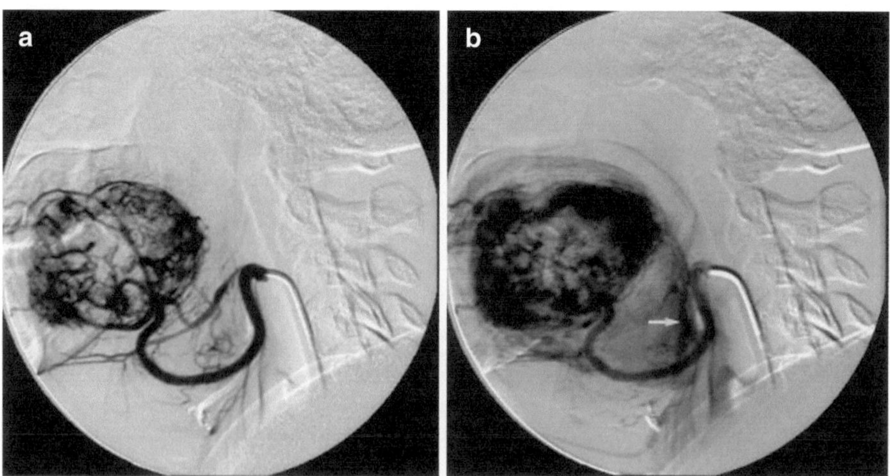

Fig. 10.11 Lateral-projection angiograms acquired during mid- (**a**) and late (**b**) arterial phases show a hypervascular mass with irregular, tortuous tumor vessels and persistent tumor blush. An early draining vein is seen at the base of tongue (*white arrow*)

carcinoma. These neoplasms are easily differentiated from ASPS on the basis of CT and MR findings. Lingual thyroid typically occurs in the posterior oral tongue and does not have areas of necrosis or flow voids.

Although rare, dermoids of the tongue appear as hypoattenuated and well-circumscribed masses on CT images that may contain fat and typically show peripheral enhancement of the cystic wall. Squamous cell carcinoma of the tongue accounts for nearly one quarter of oral cavity cancer but typically does not have well-circumscribed borders, flow voids, intense enhancement, and hyperintense signal on T2-weighted images as seen in ASPS [24].

10.3.2.6 Histopathology

Histological features of ASPS are deceptively benign histologically with no atypical mitotic figures or nuclear pleomorphism. Demonstration of PAS-positive diastase-resistant crystals with the appropriate clinical history confirms the diagnosis [25].

10.3.2.7 Management

Aggressive surgical excision is recommended, because local recurrence is common. Massive bleeding during surgical resection of ASPS has been reported and when located posteriorly in the tongue may be difficult to control at surgery [19, 25]. Preoperative embolization for ASPS is useful to control blood loss and the need for transfusion therapy [22].

10.3.2.8 Prognosis

Five-year and 20-year survival rates of 59% and 15%, respectively, have been reported, with local recurrence and distant metastasis primarily responsible for the poor prognosis of this neoplasm [20, 26].

10.3.3 Synovial Sarcoma of the Tongue

Synovial sarcoma is a soft tissue sarcoma with characteristic morphological and genetic features.

10.3.3.1 Incidence: Location

It often occurs in the limbs near the joints, and the head and neck, including the parapharyngeal space and parotid gland. In the oral cavity, synovial sarcomas can occur in the buccal mucosa, gingivobuccal sulcus, soft and hard palates, floor of the mouth, retromolar region, submental region, and tongue [27]. However, synovial sarcomas of the tongue are extremely rare; only 15 cases of synovial sarcoma originating in the tongue have been reported [28–37].

10.3.3.2 Clinical Manifestations

There is a striking male predilection. Approximately, 81.25% patients are male with an average *age* of 27 years. The base of the tongue appears to be the most frequent site for synovial sarcoma (62.5%). Early tumor growth is slow and the location is deep. A sudden increase in symptoms is often noted many years after tumour initiation. Clinical manifestations are related to the site of the tumor and include a tumour mass, dysphagia, pain, hoarseness, headache, and hearing loss.

10.3.3.3 Investigations: Diagnosis

10.3.3.3.1 Tumor Markers

Synovial sarcoma has no characteristic diagnostic markers. Thus, several antibody markers are often used to exclude many morphologically similar sarcomas or carcinomas.

10.3.3.3.2 Imaging

MRI is the most commonly used imaging method for the diagnosis of soft tissue tumors and the boundaries of soft tissue tumors are depicted. Synovial sarcoma imaging is *not* specific, but MRI is significant for determining the primary site and presence of adjacent tissue infiltration and LN metastasis [38, 39].

10.3.3.3.3 Histopathology

Histologically, synovial sarcoma is mainly described as biphasic (25%), monophasic fibrous, or monophasic epithelial (70%), poorly differentiated (less than 5%), or as a myxoid variant [40]. These tumors present *microscopically* with two distinct cell populations, contain epithelial-like cells in glandular structures and spindle cells, and exhibit biphasic differentiation. Migration is noted between spindle cells and epithelial-like cells.

Immunohistochemical (IHC) staining is necessary for the accurate diagnosis of synovial sarcoma. According to several reports, 90% of synovial sarcomas stain positive for focal *cytokeratins and EMA*.

EMA is the most sensitive indicator of synovial sarcoma expression markers with a sensitivity of 91% (74% of which is clearly stained) and specificity of 82%. The overall sensitivity of *cytokeratins* was 70% and specificity was 68% [41]. Negative IHC staining also has a diagnostic value in excluding morphological similar tumors. Immunoreactivity for cytokeratins, smooth muscle actin, desmin and myogenin has not been described. Synovial sarcomas yield variable results with immunohistochemical staining, but *chromosomal studies* revealed that the balanced reciprocal translocation t(X; 18) (p11.2q;q11.2) is found in >90% of all synovial sarcoma subtypes [42]. This translocation results in a fusion of the *SYT* or *SSXT* gene from chromosome 18 to the *SSX1*, *SSX2,* or *SSX4* genes from the X-chromosome. The SYT-SSX fusion transcript has high diagnostic value in synovial sarcoma.

10.3.3.4 Management

Surgical resection is recommended, followed by consideration of adjuvant radiotherapy with or without chemotherapy [43].

10.3.3.4.1 Surgery

Surgery is the key to reducing recurrence and metastasis; however, the recurrence rate (RR) has been reported to be very high (>70%) [44]. Lack of capsule formation leads to incomplete surgical removal. Moreover, Wide excision of the tumor may result in dysfunction or even death. The tumour is easily misdiagnosed, which causes repeated recurrence after surgery, thereby increasing the risk of LN and distant metastases, eventually leading to treatment failure. The majority of scholars believe that the surgical margin and tumour size are key factors that affect prognosis [35, 45]. Reduced LN metastases are noted in synovial sarcoma of the head and neck, and unless distinct enlarged LNs are present, prophylactic cervical LN dissection is not recommended [45].

10.3.3.4.2 Chemoradiotherapy

Fayda et al., believe that chemoradiotherapy is a better option for treating head and neck synovial sarcoma in general. The recommended total dose is 65 Gy and ifosfamide is the main chemotherapy [46, 47].

10.3.3.4.3 Radiotherapy (RT)

Radiotherapy (RT) improves the disease-free survival in the majority of patients with synovial sarcoma [48]. According to the 2017 NCCN Clinical Practice Guidelines in Oncology of soft tissue sarcoma (version 2) [49], postoperative RT in the range of 45 Gy for a low-dose rate or a high-dose equivalent is recommended. If the dose is too high, it will lead to adverse effects, such as radiation mucositis, ulceration, and osteoradionecrosis [50, 51].

10.3.4 Myoblastic (Myofibroblastic) Sarcoma

Low-grade myofibroblastic sarcoma (LGMS) is known to be a rare tumor [52–54]. Atypical myofibroblasts have been shown to be involved in LGMS, such as in the femur [52], vulva [53], and phalanx [54]. In the head and neck region, LGMS frequently occurs in the tongue [55], especially at the lateral edge [56]. A myoblastic sarcoma occurring at the tip of the tongue had been recently reported by Mikami et al. [57].

10.3.4.1 Pathology

Myofibroblasts, which show characteristics of both fibroblasts and smooth muscle cells, were firstly identified in granulation tissue in 1971 [58]. Fibroblasts differentiate into myofibroblasts during wound healing and tissue repair [59]. According to the 2013 World Health Organization (WHO) classification [60], LGMS is categorized as a fibroblastic/myofibroblastic tumor; mainly composed of atypical myofibroblasts intermediate-rarely metastasizing tumor.

Immunohistochemically, LGMS tumor cells are positive for at least one myogenic marker, such as alpha-smooth muscle actin (α-SMA), desmin, or muscle actin

(HHF-35). As no definitive markers of LGMS have been found to date, it is difficult to make a diagnosis based on the pathological findings alone. In addition, whether or not the genetic mutations of cancer-related genes shown in sarcomas are involved in LGMS is unclear.

Myofibroblasts share immunohistochemical and ultrastructural features of both fibroblasts and smooth muscle cells and play a role in wound and tissue repair [61]. However, the function of myofibroblasts in LGMS has been unclear. Low-grade myofibroblastic sarcoma tends to be found in local recurrence rather than metastasis [62].

10.3.4.2 Clinical Behavior

Clinically, LGMS has a propensity for local recurrence and is associated with a low risk of metastatic spread.

10.3.4.3 Differential Diagnosis

The differential diagnosis of LGMS should include other spindle cell tumors, such as benign tumors; inflammatory myofibroblastic tumors and nodular fasciitis, such as intermediate tumor; and desmoplastic fibroma or malignant tumors, such as synovial sarcoma [63], leiomyosarcoma, and osteosarcoma [52].

Inflammatory myofibroblastic tumor shows infiltration of inflammatory cells. The genomic rearrangement of *MYH9-USP6s* (*MYH9* exon 1 and *USP6* exon 1 or *MYH9* exon 1 and USP6 exon 2) is frequently observed in nodular fasciitis [64]. Synovial sarcoma would be ruled out by the reduced expression of BAF47 (INI1 gene product) protein [65]. Many cases of leiomyosarcoma [66] and osteosarcoma [67] have been reported to have a gene mutation in *p53*, and desmoplastic fibroma has a point mutation in *CTNNB1*. Therefore, point mutations of the investigated genes might not be involved in intravascular invasion of myofibroblasts in LGMS.

10.3.4.4 Treatment

Because there are no established treatments for LGMS at present, the mechanism underlying the invasion of atypical myofibroblasts into vascular tissue should be clarified in the future. Surgical resection with a safety margin is the treatment of choice if feasible.

10.3.5 Spindle Cell Sarcoma (SCS)

10.3.5.1 Introduction

Spindle cell sarcoma (SCS) is a type of connective tissue cancer in which the cells are spindle-shaped when examined under a microscope. Spindle cell neoplasms are diverse in nature with clinicopathological and tumor biological heterogeneity [68]. SCS is a type of connective tissue tumor and generally begins in layers of connective tissue such as that under the skin, between muscles, and surrounding organs. *Primary SCS* is an extremely rare entity and one of the least reported tumors [69–71], rendering it a diagnostic and therapeutic challenge [72, 73].

At the early stage, the clinical presentation of SCS is similar to the benign lesion [73, 74]. Like other sarcoma, SCS were treated aggressively with surgical therapy as a mainstay in the management and adjuvant chemoradiotherapy was implemented for patients with high risk behavior [69, 71, 72, 74–78].

Nowadays, the sophisticated molecular pathological diagnostic techniques have made the diagnosis of SCS accurate and reliable [69]. However, owing to the rarity of spindle cell sarcoma, there is lack of basic information regarding the exact tumor incidence, distinctive clinical characteristics, and treatment options and outcome as well as disease-specific prognostic factors

10.3.5.2 Etiology: Pathogenesis

Spindle cell sarcoma can develop for a variety of reasons, including genetic predisposition and a combination of other factors such as injury and inflammation in patients that are already thought to be predisposed to such tumors. Spindle cells are a naturally occurring part of the body's response to injury, infection, or other immune response where the connective tissues will begin dividing to heal the affected area. If cellular turnover becomes high, it may result in the formation of a cancerous tumor.

10.3.5.3 Stages of SCS

According to the number system of spindle cell sarcoma (SCS), it is divided into four stages as summarized and described in Table 10.2.

10.3.5.4 Clinical Presentation: Treatment

Similar to soft tissue sarcomas [79], SCS affects people of almost all ages. It occurs more commonly in middle and old age adult groups. A retrospective study was recently carried out by Feng et al. [80] with a study population from Surveillance, Epidemiology, and End Results (SEER) database. A total of 3299 cases were identified. The average follow-up time was 43 months, with a median follow-up of 15

Table 10.2 Staging of spindle cell sarcoma (SCS)

Stage	Description
Stage 1	Cancer cells are in the slow mitotic rate grade or grade 1 and it may be in the deep tissues or in the superficial tissues without signs of metastases • Stage 1A: the tumor is small (<5 cm) • Stage 1B: the tumor is large (>5 cm)
Stage 2	Cancer cells are in the medium grade (grade 2) or the high grade (grade 3) and it may be in the deep tissues or in the superficial tissues without signs of metastases. • Stage 2A: the tumor is small (<5 cm) • Stage 2B: the tumor is large (>5 cm)
Stage 3	Cancer cells are in grade 3, in which the cells have rapid mitotic division. The tumor is large and it may be found in the deep or superficial tissues. Cancer cells have already metastasized to lymph nodes (LNs)
Stage 4	The tumor has already metastasized to another site in the body, as well as LNs i.e. there is already formation of secondary tumors. Since there are already one or more tumors in the body, the tumor varies in size and grade

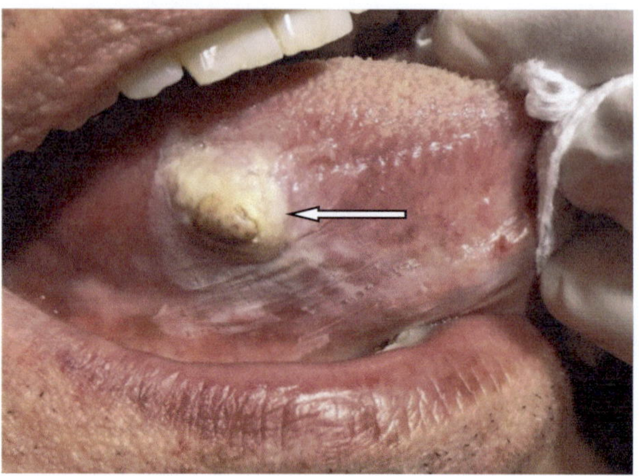

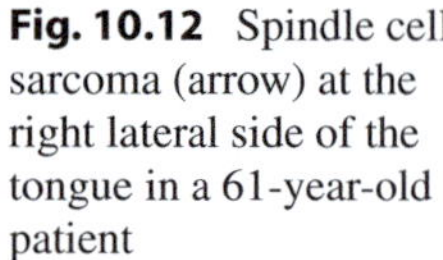

Fig. 10.12 Spindle cell sarcoma (arrow) at the right lateral side of the tongue in a 61-year-old patient

months (range, 14–81 months). Of these patients, the mean *age* at diagnosis was 61 ± 19 years (range: birth-103 years). The incidence peaked during the seventh decade of life and the majority of cases were *white* people (80.9%). There was no significant difference for *gender* distribution including 1605 females and 1694 males. According to this dataset, SCS could occur at almost any site of the body including the tongue (Fig. 10.12). The incidence was higher in superficial primary tumor site than internal site (2041 versus 1151). Superficial sites included the skin and subcutaneous soft tissue in head and neck, upper limb, shoulder, lower limb, thorax, breast, abdomen, pelvis, and trunk. Interior sites included bone or viscera of the digestive, respiratory, reproductive, urinary, nervous, endocrine, and circulatory systems.

The tumors start as a small lump with inflammation that grows. At first, the lump is self-contained as the tumor exists in its stage 1 state, and will not necessarily expand beyond its encapsulated form. However, it may develop cancerous processes that can only be detected through microscopic examination. As such, at this level, the tumor is usually treated by excision with a wide safety margin, followed by biopsy and additional excision if necessary. Surgical resection remains the mainstay of treatment for SCS. However, the value of extensive radical operation and lymphadenectomy is still ambiguous [80].

10.3.5.5 Prognosis

The prognosis of a stage-1 tumor excision is usually fairly positive, but if the tumors progress to stages 2 and 3, prognosis is worse because tumor cells have likely spread to other locations. These locations can either be nearby tissues or system-wide locations that include the lungs, kidneys, and liver. In these cases, chemotherapy and radiation are the only methods of controlling the cancer.

Survival analysis [81, 82] showed that the significant factors that affected overall survival and disease-free survival (DFS) were age, marital status, pathological grade, AJCC stage, T stage, N stage, M stage, tumor site *(superficial sites have a better prognosis),* and treatment modality [83].

10.3.6 Kaposi Sarcoma (KS)

10.3.6.1 Introduction

Kaposi's sarcoma (KS) is a type of cancer that can form masses in the skin, lymph nodes (LNs), or other organs [84]. The skin lesions are usually purple in color [84], and may be flat or raised [85]. Lesions can occur singularly, in a limited area, or be widespread. Progress of the disease is either slow or rapid [85]. Risk factors include poor immune function and chronic lymphedema [84, 85].

The condition is relatively common in people with HIV/AIDS and following organ transplant as of 2017 [85, 86]. Over 35% of people with AIDS may be affected [87]. It was first described by Moritz Kaposi in 1872 [88, 89]. It became more widely known as one of the AIDS-defining illnesses in the 1980s [88]. The virus associated with this cancer was discovered back in 1994 [88, 89].

10.3.6.2 Epidemiology

With the decrease in the death rate among people with HIV/AIDS receiving new treatments in the 1990s, the rates and severity of epidemic KS also decreased. However, the number of people living with HIV/AIDS is increasing in the United States, and it is possible that the number of people with AIDS-associated Kaposi sarcoma will again rise as these people live longer with HIV infection.

10.3.6.3 Etiology

Kaposi's sarcoma-associated herpes virus (KSHV), also called HHV-8, is present in almost 100% of KS lesions, whether HIV-related, classic, endemic, or iatrogenic [90]. KSHV encodes oncogenes, micro-RNAs, and circular RNAs that promote cancer cell proliferation and escape from the immune system.

10.3.6.3.1 Transmission

In Europe and North America, KSHV is transmitted through saliva. Thus, kissing is a theoretical risk factor for transmission. Higher rates of transmission among gay and bisexual men have been attributed to "deep kissing" sexual partners with KSHV [91]. Another alternative theory suggests that use of saliva as a sexual lubricant might be a major mode for transmission. Prudent advice is to use commercial lubricants when needed and avoid deep kissing with partners with KSHV infection or whose status is unknown. KSHV is also transmissible via both organ transplantation [92] and blood transfusion [93]. Testing for the virus before these procedures is likely to effectively limit iatrogenic transmission.

10.3.6.4 Pathology

Despite its name, in general it is not considered a true sarcoma [94, 95], which is a tumor arising from mesenchymal tissue. The histogenesis of KS remains controversial [96]. It may arise as a cancer of the lymphatic endothelium [97] and forms vascular channels that fill with blood cells, giving the tumor its characteristic bruise-like appearance. KSHV proteins are uniformly detected in KS cancer cells. The most typical feature of Kaposi sarcoma is the presence of *spindle cells* forming slits

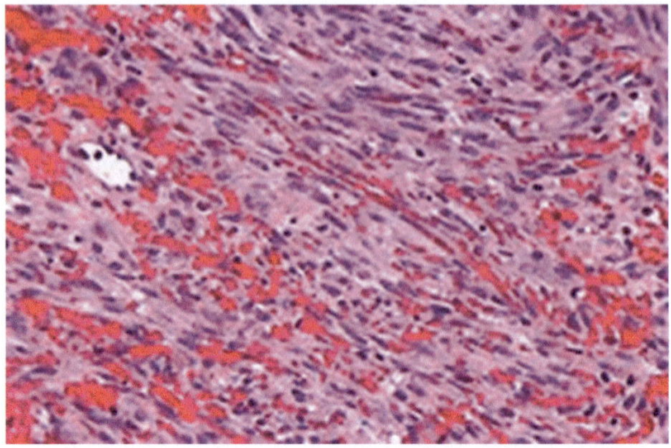

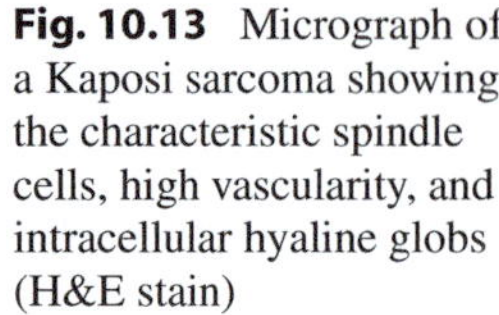

Fig. 10.13 Micrograph of a Kaposi sarcoma showing the characteristic spindle cells, high vascularity, and intracellular hyaline globs (H&E stain)

containing red blood cells (Fig. 10.13). Mitotic activity is only moderate and pleomorphism is usually absent [98]. The tumor is highly vascular, containing abnormally dense and irregular blood vessels, which leak red blood cells into the surrounding tissue and give the tumor its dark color. Inflammation around the tumor may produce swelling and pain. Variously sized PAS positive hyaline bodies are often seen in the cytoplasm or sometimes extracellularly. The spindle cells of KS differentiate toward endothelial cells, probably of lymph vessel rather than blood vessel origin [99]. The consistent immuno-receptivity for *podoplanin* supports the lymphatic nature of the lesion.

10.3.6.5 Clinical Picture

Kaposi sarcoma lesions are nodules or blotches that may be red, purple, brown, or black, and are usually papular. They are typically found on the skin, but spread elsewhere is common, especially the mouth, gastrointestinal tract (GIT) and respiratory tract. Growth ranges from very slow to explosively fast, and is associated with significant mortality and morbidity [100]. The lesions are painless, but become cosmetically disfiguring or interruptive to organs [101].

10.3.6.5.1 Skin

Commonly affected areas include the lower limbs, back, face, mouth, and genitalia. The lesions are usually reddish-brown or purple), but may occasionally be plaque-like (often on the soles of the feet) or even involved in skin breakdown with resulting fungating lesions. Associated swelling may result from local inflammation or lymphedema due to obstruction of local lymphatic vessels by the lesion. Skin lesions may be quite disfiguring for the sufferer, and a cause of much psychosocial disturbances [102].

10.3.6.5.2 Mouth

The mouth is involved with Kaposi sarcoma in approximately 30% of cases, and is the initial site in 15% of AIDS-related KS. In the mouth, the hard palate is most

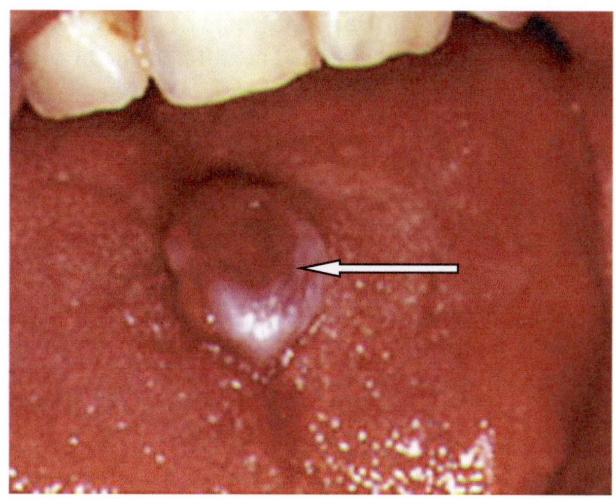

Fig. 10.14 Nodular lesion of Kaposi sarcoma affecting the dorsum of the anterior two-thirds of the tongue (arrow)

frequently affected, followed by the gums and tongue (Fig. 10.14). Lesions in the mouth may be easily damaged by chewing and bleed or suffer secondary infection, and even interfere with swallowing or speech [103].

10.3.6.5.3 Gastrointestinal Tract

Involvement can be common in those with transplant-related or AIDS-related KS, and it may occur in the absence of skin involvement. The gastrointestinal lesions may be silent or cause weight loss, pain, nausea/vomiting, diarrhea, bleeding (hematemesis, melena or bleeding per rectum), malabsorption, or intestinal obstruction [104].

10.3.6.5.4 Respiratory Tract

Involvement of the airway can present with shortness of breath, fever, cough, hemoptysis, or chest pain, or as an incidental finding on chest X-ray [105]. Diagnosis is usually confirmed by bronchoscopy, when the lesions are directly seen and often biopsied. Kaposi's sarcoma of the lung has a poor prognosis.

10.3.6.6 Diagnosis

The *diagnosis* of Kaposi sarcoma is by tissue biopsy while the *extent* of disease may be determined by medical imaging.

Although Kaposi sarcoma may be suspected from the appearance of lesions and the patient's risk factors, definite diagnosis can be made only by *biopsy* and microscopic examination. Detection of the KSHV protein LANA in tumor cells confirms the diagnosis. In the differential diagnosis, arteriovenous malformations, pyogenic granuloma, and other vascular proliferations can be microscopically confused with KS [106].

10.3.6.7 Differential Diagnosis of Kaposi Sarcoma

Kaposi sarcoma lesions should be differentiated from the following:

1. Nevus
2. Histiocytoma
3. Cryptococcosis
4. Histoplasmosis
5. Leishmaniasis
6. Pneumocystis lesions
7. Dermatophytosis
8. Angioma
9. Bacillary angiomatosis
10. Pyogenic granuloma
11. Melanoma

10.3.6.8 Classification

HHV-8 is responsible for all varieties of KS. Since *Moritz Kaposi* first described this cancer, the disease has been reported in 4 separate clinical settings, with different presentations, epidemiology, and prognoses [84, 107]. All of these forms are infected with KSHV and are different manifestations of the same disease, but have differences in clinical aggressiveness, prognosis and treatment.

- *Classic Kaposi sarcoma* most commonly appears early on the toes and soles as reddish, violaceous, or bluish-black macules and patches that spread and coalesce to form nodules or plaques [107]. A small percentage of these patients may have visceral lesions. In most cases, treatment involves surgical excision of the lesion. The condition tends to be indolent and chronic [84], affecting elderly men from the Mediterranean region, Arabian countries [108] or of Eastern European descent. Countries bordering the Mediterranean basin have higher rates of KSHV/HHV-8 infection than the remainder of Europe [109, 110].
- *Endemic KS*, which has two types. Although this may be present worldwide, it has been originally described later in young African people, mainly from sub-Saharan Africa [84].This variant is not related to HIV infection [111, 112] and is a more aggressive disease that infiltrates the skin extensively [111].
  - *African lymphadenopathic Kaposi sarcoma* is aggressive, occurring in children under 10 years of age, presenting with LN involvement, with or without skin lesions [107].
  - *African cutaneous Kaposi sarcoma* presents with nodular, infiltrative, vascular masses on the extremities, mostly in men between the ages of 20–50 years, and is endemic in tropical Africa [107].
- *Immunosuppression-associated Kaposi sarcoma* had been rarely described, until the advent of immunosuppressants (such as cyclosporine-A) for transplant patients in the 1980s, when its incidence grew rapidly. The tumor arises either when an HHV 8-infected organ is transplanted into someone who has not been exposed to the virus or when the transplant recipient already harbors preexisting

HHV 8 infection [113, 114]. Unlike classic Kaposi sarcoma, the site of presentation is more variable [107].

- *AIDS-associated Kaposi sarcoma* (*Epidemic KS*) typically presents with cutaneous lesions that begin as one or several red to purple-red macules, rapidly progressing to papules, nodules, and plaques, with a predilection for the head, back, neck, trunk, and mucous membranes. In more advanced cases, lesions can be found in the stomach and intestines, the lymph nodes, and the lungs [107]. Compared to other forms of KS, KS-AIDS stimulated more interest in KS research, as it was one of the first illnesses associated with AIDS and first described in 1981 [115–117]. This form of KS is over 300 times more common in AIDS patients than in renal transplant recipients. In this case, HHV 8 is sexually transmitted among people also at risk for sexually transmitted HIV infection [118].

10.3.6.9 Prevention

Blood tests to detect antibodies against KSHV have been developed and can be used to determine whether a person is at risk for transmitting infection to their sexual partner, or whether an organ is infected prior to transplantation. However, these tests are not available except as research tools, and, thus, there is little screening for persons at risk for becoming infected with KSHV, such as people following a transplant.

10.3.6.10 Treatment

Kaposi sarcoma is *not* curable, but it can often be treatable for many years. Treatment is based on the subtype (whether the condition is localized or widespread), and the person's immune function [85].

In KS associated with immunodeficiency or immunosuppression, treating the cause of immunity dysfunction can slow or stop the progression of KS.

In 40% or more of people with *AIDS-associated KS*, the Kaposi lesions will shrink upon first starting highly active antiretroviral therapy (HAART). Therefore, HAART is considered the cornerstone of therapy in AIDS-associated KS. However, KS may recur after a number of years on HAART, especially if HIV is not completely suppressed.

Patients with a few local lesions can often be treated with local measures such as radiation therapy or *cryosurgery* [119, 120]. Weak evidence suggests that antiretroviral therapy in combination with *chemotherapy* is more effective than either of those two therapies given individually [121]. Limited basic and clinical evidence suggest that topical *beta-blockers*, such as *timolol*, may induce regression of localized lesions in classic as well as HIV-associated KS [122, 123]. In general, *surgery is not recommended*, as KS can appear in wound edges. More widespread disease, or disease affecting internal organs, is treated with systemic therapy with *interferon alpha* (IFN-∞), liposomal *anthracyclines* (e.g. *liposoma doxorubicin* or *daunorubicin*), *thalidomide*, or *paclitaxel* [124, 125].

Alitretinoin, applied to the lesion, may be used when the lesions are not getting better with standard treatment of HIV/AIDS and chemotherapy or radiation therapy cannot be used [126].

References

1. Bouquot JE, Nikai H. Lesions of the oral cavity. In: Gnepp DR, editor. Diagnostic surgical pathology of the head and neck. Philadelphia: Saunders; 2001. p. 141.
2. Gardner ES, Goldberg LH. Granular cell tumor treated with Mohs micrographic surgery: report of a case and review of the literature. Dermatol Surg. 2001;27(8):772–4.
3. Mooney MA, Janniger CK. Pyogenic granuloma. Cutis. 1995;55(3):133–6.
4. Castro TMPPG, Filho IB. Prevalence of human papillomavirus (HPV) in oral cavity and oropharynx. Braz J Otorhinolaryngol. 2006;72(2):272–82.
5. Castro TMPPG, Neto CER, Scala KA, et al. Oral manifestations related to papillomavirus. Braz J Otorhinolaryngol. 2004;70(4):546–50.
6. Jaju PP, Suvarna PV, Desai RS. Squamous papilloma: case report and review of literature. Int J Oral Sci. 2010;2(4):222–5.
7. Carneiro TE, Marinho SA, Verli FD, et al. Oral squamous papilloma: clinical, histologic and immunohistocheamecal analyses. J Oral Sci. 2009;51(3):367–72.
8. Mannarini L, Kratochivil V, Calabrese L, et al. Human papilloma virus (HPV) in head and neck region: review of literature. Acta Otorhinolaryngol Ital. 2009;29:119–26.
9. Williams JD, Sclafani AP, Slupchinskij O, Douge C. Evaluation and management of the lingual thyroid gland. Ann Otol Rhinol Laryngol. 1996;105(4):312–6.
10. Kansal P, Sakati N, Rifai A, Woodhouse N. Lingual thyroid. Diagnosis and treatment. Arch Intern Med. 1987;147(11):2046–8.
11. Taibah K, Ahmed M, Baessa E, Saleem M, Rifai A, al-Arifi A. An unusual cause of obstructive sleep apnoea presenting during pregnancy. J Laryngol Otol. 1998;112(12):1189–91.
12. Neville BW, Damm DD, Allen CM. Oral and maxillofacial pathology. 2nd ed. Philadelphia: WB Saunders; 2002.
13. Avila ED, Molon RS, Conte Neto N, Gabrielli MA, Hochuli-Vieira E. Lip cavernous hemangioma in a young child. Braz Dent J. 2010;21:370–4.
14. Okoji VN, Alonge TO, Olusanya AA. Intra-tumoral ligation and the injection of sclerosant in the treatment of lingual cavernous hemangioma. Niger J Med. 2011;20:172–5.
15. Sakoda S, Kodama Y, Shiba R. Lymphoepithelial cyst of oral cavity. Report of a case and review of the literature. Int J Oral Surg. 1983;12(2):127–31.
16. Llewellyn CD, Johnson NW, Warnakulasuriya KA. Risk factors for squamous cell carcinoma of the oral cavity in young people - a comprehensive literature review. Oral Oncol. 2001;37(5):401–18.
17. Sherin N, Simi T, Shameena P, Sudha S. Changing trends in oral cancer. Indian J Cancer. 2008;45(3):93–6.
18. Jones AS, Rafferty M, Fenton JE, Jones TM, Husband DJ. Treatment of squamous cell carcinoma of the tongue base: irradiation, surgery, or palliation? Ann Otol Rhinol Laryngol. 2007;116(2):92–9.
19. Ordonez NG, Mackay B. Alveolar soft-part sarcoma: a review of the pathology and histogenesis. Ultrastruct Pathol. 1998;22:275–92.
20. Lorigan JG, O'Keeffe FN, Evans HL, Wallace S. The radiologic manifestations of alveolar soft-part sarcoma. AJR Am J Roentgenol. 1989;153:335–9.
21. Mulliken JB, Glowacki J. Hemangiomas and vascular malformations in infants and children: a classification based on endothelial characteristics. Plast Reconstr Surg. 1982;69:412–20.
22. Donald PJ. Alveolar soft part sarcoma of the tongue. Head Neck Surg. 1987;9:172–8.
23. Iwamoto Y, Morimoto N, Chuman H, et al. The role of MR imaging in the diagnosis of alveolar soft part sarcoma: a report of 10 cases. Skelet Radiol. 1995;24:267–70.
24. Hunter BC, Ferlito A, Devaney KO, Rinaldo A. Clinicopathological consultation: alveolar soft part sarcoma of the head and neck region. Ann Otol Rhinol Laryngol. 1998;107:810–4.
25. Ordónez NG. Alveolar soft part sarcoma: a review and update. Adv Anat Pathol. 1999;6:125–39.

26. Aiken AH, Jeffrey A. Stone alveolar soft-part sarcoma of the tongue. Case report. AJNR Am J Neuroradiol. 2003;24:1156–8.
27. Al-Daraji W, Lasota J, Foss R, Miettinen M. Synovial sarcoma involving the head: analysis of 36 cases with predilection to the parotid and temporal regions. Am J Surg Pathol. 2009;33(10):1494–503.
28. Engelhardt J, Leafstedt SW. Synovial sarcoma of tonsil and tongue base. Case Rep Dermatol. 1983;76(2):243–4.
29. Fortuño-Mar A, Mayayo E, Guiral H, et al. Synovial sarcoma of the tongue: case report and review of the literature. An Otorrinolaringol Ibero Am. 2000;27(4):323–31.
30. Carrillo R, El-Naggar AK, Rodriguez-Peralto JL, Batsakis JG. Synovial sarcoma of the tongue: case report and review of the literature. J Oral Maxillofac Surg. 1992;50(8):904–6.
31. Ghodsi S, Sadr AM, Moussavi A. Synovial sarcoma of the tongue: report of a case. Acta Med Iran. 1974;17(3-4):155–60.
32. Guzman PC, Ortiz TH, Garza GR. Synovial sarcoma of the oral cavity (foramen caecum): report of a case and review of the literature. Prensa Med Mex. 1975;19:215–20.
33. Holtz F, Magielski JE. Synovial sarcomas of the tongue base: the seventh reported case. Arch Otolaryngol. 1985;111(4):271–2.
34. Bridge JA, Bridge RS, Borek DA, et al. Translocation t(X; 18) in orofacial synovial sarcoma. Cancer. 2015;62:935–7.
35. Komis C, Lagogiannis GA, Faratzis G, Rapidis AD. Synovial sarcoma of the tongue: report of a case and review of the literature. J Oral Maxillofac Surg. 2008;66:154–60.
36. Novotny GM, Fort TC. Synovial sarcoma of the tongue. Arch Otolaryngol. 1971;94(1):77–9.
37. Shmookler BM, Enzinger FM, Brannon RB. Orofacial synovial sarcoma: a clinicopathologic study of 11 new cases and review of the literature. Cancer. 1982;50(2):269–76.
38. Murphey MD, Smith WS, Smith SE, et al. Imaging of musculoskeletal neurogenic tumors: radiologic-pathologic correlation. Radiographics. 1999;19:1253–80.
39. Hirsch RJ, Yousem DM, Loevner LA, et al. Synovial sarcomas of the head and neck: MR findings. Am J Roentgenol. 1997;169(4):1185–8.
40. Villaroel-Salinas J, Campos-Martinez J, Ortiz-Hidalgo C. Synovial sarcoma of the tongue confirmed by molecular detection of the SYT-SSX2 fusion gene transcript. Int J Surg Pathol. 2012;20:386–9.
41. Olsen SH, Thomas DG, Lucas DR. Cluster analysis of immunohistochemical profiles in synovial sarcoma, malignant peripheral nerve sheath tumor, and Ewing sarcoma. Mod Pathol. 2006;19:659–68.
42. Naka N, Takenaka S, Araki N, Toshitada M, Nobuyuki H, Kiyoko Y. Synovial sarcoma is a stem cell malignancy. Stem Cells. 2010;28(7):1119–31.
43. Basile LE, Hoch B, Dillon JK. Synovial sarcoma of the tongue: report of a case. J Oral Maxillofac Surg. 2016;74(1):95–103.
44. Lagrange JL, Ramaioli A, Chateau MC, Marchal C, Resbeut M, Richaud R, et al. Sarcoma after radiation therapy: retrospective multiinstitutional study of 80 histologically confirmed cases. Radiology. 2000;216(1):197–205.
45. Agarwal AP, Shet TM, Joshi R, Desai SB, Chinoy RF, et al. Monophasic synovial sarcoma of tongue. Indian J Pathol Microbiol. 2009;52:568–70.
46. Bilgic B, Mete Ö, Öztürk AS, Demiryont M, Keles N, Basaran M. Synovial sarcoma: a rare tumor of larynx. Pathol Oncol Res. 2003;9:242–5.
47. Fayda M, Aksu G, Agaoglu FY, Karadeniz A, Darendeliler E, Altun M, et al. The role of surgery and radiotherapy in treatment of soft tissue sarcomas of the head and neck region: review of 30 cases. J Craniomaxillofac Surg. 2009;37(1):42–8.
48. Yang JC, Chang AE, Baker AR, Sindelar WF, Danforth DN, Topalian SL, et al. Randomized prospective study of the benefit of adjuvant radiation therapy in the treatment of soft tissue sarcomas of the extremity. J Clin Oncol. 1998;16(1):197–203.
49. National Comprehensive Cancer Network, version 2.2017. Fort Washington: NCCN, 2017.

50. Meer S, Coleman H, Altini M. Oral synovial sarcoma: a report of 2 cases and a review of the literature. Oral Surg Oral Med Oral Pathol Oral Radiol Endod. 2003;96(3):306–15.
51. Su Z, Zhang J, Gao P, Shi J, Qi M, Chen L, Wang X. Synovial sarcoma of the tongue: report of a case and review of the literature. Ann R Coll Surg Engl. 2018;100(5):118–22.
52. Saito T, Mitomi H, Kurisaki A, Torigoe T, Takagi T, Suehara Y, et al. Low-grade myofibroblastic sarcoma of the distal femur. Int J Surg Case Rep. 2013;4:195–9.
53. Roth TM, Fratkin J, Woodring TC, McGehee RP. Low-grade myofibroblastic sarcoma of the vulva. Gynecol Oncol. 2004;92:361–4.
54. Miguel San P, Fernández G, Ortiz-Rey JA, Larrauri P. Low-grade myofibroblastic sarcoma of the distal phalanx. J Hand Surg Am. 2004;29:1160–3.
55. Yamada T, Yoshimura T, Kitamura N, Sasabe E, Ohno S, Yamamoto T. Low-grade myofibroblastic sarcoma of the palate. Int J Oral Sci. 2013;4:170–3.
56. Demarosi F, Bay A, Moneghini L, Carrassi A. Low-grade myofibroblastic sarcoma of the oral cavity. Oral Surg Oral Med Oral Pathol Oral Radiol Endod. 2009;108:248–54.
57. Mikami Y, Fujii S, Kohashi K, Yamada Y, Moriyama M, Kawano S, Nakamura S, Oda Y, Kiyoshima T. Low-grade myofibroblastic sarcoma arising in the tip of the tongue with intravascular invasion: a case report. Oncol Lett. 2018;16(3):3889–94.
58. Gabbiani G, Ryan GB, Majne G. Presence of modified fibroblasts in granulation tissue and their possible role in wound contraction. Experientia. 1971;27:549–50.
59. Follonier L, Schaub S, Meister JJ, Hinz B. Myofibroblast communication is controlled by intercellular mechanical coupling. J Cell Sci. 2008;121:3305–16.
60. Mentzel T. Low-grade myofibroblastic sarcoma. In: Fletcher CDM, Bridge JA, Hogendoorn PCW, Mertens F, editors. World Health Organization classification of tumours: pathology and genetics of tumours of soft tissue and bone. Lyon: IARC Press; 2013. p. 85–6.
61. Tomasek JJ, Gabbianr G, Hinz B, Chaponnier C, Brown RA. Myofibroblasts and mechanoregulation of connective tissue remodelling. Nat Rev Mol Cell Biol. 2002;3:349–63.
62. Niedzielska I, Janic T, Mrowiec B. Low-grade myofibroblastic sarcoma of the mandible: a case report. J Med Case Rep. 2009;3:8458.
63. Oda Y, Sakamoto A, Saito T, Kawauchi S, Iwamoto Y, Tstuneyoshi M. Molecular abnormalities of p53, MDM2, and H-ras in synovial sarcoma. Mod Pathol. 2000;13:994–1004.
64. Erickson-Johnson MR, Chou MM, Evers BR, Roth CW, Seys AR, Jin L, et al. Nodular fasciitis: a novel model of transient neoplasia induced by MYH9-USP6 gene fusion. Lab Investig. 2011;91:1427–33.
65. Kohashi K, Oda Y, Yamamoto H, Tamiya S, Matono H, Iwamoto Y, et al. Reduced expression of SMARCB1/INI1 protein in synovial sarcoma. Mod Pathol. 2010;23:981–90.
66. Lee PJ, Yoo NS, Hagemann IS, Pfeifer JD, Cottrell CE, Abel HJ, et al. Spectrum of mutations in leiomyosarcomas identified by clinical targeted next-generation sequencing. ERP Mol Pathol. 2017;102:156–61.
67. Overholtzer M, Rao PH, Favis R, Lu XY, Elowitz MB, Barany F, et al. The presence of p53 mutations in human osteosarcomas correlates with high levels of genomic instability. Proc Natl Acad Sci U S A. 2003;100:11547–52.
68. Cerio R. Spindle cell neoplasms. J Eur Acad Dermatol Venereol. 1998;11:52.
69. Jo VY, Fletcher CD. WHO classification of soft tissue tumours: an update based on the 2013. Pathology. 2014;46:95–104.
70. Teleb M, Olivas CC, Kanu O, Ramos LD, Sumayin N, Albaghdadi A, et al. Spindle-cell sarcoma involving the major pulmonary arteries. PRO. 2017;30:311–3.
71. Siyad AK, Gopi P, Jayan NP, Augustine J. Spindle cell sarcoma of thyroid: a case report. Indian J Surg Oncol. 2014;5:312–4.
72. Fletcher CD. The evolving classification of soft tissue tumours–an update based on the new 2013 WHO classification. Histopathology. 2014;64:2–11.
73. Bills V, Iqbal R, Haqqani M, Clague JE. Spindle cell sarcoma: a rare cause of a large abdominal mass. Age Ageing. 2005;34:88–9.

74. Mehra S, Ibrahim O, Moshiri M, Cahill J, Bhargava P. Spindle-cell sarcoma of the heart: a rare cause for a cardiac mass. Radiol Case Rep. 2012;7:792.
75. Patel KN, Jha RK, Pandya SJ. Surgical management of primary spindle cell sarcoma of prostate. Urology. 2017;105:7–8.
76. Muturi A, Kotecha V, Ruturi J, Muhinga M, Waweru W. High-grade spindle cell sarcoma of the heart: a case report and review of literature. J Cardiothorac Surg. 2015;10:46.
77. Lokesh V, Naveen T, Pawar YS. Spindle cell sarcoma of esophagus: a rare case presentation. J Cancer Res Therap. 2010;6:100–1.
78. Bhaumik G, Chatterjee K. Spindle cell sarcoma of the maxillary antrum. J Indian Med Assoc. 2012;110:657–8.
79. Borden EC, Baker LH, Bell RS, Bramwell V, Demetri GD, Eisenberg BL, et al. Soft tissue sarcomas of adults: state of the translational science. Clin Cancer Res. 2003;9:1941–56.
80. Feng L, Wang M, Yibulayin F, Zhang H, Yang Y, Ren F, Wushou A. Spindle cell sarcoma: a SEER population-based analysis. Sci Rep. 2018;8:5024.
81. Wushou A, Jiang YZ, Liu YR, Shao ZM. The demographic features, clinicopathologic characteristics, treatment outcome and disease-specific prognostic factors of solitary fibrous tumor: a population-based analysis. Oncotarget. 2015;6:41875–83.
82. Feng L, Cai D, Muhetaer A, Yang YL, Ren F, Yishake M, et al. Spindle cell carcinoma: the general demographics, basic clinico-pathologic characteristics, treatment, outcome and prognostic factors. Oncotarget. 2017;8:43228–36.
83. Collini P, Sorensen PHB, Patel S, Blay JY, Issels RD, Maki RG, et al. Sarcomas with spindle cell morphology. Semin Oncol. 2009;36:324–37.
84. Kaposi sarcoma treatment. National Cancer Institute. 2017.
85. Schwartz RA, Micali G, Nasca MR, Scuderi L. Kaposi sarcoma: a continuing conundrum. J Am Acad Dermatol. 2008;59(2):179–206.
86. Hoffmann C, Sabranski M, Esser S. HIV-associated Kaposi's sarcoma. Oncol Res Treat. 2017;40(3):94–8.
87. Ferri, Fred F. Ferri's clinical advisor. 2018 E-Book: 5 Books in 1. Elsevier Health Sciences. 2017. p. 735.
88. Kaposi Sarcoma Treatment. National Cancer Institute. 2015.
89. Kaposi M. Idiopathisches multiples Pigmentsarkom der Haut. Arch Dermatol Syph. 1872;4(2):265–73.
90. Ablashi DV, Chatlynne LG, Whitman JE, Cesarman E. Spectrum of Kaposi's sarcoma-associated herpesvirus, or human herpesvirus 8, diseases. Clin Microbiol Rev. 2002;15(3):439–64.
91. Pauk J, Huang ML, Brodie SJ, Wald A, Koelle DM, Schacker T, et al. Mucosal shedding of human herpesvirus 8 in men. N Engl J Med. 2000;343(19):1369–77.
92. Parravicini C, Olsen SJ, Capra M, Poli F, Sirchia G, Gao SJ, et al. Risk of Kaposi's sarcoma-associated herpes virus transmission from donor allografts among Italian posttransplant Kaposi's sarcoma patients. Blood. 1997;90(7):2826–9.
93. Hladik W, Dollard SC, Mermin J, Fowlkes AL, Downing R, Amin MM, et al. Transmission of human herpesvirus 8 by blood transfusion. N Engl J Med. 2006;355(13):1331–8.
94. Coffin JM, Hughes SH, Varmus HE. Retroviruses. Cold Spring Harbor: Cold Spring Harbor Laboratory Press; 1997.
95. Ensoli B, Sirianni MC. Kaposi's sarcoma pathogenesis: a link between immunology and tumor biology. Crit Rev Oncog. 1998;9(2):107–24.
96. Gurzu S, Ciortea D, Munteanu T, Kezdi-Zaharia I, Jung I. Mesenchymal-to-endothelial transition in Kaposi sarcoma: a histogenetic hypothesis based on a case series and literature review. PLoS One. 2008;8(8):e71530.
97. Beckstead JH, Wood GS, Fletcher V. Evidence for the origin of Kaposi's sarcoma from lymphatic endothelium. Am J Pathol. 1985;119(2):294–300.
98. Rosai J. Rosai and Ackerman's surgical pathology. 10th ed. St. Louis: Mosby; 2011.

99. Weninger W, et al. Expression of vascular endothelial growth factor receptor-3 and podoplanin suggest a lymphatic endothelial origin of Kaposi's sarcoma tumor cells. Lab Investig. 1999;79:243–51.
100. Dezube BJ. Clinical presentation and natural history of AIDS–related Kaposi's sarcoma. Hematol Oncol Clin North Am. 1996;10(5):1023–9.
101. Kaposi's Sarcoma. Taber's cylcopedic medical dictionary, vol. 21. Philadelphia: FA Davis Company; 2009. p. 1256.
102. Soyer HP, Jakob L, Metzler G, Chen KM, Garbe C. Non-AIDS associated Kaposi's sarcoma: clinical features and treatment outcome. PLoS ONE. 2011;6(4):e18397.
103. Nichols CM, Flaitz CM, Hicks MJ. Treating Kaposi's lesions in the HIV-infected patient. JADA. 1993;124(11):78–84.
104. Danzig JB, Brandt LJ, Reinus JF, Klein RS. Gastrointestinal malignancy in patients with AIDS. Am J Gastroenterol. 1991;86(6):715–8.
105. Garay SM, Belenko M, Fazzini E, Schinella R. Pulmonary manifestations of Kaposi's sarcoma. Chest. 1987;91(1):39–43.
106. Blumenfeld W, et al. Differential diagnosis of Kaposi's sarcoma. Arch Pathol Lab Med. 1985;109:123–7.
107. James W, Berger T. Elston D Andrews' diseases of the skin: clinical dermatology. 10th ed. Philadelphia: WB Saunders; 2005.
108. Kumar P. Classic Kaposi's sarcoma in Arabs-widening ethnic involvement. J Cancer Res Therap. 2011;7(1):92–4.
109. Iscovich J, Boffetta P, Winkelmann R, Brennan P, Azizi E. Classic Kaposi's sarcoma in Jews living in Israel, 1961-1989: a population-based incidence study. AIDS. 1998;12(15):2067–72.
110. Fenig E, Brenner B, Rakowsky E, Lapidoth M, Katz A, Sulkes A. Classic Kaposi sarcoma: experience at Rabin Medical Center in Israel. Am J Clin Oncol. 1998;21(5):498–500.
111. Cook-Mozaffari P, Newton R, Beral V, Burkitt DP. The geographical distribution of Kaposi's sarcoma and of lymphomas in Africa before the AIDS epidemic. Br J Cancer. 1998;78(11):1521–8.
112. Olsen SJ, Chang Y, Moore PS, Biggar RJ, Melbye M. Increasing Kaposi's sarcoma-associated herpesvirus seroprevalence with age in a highly Kaposi's sarcoma endemic region, Zambia in 1985. AIDS. 1998;12(14):1921–5.
113. Qunibi W, Al-Furayh O, Almeshari K, Lin SF, Sun R, Heston L, Ross D, Rigsby M, Miller G. Serologic association of human herpesvirus eight with posttransplant Kaposi's sarcoma in Saudi Arabia. Transplantation. 1998;65(4):583–5.
114. Luppi M, Barozzi P, Schulz TF, Setti G, Staskus K, Trovato R, et al. Bone marrow failure associated with human herpesvirus 8 infection after transplantation. N Engl J Med. 2000;43(19):1378–85.
115. Borkovic SP, Schwartz RA. Kaposi's sarcoma presenting in the homosexual man - a new and striking phenomenon. Ariz Med. 1981;38(12):902–4.
116. Hausen HZ. Rhadinoviruses. Infections causing human cancer. Weinheim: Wiley; 2006.
117. Drabell FG. Kaposi's sarcoma and renal diseases. New topics in cancer research. New York: Nova Biomedical Books; 2006.
118. Beral V, Peterman TA, Berkelman RL, Jaffe HW. Kaposi's sarcoma among persons with AIDS: a sexually transmitted infection? Lancet. 1990;335(8682):123–8.
119. Tappero JW, Berger TG, Kaplan LD, Volberding PA, Kahn JO. Cryotherapy for cutaneous Kaposi's sarcoma (KS) associated with acquired immune deficiency syndrome (AIDS): a phase II trial. AIDS. 1991;4(9):839–46.
120. Zimmerman EE, Crawford P. Cutaneous cryosurgery. Am Fam Physician. 2012;86(12):1118–24.
121. Anglemyer A, Agrawal AK, Rutherford GW. Treatment of Kaposi sarcoma in children with HIV-1 infection. Cochrane Database Syst Rev. 2014;1(1):CD009826.
122. McAllister SC, Hanson RS, Manion RD. Propranolol decreases proliferation of endothelial cells transformed by Kaposi's sarcoma-associated herpesvirus and induces lytic viral gene expression. J Virol. 2015;89(21):11144–9.

123. Abdelmaksoud A, Filoni A, Giudice G, Vestita M. Classic and HIV-related Kaposi sarcoma treated with 0.1% topical timolol gel. JADA. 2017;76(1):153–5.
124. Gill PS, Tulpule A, Espina BM, Cabriales S, Bresnahan J, Ilaw M, et al. Paclitaxel is safe and effective in the treatment of advanced AIDS-related Kaposi's sarcoma. J Clin Oncol. 1999;17(6):1876–83.
125. Sgadari C, Toschi E, Palladino C, Barillari G, Carlei D, Cereseto A, et al. Mechanism of paclitaxel activity in Kaposi's sarcoma. J Immunol. 2000;165(1):509–17.
126. Summary of product characteristics. EMA.

Tongue Manifestations of Systemic Diseases

11

11.1 Overview

Oral manifestations of systemic diseases, including those involving the tongue, are common and diverse. They may be the direct result of disease pathology, secondary infiltrative processes, or treatment-related adverse effects. Oral manifestations may be (1) the first, only, or most severe feature of systemic disease, (2) the principal focus of therapy, and/or (3) the dominant cause of affecting the person's quality of life.

The appearance of the tongue may serve as an indicator of the general health of the individual. Tongue manifestations, including change in color and texture, can be the presenting symptom of many systemic diseases and can be helpful in the diagnosis and management of the underlying disorder. Thus, a careful medical and social history is critical to ensure that diagnosis and treatment are not delayed. Furthermore, many of the tongue pathologies cause pain and discomfort and are likely to cause changes in taste, all of which not only negatively impact patients' quality of life but may also lead to inadequate food and water intake. Thus, oral manifestations in general and tongue manifestations in particular must be promptly recognized and appropriately treated.

This chapter provides a general overview of tongue manifestations (as part of oral manifestations) of systemic diseases. It is not intended to provide details about the diagnosis and management of these conditions. The different systemic diseases with examples of the disorders of each system are summarized in Table 11.1.

© The Author(s), under exclusive license to Springer Nature Switzerland AG 2022

M. F. Sakr, *Tongue Lesions*, https://doi.org/10.1007/978-3-031-08198-9_11

Table 11.1 Systemic conditions with tongue manifestations

Systemic disease	Examples
Gastrointestinal diseases	• Inflammatory bowel disease (IBD): ulcerative colitis, Crohn's disease • Pyostomatitis vegetans • Chronic liver disease (CLD)—hepatitis C • Celiac disease
Nutritional diseases	• Water-soluble vitamin deficiency • Fat-soluble vitamin deficiency • Mineral deficiency
Hematologic disorders	• WBC disorders: leukemia, lymphoma, cyclic neutropenia • Platelet disorders: thrombocytopenia • RBC disorders: anemias, hemochromocytosis, congenital erythropoietic porphyria, thalassemias (sickle cell disease, polycythemia vera)
Autoimmune disorders	• Sjogren's syndrome • Kawasaki disease • Systemic lupus erythematosis (SLE) • Scleroderma (systemic sclerosis)
Pulmonary conditions	• Granulomatosis with polyangitis • Sarcoidosis
Multisystem conditions	• Amyloidosis
Immune system disorders	• HIV diseases: candidiasis, herpes simplex (HS), hairy leukoplakia, Kaposi sarcoma, cytomegalovirus (CMV), human papilloma virus (HPV), aphthous-like ulcerations
Cutaneous diseases	• Psoriasis • Acanthosis Negricans
Neurological diseases	• Neurofibromatosis (types 1 and 2)
Endocrine diseases	• Diabetes mellitus (DM) • Thyroid gland disorder • Parathyroid gland (PTG) disorders • Adrenal disorders
Renal diseases	• Uremic stomatitis • Diseases related to immunosuppressants after transplantation
Drug-induced conditions	• Aphthus stomatitis • Dry mouth • Lichen planus • Conditions due to inhalational steroids
Psychiatric disorders	• Anorexia nervosa • Bulimia nervosa

11.2 Gastrointestinal (GI) Diseases

11.2.1 Inflammatory Bowel Disease (IBD)

While *Crohn's disease* can affect any part of the GI tract (from the oral cavity to the anus), inflammation in ulcerative colitis is generally restricted to the colon and is specifically limited to the mucosa and submucosa. In *ulcerative colitis*, aphthous ulcers in the oral cavity or angular stomatitis occur in as many as 5–10% of patients,

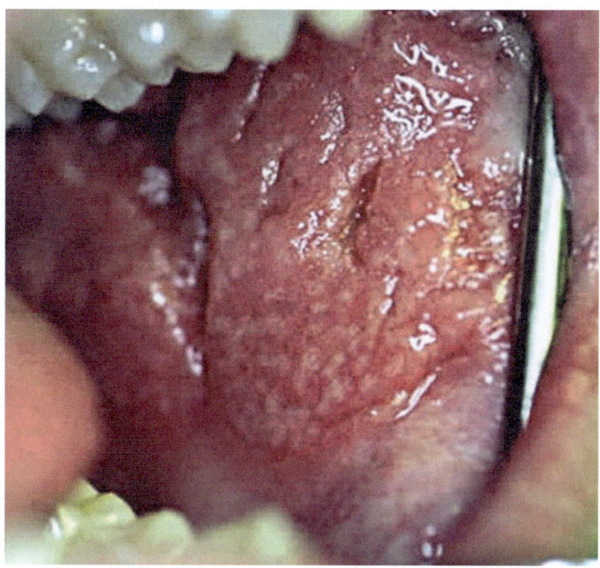

Fig. 11.1 The tongue of a patient with ulcerative colitis who developed pyostomatitis vegetans (PSV) presenting with pustules with a "snail track" appearance, multiple erosions, and vegetations

although hemorrhagic ulcers can also occur [1]. Rarely, patients can develop pyostomatitis vegetans (PSV) (Fig. 11.1).

Intra-oral involvement occurs in up to 50% of patients with *Crohn's disease* and may precede intestinal involvement [2]. The severity of oral lesions may indicate the severity of the systemic disease and, as such, may be used as a marker for intestinal impairment [3]. Specific oral findings of Crohn's disease include diffuse lip, gingival, or mucosal swelling; cobble stoning of the buccal mucosa and gingiva; mucosal tags; and fissures at the angles of the mouth [4, 5]. These lesions are considered *specific*, because histological examination reveals evidence of the characteristic noncaseating granulomatous change [4–6].

Nonspecific oral findings of Crohn's disease (i.e. lesions for which histology does not reveal granulomatous change) are more common than the specific oral findings [5] and include glossitis (Fig. 11.2) and aphthous ulcers. Approximately 5% of patients with Crohn's disease have aphthous ulcers, which are indistinguishable from classic aphthae [6]. Patient symptoms may include significant pain, impaired speech, or difficulty eating secondary to gingival and mucosal swelling, ulcers, or fissures. Patients who present with oral findings suggestive of Crohn's disease warrant a full systemic evaluation, including colonoscopy and biopsy with histopathological correlation.

11.2.2 Pyostomatitis Vegetans (PSV)

Pyostomatitis vegetans (PVS) is considered a rare specific finding of IBD, and its presence can precede GI symptoms by months or years [7]. It presents as pustules with a "snail track" appearance, erosions (Fig. 11.3), and vegetations involving the labial mucosa of the upper and lower lips, buccal mucosa, and gingival mucosa.

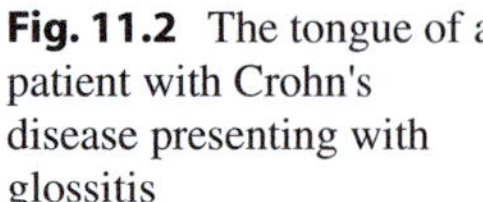

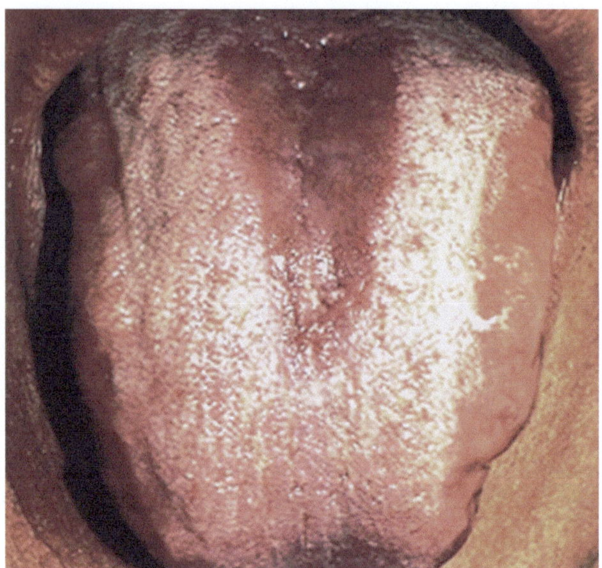

Fig. 11.2 The tongue of a patient with Crohn's disease presenting with glossitis

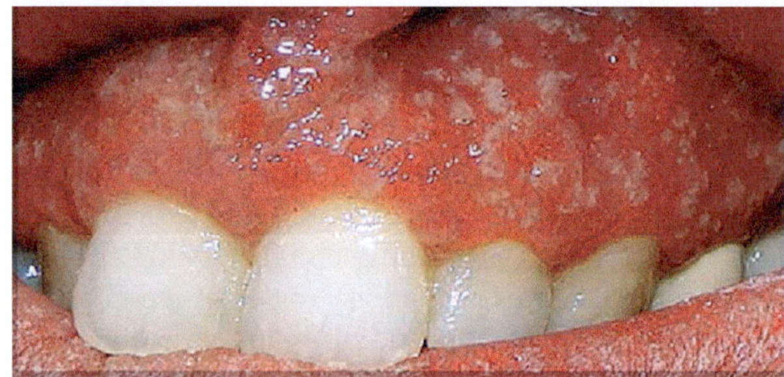

Fig. 11.3 Pyostomatitis vegetans (PVS) presenting with multiple tongue erosions

While the tongue and floor of the mouth are generally spared, the filiform and fungiform lingual papillae may be atrophic [5, 6, 8]. Moreover, PSV also affects the mucosal membranes in the vagina, nasal passages, and periocular region [5]. Symptoms such as pain and burning may be severe or negligible [6]. Histological examination reveals both intraepithelial and subepithelial eosinophilic miliary abscesses [6].

11.2.3 Chronic Liver Disease (CLD)

The systemic manifestations of CLD are numerous and can be classified as those due to (1) synthetic dysfunction (e.g. coagulopathies, hypoalbuminemia), (2) portal hypertension (e.g. ascites, esophageal varices, hemorrhoids), (3) bilirubin secretion (e.g. jaundice), (4) increased circulating estrogen (e.g. gynecomastia, testicular atrophy), as well as more complex syndromes including hepatorenal syndrome and hepatopulmonary syndrome [9, 10].

Cutaneous manifestations due to CLD include spider nevi due to estrogen excess, easy bruising or petichiae secondary to coagulopathies, jaundice, or caput medusa, which is pathognomonic for portal hypertension [11]. Oral manifestations are also common in patients with CLD. For example, due to coagulopathies, patients may have petichiae on the mucous membranes or excessive gingival bleeding with minor trauma, often in the absence of inflammation [12]. Jaundice may also appear in the oral mucosa due to the yellow pigmentation that results from deposition of bilirubin into the submucosa [13]. Because the sublingual and soft palate mucosae are very thin, they are often first to show a yellow hue [13].

Hepatitis C virus (HCV) is one of the leading causes of CLD worldwide [14–16] and those patients with CLD have a 2.5- to 4.5-fold increased risk of developing lichen planus (LP) [14, 15]. Oral LP may be classified based on clinical presentation. *Reticular LP*, the most common form, presents as white papules or plaques on a bed of erythema with Wickham striae [17, 18]. The buccal mucosa, tongue, and gingivae may be involved. It is generally asymptomatic [17]. Other less common forms of LP include erosive LP, erythematous (atrophic) LP, and papular (plaque-like) LP [17, 18]. Rarely, bullous LP may be observed [18]. Histology reveals a band-like lymphocytic infiltrate with a saw-tooth appearance of the rete ridges, as well as parakeratosis, acanthosis, and orthokeratotic hyperkeratosis [19]. Colloid bodies and Max-Joseph spaces are also classic findings more specific to LP [19].

11.2.4 Celiac Disease

Celiac disease is a chronic intestinal disease caused by intolerance to gluten associated with poor digestion and absorption of the majority of nutrients and vitamins, which may affect both developing dentition and oral mucosa. Enamel hypoplasia is the most common manifestation in untreated celiac children and adolescents. It results from hypocalcemia during enamel formation and other systemic factors such as malnutrition and vitamin D and A deficiency. The main oral manifestations associated with celiac disease are angular chelitis, glossitis, depapillated tongue (Fig. 11.4), and dry mouth. Ulcers are the most common type of oral lesions presenting in a papular or erosive form, generally with an erythematous margin.

11.3 Nutritional Diseases

Nutritional deficiencies often result in impairments in the integrity of skin and mucous membranes [20]. They may result from (1) a reduced intake due to poor diet, fatty diets, alcohol or drug addiction, and psychiatric disease (2) failure to absorb ingested vitamins and minerals due to pancreatic insufficiency, infectious agents, enzyme deficiencies, GI disease, systemic diseases, and intestinal resection or radiation, or (3) increased host demand (e.g. gravid women).

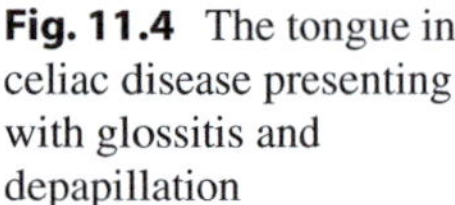

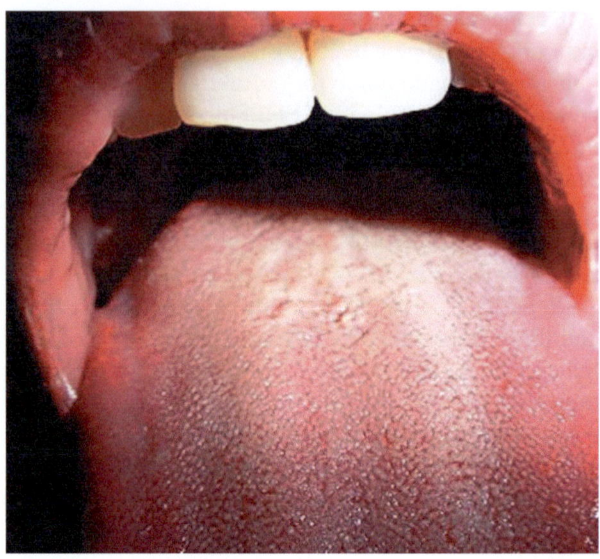

Fig. 11.4 The tongue in celiac disease presenting with glossitis and depapillation

11.3.1 Water-Soluble Vitamin Deficiency

Water-soluble vitamins include vitamin B-2 (riboflavin), B-3 (niacin), B-5 (pantothenic acid), B-6 (pyridoxine), B-7 (biotin, vitamin H), B-9 (folic acid), B-12 (cobalamin), and vitamin C (L-ascorbic acid) [21]. These vitamins are stored in the body in limited quantities and therefore require regular replenishment through dietary intake. Water-soluble vitamin deficiencies with oral manifestations including the tongue are listed in Table 11.2. Currently, there are no known oral manifestations of vitamin B-5 (pantothenic acid) or B-7 (biotin, vitamin H) deficiencies (Figs. 11.5 and 11.6).

11.3.2 Fat-Soluble Vitamin Deficiency/Toxicity

Vitamins A, D, E, and K are fat soluble and thus are readily stored in the body [27]. While these reservoirs successfully prevent against deficiencies, the resultant risk of hypervitaminosis is increased. There are no oral manifestations of vitamins E, D, or K toxicity or vitamin E deficiency. Oral manifestations of fat-soluble vitamin deficiencies and toxicities are summarized in Table 11.3.

Table 11.2 Oral manifestation of water-soluble vitamin deficiencies

Vitamin Deficiency	Oral Manifestations	References
Vitamin B-2 (riboflavin, lactoflavin) deficiency	• Erythema of pharyngeal and oral mucosa • Atrophic glossitis, often with a magenta hue • Glossodynia • Cheilosis and angular cheilitis	Schlosser et al. [20]
Vitamin B-3 (niacin, nicotinic acid) deficiency (pellagra)	• Mucosal edema • Cheilosis and angular cheilitis • Bright red glossitis • Burning mouth • Gingival erythema • Dental caries	Schlosser et al. [20], Boyd and Palmer [22]
Vitamin B-6 (pyridoxine, pyridoxal, pyridoxamine) deficiency	• Atrophic glossitis • Cheilosis • Angular stomatitis • Gingival erythema	Schlosser et al. [20]
Vitamin B-9 (folic acid, folate) deficiency	• Atrophic glossitis with erythema and swelling of the tongue • Angular cheilitis • Glossodynia • Dysphagia • Recurrent aphthous stomatitis	Schlosser et al. [20], Kozlak et al. [23]
Vitamin B-12 (cobalamin, cyanocobalamin) deficiency	• Generalized stomatitis • Taste disturbance • Red, atrophic, beefy, burning tongue (Fig. 11.5) with bald appearance due to loss of filiform papillae (Fig. 11.6) • Recurrent aphthous stomatitis	Schlosser et al. [20], Kozlak et al. [23], Field et al. [24]
Vitamin C (ascorbic acid, L-ascorbic acid, ascorbate) deficiency, also known as scurvy	• Mucosal petichiae • Hemorrhagic gingivitis • Gingival bleeding • Gingival hypertrophy • Interdental infarcts • Loosening or loss of teeth	Schlosser et al. [20], Leggott et al. [25], Yasui et al. [26]

11.3.3 Mineral Deficiencies

Minerals are crucial to numerous cellular functions and deficiencies have been associated with many systemic diseases. Minerals such as calcium and magnesium have been associated with periodontal disease [30]. Additional oral manifestations of mineral deficiencies are listed in Table 11.4.

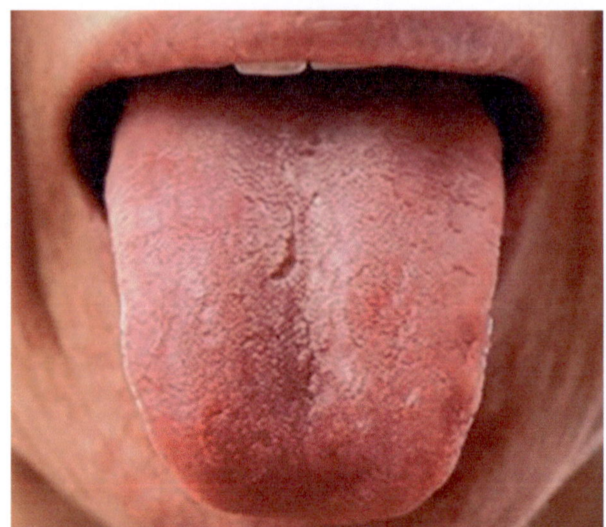

Fig. 11.5 The tongue of a patient with vitamin B-12 deficiency showing a characteristic red, atrophic, beefy appearance

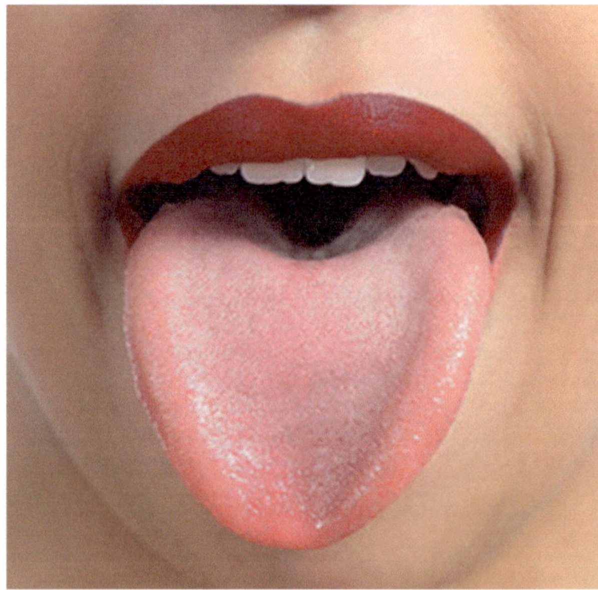

Fig. 11.6 The tongue of a patient with vitamin B-12 deficiency showing a bald appearance due to loss of filiform papillae

Table 11.3 Oral manifestation of fat-soluble vitamin deficiencies and toxicities

Vitamin deficiency/toxicity	Oral manifestations	References
Vitamin A (retinol) deficiency	• Xerostomia • Periodontal disease • Increased intraoral infection • Impaired tooth development in children	Schlosser et al. [20]
Vitamin A (retinol) toxicity	• Cheilitis • Gingivitis • Impaired healing	Schlosser et al. [20]
Vitamin D (calciferol, cholecalciferol, ergocalciferol) deficiency	• Periodontal attachment • Recurrent aphthous stomatitis	Schlosser et al. [20], Khabbazi et al. [28], Holick and Chen [29]
Vitamin K (phylloquinone) deficiency	• Submucosal hemorrhage • Gingival bleeding	Schlosser et al. [20]

Table 11.4 Oral manifestation of mineral deficiencies

Mineral deficiency	Oral manifestations	References
Iron deficiency	• Angular cheilitis • Atrophic glossitis • Glossodynia • Recurrent aphthous stomatitis	Schlosser et al. [20], Sun et al. [31], Zimmermann and Hurrell [32]
Zinc deficiency	• Burning mouth syndrome • Recurrent aphthous stomatitis • Perioral or intra-oral erosions • Dysgeusia (taste alteration)	Cho et al. [33], Orback et al. [34], Nakano et al. [35], Epstein and Barasch [36], Hambidge and Krebs [37]

11.4 Hematological Disorders

11.4.1 White Blood Cell (WBC) Disorders

11.4.1.1 Leukemia

Leukemias are classified by their clinical course (acute or chronic) and the progenitor cell lineage primarily effected (lymphoid or myeloid) [38, 39]. Systemically, dysregulated leukocyte proliferation results in suppressed hematopoiesis, often leading to anemia and thrombocytopenia. Since leukocytes are a critical component of the immune system, patients with leukemias are also at increased risk of infection. Cutaneous manifestations include leukemic skin infiltrations (leukemia cutis), as well as nonspecific lesions (e.g., cutaneous infections, vasculitis, purpura, paraneoplastic pemphigus, Sweet syndrome) or therapy-induced lesions (e.g., drug reactions, graft vs. host disease) [40, 41].

Oral manifestations are more common in acute leukemias than in chronic leukemias [42]. Gingival hypertrophy and hyperplasia are most commonly associated with acute myelogenous leukemia and acute promyelocytic leukemia [43]. Thrombocytopenia commonly manifests as petichiae and ecchymoses on the mucosal surfaces of the mouth, as well as spontaneous gingival bleeding [44]. Chemotherapeutic drugs may cause diffuse oral ulceration (mucositis), which should be differentiated from herpes simplex virus (HSV) or cytomegalovirus (CMV) infection [45]. Chemotherapeutics often cause immunosuppression and, thus, increase the risk for secondary viral, fungal, and bacterial infections in the oral cavity [42].

11.4.1.2 Lymphoma

Oral manifestations of Hodgkin lymphoma are uncommon, although they may develop secondary to chemotherapeutic agents. Certain subtypes of non-Hodgkin lymphoma (NHL), such as cutaneous T-cell lymphoma, Burkett lymphoma, and AIDS-associated lymphoma, are commonly associated with both cutaneous and oral manifestations. Lymphomas in the oral cavity are generally described as painless soft masses, with or without traumatic ulceration (Fig. 11.7) [20].

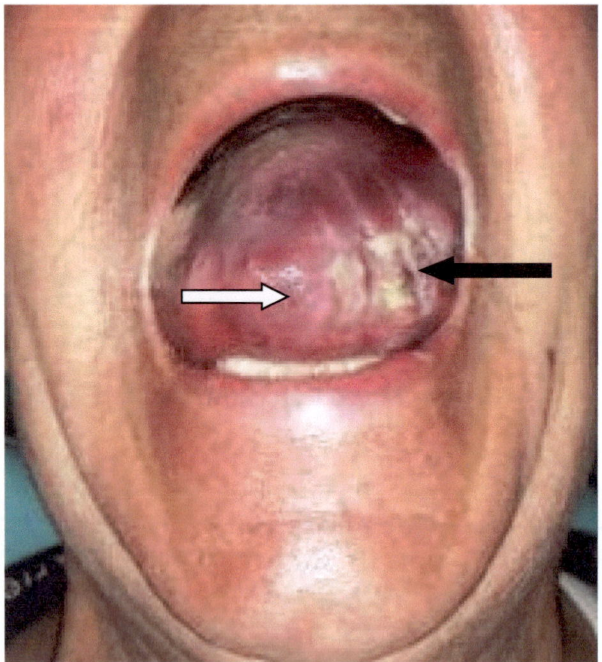

Fig. 11.7 The tongue of a 52-year-old patient with non-Hodgkin lymphoma showing a soft mass (white arrow) with traumatic ulcerations (black arrow)

Although cutaneous and lymph node involvement is most common in *cutaneous T-cell lymphoma*, oral lesions have been observed in a minority of patients and include ulcerated plaques or solid tumors on the gingiva, palate, or tongue [46]. Histological examination reveals a dense inflammatory infiltrate with atypical lymphocytes and Darier-Pautrier microabscesses [46]. Oral lesions represent advanced disease and indicate a poor prognosis [46].

An aggressive B-cell lymphoma, *Burkitt lymphoma* is associated with Epstein-Barr virus (EBV) and can be classified as one of three subtypes: endemic, sporadic, or immunodeficiency-related. Burkett lymphoma generally presents as a rapidly enlarging mass, frequently involving the head and neck [47]. Oral involvement in *AIDS-associated lymphoma* occurs in approximately 3% of cases and may present with masses or ulcers that involve the gingiva, palate, tonsils, tongue, and lower jaw [48, 49].

11.4.1.3 Cyclic Neutropenia

Cyclic neutropenia is a rare disorder due to an inherited or sporadic mutation in the neutrophil elastase gene (*ELANE*), which is located on band 19p13.3 [50, 51]. It is characterized by periodic (21-day cycles) failures of hematopoiesis, leading to neutropenia, as well as decreased monocyte, eosinophil, lymphocyte, platelet, and reticulocyte counts [52–54]. These failures lead to transient recurrent fevers, malaise, and recurrent infections that may be life- threatening [20]. Onset of symptoms occurs in childhood and may improve as the patient approaches adulthood [53].

Oral manifestations are present in over 90% of patients with cyclic neutropenia [55]. In one series, investigators reported that 94% of patients had recurrent ulcers similar to recurrent aphthous stomatitis [55]. These ulcers vary in size and may be found on the buccal mucosa, lips, tongue, and pharynx [55, 56]. They generally present during periods of neutropenia and resolve within 1–2 days once neutrophil counts rebound [56]. Granulocyte colony-stimulating factor (G-CSF) can be used to improve neutrophil counts and reduce morbidity [57]. Patients should also be diligent about oral hygiene to reduce the risk of intra-oral infection.

11.4.2 Platelet Disorders

Thrombocytopenia is defined as a reduced number of circulating platelets, generally below 150,000/μL [58]. Since platelets play an integral role in the maintenance of hemostasis, thrombocytopenia leads to an increased risk of bleeding. There are numerous causes of thrombocytopenia, including autoimmune destruction, splenic sequestration, bone marrow infiltration by tumor cells, infection, and drug reactions [20].

In the oral cavity, petichiae and ecchymoses may be visible on the soft palate and buccal mucosa [20]. Gingival bleeding is common and often spontaneous [20]. Hemorrhagic bullae that appear as deep red-to-violaceous or black blisters may appear on mucosal surfaces in cases of severe thrombocytopenia (<50,000/μL) [59].

11.4.3 Red Blood Cell (RBC) Disorders

11.4.3.1 Anemias

Common anemias associated with tongue manifestations include iron-deficiency anemia (atrophic glossitis and Glossodynia) and macrocystic anemia secondary to B-12 deficiency(red, atrophic, beefy, burning tongue with bald appearance due to loss of filiform papillae. Of note, all forms of anemia can result in mucosal pallor.

11.4.3.2 Hemochromatosis

Hemochromatosis, a syndrome of systemic iron overload, may be caused by hereditary hemochromatosis, transfusional iron overload, chronic hemolysis, or excess dietary iron [60]. Common systemic sequelae include liver cirrhosis, cardiomyopathy, arthritis, and various endocrinopathies [61]. Cutaneous manifestations include skin hyperpigmentation resulting in the classic "bronzed" appearance [61]. Oral manifestations are observed in approximately 15–25% of patients in the form of a blue-gray hyperpigmentation of the oral mucosa [62]. The most commonly affected sites are the buccal mucosa and gingiva, although a minority of patients have diffuse, homogenous pigmentation of the oral cavity [20, 61, 62]. Histological examination with Prussian blue stain reveals iron mineral deposits [20].

11.4.3.3 Congenital Erythropoietic Porphyria (CEP)

Congenital erythropoietic porphyria (CEP) is a rare, autosomal recessive disease caused by a mutation in the *UROS* gene, which encodes uroporphyrinogen III synthase [63]. This enzyme defect disrupts heme biosynthesis and leads to an accumulation of uroporphyrin in erythrocytes, which, in turn, increases their osmotic fragility and results in hemolysis [20]. In the oral cavity, erythrodontia, a red-brown discoloration of the teeth, is pathognomonic for congenital erythropoietic porphyria [20, 64]. Teeth appear bright red with exposure to UV fluorescence [63].

11.4.3.4 Thalassemias

11.4.3.4.1 Sickle Cell Disease (SCD)

Sickle cell disease (SCD) is an autosomal recessive hemoglobinopathy that causes erythrocyte malformation [20, 65–67]. The clinical manifestations of SCD are diverse, but often relate to the vaso-occlusive events, microvascular infarctions, hemolysis, and increased infectious susceptibility. Pain crises, acute chest syndrome, priapism, dactylitis, osteomyelitis, and strokes represent some of the most common sequelae of SCD [67]. Cutaneous manifestations include ulcers (mostly commonly leg ulcers) and pseudo-xanthoma elasticum–like lesions [68]. Pallor and jaundice of the oral mucosa secondary to anemia and hemolysis are the most common oral manifestations of SCD [20]. Patients with SCD may also experience mental nerve neuropathy secondary to infarction of nerve branches, which may cause numbness of the chin, lips, gingiva, mucosa, and even teeth [20, 65].

11.4.3.4.2 Polycythemia Vera

The clinical signs of polycythemia vera include elevated hematocrit, thrombocytosis, and leukocytosis [69]. Patients are at significantly increased risk of thrombosis [69, 70]. Common systemic manifestations include microvascular abnormalities, erythromegaly, and splenomegaly [70, 71]. Patients often experience constitutional symptoms, such as fatigue and headache [70, 71]. Cutaneous manifestations include aquagenic pruritus and evidence of bleeding complications such as ecchymoses [70, 71]. Rarely, polycythemia vera can manifest orally with petichial hemorrhages, easy bruising, and gingival bleeding with minor trauma [72, 73]. A deep red, violaceous hue may be present on the tongue, gingiva, and other mucosal surfaces [72–74].

11.5 Autoimmune Diseases

11.5.1 Sjogren's Syndrome (SS)

Sjogren's syndrome (SS) is an autoimmune disease in which the salivary and lacrimal glands are targeted. It is the second most common autoimmune disease, affecting as many as 3% of women aged 50 years or older. Over 85% of patients are female [75]. Systemically, SS is characterized by sicca syndrome, including keratoconjunctivitis sicca and xerostomia [76]. Cutaneous manifestations include xerosis, angular cheilitis, eyelid dermatitis, annular erythema, and vascular lesions, such as palpable purpura and urticarial vasculitis [77].

In SS, saliva can be thick, ropey, and mucinous, or it may be altogether absent [78]. Oral mucosal changes are those typical of xerostomia. They include dry, red, and wrinkled mucosa and a cobblestone-like appearance of the tongue (Fig. 11.8),

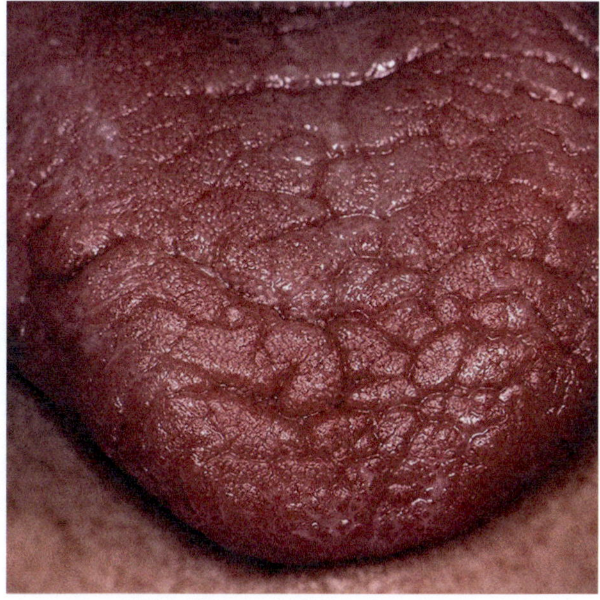

Fig. 11.8 Oral dryness secondary to Sjogren's syndrome—the tongue has cobblestone-like appearance. It is notably fissured and also has signs of mild oral lichen planus

owing to atrophy of the papillae [79]. Tongue fissuring and angular cheilitis are also common [79]. Candidiasis is common [80] and an increased incidence of dental caries is also seen in SS [80, 81]. Common symptoms include odynophagia, dysphagia, disturbances in taste, and difficulty speaking secondary to decreased salivary production [79, 82–84]. Certain medications can maximize saliva production from the remaining functional glands. Good oral hygiene and frequent dental visits are essential to minimize the deleterious effects of compromised salivary flow.

11.5.2 Kawasaki Disease

Kawasaki disease, or mucocutaneous lymph node syndrome, is a vasculitis that primarily affects medium and large vessels. Kawasaki disease generally affects children younger than 5 years and has replaced rheumatic fever as the primary cause of childhood heart disease in the United States [85]. Diagnostic criteria include a fever lasting 5 days or more, and at least four of the five following findings: (1) acute cervical lymphadenopathy, (2) peripheral extremity edema, erythema, or desquamation, (3) bilateral painless conjunctival injection, (4) polymorphous exanthema, and (5) oral mucosae erythema or strawberry tongue [86]. Cardiac sequelae of the vasculitis include aneurysms and myocardial infarction [86, 87]. Myocarditis commonly occurs within a week following fever resolution [86].

Oral findings, one of the five diagnostic criteria, include swelling of papillae on the surface of the tongue (strawberry tongue) (Fig. 11.9) and intense erythema of the mucosal surfaces [88]. Ulceration in the oral cavity is a common presenting sign [89]. In addition, lips may appear cracked, cherry red, swollen, or hemorrhagic [78].

11.5.3 Systemic Lupus Erythematosus (SLE)

Systemic lupus erythematosus (SLE) is an autoimmune connective-tissue disorder that affects numerous organ systems, including the musculoskeletal system, lungs, heart, and kidneys. It is more common in women, particularly women of African American descent [90]. The prevalence is estimated to be 40–50 cases per 100,000 population [90].

Oral manifestations of SLE are found in 5–25% of patients and include ulcers in the *tongue*, palate, and buccal mucosa [70]. Cheilitis involving the lower lip vermilion is also seen in patients with SLE and is referred to as *lupus cheilitis* [78]. Xerostomia can also occur, with resultant increased risk for candidiasis and periodontal disease [78]. Lourenço et al. study revealed a lichenoid mucositis with an inflammatory infiltrate, primarily composed of T cells [91]. The basement membrane zone has linear deposits of IgG and C3 visualized by direct immunofluorescence [91].

A form of SLE known as *discoid lupus erythematous* (DLE) is limited to the skin and mucous membranes. Oral manifestations appear with cutaneous lesions and are clinically and histologically similar to oral lichen planus [78]. Lesions appear as

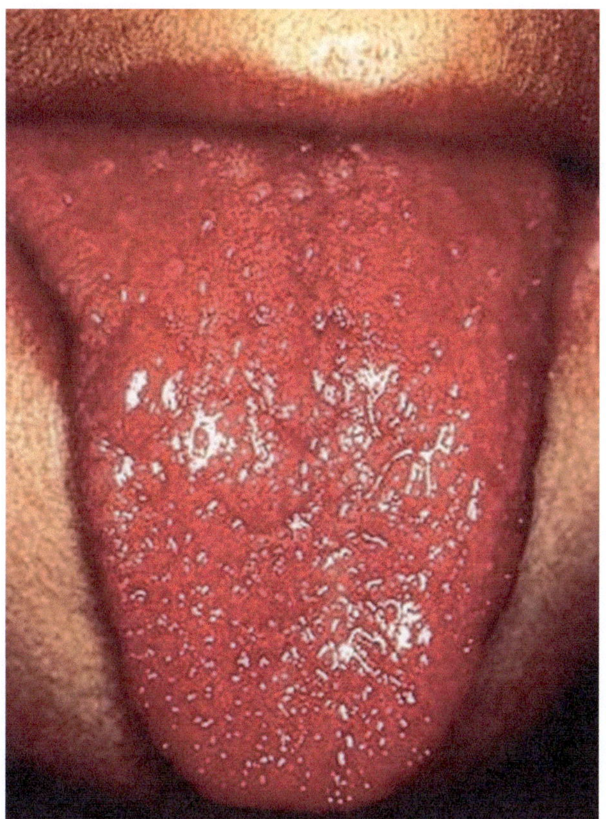

Fig. 11.9 Kawasaki disease: swelling of papillae on the surface of the tongue (strawberry tongue) and intense erythema of the mucosal surface

well-demarcated ulcerations or erythematous plaques with atrophy encircled by white, radiating striae [78]. The sunburst pattern is typically unilateral as compared with the reticulated red and white plaques of lichen planus.

11.5.4 Scleroderma

Scleroderma is a rare autoimmune disease characterized by progressive fibrosis in numerous organ systems. The prevalence is estimated at 50–300 cases per 1 million persons, and women are at a 3- to 14-fold increased risk [92]. *Limited scleroderma*, commonly known as CREST (calcinosis, Raynaud's phenomenon, esophageal involvement, sclerodactyly, and telangiectasias) syndrome, has minimal oral involvement, although intra-oral and perioral telangiectasias may be present [93].

Diffuse scleroderma is a rapidly progressing disease with significant systemic manifestations involving nearly any internal organ by the pathologic fibrosis [92]. Cutaneous involvement is marked by significant skin fibrosis, pigmentary changes, and shiny skin [94]. Oral manifestations can be profound in diffuse scleroderma. From 70–80% of patients experience microstomia, a phenomenon in which the opening to the oral cavity reduces in size secondary to perioral collagen deposition [78, 93]. Xerostomia occurs as a result of progressive fibrosis of the salivary glands, and it often mirrors the progression of microstomia [95]. Other oral manifestations of diffuse scleroderma include telangiectasias and atrophy of the oral mucosa [95]. Histology generally reveals extensive fibrosis, as well as endothelial cell and capillary basal cell damage [95].

11.6 Pulmonary Conditions

11.6.1 Granulomatosis with Polyangitis (GPA)

Granulomatosis with polyangitis (GPA), formerly known as "Wegener granulomatosis," is a necrotizing vasculitis of small- to medium-sized vessels associated with necrotizing granulomas of the upper and lower airways and necrotizing glomerulonephritis [96, 97]. The prevalence of GPA is between 20 and 160 cases per million persons, and evidence suggests it is more common in Northern European countries [98].

Although classically associated with pulmonary and renal pathology, GPA can also affect the eyes, ears, heart, central nervous system, peripheral nervous system, pharynx, and sinuses [99]. Cutaneous manifestations include leukocytoclastic vasculitis, subcutaneous nodules, ulcers, and gangrenous necrosis [99].

Oral cavity is affected in nearly all cases of GPA [100]. Oral lesions include ulcerations and gingival enlargement [96]. The characteristic gingival appearance in GPA is a pathognomonic finding known as strawberry gingivitis [101, 102]. Involvement may eventually include the lingual and palatal mucosa [100]. Oral and skin manifestations may correlate with disease progression and thereby have a prognostic value. Pathological findings consistent with GPA (necrotizing vasculitis with accompanying granulomatous inflammation) combined with a positive antineutrophil cytoplasmic antibody (ANCA) testing are diagnostic [97].

11.6.2 Sarcoidosis

Sarcoidosis is an idiopathic systemic disease characterized by bilateral hilar lymphadenopathy and noncaseating granulomas in the lungs. It can involve nearly any organ, including the liver, heart, spleen, kidneys, and lymph system [103]. Pulmonary manifestations are the most common and include dyspnea with exertion, nonproductive cough, chest pain, wheezing, nasal congestion, and hemoptysis [103]. Ocular and cutaneous manifestations are also common [103].

Oral manifestations may include brown or purple papules and nodules or painless nonspecific ulcerations of the gingiva, buccal mucosa, labial mucosae, and palate [103]. Between 19% and 59% of patients may also experience tumor-like swellings on the mucosa of salivary glands [103]. Rarely, sarcoidosis may involve the tongue, including swelling, enlargement, and ulcerations. Involvement of the tongue is an uncommon oral manifestation of sarcoidosis, but in rare cases may be the presenting sign of the disease [104]. Histological analysis reveals noncaseating granulomas surrounded by multinucleate giant cells along with lymphocytic infiltrate [103]. Treatment with systemic corticosteroids may be useful, but symptoms may resolve spontaneously or progress despite treatment [105].

11.7 Multi-system Conditions

11.7.1 Amyloidosis

Amyloidosis is the deposition of amyloid protein in the body's tissues leading to tissue damage, commonly affecting the heart, kidneys, and GI tract. The most common oral manifestation of primary systemic amyloidosis is macroglossia, which occurs in 12–40% of patients [78]. The enlarged tongue demonstrates lateral ridging secondary to teeth indentation [106]. Grossly, the tongue may be firm and appear relatively normal, or it may have nodules, fissures, or ulcerations, often on the lateral surface (Fig. 11.10) [107, 108].

Submandibular lymphadenopathy occurs subsequent to tongue enlargement, and both can lead to respiratory obstruction [109]. Although pain is not usually present, loss of mobility is common. Interference with taste has also been reported in some patients. In addition, hyposalivation may result from amyloid deposition in the salivary glands [108].

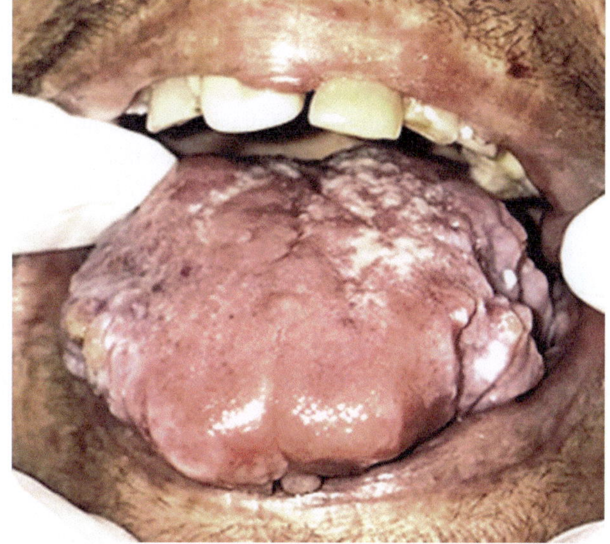

Fig. 11.10 Primary systemic amyloidosis presenting with macroglossia that demonstrates nodules, fissures, and ulcerations on the lateral surface of the tongue

The amorphous, fissured appearance of deposited amyloid can be seen with microscopic examination of a biopsy sample from an enlarged tongue [108]. A characteristic green negative birefringence is seen when polarized light is shone on tissue stained with Congo red [108].

11.7.2 Human Immunodeficiency Virus (HIV) Disease

Human immunodeficiency virus (HIV) targets critical components of the human immune system, leading to acquired immunodeficiency syndrome (AIDS). In 2014, the World Health Organization (WHO) estimated that there were 36.9 million people living with HIV worldwide, noting that approximately 54% of individuals are unaware of their HIV-positive status [110].

Patients with HIV/AIDS are highly susceptible to infections (many of which are rare in immunocompetent hosts) and malignancies [111, 112]. HIV infection has been associated with numerous oral lesions and diseases [113]. In general, these conditions only occur when CD4 lymphocyte counts drop below 400 cells/μL and many have a positive predictive value for immune decline [114–119]. Treatment of HIV is based around "highly active antiretroviral therapy" (HAART), which has been proven to significantly lower the prevalence of oral lesions, particularly oral candidiasis and oral hairy leukoplakia.

11.7.2.1 Candidiasis

Oral candidiasis is often the first presenting sign of HIV infection occurring in as many as 50–90% of patients [113, 120]. HIV infection should be considered in patients presenting with repeated oral candidiasis in the absence of other associated risk factors, such as steroid or antibiotic use. The frequency of candidal infection increases as HIV disease progresses (i.e. as viral loads increase and CD4 lymphocyte counts decline).

The four common classifications of candidal infections are pseudomembranous candidiasis, erythematous candidiasis, angular cheilitis, and hyperplastic candidiasis. Erythematous candidiasis manifests as nonspecific areas of erythema and atrophy, commonly on the palate or dorsum of the tongue (or both as a result of autoinoculation) [113].

HIV-positive patients adhering to the "highly active antiretroviral therapy" (HAART) regimen have a significantly reduced incidence of oral candidiasis [113]. Treatment with antifungal drugs is recommended; however, oral candidiasis can be difficult to eradicate in immunocompromised patients. Fungal resistance to azole drugs (e.g. fluconazole) is increased among HIV-infected patients [121].

11.7.2.2 Herpes Simplex Virus (HSV)

Herpes simplex virus (HSV) is a double-stranded DNA virus that has two subtypes: HSV-1 and HSV-2 [122]. Stress, fever, sunlight, or decreased immunity may precipitate reactivation of HSV, enabling the virus to travel down peripheral nerves and produce lesions [122]. In rare cases, HSV can cause a systemic infection, although

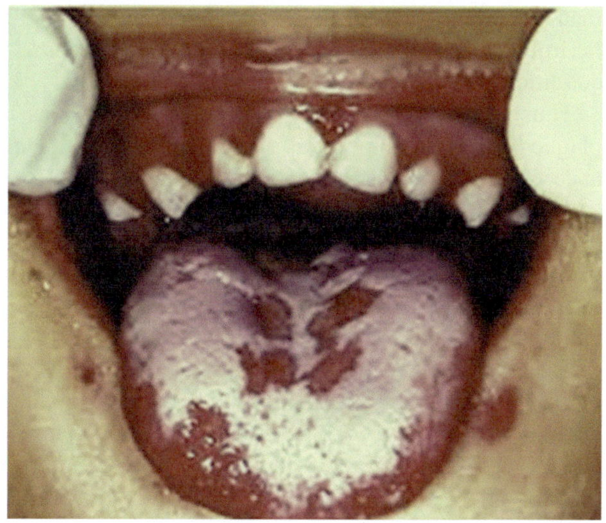

Fig. 11.11 The inflamed, erythematous tongue of an HIV-patient with herpes simplex virus infection. It shows weeping ulcerations on the dorsal surface of the tongue

in healthy hosts its presentation is generally limited to a mucocutaneous vesicular eruption, most commonly on the vermilion of the lips, sometimes preceded by a burning or tingling sensation [123, 124]. These vesicles rupture and leave behind painful, weeping ulcerations (Fig. 11.11) that are highly infectious for about 3–5 days, until they form an overlying crust. In immunocompetent individuals, the normal duration of lesions is 7–10 days [123, 124].

Immunodeficiency, as seen with HIV infection, permits reactivation of latent herpes infections [122, 125], which are often more aggressive, prolonged, and diffuse than in an immunocompetent individual [122, 123]. For example, intra-oral HSV lesions generally occur on keratinized mucosa, such as the dorsal aspect of the tongue, gingiva, and hard palate [124]. However, in immunocompromised hosts, HSV lesions can manifest on nonkeratinized surfaces, including the labial mucosa, ventral tongue, floor of the mouth, buccal mucosa, and the soft palate [125]. Herpetic lesions may extend to other areas, including the tonsillar pillars and esophagus [126].

Diagnosis is made by physical examination and a history of prodrome at the site of the vesicles. A Tzanck smear demonstrating multinucleate giant cells is highly suggestive of HSV infection, but culture and antibody staining results are diagnostic. Tissue biopsy may also be used to obtain a definitive diagnosis. Thymidine kinase inhibitors are the most commonly used antivirals to treat HSV infections [127]. These include acyclovir, valacyclovir, and famciclovir. However, acyclovir-resistant strains are more common among HIV-infected individuals [127]. In these instances, infections are treated aggressively with intravenous foscarnet [127].

11.7.2.3 Hairy Leukoplakia (HL)

Hairy leukoplakia (HL) is caused by the activity of the Epstein-Barr virus (EBV) within the epithelial cells [128, 129]. In the early 1980s, HL was identified and characterized in HIV-positive patients [129, 130]. It still remains the most specific manifestation of HIV disease occurring in the mouth, and its presence has prognostic implications for the progression to AIDS because patients rarely manifest the condition with CD4 counts more than 200 cells/μL [131].

Hairy leukoplakia most commonly manifests as corrugated white verrucous plaques on the lateral portions of the tongue. These plaques range in size and appearance from thin and homogenous to thickened and rough, mimicking hyperplastic candidiasis [128, 129]; a biopsy should be performed for definitive diagnosis [129]. Histological examination reveals hair-like projections, which demonstrate hyperparakeratosis, acanthosis, groups of ballooning cells, and a limited inflammatory infiltrate [132, 133]. Definitive diagnosis may be made with in situ hybridization of the DNA from EBV in surface epithelial cells [133].

Because HL is usually asymptomatic, treatment is elective. Common treatment regimens include 25% podophyllin resin, a 25% podophyllin resin with a 1% penciclovir cream, and a 25% podophyllin resin with a 5% acyclovir cream [134]. If a patient reports symptoms associated with HL, the lesions are most likely superinfected with *Candida* species. Antifungal treatment usually ameliorates these symptoms.

11.7.2.4 Kaposi Sarcoma (KS)

Kaposi sarcoma (KS) is the second most common malignancy in patients who are HIV positive and is considered an AIDS-defining illness [135]. It presents as angioproliferative tumors on visceral organs or the skin [135]. Oral involvement is seen in approximately 50% of AIDS-KS cases and may be present at the time of HIV diagnosis in up to 20% of patients [113, 136]. Intra-orally, KS appears as brown, blue, purple, or red patches and papules on the hard palate, mucosa, and gingiva [113, 137]. While early lesions appear as flat macules or patches on the mucosal surface, over time they become nodular, with a predilection to ulcerate and bleed. [137]. Kaposi sarcoma can also affect the salivary glands and may cause head and neck lymphadenopathy [138, 139].

A biopsy should be performed to definitively diagnose KS. Histologically, KS is characterized by increased vascularity, spindle-shaped cells with minimal mitotic activity, and hemosiderin deposition [140]. Treatment is accomplished through a variety of methods, including surgical excision, cryotherapy, sclerotherapy, radiotherapy, laser therapy, and topical or intralesional chemotherapy [140].

11.7.2.5 Cytomegalovirus (CMV)

Cytomegalovirus (CMV) is a double-stranded DNA virus. In the United States, data indicate that 30–70% of people are seropositive [141]. In HIV-positive patients CMV may cause retinitis, pneumonia, and encephalitis and is associated with significant morbidity and mortality [142]. Even in immunocompromised patients, CMV infection rarely manifests intra-orally. However, in these rare cases, CMV infection produces deep, penetrating oral ulcerations on the lips, tongue, or pharynx [143–145]. The aphthous-like ulcerations have a punched-out look with rolled, erythematous borders [143, 144]. Diagnosis can be confirmed histologically, with identification of the characteristic “owl’s-eye” appearance of cellular inclusions [146]. CMV infection is treated with intravenous agents such as ganciclovir or cidofovir [145].

11.7.2.6 Human Papillomavirus (HPV)

Human papillomavirus (HPV) is a DNA virus that affects both immunocompetent and immunocompromised individuals [147, 148]. As of 2010, the prevalence of oral HPV in adolescents and adults (aged 15–69 years) in the United States was 6.9%. Estimates of the genital HPV prevalence is much higher; nearly 43% in females aged 18–59 [149]. However, the prevalence of HPV has been decreasing since the advent of the quadrivalent vaccine [150].

The most common oral manifestation of HPV is oral warts (papillomas or condylomas) that are soft, pink masses with a characteristic papillary texture that usually appear on the gingiva, lips, and labial mucosa [147]. HPV-associated oral squamous cell carcinomas may present as a nonhealing ulcer with signs of bleeding, loosening of teeth, neck masses (lymphadenopathy), and symptoms that include dysphagia, dysarthria, and odynophagia [151]. Such malignancies may derive from asymptomatic, precancerous lesions on the oral mucosa; leukoplakia or erythroplakia [151]. Therapeutic options for HPV-associated oral warts include excision, laser ablation, cryotherapy, or topical 5-fluorouracil or imiquimod [147, 152].

11.7.2.7 Aphthous-Like Ulcerations

Aphthous ulcerations are ulcerations of the oral cavity that are not caused by an infectious agent. Three forms of recurrent aphthous ulcerations are recognized: minor, major, and herpetiform. Similar ulcerations can occur in the GI tract or on genital mucosal surfaces.

Aphthous lesions manifest as yellow-gray areas of ulceration ranging in size from a few millimeters to larger than a centimeter [153]. These ulcerations are characteristically surrounded with a halo of erythema and are usually very painful [153]. In immunocompetent individuals, aphthous ulcerations affect only nonkeratinized surfaces within the oral cavity [153]. However, in immunocompromised hosts, these ulcerations can appear anywhere in the oral cavity including the tongue [154]. The recurrent appearance of these lesions in an HIV-infected patient is a reliable indicator of severe immunodeficiency and disease progression [154].

Biopsy is indicated for definitive diagnosis of all HIV-related ulcerations because bacterial, viral, and fungal pathogens, as well as HIV medications, may cause atypical oral ulcerations. Numerous treatment modalities are available including topical, intralesional, and systemic therapies [153]. In the HIV-positive population, immunosuppressants should be prescribed with particular care, owing to the associated risk of other intraoral infections, such as with *Candida* species. Thalidomide and amlexanox are currently the only US Food and Drug Administration–approved treatments for aphthae, with thalidomide specifically designated for HIV-associated aphthous ulceration [155–159].

11.8 Cutaneous Diseases

11.8.1 Psoriasis

Psoriasis is a chronic papulosquamous inflammatory condition of the skin that affects approximately 2% of the US population [160]. The precise etiology of psoriasis remains unknown. Clinically, its extent and severity can vary greatly. Characteristic scaly, white, well-demarcated plaques typically affect the scalp, elbows, and knees [160, 161]. When the silvery scale is elevated or scratched, bleeding points are evident (Auspitz sign). In moist intertriginous areas, such as the axillae and groin, well-demarcated erythematous patches and plaques, without the presence of slivery scale, predominate [160, 161].

Although controversial, psoriasis can manifest in the oral cavity [162–166]. Intra-orally, sites affected include the palate, buccal mucosa, gingiva, and tongue with nonspecific inflammatory plaques. Geographic tongue and fissured tongue (Fig. 11.12) have an increased incidence in patients with psoriasis [166, 167]. Pindborg and van der Waal identified three findings suggestive of oral psoriasis: (1) small, white papules that yield bleeding points upon scraping, (2) red and white plaques that follow skin lesions, and (3) bright-red patches [168].

Since oral psoriasis rarely manifests without cutaneous involvement, definitive oral diagnosis is made with the finding of corresponding cutaneous lesions and is confirmed with biopsy results. Histological findings show parakeratosis and hyperplasia of the epidermis, elongation of rete ridges, a thinned stratum granulosum, Munro microabscesses of neutrophils superficially, and chronic inflammation of the epidermis and the dermis with polymorphonuclear leukocytes, lymphocytes, and

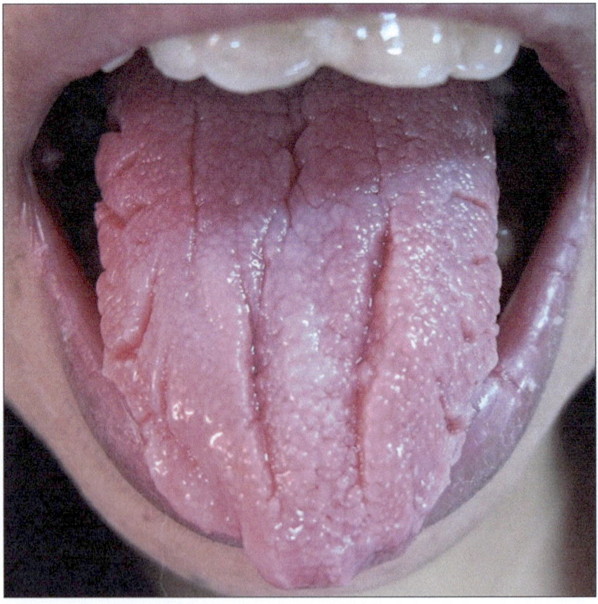

Fig. 11.12 Multiple longitudinal fissures seen on the dorsal surface of the tongue in a patient with psoriasis

histiocytes [161]. Dilated and tortuous blood vessels high in the submucosa may also be present. Although these are the characteristic psoriatic histological findings, they are identical to geographic tongue, so a careful clinical history and physical examination are important to make a diagnosis [161].

11.8.2 Acanthosis Negricans (AN)

Acanthosis Negricans (AN) is a cutaneous disorder of hyperpigmentation and papillomatosis. It is generally associated with fibroblast growth factor receptor mutations and genetic or acquired insulin resistance [169]. The prevalence of acanthosis negricans positively correlated with the number of diabetes risk factors (i.e. dyslipidemia, hypertension, weight, family history) possessed by the patient [170].

Patients generally present in childhood or adolescence with hyperpigmented, velvety, papillated plaques in flexural areas, such as the neck, axilla, groin, and fingers [169, 171]. Rarely, *benign AN* manifests in an exuberant fashion, with involvement of the umbilicus, areolae, and oral cavity [171, 172]. *Malignancy-associated AN* (MAN) is a mucocutaneous paraneoplastic disorder of hyperpigmentation and exuberant papillomatosis, and may present in conjunction with tripe palms (hyperkeratosis of the palms and soles) and the Leser-Trélat sign (a sudden eruption of seborrheic keratosis) [173]. Recognition of these lesions could facilitate the early diagnosis of a potentially fatal malignancy.

Oral manifestations have been noted in 25–50% of patients with MAN, in contrast to the benign form in which oral involvement is rare [174]. In oral MAN, the tongue, lips, palate, and gingiva may be involved. Nonpigmented hypertrophy of the papillae along the tongue's dorsal surface and lateral edge yield a characteristic shaggy, fissured texture (Fig. 11.13) [175]. The lips are also subject to these

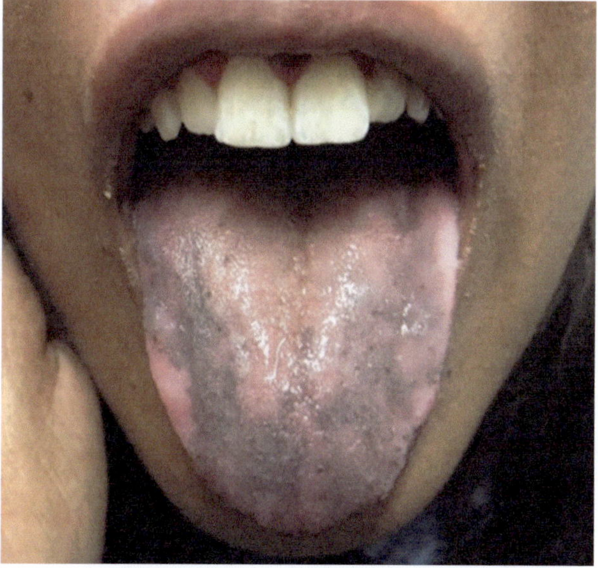

Fig. 11.13 Hyperpigmentation of the dorsal surface of the tongue with hypertrophy of the papillae and a characteristic shaggy texture

papillomatous growths and often exhibit profound swelling [176]. While the buccal mucosa may have similar papillae; it is more common to see velvety white plaques and an uneven appearance. Gingival hyperplasia may be prominent, with interdental gingiva so hyperplastic as to cover teeth and interfere with eating [177].

Histologically, oral MAN shows acanthosis and epithelial papillary hyperplasia with minimal inflammatory infiltrate [175]. While cutaneous "AN" shows increased melanin deposition in the basal cell layer, oral lesions do *not* share this characteristic feature [175].

11.9 Neurological Diseases

11.9.1 Neurofibromatosis (NF) Types 1 and 2

Neurofibromatosis type 1 (NF1) (von Recklinghausen disease) is a neurocutaneous syndrome caused by an inherited or de novo mutation in the *NF1* gene. This gene is a tumor-suppressor gene located in the pericentromeric region of chromosome 17 [178]. NF1 is classically characterized by cutaneous neurofibromas, plexiform neurofibromas, café-au-lait macules, axillary or inguinal freckling, iris hamartomas (Lisch nodules), and optic gliomas [178].

Neurofibromatosis type 2 (NF2) is caused by a mutation in a different gene, *NF2*, which is located on a separate chromosome [179]. It can also be inherited in an autosomal dominant fashion or by de novo mutation and is characterized by vestibular schwannomas and other benign tumors of neural tissue such as meningiomas and gliomas [179]. Patients with NF2 generally do *not* exhibit the same degree of cutaneous involvement as patients with NF1, although cutaneous neurofibromas are typical and café-au-lait macules occur at rates higher than the general population [179].

Geist et al., reported that the majority of patients with oral lesions had NF1, and documented intra-oral neurofibromas on the lips, palate, buccal mucosa, gingiva, and tongue (Fig. 11.14) [180]. More recent studies looking at NF1 specifically

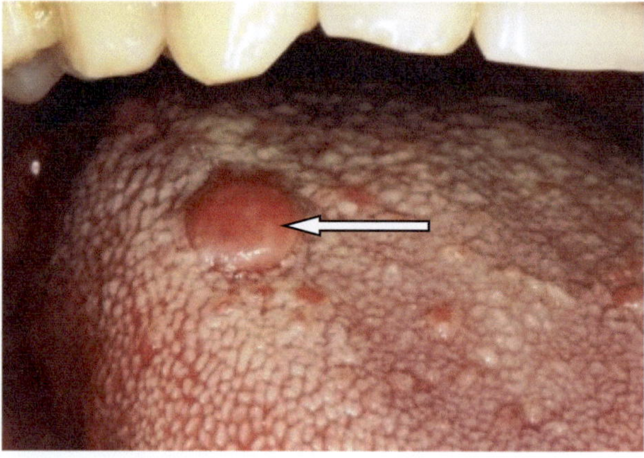

Fig. 11.14 Neurofibroma of the tongue in a patient with neurofibromatosis type 1 (NF1) (arrow)

confirmed previous observations that the tongue is the most common site of intraoral involvement [181, 182]. Although most lesions of the tongue are nodular, diffuse macroglossia and enlargement of the fungiform papillae have also been noted [180, 182]. Hyperpigmentation and enlargement of the gingiva may also be seen in NF1 [181]. Osseous manifestations occur in almost 40% of patients and include lesions of the cranial and jaw bones, while dental abnormalities such as impacted teeth, supernumerary teeth, overgrowth of the alveolar process, and a possible increased risk of caries have been described. An increased prevalence of malignancy has been documented in patients affected by NF1 [183–185].

The early diagnosis of asymptomatic neurofibromas of the tongue requires a high index of clinical suspicion. Symptomatic lesions are more readily diagnosed when a patient complains of mass or other discomfort, which will direct the clinician to the primary lesion.

A significant correlation is also found between delay in diagnosis and the location of a lesion in the oral cavity. When symptoms associated with lesions of the base of the tongue are reported, a neck mass, odynophagia, dysphagia, voice changes, and ear pain can be noted.

Differential diagnosis of enlarging tongue masses includes lipoma, angiolipoma, chondroid lipoma, myolipoma, hamartomatous lesions, schwannoma, lymphangioma, granular cell tumor, fibroma, leiomyoma, rhabdomyosarcoma, hemangioma, neurofibroma, plexiform neurofibromas.

11.10 Endocrine Diseases

11.10.1 Diabetes Mellitus (DM)

Diabetes mellites (DM) is associated with numerous diseases and lesions of the oral cavity. Mucosal manifestations include fissured tongue, benign migratory glossitis, coated tongue, irritation fibroma, traumatic ulcers, and recurrent aphthous ulcers [186, 187]. Some studies also indicate increased prevalence of lichen planus, although this remains highly controversial [187]. Premalignant conditions such as leukoplakia, erythroplakia, and actinic cheilitis may also be more prevalent in patients with DM [187, 188]. Salivary dysfunction, with or without signs of salivary gland enlargement, burning mouth syndrome, and taste disturbances are also common in diabetes, likely owing to secondary neuropathy [189, 190]. Diabetic patients are also at an increased risk of oral fungal infections, specifically candidiasis [190, 191]. Similarly, dental caries, periodontitis, and gingivitis are also more common in persons with diabetes [190, 191]. In addition to general diabetes therapies, oral hygiene is critical to reduce the risk of these complications [186].

11.10.2 Thyroid Gland Disorders

Hypothyroidism has a prevalence of 1–2%; while hyperthyroidism has a prevalence of 0.5–2% in women, but it is 10 times less common in men [192]. Systemic manifestations of hypothyroidism include cold intolerance, constipation, weight gain, and lethargy, while cutaneous manifestations include dry skin and hair [193]. On the other hand, common manifestations of hyperthyroidism include heat intolerance, abdominal pain, weight loss, and tachycardia, while cutaneous manifestations include fine hair and warm, smooth skin [193].

Oral manifestations are more common in hypothyroidism and generally relate to its severe form; *myxedema*. In these cases, deposition of glycosaminoglycans results in diffuse swelling of the lips and tongue [151]. Patients with hyperthyroidism have an increased susceptibility to caries, periodontal disease, and burning mouth syndrome [193, 194]. Sjogren's syndrome is also more common in these patients [193, 194]. It is noteworthy that congenital hypothyroidism is characterized by thick lips, macroglossia, delayed tooth eruption, and dysgeusia, as well as severe intellectual delay [193, 194].

11.10.3 Parathyroid Gland (PTG) Disorders

Parathyroid hormone (PTH), produced by the PTGs, is critical to the maintenance of calcium and phosphate homeostasis in the body. Hypoparathyroidism is characterized by low levels of calcium, and systemic manifestations include paresthesias, increased neuromuscular irritability, laryngospasm and bronchospasm, cataracts, personality alterations, seizures, and cardiac involvement (prolonged QT and arrhythmias) [195]. Cutaneous manifestations include xerotic skin, skin pigmentation, and changes in the hair and nails [196]. Oral manifestations of hyperparathyroidism usually spare the tongue. They include loss of the lamina dura of roots of the teeth; an abnormal trabecular pattern in the bones; and the well-demarcated, unilocular, radiolucent "brown" tumors that can effect jawbones [197, 198]. If hypoparathyroidism develops early in life, oral manifestations include failure of tooth eruption or a pitting enamel hypoplasia [78].

11.10.4 Adrenal Gland Disorders

The adrenal glands are responsible for the production of numerous steroid hormones, including the glucocorticoid cortisol that plays a critical role in the regulation of metabolism and the immune system. In *hypocorticalism* (adrenal insufficiency), hyperpigmentation may been seen on the tongue and on the periodontal and buccal mucosa [199, 200]. There may also be hyperpigmentation of the vermillion border, in addition to common cutaneous sites of hyperpigmentation, such as the flexural creases and recent scars [199, 200]. On the other hand, *hypercortisolism* (Cushing syndrome) does not seem to affect the tongue as oral manifestations generally relate to jaw-bone fractures, secondary to skeletal fragility, and slow healing lesions, secondary to impaired wound healing [78].

11.11 Renal Diseases

There are a number of oral complications following renal transplantation. The immunosuppressant cyclosporine is used to prevent rejection of the transplanted kidney. Due to the immunosuppression, these patients are more likely to suffer from gingival hyperplasia, aphthous ulceration, herpes simplex virus (HSV) infection, oral leucoplakia; which may transform into squamous cell carcinoma, candidiasis infection, or Kaposi's sarcoma.

In patients with chronic renal disease, patients may suffer from uremic stomatitis, which manifests with painful plaques and crusts on the buccal mucosa and dorsum of the tongue. The floor of the mouth is covered with pseudomembranes (Fig. 11.15) and painful ulcers

11.12 Drug-Induced Conditions

Many lesions and disorders of the oral cavity involving the tongue may be caused by medical therapies. As such, thorough medication reconciliation is essential for any patient presenting with an oral pathology. Below, common oral pathologies and the major pharmacological agents that either cause or are associated with these conditions are reviewed.

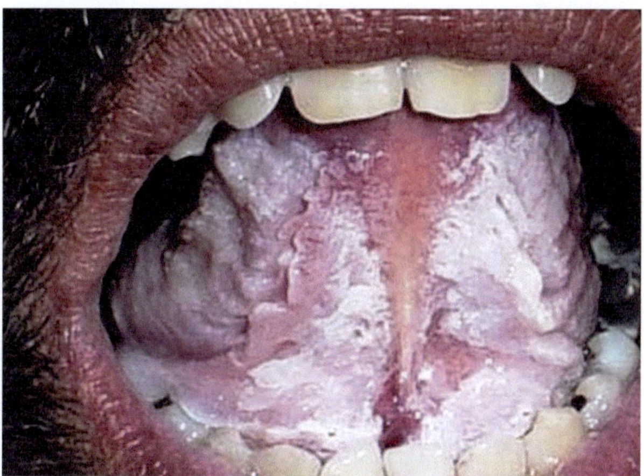

Fig. 11.15 Adherent white patches on the ventral surface of the tongue and floor of the mouth in a patient with uremic stomatitis

11.12.1 Aphthous Stomatitis

Pharmacological agents are among the most common causes of recurrent aphthous ulcers. These ulcerations are round, crater form, white-yellow depressions surrounded by a rim of erythema. The size of an aphthous ulcer may vary from 1–3 mm (aphthous minor, approximately 80% of cases) to larger than 1 cm (aphthous major, approximately 15% of cases) [201]. Patients may have outbreaks of multiple ulcerations at one time [201]. These are usually quite painful, but typically are self-limiting and resolve in 7–10 days for aphthous minor and 14–21 days for aphthous major lesions [201]. Offending drugs may include nonsteroidal anti-inflammatory drugs (NSAIDs), nicorandil, ACE inhibitors, or bisphosphonates, but any drug can potentially produce an aphthous-like reaction [202].

11.12.2 Dry Mouth (Hyposalivation or Xerostomia)

Dry mouth (hyposalivation or xerostomia) could be an adverse effect of many medications. These include (1) dehydrating agents(diuretics), (2) anticholinergic agents (tricyclic antidepressants, muscarinic agonists, alpha-receptor antagonists, antipsychotics, and antihistamines), (3) sympathetic effectors (antihypertensives, appetite suppressants, decongestants, bronchodilators, muscle relaxants, and antimigraine medications), (4) drugs of abuse (opioids, benzodiazepines, and cannabis), (5) and others (anti-HIV drugs, retinoids, cytotoxic drugs, proton-pump inhibitors and H2-receptor antagonists, and caffeinated and alcoholic beverages/products) [203].

Dry mouth may cause altered taste, increased risk of fungal infection and caries, and increased prevalence of traumatic ulceration due to lack of lubrication [204]. Patients with severely impaired salivary flow also have difficulty with eating, swallowing, and speech [203]. Many management options are available for decreased salivation ranging from simple solutions, such as increased hydration, to systemic procholinergic agents to increase salivation [203].

11.12.3 Lichen Planus (LP)

As discussed above, lichen planus (LP) is a mucocutaneous disorder with a prevalence of 0.4–4% in the general population [19]. The prevalence of oral lichen planus (OLP) is unknown, but both forms may be triggered by pharmacological agents [19].

Drug-associated OLP, or oral lichenoid drug reactions (OLDRs), generally present in the oral cavity as the classic reticular form; however, ulcerated or eroded forms have also been described [205]. In addition to a clinical evaluation, a biopsy is warranted to verify diagnosis. Histopathology reveals a dense lichenoid infiltrate along the dermoepidermal junction and a saw-toothed rete-ridge pattern with Max-Joseph spaces [205]. A small subset of OLP cases, specifically the erosive types, have been linked to the development of squamous cell carcinoma [206].

Table 11.5 Oral mucosal white patches associated with systemic disease

White plaques	Causes
Nonadherent	• Pseudomembranous candidiasis (thrush) • Other mycoses • Food debris • Furred tongue • Drug-associated necrotic debris (e.g. aspirin, cocaine)
Adherent	• Papillomas • White sponge nevus • Geographic tongue (erythema migrans—psoriasis) • Frictional keratosis (e.g. due to abnormal orofacial movement) • Lichen planus • Lupus disorders • Oral hairy leukoplakia • Chronic mucocutaneous candidiasis

Currently, over 200 agents have been implicated in OLDRs [207]. Well-documented drugs known to trigger OLDRs include ACE inhibitors, beta-blockers, NSAIDs, diuretics, hydroxychloroquine, and zidovudine [208]. Many vaccines, most notably the hepatitis B vaccine, have also been known to cause LP [209–211]. A thorough medication history may be required to identify the causative agent; although the average time span between drug intake and an OLDR is 2–3 months [19].

11.12.4 Candidiasis (Secondary to Inhaled Steroids)

Patients using inhaled corticosteroids (ICS) experience a 2- to 4-fold increased risk of contracting oral candidiasis (thrush) [212, 213]. Rates of oral candidiasis subsequent to ICS vary, but they may be over 15% [213, 214]. Some studies suggest that the use of Rotacaps inhalers confers a higher risk than use of metered-dose inhalers with a spacer [214].

Oral candidiasis is characterized by small, curdy-appearing white papules and plaques that are easily wiped from the mucosa [212, 215]. The tissue beneath these plaques is often inflamed and may bleed [212, 215]. Causes of white patches in the oral mucosa are summarized in Table 11.5. The infection is usually self-limiting, so steroid use can continue. To prevent further exacerbations, adding a spacer to the inhaler, decreasing the frequency of steroid use, and using anticandidal mouthwashes after taking the steroids are recommended [214, 215].

11.13 Psychiatric Disorders

Eating disorders are a psychiatric problem, which has an impact on the gastrointestinal tract. Two common eating disorders are "anorexia nervosa" and "bulimia nervosa." Anorexia nervosa is a refusal to maintain a "normal" body weight with a fear of weight gain and distorted perception of body image. Bulimia nervosa is binge-eating followed by attempts to restrict weight gain and can include purging [216]. Oral manifestations of eating disorders are usually severe palatal erosions due to frequent vomiting. There is also occlusal erosion of the maxillary teeth causing the incised edges of the incisors to be thin and knife-edged and predisposing the tongue to frequent and recurrent injuries. Extraorally eating disorders may present with swollen parotid glands [216].

References

1. Boirivant M, Cossu A. Inflammatory bowel disease. Oral Dis. 2012;18(1):1–15.
2. Katsanos KH, Torres J, Roda G, Brygo A, Delaporte E, Colombel JF. Review article: non-malignant oral manifestations in inflammatory bowel diseases. Aliment Pharmacol Ther. 2015;42(1):40–60.
3. Halme L, Meurman JH, Laine P, von Smitten K, Syrjänen S, Lindqvist C, et al. Oral findings in patients with active or inactive Crohn's disease. Oral Surg Oral Med Oral Pathol. 1993;76(2):175–81.
4. Plauth M, Jenss H, Meyle J. Oral manifestations of Crohn's disease. An analysis of 79 cases. J Clin Gastroenterol. 1991;13(1):29–37.
5. Lankarani KB, Sivandzadeh GR, Hassanpour S. Oral manifestation in inflammatory bowel disease: a review. World J Gastroenterol. 2013;19(46):8571–9.
6. Mirowski GW, LeBlanc J, Mark LA. Oral disease and oral-cutaneous manifestations of gastrointestinal and liver disease. In: Friedman LS, Brandt LJ, editors. Feldman, Sleisenger and Fordtran's gastrointestinal and liver disease: pathophysiology/diagnosis/management. 10th ed. Philadelphia: Elsevier; 2016. p. 377–96.
7. Marzano AV, Borghi A, Stadnicki A, Crosti C, Cugno M. Cutaneous manifestations in patients with inflammatory bowel diseases: pathophysiology, clinical features, and therapy. Inflamm Bowel Dis. 2014;20(1):213–27.
8. Hegarty AM, Barrett AW, Scully C. Pyostomatitis vegetans. Clin Exp Dermatol. 2004;29(1):1–7.
9. Karnath B. Stigmata of chronic liver disease. Turner-White communications. 2003. Available at http://www.turner-white.com/pdf/hp_jul03_stigmata.pdf. Accessed July 18, 2016.
10. Schuppan D, Afdhal NH. Liver cirrhosis. Lancet. 2008;371(9615):838–51.
11. Ghosn SH, Kibbi AG. Cutaneous manifestations of liver diseases. Clin Dermatol. 2008;26(3):274–82.
12. Amitrano L, Guardascione MA, Brancaccio V, Balzano A. Coagulation disorders in liver disease. Semin Liver Dis. 2002;22(1):83–96.
13. Daley TD, Armstrong JE. Oral manifestations of gastrointestinal diseases. Can J Gastroenterol. 2007;21(4):241–4.
14. Lodi G, Pellicano R, Carrozzo M. Hepatitis C virus infection and lichen planus: a systematic review with meta-analysis. Oral Dis. 2010;16(7):601–12.
15. Shengyuan L, Songpo Y, Wen W, Wenjing T, Haitao Z, Binyou W. Hepatitis C virus and lichen planus: a reciprocal association determined by a meta-analysis. Arch Dermatol. 2009;145(9):1040–7.
16. Mohd Hanafiah K, Groeger J, Flaxman AD, Wiersma ST. Global epidemiology of hepatitis C virus infection: new estimates of age-specific antibody to HCV seroprevalence. Hepatology. 2013;57(4):1333–42.
17. Eisen D. The clinical features, malignant potential and systemic associations of oral lichen planus: a study of 723 patients. J Am Acad Dermatol. 2002;46(2):207–14.
18. Wagner G, Rose C, Sachse MM. Clinical variants of lichen planus. J Dtsch Dermatol Ges. 2013;11(4):309–19.

19. Schlosser BJ. Lichen planus and lichenoid reactions of the oral mucosa. Dermatol Ther. 2010;23(3):251–67.
20. Schlosser BJ, Pirigyi M, Mirowski GW. Oral manifestations of hematologic and nutritional diseases. Otolaryngol Clin N Am. 2011;44(1):183–203.
21. Said HM. Water-soluble vitamins. In: Bier DM, Mann J, Alpers DH, Vorster HHE, Gibney MJ, editors. Nutrition for the primary care provider, vol. 111. Basel: Karger Publishers; 2014. p. 30–7.
22. Boyd L, Palmer C. Complete review of dental hygiene. In: Brian NJ, Cooper MD, editors. Nutrition and oral health. Upper Saddle River: Prentice-Hall; 2001.
23. Kozlak ST, Walsh SJ, Lalla RV. Reduced dietary intake of vitamin B12 and folate in patients with recurrent aphthous stomatitis. J Oral Pathol Med. 2010;39(5):420–3.
24. Field EA, Speechley JA, Rugman FR, Varga E, Tyldesley WR. Oral signs and symptoms in patients with undiagnosed vitamin B12 deficiency. J Oral Pathol Med. 1995;24(10):468–70.
25. Leggott PJ, Robertson PB, Jacob RA, Zambon JJ, Walsh M, Armitage GC. Effects of ascorbic acid depletion and supplementation on periodontal health and subgingival microflora in humans. J Dent Res. 1991;70(12):1531–6.
26. Yasui K, Kurata T, Yashiro M, Tsuge M, Ohtsuki S, Morishima T. The effect of ascorbate on minor recurrent aphthous stomatitis. Acta Paediatr. 2010;99(3):442–5.
27. Albahrani AA, Greaves RF. Fat-soluble vitamins: clinical indications and current challenges for chromatographic measurement. Clin Biochem Rev. 2016;37(1):27–47.
28. Khabbazi A, Ghorbanihaghjo A, Fanood F, Kolahi S, Hajialiloo M, Rashtchizadeh N. A comparative study of vitamin D serum levels in patients with recurrent aphthous stomatitis. Egypt Rheumatol. 2015;37(3):133–7.
29. Holick MF, Chen TC. Vitamin D deficiency: a worldwide problem with health consequences. Am J Clin Nutr. 2008;87(4):1080–6.
30. Meisel P, Schwahn C, Luedemann J, John U, Kroemer HK, Kocher T. Magnesium deficiency is associated with periodontal disease. J Dent Res. 2005;84(10):937–41.
31. Sun A, Chen HM, Cheng SJ, Wang YP, Chang JY, Wu YC, et al. Significant association of deficiencies of hemoglobin, iron, vitamin B12, and folic acid and high homocysteine level with recurrent aphthous stomatitis. J Oral Pathol Med. 2015;44(4):300–5.
32. Zimmermann MB, Hurrell RF. Nutritional iron deficiency. Lancet. 2007;370(9586):511–20.
33. Cho GS, Han MW, Lee B, Roh JL, Choi SH, Cho KJ, et al. Zinc deficiency may be a cause of burning mouth syndrome as zinc replacement therapy has therapeutic effects. J Oral Pathol Med. 2010;39(9):722–7.
34. Orbak R, Cicek Y, Tezel A, Dogru Y. Effects of zinc treatment in patients with recurrent aphthous stomatitis. Dent Mater J. 2003;22(1):21–9.
35. Nakano A, Nakano H, Nomura K, Toyomaki Y, Hanada K. Novel SLC39A4 mutations in acrodermatitis enteropathica. J Invest Dermatol. 2003;120(6):963–6.
36. Epstein JB, Barasch A. Taste disorders in cancer patients: pathogenesis, and approach to assessment and management. Oral Oncol. 2010;46(2):77–81.
37. Hambidge KM, Krebs NF. Zinc deficiency: a special challenge. J Nutr. 2007;137(4):1101–5.
38. Vogel VG, Fisher RE. Epidemiology and etiology of leukemia. Curr Opin Oncol. 1993;5(1):26–34.
39. Swerdlow SH, International Agency for Research on Cancer. WHO classification of tumours of haematopoietic and lymphoid tissues. World Health Organization classification of tumours. 4th ed. Lyon: World Health Organization; 2008.
40. Yamaguchi T, Ohshima K, Karube K, Tutiya T, Kawano R, Suefuji H, et al. Clinicopathological features of cutaneous lesions of adult T-cell leukaemia/lymphoma. Br J Dermatol. 2005;152(1):76–81.
41. Desch JK, Smoller BR. The spectrum of cutaneous disease in leukemias. J Cutan Pathol. 1993;20(5):407–10.
42. Hou GL, Huang JS, Tsai CC. Analysis of oral manifestations of leukemia: a retrospective study. Oral Dis. 1997;3(1):31–8.

43. Cooper CL, Loewen R, Shore T. Gingival hyperplasia complicating acute myelomonocytic leukemia. J Can Dent Assoc. 2000;66(2):78–9.
44. Chavan M, Subramaniam A, Jhaveri H, Khedkar S, Durkar S, Agrwal A. Acute myeloid leukemia: a case report with palatal and lingual gingival alterations. Braz J Oral Sci. 2010;9(1):67–9.
45. Ponce-Torres E, Ruíz-Rodríguez Mdel S, Alejo-González F, Hernández-Sierra JF, Pozos-Guillén AJ. Oral manifestations in pediatric patients receiving chemotherapy for acute lymphoblastic leukemia. J Clin Pediatr Dent. 2010;34(3):275–9.
46. Sirois DA, Miller AS, Harwick RD, Vonderheid EC. Oral manifestations of cutaneous T-cell lymphoma. A report of eight cases. Oral Surg Oral Med Oral Pathol. 1993;75(6):700–5.
47. Molyneux EM, Rochford R, Griffin B, Newton R, Jackson G, Menon G, et al. Burkitt's lymphoma. Lancet. 2012;379(9822):1234–44.
48. Corti M, Villafañe MF, Solari R, De Carolis L, Cangelosi D, Santoro J, et al. Non-Hodgkin lymphomas of the oral cavity in AIDS patients in a reference hospital of infectious diseases in Argentina: report of eleven cases and review of the literature. J Gastrointest Cancer. 2011;42(3):143–8.
49. Bower M. Acquired immunodeficiency syndrome-related systemic non-Hodgkin's lymphoma. Br J Haematol. 2001;112(4):863–73.
50. Horwitz M, Benson KF, Person RE, Aprikyan AG, Dale DC. Mutations in ELA2, encoding neutrophil elastase, define a 21-day biological clock in cyclic haematopoiesis. Nat Genet. 1999;23(4):433–6.
51. Online Mendelian Inheritance in Man, OMIM®. MIM number: cyclic neutropenia. Available at http://omim.org/. Accessed: June 2, 2016.
52. Berliner N, Horwitz M, Loughran TP Jr. Congenital and acquired neutropenia. Hematology. 2004;2004:63–79.
53. Dale DC, Bolyard AA, Aprikyan A. Cyclic neutropenia. Semin Hematol. 2002;39(2):89–94.
54. Bellanné-Chantelot C, Clauin S, Leblanc T, Cassinat B, Rodrigues-Lima F, Beaufils S, et al. Mutations in the ELA2 gene correlate with more severe expression of neutropenia: a study of 81 patients from the French Neutropenia Register. Blood. 2004;103(11):4119–25.
55. Dale DC, Hammond WP. Cyclic neutropenia: a clinical review. Blood Rev. 1988;2(3):178–85.
56. Cohen DW, Morris AL. Periodontal manifestations of cyclic neutropenia. J Periodontol. 1961;32(2):159–68.
57. Dale DC, Bolyard AA, Kelley ML, Makaryan V, Bonilla MA, Boxer LA, et al. Long term outcomes for patients with cyclic neutropenia treated with granulocyte colony-stimulating factor (G-CSF). Blood. 2015;126(23):996.
58. George JN, Arnold DM. Approach to the adult with unexplained thrombocytopenia. UpToDate. Available at http://www.uptodate.com/contents/approach-to-the-adult-with-unexplained-thrombocytopenia. Accessed July 10, 2016.
59. James WD, Guiry CC, Grote WR. Acute idiopathic thrombocytopenic purpura. Oral Surg Oral Med Oral Pathol. 1984;57(2):149–1451.
60. Adams PC. Epidemiology and diagnostic testing for hemochromatosis and iron overload. Int J Lab Hematol. 2015;37:25–30.
61. Pietrangelo A. Hereditary hemochromatosis: pathogenesis, diagnosis, and treatment. Gastroenterology. 2010;139(2):393–408.
62. Adams PC, Reboussin DM, Barton JC, et al. Hemochromatosis and iron-overload screening in a racially diverse population. N Engl J Med. 2005;352(17):1769–78.
63. Erwin A, Balwani M, Desnick RJ. Congenital erythropoietic porphyria. GeneReviews. 2013. Available at http://www.ncbi.nlm.nih.gov/books/NBK154652/. Accessed July 10, 2016.
64. Fayle SA, Pollard MA. Congenital erythropoietic porphyria–oral manifestations and dental treatment in childhood: a case report. Quintessence Int. 1994;25(8):551–4.
65. Javed F, Correa FO, Nooh N, Almas K, Romanos GE, Al-Hezaimi K. Orofacial manifestations in patients with sickle cell disease. Am J Med Sci. 2013;345(3):234–7.
66. Online Mendelian Inheritance in Man, OMIM®. OMIM 603903. Available at http://omim.org/. Accessed May 16, 2016.

67. Rees DC, Williams TN, Gladwin MT. Sickle-cell disease. Lancet. 2010;376(9757):2018–31.
68. Jones H, Blinder M, Anadkat M. Cutaneous manifestations of sickle cell disease. Open J Blood Dis. 2013;3:94–9.
69. Tefferi A. Polycythemia vera: a comprehensive review and clinical recommendations. Mayo Clin Proc. 2003;78(2):174–94.
70. Anía BJ, Suman VJ, Sobell JL, Codd MB, Silverstein MN, Melton LJ. Trends in the incidence of polycythemia vera among Olmsted County, Minnesota residents, 1935-1989. Am J Hematol. 1994;47(2):89–93.
71. Najean Y, Rain JD, Billotey C. Epidemiological data in polycythaemia vera: a study of 842 cases. Hematol Cell Ther. 1998;40(4):159–65.
72. Lele MV. Oral manifestations of polycythaemia rubra vera. J All India Dent Assoc. 1965;37(11):345–8.
73. Ruparella PB, Ruparella KP, Shirolkar R, Tipathy A. Chronic myeloproliferative disorders: a rarest case with oral manifestations and dental management. J Indian Acta Oral Med Radiol. 2012;24(2):155–7.
74. Carlson ER, Chewning LC. Polycythemia vera in an oral surgical patient. A case report. Oral Surg Oral Med Oral Pathol. 1989;67(6):673–5.
75. Cooper GS, Stroehla BC. The epidemiology of autoimmune diseases. Autoimmun Rev. 2003;2(3):119–25.
76. Baldini C, Talarico R, Tzioufas AG, Bombardieri S. Classification criteria for Sjogren's syndrome: a critical review. J Autoimmun. 2012;39(1-2):9–14.
77. Baldini C, Bernacchi E, Talarico R. Skin manifestations and Sjögren's syndrome. In: Matucci-Cerinic M, Furst D, Fiorentino D, editors. Skin manifestations in rheumatic disease. New York: Springer; 2014. p. 207–15.
78. Islam NM, Bhattacharyya I, Cohen DM. Common oral manifestations of systemic disease. Otolaryngol Clin N Am. 2011;44(1):161–82.
79. Kassan SS, Moutsopoulos HM. Clinical manifestations and early diagnosis of Sjögren syndrome. Arch Intern Med. 2004;164(12):1275–84.
80. Rhodus NL, Bloomquist C, Liljemark W, Bereuter J. Prevalence, density, and manifestations of oral Candida albicans in patients with Sjögren's syndrome. J Otolaryngol. 1997;26(5):300–5.
81. Soto-Rojas AE, Villa AR, Sifuentes-Osornio J, Alarcon-Segovia D, Kraus A. Oral candidiasis and Sjogren's syndrome. J Rheumatol. 1998;25(5):911–5.
82. Ravald N, List T. Caries and periodontal conditions in patients with primary Sjögren's syndrome. Swed Dent J. 1998;22(3):97–103.
83. Williams RC, Gibbons RJ. Inhibition of streptococcal attachment to receptors on human buccal epithelial cells by antigenically similar salivary glycoproteins. Infect Immun. 1975;11(4):711–8.
84. Epstein JB, Truelove EL, Izutzu KT. Oral candidiasis: pathogenesis and host defense. Rev Infect Dis. 1984;6(1):96–106.
85. Taubert KA. Epidemiology of Kawasaki disease in the United States and worldwide. Prog Pediatr Cardiol. 1997;6(3):181–5.
86. Council on Cardiovascular Disease in the Young, Committee on Rheumatic Fever, Endocarditis, and Kawasaki Disease, American Heart Association. Diagnostic guidelines for Kawasaki disease. Circulation. 2001;103(2):335–6.
87. Yim D, Curtis N, Cheung M, Burgner D. Update on Kawasaki disease: epidemiology, aetiology and pathogenesis. J Paediatr Child Health. 2013;49(9):704–8.
88. Ogden GR, Kerr M. Mucocutaneous lymph node syndrome (Kawasaki disease). Oral Surg Oral Med Oral Pathol. 1989;67(5):569–72.
89. Ozdemir H, Ciftçi E, Tapisiz A, Ince E, Tutar E, Atalay S, et al. Clinical and epidemiological characteristics of children with Kawasaki disease in Turkey. J Trop Pediatr. 2010;56(4):260–2.
90. Lawrence RC, Helmick CG, Arnett FC, Deyo RA, Felson DT, Giannini EH, et al. Estimates of the prevalence of arthritis and selected musculoskeletal disorders in the United States. Arthritis Rheum. 1998;41(5):778–99.

91. Lourenço SV, de Carvalho FR, Boggio P, Sotto MN, Vilela MA, Rivitti EA, et al. Lupus erythematosus: clinical and histopathological study of oral manifestations and immunohistochemical profile of the inflammatory infiltrate. J Cutan Pathol. 2007;34(7):558–64.
92. Gabrielli A, Avvedimento EV, Krieg T. Scleroderma. N Engl J Med. 2009;360(19):1989–2003.
93. Fischer DJ, Patton LL. Scleroderma: oral manifestations and treatment challenges. Spec Care Dentist. 2000;20(6):240–4.
94. Hinchcliff M, Varga J. Systemic sclerosis/scleroderma: a treatable multisystem disease. Am Fam Physician. 2008;78(8):961–8.
95. Nagy G, Kovács J, Zeher M, Czirják L. Analysis of the oral manifestations of systemic sclerosis. Oral Surg Oral Med Oral Pathol. 1994;77(2):141–6.
96. Eufinger H, Machtens E, Akuamoa-Boateng E. Oral manifestations of Wegener's granulomatosis. Review of the literature and report of a case. Int J Oral Maxillofac Surg. 1992;21(1):50–3.
97. Patten SF, Tomecki KJ. Wegener's granulomatosis: cutaneous and oral mucosal disease. J Am Acad Dermatol. 1993;28(5):710–8.
98. Mahr AD, Neogi T, Merkel PA. Epidemiology of Wegener's granulomatosis: lessons from descriptive studies and analyses of genetic and environmental risk determinants. Clin Exp Rheumatol. 2006;24(2):82–91.
99. Tarabishy AB, Schulte M, Papaliodis GN, Hoffman GS. Wegener's granulomatosis: clinical manifestations, differential diagnosis, and management of ocular and systemic disease. Surv Ophthalmol. 2010;55(5):429–44.
100. Almouhawis HA, Leao JC, Fedele S, Porter SR. Wegener's granulomatosis: a review of clinical features and an update in diagnosis and treatment. J Oral Pathol Med. 2013;42(7):507–16.
101. Knight JM, Hayduk MJ, Summerlin DJ, Mirowski GW. "Strawberry" gingival hyperplasia: a pathognomonic mucocutaneous finding in Wegener granulomatosis. Arch Dermatol. 2000;136(2):171–3.
102. Napier SS, Allen JA, Irwin CR, McCluskey DR. Strawberry gums: a clinicopathological manifestation diagnostic of Wegener's granulomatosis? J Clin Pathol. 1993;46(8):709–12.
103. Suresh L, Radfar L. Oral sarcoidosis: a review of literature. Oral Dis. 2005;11(3):138–45.
104. Marcoval J, Mañá J. Specific (granulomatous) oral lesions of sarcoidosis: report of two cases. Med Oral Patol Oral Cir Bucal. 2010;15(3):456–8.
105. Lisowe JA, Fleck JD, Mirowski GW. Pearls in neurodermatology. Semin Neurol. 1998;18(2):243–55.
106. Falk RH, Comenzo RL, Skinner M. The systemic amyloidoses. N Engl J Med. 1997;337(13):898–909.
107. Viggor SF, Frezzini C, Farthing PM, Freeman CO, Yeoman CM, Thornhill MH. Amyloidosis: an unusual case of persistent oral ulceration. Oral Surg Oral Med Oral Pathol Oral Radiol Endod. 2009;108(5):46–50.
108. Elad S, Czerninski R, Fischman S, Keshet N, Drucker S, Davidovich T, et al. Exceptional oral manifestations of amyloid light chain protein (AL) systemic amyloidosis. Amyloid. 2010;17(1):27–31.
109. Carbone JE, Barker D, Stauffer JL. Sleep apnea in amyloidosis. Chest. 1985;87(3):401–3.
110. World Health Organization. HIV/AIDS Fact Sheet. 2015. Available at http://www.who.int/mediacentre/factsheets/fs360/en/. Accessed July 11, 2016.
111. Meyer U, Kleinheinz J, Handschel J, Kruse-Lösler B, Weingart D, Joos U. Oral findings in three different groups of immunocompromised patients. J Oral Pathol Med. 2000;29(4):153–8.
112. Zancanaro PC, McGirt LY, Mamelak AJ, Nguyen RH, Martins CR. Cutaneous manifestations of HIV in the era of highly active antiretroviral therapy: an institutional urban clinic experience. J Am Acad Dermatol. 2006;54(4):581–8.
113. Nokta M. Oral manifestations associated with HIV infection. Curr HIV/AIDS Rep. 2008;5(1):5–12.
114. Casiglia JW, Woo S. Oral manifestations of HIV infection. Clin Dermatol. 2000;18(5):541–51.
115. Centers for Disease Control and Prevention. 1993 revised classification system for HIV infection and expanded surveillance case definition for AIDS among adolescents and adults. MMWR Recomm Rep. 1992;41:1–19.

116. Greenspan JS, Barr CE, Sciubba JJ, Winkler JR. Oral manifestations of HIV infection. Definitions, diagnostic criteria, and principles of therapy. The U.S.A. Oral AIDS Collaborative Group. Oral Surg Oral Med Oral Pathol. 1992;73(2):142–4.
117. Kademani D, Glick M. Oral ulcerations in individuals infected with human immunodeficiency virus: clinical presentations, diagnosis, management, and relevance to disease progression. Quintessence Int. 1998;29(8):523–34.
118. Mirowski GW, Hilton JF, Greenspan D, et al. Association of cutaneous and oral diseases in HIV-infected men. Oral Dis. 1998;4(1):16–21.
119. Scully C, Laskaris G, Pindborg J, Porter SR, Reichart P. Oral manifestations of HIV infection and their management. I. More common lesions. Oral Surg Oral Med Oral Pathol. 1991;71(2):158–66.
120. Nweze EI, Ogbonnaya UL. Oral Candida isolates among HIV-infected subjects in Nigeria. J Microbiol Immunol Infect. 2011;44(3):172–7.
121. Armstrong-James D, Meintjes G, Brown GD. A neglected epidemic: fungal infections in HIV/AIDS. Trends Microbiol. 2014;22(3):120–1207.
122. Langenberg AG, Corey L, Ashley RL, Leong WP, Straus SE. A prospective study of new infections with herpes simplex virus type 1 and type 2. Chiron HSV Vaccine Study Group. N Engl J Med. 1999;341(19):1432–8.
123. Birek C, Ficarra G. The diagnosis and management of oral herpes simplex infection. Curr Infect Dis Rep. 2006;8(3):181–8.
124. Eisen D. The clinical characteristics of intraoral herpes simplex virus infection in 52 immunocompetent patients. Oral Surg Oral Med Oral Pathol Oral Radiol Endod. 1998;86(4):432–7.
125. Ficarra G. Oral ulcers in HIV-infected patients: an update on epidemiology and diagnosis. Oral Dis. 1997;3:183–9.
126. Génèreau T, Lortholary O, Bouchaud O, Lacassin F, Vinceneux P, De Truchis P, et al. Herpes simplex esophagitis in patients with AIDS: report of 34 cases. The Cooperative Study Group on Herpetic Esophagitis in HIV Infection. Clin Infect Dis. 1996;22(6):926–31.
127. Levin MJ, Bacon TH, Leary JJ. Resistance of herpes simplex virus infections to nucleoside analogues in HIV-infected patients. Clin Infect Dis. 2004;39:248–57.
128. Greenspan D, Greenspan JS. Significance of oral hairy leukoplakia. Oral Surg Oral Med Oral Pathol. 1992;73(2):151–4.
129. Greenspan JS, Greenspan D, Webster-Cyriaque J. Hairy leukoplakia; lessons learned: 30-plus years. Oral Dis. 2016;22:120–7.
130. Itin P, Rufli T, Rüdlinger R, Cathomas G, Huser B, Podvinec M, et al. Oral hairy leukoplakia in a HIV-negative renal transplant patient: a marker for immunosuppression? Dermatologica. 1988;177(2):126–8.
131. Chattopadhyay A, Caplan DJ, Slade GD, Shugars DC, Tien HC, Patton LL. Risk indicators for oral candidiasis and oral hairy leukoplakia in HIV-infected adults. Community Dent Oral Epidemiol. 2005;33(1):35–44.
132. Schiødt M, Greenspan D, Daniels TE, Greenspan JS. Clinical and histologic spectrum of oral hairy leukoplakia. Oral Surg Oral Med Oral Pathol. 1987;64(6):716–20.
133. Triantos D, Porter SR, Scully C, Teo CG. Oral hairy leukoplakia: clinicopathologic features, pathogenesis, diagnosis, and clinical significance. Clin Infect Dis. 1997;25(6):1392–6.
134. Moura MD, Haddad JP, Senna MI, Ferreira Ferreira E, Mesquita RA. A new topical treatment protocol for oral hairy leukoplakia. Oral Surg Oral Med Oral Pathol Oral Radiol Endod. 2010;110(5):611–7.
135. Martellotta F, Berretta M, Vaccher E, Schioppa O, Zanet E, Tirelli U. AIDS-related Kaposi's sarcoma: state of the art and therapeutic strategies. Curr HIV Res. 2009;7(6):634–8.
136. Levine AM, Tulpule A. Clinical aspects and management of AIDS-related Kaposi's sarcoma. Eur J Cancer. 2001;37(10):1288–95.
137. Ficarra G, Berson AM, Silverman S Jr, Quivey JM, Lozada-Nur F, Sooy DD, et al. Kaposi's sarcoma of the oral cavity: a study of 134 patients with a review of the pathogenesis, epidemiology, clinical aspects, and treatment. Oral Surg Oral Med Oral Pathol. 1988;66(5):543–50.

138. Yeh CK, Fox PC, Fox CH, Travis WD, Lane HC, Baum BJ. Kaposi's sarcoma of the parotid gland in acquired immunodeficiency syndrome. Oral Surg Oral Med Oral Pathol. 1989;67(3):308–12.
139. Castle JT, Thompson LD. Kaposi sarcoma of major salivary gland origin: a clinicopathologic series of six cases. Cancer. 2000;88(1):15–23.
140. Fatahzadeh M. Kaposi sarcoma: review and medical management update. Oral Surg Oral Med Oral Pathol Oral Radiol. 2012;113(1):2–16.
141. Cannon MJ, Schmid DS, Hyde TB. Review of cytomegalovirus seroprevalence and demographic characteristics associated with infection. Rev Med Virol. 2010;20(4):202–13.
142. Chakraborty A, Siddhanta S, De C, Bhattacharyya S, Guha SK, et al. Cytomegalovirus retinitis with multiple co infections in a HIV/AIDS patient having extreme low CD4 count: a case report and review of literature. J AIDS Clin Res. 2014;5:394.
143. Greenspan D, Greenspan JS. Oral manifestations of human immunodeficiency virus infection. Dent Clin N Am. 1993;37(1):21–32.
144. Itin PH, Lautenschlager S, Flückiger R, Rufli T. Oral manifestations in HIV-infected patients: diagnosis and management. J Am Acad Dermatol. 1993;29(5):749–60.
145. Mathur S, Jani M, Thakkar P, Shah A. Oral manifestations of HIV infection. Int J Dent Med Res. 2014;1(4):139.
146. Mattes FM, McLaughlin JE, Emery VC, Clark DA, Griffiths PD. Histopathological detection of owl's eye inclusions is still specific for cytomegalovirus in the era of human herpesviruses 6 and 7. J Clin Pathol. 2000;53(8):612–4.
147. Kreimer AR, Alberg AJ, Daniel R, Gravitt PE, Viscidi R, Garrett ES, et al. Oral human papillomavirus infection in adults is associated with sexual behavior and HIV serostatus. J Infect Dis. 2004;89(4):686–98.
148. Brickman C, Palefsky JM. Human papillomavirus in the HIV-infected host: epidemiology and pathogenesis in the antiretroviral era. Curr HIV/AIDS Rep. 2015;12(1):6–15.
149. Devarakonda S, Neppalli A, Liu L, Shi R. Risk factors and prevalence of genital HPV infection among adult females in US between 2003-2010: data from NHANES study. Cancer Res. 2014;74(19):278.
150. Markowitz LE, Hariri S, Lin C, Dunne EF, Steinau M, McQuillan G, et al. Reduction in human papillomavirus (HPV) prevalence among young women following HPV vaccine introduction in the United States, National Health and Nutrition Examination Surveys, 2003-2010. J Infect Dis. 2013;208(3):385–93.
151. Neville BW, Day TA. Oral cancer and precancerous lesions. CA Cancer J Clin. 2002;52(4):195–215.
152. Syrjanen S, Termine N, Capra G, Paderni C, Panzarella V, Campisi G. Oral HPV infection: current strategies for prevention and therapy. Curr Pharm Des. 2012;18(34):5452–69.
153. Chavan M, Jain H, Diwan N, Khedkar S, Shete A, Durkar S. Recurrent aphthous stomatitis: a review. J Oral Pathol Med. 2012;41(8):577–83.
154. Muzyka BC, Glick M. Major aphthous ulcers in patients with HIV disease. Oral Surg Oral Med Oral Pathol. 1994;77(2):116–20.
155. Randall P. Thalidomide effective treatment for AIDS-related mouth ulcers. NIAID AIDS Agenda. 1995;2:11363350.
156. Khandwala A, Van Inwegen RG, Alfano MC. 5% amlexanox oral paste, a new treatment for recurrent minor aphthous ulcers: I. Clinical demonstration of acceleration of healing and resolution of pain. Oral Surg Oral Med Oral Pathol Oral Radiol Endod. 1997;83(2):222–30.
157. Meng W, Dong Y, Liu J, Wang Z, Zhong X, Chen R, et al. A clinical evaluation of amlexanox oral adhesive pellicles in the treatment of recurrent aphthous stomatitis and comparison with amlexanox oral tablets: a randomized, placebo controlled, blinded, multicenter clinical trial. Trials. 2009;10:30.
158. Jacobson JM, Greenspan JS, Spritzler J, Ketter N, Fahey JL, Jackson JB, et al. Thalidomide for the treatment of oral aphthous ulcers in patients with human immunodeficiency virus infection. National Institute of Allergy and Infectious Diseases AIDS Clinical Trials Group. N Engl J Med. 1997;336(21):1487–93.

159. Challacombe SJ, Alsahaf S, Tappuni A. Recurrent aphthous stomatitis: towards evidence-based treatment? Curr Oral Health Rep. 2015;2:158–67.
160. Langley RG, Krueger GG, Griffiths CE. Psoriasis: epidemiology, clinical features, and quality of life. Ann Rheum Dis. 2005;64(Suppl 2):118–23.
161. Johnson MA, Armstrong AW. Clinical and histologic diagnostic guidelines for psoriasis: a critical review. Clin Rev Allergy Immunol. 2013;44(2):166–72.
162. Eastman JR, Goldblatt LI. Psoriasis. Palatal manifestations and physiologic considerations. J Periodontol. 1983;54(12):736–9.
163. Morris LF, Phillips CM, Binnie WH, Sander HM, Silverman AK, Menter MA. Oral lesions in patients with psoriasis: a controlled study. Cutis. 1992;49(5):339–44.
164. Richardson LJ, Kratochvil FJ, Zieper MB. Unusual palatal presentation of oral psoriasis. J Can Dent Assoc. 2000;66(2):80–2.
165. Zhu JF, Kaminski MJ, Pulitzer DR, Hu J, Thomas HF. Psoriasis: pathophysiology and oral manifestations. Oral Dis. 1996;2(2):135–44.
166. Mattsson U, Warfvinge G, Jontell M. Oral psoriasis-a diagnostic dilemma: a report of two cases and a review of the literature. Oral Surg Oral Med Oral Pathol Oral Radiol. 2015;120(4):183–9.
167. Germi L, De Giorgi V, Bergamo F, Niccoli MC, Kokelj F, Simonacci M, et al. Psoriasis and oral lesions: multicentric study of Oral Mucosa Diseases Italian Group (GIPMO). Dermatol Online J. 2012;18(1):11.
168. van der Waal I, Pindborg JJ. Diseases of the tongue. Chicago: Quintessence Publishing; 1986. p. 103–4.
169. Higgins SP, Freemark M, Prose NS. Acanthosis nigricans: a practical approach to evaluation and management. Dermatol Online J. 2008;14(9):2.
170. Kong AS, Williams RL, Rhyne R, Urias-Sandoval V, Cardinali G, Weller NF, et al. Acanthosis Nigricans: high prevalence and association with diabetes in a practice-based research network consortium–a PRImary care Multi-Ethnic network (PRIME Net) study. J Am Board Fam Med. 2010;23(4):476–85.
171. Schwartz RA. Acanthosis nigricans. J Am Acad Dermatol. 1994;31(1):1–19.
172. Sedano HO, Gorlin RJ. Acanthosis nigricans. Oral Surg Oral Med Oral Pathol. 1987;63(4):462–7.
173. Pentenero M, Carrozzo M, Pagano M, Gandolfo S. Oral acanthosis nigricans, tripe palms and sign of leser-trélat in a patient with gastric adenocarcinoma. Int J Dermatol. 2004;43(7):530–2.
174. Nomachi K, Mori M, Matsuda N. Improvement of oral lesions associated with malignant acanthosis nigricans after treatment of lung cancer. Oral Surg Oral Med Oral Pathol. 1989;68(1):74–9.
175. Ramirez-Amador V, Esquivel-Pedraza L, Caballero-Mendoza E, Berumen-Campos J, Orozco-Topete R, Angeles-Angeles A. Oral manifestations as a hallmark of malignant acanthosis nigricans. J Oral Pathol Med. 1999;28(6):278–81.
176. Mostofi RS, Hayden NP, Soltani K. Oral malignant acanthosis nigricans. Oral Surg Oral Med Oral Pathol. 1983;56(4):372–4.
177. Cairo F, Rubino I, Rotundo R, Prato GP, Ficarra G. Oral Acanthosis nigricans as a marker of internal malignancy. A case report. J Periodontol. 2001;72(9):1271–5.
178. Friedman JM. Neurofibromatosis 1. GeneReviews. 2014. Available at http://www.ncbi.nlm.nih.gov/books/NBK1109/. Accessed July 10, 2016.
179. Evans DG. Neurofibromatosis 2. GeneReviews. 2011. Available at http://www.ncbi.nlm.nih.gov/books/NBK1201/. Accessed July 10, 2016.
180. Geist JR, Gander DL, Stefanac SJ. Oral manifestations of neurofibromatosis types I and II. Oral Surg Oral Med Oral Pathol. 1992;73(3):376–82.
181. Javed F, Ramalingam S, Ahmed HB, Gupta B, Sundar C, Qadri T, et al. Oral manifestations in patients with neurofibromatosis type-1: a comprehensive literature review. Crit Rev Oncol Hematol. 2014;91(2):123–9.
182. Bongiorno MR, Pistone G, Aricò M. Manifestations of the tongue in Neurofibromatosis type 1. Oral Dis. 2006;12(2):125–9.

183. Tsang ES, Birch P, Friedman JM, Johnston D, Tucker T, Armstrong L. Prevalence of dental caries in children with neurofibromatosis 1. Clin Oral Investig. 2010;14(4):479–80.
184. D'Ambrosio JA, Langlais RP, Young RS. Jaw and skull changes in neurofibromatosis. Oral Surg Oral Med Oral Pathol. 1988;66(3):391–6.
185. Cunha KS, Barboza EP, Dias EP, Oliveira FM. Neurofibromatosis type I with periodontal manifestation. A case report and literature review. Br Dent J. 2004;196(8):457–60.
186. Leite RS, Marlow NM, Fernandes JK. Oral health and type 2 diabetes. Am J Med Sci. 2013;345(4):271–3.
187. Bastos AS, Leite AR, Spin-Neto R, Nassar PO, Massucato EM, Orrico SR. Diabetes mellitus and oral mucosa alterations: prevalence and risk factors. Diabetes Res Clin Pract. 2011;92(1):100–5.
188. Dikshit RP, Ramadas K, Hashibe M, Thomas G, Somanathan T, Sankaranarayanan R. Association between diabetes mellitus and pre-malignant oral diseases: a cross sectional study in Kerala, India. Int J Cancer. 2006;118(2):453–7.
189. Quirino MR, Birman EG, Paula CR. Oral manifestations of diabetes mellitus in controlled and uncontrolled patients. Braz Dent J. 1995;6(2):131–6.
190. Lamster IB, Lalla E, Borgnakke WS, Taylor GW. The relationship between oral health and diabetes mellitus. J Am Dent Assoc. 2008;139:19–24.
191. Murrah VA. Diabetes mellitus and associated oral manifestations: a review. J Oral Pathol. 1985;14(4):271–81.
192. Vanderpump MPJ, Tunbridge WMG. The epidemiology of thyroid diseases. In: Werner SC, Ingbar SH, Braverman LE, Utiger RD, editors. Werner & Ingbar's the thyroid: a fundamental and clinical text. 9th ed. Philadelphia: Lippincott Williams & Wilkins; 2005. p. 398–406.
193. Pinto A, Glick M. Management of patients with thyroid disease: oral health considerations. J Am Dent Assoc. 2002;133(7):849–58.
194. Chandna S, Bathla M. Oral manifestations of thyroid disorders and its management. Indian J Endocrinol Metab. 2011;15(2):113–6.
195. Wheeler AL, Shoback DM. Clinical presentation of hypoparathyroidism. In: Brandi ML, Brown EM, editors. Hypoparathyroidism. Milan: Springer; 2015. p. 155–65.
196. Sarkar S, Mondal M, Das K, Shrimal A. Mucocutaneous manifestations of acquired hypoparathyroidism: an observational study. Indian J Endocrinol Metab. 2012;5:819–20.
197. Fletcher PD, Scopp IW, Hersh RA. Oral manifestations of secondary hyperparathyroidism related to long-term hemodialysis therapy. Oral Surg Oral Med Oral Pathol. 1977;43(2):218–26.
198. Triantafillidou K, Zouloumis L, Karakinaris G, Kalimeras E, Iordanidis F. Brown tumors of the jaws associated with primary or secondary hyperparathyroidism. A clinical study and review of the literature. Am J Otolaryngol. 2006;27(4):281–6.
199. Nieman LK, Chanco Turner ML. Addison's disease. Clin Dermatol. 2006;24(4):276–80.
200. Eisen D. Disorders of pigmentation in the oral cavity. Clin Dermatol. 2000;18(5):579–87.
201. Scully C, Felix DH. Oral medicine–update for the dental practitioner. Aphthous and other common ulcers. Br Dent J. 2005;199(5):259–64.
202. Casiglia JM. Recurrent aphthous stomatitis: etiology, diagnosis, and treatment. Gen Dent. 2002;50(2):157–66.
203. Scully C. Drug effects on salivary glands: dry mouth. Oral Dis. 2003;9(4):165–76.
204. Kharazmi M, Sjöqvist K, Rizk M, Warfvinge G. Oral ulcer associated with alendronate: a case report. Oral Surg Oral Med Oral Pathol Oral Radiol Endod. 2010;110(6):11–3.
205. Lehman JS, Tollefson MM, Gibson LE. Lichen planus. Int J Dermatol. 2009;48(7):682–94.
206. Fitzpatrick SG, Hirsch SA, Gordon SC. The malignant transformation of oral lichen planus and oral lichenoid lesions: a systematic review. J Am Dent Assoc. 2014;145(1):45–56.
207. Litt JZ. Litt's drug eruption and reaction manual. 21st ed. Boca Raton: CRC Press; 2015.
208. Arirachakaran P, Hanvanich M, Kuysakorn P, Thongprasom K. Antiretroviral drug-associated oral lichenoid reaction in HIV patient: a case report. Int J Dent. 2010;2010:291072.
209. Calista D, Morri M. Lichen planus induced by hepatitis B vaccination: a new case and review of the literature. Int J Dermatol. 2004;43(8):562–4.

210. Agrawal A, Shenoi SD. Lichen planus secondary to hepatitis B vaccination. Indian J Dermatol Venereol Leprol. 2004;70(4):234–5.
211. Akay BN, Arslan A, Cekirge S, Erkin G, Anadolu-Brasie R. The first reported case of lichen planus following inactivated influenza vaccination. J Drugs Dermatol. 2007;5:536–8.
212. Hanania NA, Chapman KR, Kesten S. Adverse effects of inhaled corticosteroids. Am J Med. 1995;98(2):196–208.
213. van Boven JF, den Berg LT, Vegter S. Inhaled corticosteroids and the occurrence of oral candidiasis: a prescription sequence symmetry analysis. Drug Saf. 2013;36(4):231–6.
214. Ullah A, Iqbal Z, Anwar A. Frequency of oral candidiasis in asthma patients using inhaled corticosteroids by different inhaler devices. Pak J Chest Med. 2016;22(1):8–11.
215. Williams DW, Kuriyama T, Silva S, Malic S, Lewis MA. Candida biofilms and oral candidosis: treatment and prevention. Periodontol. 2011;55(1):250–65.
216. Milosevic A. Eating disorders and the dentist. Br Dent J. 1999;186(3):109–13.

Tongue Discoloration 12

12.1 Black Hairy Tongue (BHT)

12.1.1 Definition

Black hairy tongue (BHT) is a "condition where the surface of the tongue takes a blackish discoloration (Fig. 12.1) and furry appearance due to abnormally hypertrophied and elongated filiform papillae" (Fig. 12.2).

12.1.2 Synonyms

Originally described by Amatus Lusitanus in 1557 as "hairs on the tongue that would regrow upon being removed," black hairy tongue has also been referred to as "hyperkeratosis of the tongue," "lingua villosa nigra," "nigrites linguae," "keratomycosis linguae," and "melanotrihia lingua" [1–4].

12.1.3 Epidemiology

Review of the medical literature shows that BHT is not uncommon. According to the American Academy of Oral Medicine, BHT is thought to affect around 13% of the population. A large cross-sectional study of 5150 Turkish dental outpatients reported a prevalence of 11.3% with increased rates in men (18%) compared to women (6%) [5]. However, a cross-sectional study of 1901 Iranian dental patients reported a prevalence of only 1.2% [6], and Sarti et al. [7] and Neville et al. [8] reported that hairy tongue occurs in about 0.5% of adults. Moreover, BHT occurred in 0.6% of Minnesota school-aged children in contrast to 8.4% of patients in a young Finnish population [9–11]. Discordance of the observed rates may stem from different patient demographics (age, sex, ethnicity, practices, and habits) and interobserver variability in defining lesions in corresponding study populations.

© The Author(s), under exclusive license to Springer Nature Switzerland AG 2022

M. F. Sakr, *Tongue Lesions*, https://doi.org/10.1007/978-3-031-08198-9_12

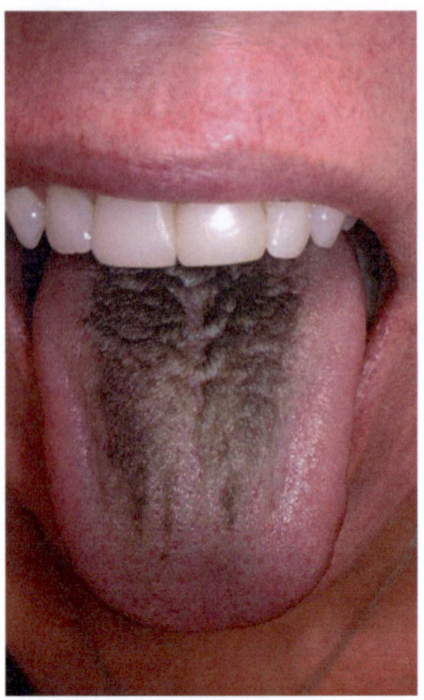

Fig. 12.1 Classic appearance of black hairy tongue (BHT)

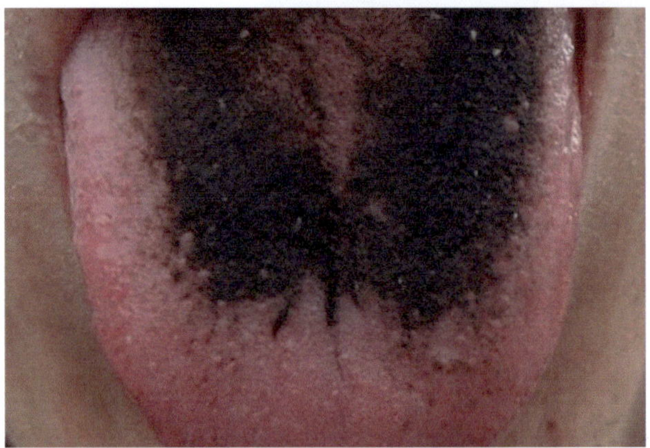

Fig. 12.2 Black hairy tongue. Note the black discoloration and furry appearance of the dorsum of the tongue (BHT)

Selected populations are at a higher risk of developing BHT, such as those with oncological disorders, smokers, black tea drinkers, and those with poor oral hygiene [5].

Black hairy tongue also shows clear *gender and age* predilection. Men are more commonly affected than women with a ratio of 3:1 [5, 6, 12]. This can be attributed to greater prominence of smoking and higher rates of poor oral hygiene among males. This difference is offset in Finland, where smoking rates have been declining among men and young women are slightly more likely to be affected with BHT [9, 13]. In addition, the chances of hairy tongue developing increase with age, as the effects of risk factors, such as tobacco use, have more time to accumulate. Some studies showed a prevalence of approximately 40% in patients over the age of 60 years [5], though cases have been reported in children as young as 2 months old [14, 15].

In addition to advanced age, poor general condition and certain neurological disorders affecting tongue movement and mastication place a patient at a higher risk of developing BHT, mainly due to the limited effective friction that results in desquamation of the keratinized layers of the filiform papillae.

Finally, it has been reported that there may also be global geographic deviations in the prevalence of BHT due to differences in oral hygiene habits and dietary patterns and variation in oral flora [16].

12.1.4 Pathogenesis

To date, the pathogenesis of BHT has not been fully elucidated. The upper surface of the tongue is rough in texture because it is covered with tiny protrusions called papillae, the most numerous of which are the filiform papillae. These are elongated, cone-shaped protrusions responsible for the gripping of food on the surface of the tongue. These structures usually grow to about 1 mm in length before they are shed from the tongue, allowing new ones to grow [17].

Hairy tongue occurs when these filiform papillae do not shed properly and start to grow. The elongated papillae can reach a length of 12–18 mm and width of 2 mm (simulating small hairs) [1, 5, 18]. These then secondarily collect fungi, bacteria, and debris [19]. This collection can include residue from tobacco, coffee, tea, other foods, and porphyrin-producing chromogenic organisms in the oral flora, which lend the lesion its characteristic hue [3, 19]. Using anti-keratin probes on BHT epithelium, Manabe et al. [20] confirmed that the "hairs" are highly elongated cornified spines that result from delayed desquamation of the cells in the central column of filiform papillae and marked retention of secondary papillary cells that expressed hair-type keratins [20].

12.1.5 Etiology

The etiology of BHT remains unclear and is likely multifactorial, resulting from a combination of local and systemic insults [8, 16]. Various appearances of BHT likely originate from differences in the potentially contributing extrinsic (environmental) and intrinsic (chromogenic oral microflora) factors [14]. Particular care should be delegated in identifying local inciting factors in the development of BHT. The different factors that can trigger the onset of BHT include the following [2, 5, 11, 21]:

12.1.5.1 Soft Diet

A lack of stimulation for abrasion to the surface of the tongue (by soft diet) can prevent sufficient shedding of the papillae or prevent keeping them short [7].

12.1.5.2 Tobacco, Tea, and Coffee Consumption

Although casual smoking poses a slightly increased risk of having BHT compared to nonsmokers (15% to 10% in men, 5.5% to 5.2% in women), heavy use of tobacco leads to a high prevalence of 58% in men and 33% in women [5, 8, 21]. Similarly, heavy black tea or coffee consumption leads to increased prevalence of BHT in both male and female patients [5].

12.1.5.3 Alcohol Intake and Intravenous (IV) Drug Use

Excessive alcohol intake and IV drug addiction have also been claimed to increase the risk of developing BHT.

12.1.5.4 Poor Oral Hygiene

Poor oral hygiene can cause a build-up of bacteria or fungi and thus contribute to the development of hairy tongue [8].

12.1.5.5 Hyposalivation or Dry Mouth

Lack of moisture in the mouth can make a person more prone to having hairy tongue [17].

12.1.5.6 Overgrowth of Microorganisms

Dietary consumption of herbal tea and sugars may lead to lowering pH on the dorsum of the tongue, promoting fungal and chromogenic bacterial overgrowth [8, 14].

12.1.5.7 Certain Diseases and General Debilitation [8]

Recently, a number of cases of BHT have been reported after allogenic *stem cell transplantation* as a cutaneous presentation of graft-versus-host disease [22]. Moreover, the prevalence of BHT is increased in the case of advanced cancer, with one study showing rates as high as 30% in men and 18% in women [23]. Other medical conditions associated with BHT include general body illness [2, 23], human immunodeficiency virus (HIV) infection [2, 23], and trigeminal neuralgia [24]. This painful condition, associated with poor oral intake and decreased mastication, is thought to limit tongue movement, resulting in decreased tongue friction with food, palate, and teeth and ultimately hindering normal desquamation of the keratinized filiform papillae, thus leading to the development of BHT [24]. Pellagra (niacin deficiency) may also cause a thick grayish fur to develop on the dorsal tongue, along with other oral signs [25].

12.1.5.8 Certain Medications

The use of systemic and local medications has been commonly implicated in the development of BHT. Antibiotics, including penicillin, aureomycin, erythromycin, doxycycline, and neomycin, are most often associated with this disorder [1, 2, 18, 26, 27]. However, it should be noted that the cause and effect factor between antibiotics and development of BHT needs to be further elucidated. Specifically, local or systemic antibiotic use may significantly alter oral flora, thus potentially predisposing the patient to develop BHT. On the other hand, pronounced anatomical alteration in the filiform papillae may predispose the patient to trap foreign material and stimulate local microbial overgrowth that leads to typical color changes seen in patients with this condition.

Xerostomic agents, including antipsychotics (olanzapine and chlorpromazine), may predispose patients to develop BHT [28, 29]. Interestingly, a case of BHT was also reported after 4 days of erlotinib (Tarceva) treatment in a patient with advanced lung cancer, possibly due to an unclear interruption of epidermal grown factor and its receptor in the lingual epithelium [30]. It is also used for treatment of pancreatic cancer. Other examples include isthmus salicylate (Pepto-Bismol), which is an antacid medication used to treat temporary discomforts of the stomach and gastrointestinal tract, such as diarrhea, indigestion, heartburn, and nausea [8].

12.1.5.9 Radiotherapy

Recent radiation therapy to the head and neck region has been reported to increase the risk of BHT [8].

12.1.5.10 Oral Hygiene Products

Prolonged use of certain tooth pastes [2] or oxidizing mouthwashes [7] containing sodium perborate, sodium peroxide, and hydrogen peroxide has also been associated with the development of BHT.

12.1.5.11 Melanoglossia

Transient surface discoloration of the tongue and other soft tissues in the mouth can occur in the absence of hairy tongue (melanoglossia). Causes of melanoglossia include smoking (or betel chewing) [17], some foods and beverages (e.g., coffee, tea, or licorice) [17], certain medications (e.g., chlorhexidine) [17], iron salts [17], and bismuth subsalicylate (e.g., Pepto-Bismol) [2, 31].

12.1.6 Clinical Presentation

12.1.6.1 Symptoms and Local Examination

A typical patient with BHT is an elderly male smoker on antibiotics or antipsychotics with poor oral hygiene, who presents with painless black hair-like lesion on the central part of the dorsum of the tongue anterior to the circumvallate papillae, although sometimes the entire dorsal surface may be involved [7, 8]. Discoloration usually accompanies hairy tongue and may be yellow, brown, green, blue, or black [3, 8, 11]. The unpleasant appearance of hairy tongue may cause some psychological discomfort or embarrassment, but it is usually a harmless condition with no other symptoms.

In addition to change in appearance, it is possible for other symptoms of BHT to develop including the following [8, 32, 33]:

- Dysgeusia (distortion of taste sensation, also known as parageusia)
- Burning sensation on the tongue—burning mouth

- Tickling on the roof of the mouth when swallowing
- Gagging sensation
- Halitosis (bad breath)
- Metallic taste in the mouth
- Nausea
- Submandibular or other cervical lymphadenopathy (may occasionally be present in some cases) [14]

12.1.6.2 General Examination

Review of systems may be significant for chronic pain, major physical disabilities, psychiatric illnesses, or other debilitating symptoms that preclude the maintenance of proper oral hygiene and normal tongue movement. Other associated clinical conditions include advanced malignancy, psychiatric conditions, and trigeminal neuralgia. Physical exam is usually unremarkable aside from the hairy-appearing tongue lesion itself.

12.1.7 Diagnosis

Diagnosis is usually made by visual *intraoral examination* showing the characteristic appearance of the lesion with a predilection for the dorsal tongue, anterior to the circumvallate papillae and sulcus terminalis. Careful review of known precipitating factors and recent medication changes is also fundamental to reach the diagnosis of BHT.

Tissue biopsy is usually *not* needed, but may be used as an adjunct to diagnosis [8]. It will demonstrate marked elongation (more than 3 mm in length) and hyperparakeratosis of the filiform papillae and numerous bacteria growing on the epithelial surface [8].

Cultures may be considered to rule out superimposed bacterial or fungal infections associated with BHT [34]. Thus, associated *laboratory* findings may include positive fungal cultures, HIV test, and blood and urine toxicology studies.

12.1.8 Differential Diagnosis

Classic BHT presents as a black, hairy-appearing lesion on the dorsum of the tongue. Differential diagnosis includes "pseudo-hairy tongue," oral hairy leukoplakia, pigmented fungiform papillae of the tongue, and acanthosis nigricans [33].

Detailed history-taking and physical examination are essential to arriving at the correct diagnosis, with particular emphasis on identifying known etiologic factors. Biopsy specimens may be required to rule out "mimicking" conditions and confirm diagnosis. In infants, congenital lingual melanotic macules and congenital melanocytic nevi should be sought for and diligently excluded [14].

12.1.8.1 Pseudo-Black Hairy Tongue

Pseudo-black hairy tongue (Fig. 12.3) appears as a darkly stained tongue in the absence of elongated filiform papillae seen in BHT. Certain foods, tobacco, and drugs, including antibiotics, antidepressants, and bismuth salicylate, can cause this condition [2, 27, 35–37].

12.1.8.2 Oral Hairy Leukoplakia

Hairy tongue may be confused with "oral hairy leukoplakia"; however, the latter usually occurs on the dorsal and ventral surfaces of the tongue, as well as sides of the tongue, buccal mucosa, and gingiva, and is associated with an opportunistic viral infection with Epstein-Barr virus (EBV) on a background immunocompromise infection (almost always HIV, but rarely other conditions which suppress the immune system) [8]. Oral hairy leukoplakia can also cause the tongue to have white patches that look hairy in appearance upon close inspection [38].

12.1.8.3 Pigmented Fungiform Papillae

Pigmented fungiform papillae of the tongue (due to melanin laden macrophages) are rare. They are, characterized by isolated hypertrophied lesions primarily on the lateral aspect and apex of the tongue that has a predilection to dark-skinned patients.

12.1.8.4 Acanthosis Nigricans

Acanthosis nigricans in the oral cavity manifests as multiple dark and demarcated papillary lesions on the dorsum and lateral sides of the tongue. Labial involvement is frequent. Acanthosis nigricans may be associated with an underlying malignancy [33].

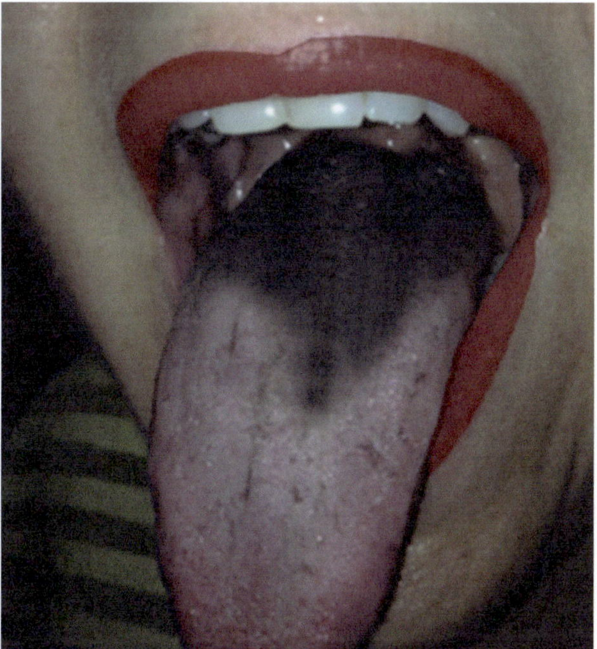

Fig. 12.3 Pseudo-black hairy tongue caused by the use of bismuth salicylate antacid

12.1.9 Prevention and Treatment

Proper patient reassurance to the benign nature of BHT is important, both to decrease the level of aesthetic anxiety and to promote appropriate treatment [8]. The patient should be educated of this condition as a potential side effect of antibiotic and antipsychotic medications. Practicing good oral hygiene, and gentle tongue brushing, may help to prevent (and treat) BHT [2, 17]. Treatment and prevention are typically achieved through changes to a person's lifestyle that may have triggered the onset of this condition. It is also essential to maintain a nutritious and well-balanced diet, containing a good balance of fresh fruits, vegetables, grains, and minimal sugar to promote oral health and may help improve this condition by facilitating the roughage on the tongue [28]. Consuming a sufficient amount of water throughout the day will also help to keep the mouth clean [2, 17].

The goal of therapy is the discontinuation of potential offending agents (including dietary or medicinal causes) and modifying predisposing factors (smoking, black tea consumption, neurological conditions, general debilitation), followed by maintaining good oral hygiene and gentle debridement with a soft tooth brush or tongue scraper to promote desquamation of the hyperkeratotic papillae.

Therapeutic approaches may thus include the following:

- *Avoiding* or *limiting* the consumption of substances that are associated with hairy tongue, such as coffee, tea, alcohol, or tobacco.
- *Brushing the tongue* or using a specialized tongue scraper to help with oral hygiene [17]. Keratolytic agents (chemicals to remove keratin) such as podophyllin are successful but carry safety concerns [8].
- *Medications*: Switching medications suspected to trigger BHT or starting antibiotics or antifungal drugs may be required [2].
- *Topical application* of baking soda or rinsing with diluted hydrogen peroxide solution may help improve desquamation of the keratinized filiform papillae and bleach the color.
- *Anecdotal use* of antimicrobial therapies, topical triamcinolone acetonide, gentian violet, salicylic acid, vitamin B complex, thymol, and topical or oral retinoids (e.g., isotretinoin), as well as keratolytics (podophyllin), topical 30% urea solution, and trichloroacetic acid have been reported in the literature, although potential side effects from local irritation and possible systemic absorption are important factors to consider [7, 14, 39–43].
- *Other reported successful measures* include eating pineapple, sucking on a peach stone, and chewing gum [17]. Yogurt and probiotic supplementation may be employed with various degree of success.
- *Resistant BHT* may require surgical removal of the filiform papillae (mechanical debridement) or clipping or removal of the papillae by electrodesiccation or carbon dioxide laser [33].

12.1.10 Complications

Typically, BHT is a self-limiting disorder, and the development of this condition commonly precipitates only aesthetic concern. Rarely, patients may report irritation, nausea, and gagging sensation mainly due to the size of unusually elongated papillae. Others may experience a disabling metallic taste, general dysgeusia, and perceived halitosis [7]. Bacterial or fungal superinfection is an important consideration, and proper recognition and treatment may preclude progression to glossopyrosis or burning mouth syndrome.

12.1.11 Prognosis

The long-term outcomes for BHT are excellent as the disease is benign and may even improve spontaneously. However, people who are affected with BHT may be distressed at the appearance and possible halitosis, and therefore treatment is indicated [8, 16, 44]. Prompt resolution occurs within days to few weeks after mechanical debridement and removal of a suspected precipitating agent. Patient education on proper oral hygiene and lifestyle modifications including smoking cessation and alcohol abstinence are vital to preventing recurrence. The development of BHT does not typically cause any sequelae.

Other coexisting clinical conditions associated with BHT (xerostomia, HIV, cancer, and trigeminal neuralgia) should be sought for and managed appropriately as well to reduce the risk of BHT reappearance.

12.1.12 Pearls for Clinical Practice

- Black hairy tongue (BHT) is a relatively common disease that classically manifests as a black and hairy-appearing lesion on the dorsum of the tongue due to abnormally hypertrophied and elongated filiform papillae.
- This benign condition is usually asymptomatic and typically triggers only local aesthetic concerns. Rarely, BHT can be accompanied by metallic taste, halitosis, burning mouth, and gagging. Its etiology and pathophysiology continue to be evolving and are undoubtedly multifactorial.
- Male gender, advanced age, smoking, alcohol abuse, excessive black tea or coffee consumption, HIV, debilitated general condition, and malignancy place patients at a higher risk for developing BHT.
- Visual inspection and thorough medical history establishes correct diagnosis, although microscopic examination, cultures of tongue swabs, and tongue biopsies may be of additional value in challenging cases.
- Management is primarily focused on mechanical debridement, maintenance of proper oral hygiene, and removal of potential causative agents.
- Overall clinical prognosis of BHT is excellent.

12.2 Orange Tongue

Fortunately, an orange tongue is usually caused by *certain foods* rich in beta-carotene (e.g., carrots), orange, gelatin, hard candy, or another type of food containing artificial coloring (Fig. 12.4). Otherwise, an orange tongue can indicate an underlying *medical condition.*

12.2.1 Etiology

The following conditions and factors may turn the tongue orange [45].

12.2.1.1 Poor Oral Hygiene: Food Debris

If a person does not regularly brush their teeth and tongue, food and other debris can build up. Using tobacco and drinking coffee or tea can make the tongue appear orange if a person does not brush their teeth afterward. Severe dry mouth, or xerostomia, can also turn the tongue orange. Dry mouth prevents bacteria from being flushed away as usual. This can lead to oral decay.

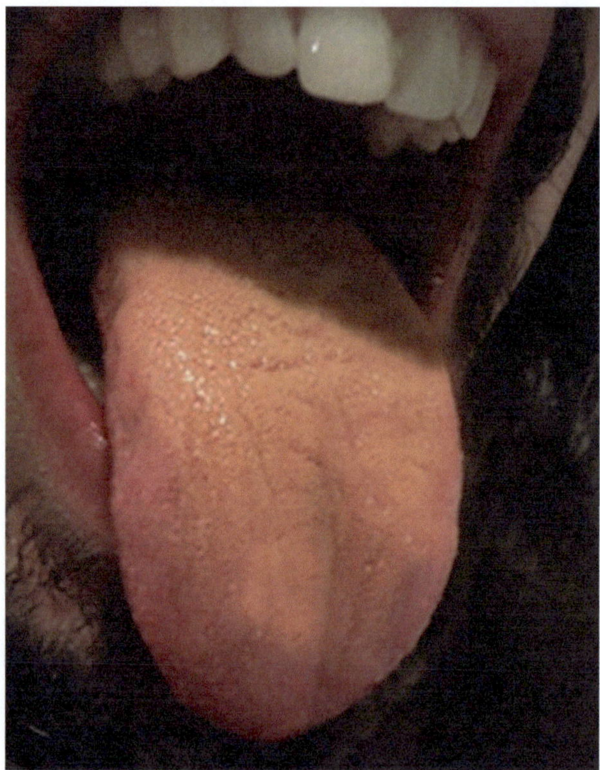

Fig. 12.4 A 23-year-old gentleman with orange discoloration of the tongue (orange tongue)

12.2.1.2 Overgrowth of Fungi (Oral Thrush) and Bacteria

Oral thrush or oral fungal infection (*Candida*) can cause the tongue to appear yellow or orange. It affects people of all ages. However, it is especially prevalent in people who are immunocompromised or receiving steroid medications. Infants are also prone to oral thrush, especially if they are on antibiotics, which can kill the bacteria that protect against overgrowth of fungi.

12.2.1.3 Certain Medications

Some medications contain certain ingredients that can temporarily turn the tongue orange. One example is rifampin (antituberculous). Other medications that can lead to an orange tongue include amiodarone, bleomycin, chloroquine, chlorpromazine, doxorubicin, hydroxy-chloroquine, minocycline, quinacrine, and quinidine. Antibiotics can cause an imbalance in a natural flora that could be a cause of orange coating on tongue. After taking the medication and having something to drink or brushing the teeth, the orange tint will usually disappear within a few hours.

12.2.1.4 Acid Indigestion/Heartburn

Acid ingestion is usually a main cause that a tongue looks orange. It is an imbalance of microorganisms that live on the mouth especially on the tongue. A treatment advisable for this is brushing and taking antacids. Reducing the intake of acidic foods or starting a low-acid diet could also be a way to prevent this.

12.2.1.5 Mold in the Environment

Living in the environment with molds could also lead to an orange tongue; it could be on the environment at home or at work. To avoid this, mold in the environment should be controlled and natural remedies started such as gargling or taking grapefruit seeds orally.

12.2.1.6 Excess Beta-Carotene (Carotenemia)

Beta-carotene is the compound that gives carrots their orange color. Excessive eating foods rich in this substance can cause orange discoloration of the skin and tongue (carotenemia) [46].

Carotenemia is most common in infants and young children, who often eat a lot of mashed carrots [47–50]. It is harmless but simulates jaundice [51]. However, the sclera turns yellow in the case of jaundice but not in people with carotenemia. Foods that contain high amounts of beta- carotene include carrots, sweet potatoes, cantaloupes, papayas, pumpkins, and mangoes [52–54].

The treatment for carotenemia is simply to eat fewer of these foods that cause orange discoloration. It is noteworthy that it may take several weeks or months for the skin and tongue to return to a normal color.

12.2.2 Clinical Presentation

Orange tongue can have different shades and shapes. It often affects young children, even toddlers and babies and especially adults. This usually happens during bedtime and waking up in the morning.

Common associated symptoms include the following:

- Unpleasant taste in the mouth
- Tongue dryness
- Bad breath (halitosis)
- Mouth itching or sore

Worst symptoms may include the following:

- Burning sensation on the throat
- Orange saliva
- Allergy or cold symptoms like sore throat, runny nose, stuffy nose, etc.
- Stomach upset
- Fatigue or weakness

An exception of a symptom of this condition is having eaten too much of a certain type of food such as carrots or tomatoes or having consumed something that is colored orange.

12.2.3 Treatment

If *poor oral hygiene* is causing an orange tongue, a person should take steps to improve their dental care routine. This should involve brushing twice a day. Using a tongue scraper will help remove excess bacteria and particle buildup.

Treatment of orange tongue caused by certain *medications* involves (1) restoring the balance of the healthy oral flora; (2) taking probiotics twice daily with food: this helps in growth of new colonies in the mouth and the gut; (3) taking antifungal herbs to keep bacteria level in balance: this includes garlic and oregano to keep fungus and virus under control; (4) receiving amino acid L-lysine is also good for the condition; and (5) taking a herbal tea containing lemon grass in between meals to help restore the balance in the mouth (honey, milk, or sugar should not be added in the tea).

For *oral thrush*, a mouthwash containing nystatin, diphenhydramine, lidocaine, and triamcinolone is indicated, 2–3 times/day. Oral antifungal medications may be necessary as well. Brushing the surface of the tongue stroking forward from the back toward its tip for at least twice a day is also useful.

Change diet: Foods that promote fungal growth or cause acid reflux should be avoided. These foods include coffee, candy, alcohol, white bread, or any sugary food, as well as excessive use of spices. Reducing carbohydrate consumption with an exception of yucca, potatoes, oatmeal, bananas, plantains, and dairy products (except yoghurt) is very helpful. For carotenemia, foods that contain beta-carotene should be reduced [50].

12.3 Strawberry (Bright Red) Tongue

12.3.1 Introduction

A healthy tongue is pink in color and is covered with small papillae. Bright red tongue (strawberry tongue) is a term used to describe a typically red tongue that is swollen and bumpy. The color and the taste bud bumping on the dorsal surface of the tongue may make it look like a strawberry or raspberry (Fig. 12.5). It may also affect the ventral surface of the tongue. Occasionally, the tongue may be white over a few days, after which it will turn red. Strawberry tongue is *not* a condition in itself, but rather a symptom that is a result of another disorder or condition. It may be a symptom of a food or drug allergy. It can indicate the presence of scarlet fever or Kawasaki disease, especially in a child. It may also be caused by glossitis [55].

12.3.2 Symptoms

If a person has a strawberry tongue, the tongue may look reddish (Fig. 12.6) or red with white patches (Fig. 12.7), swollen, enlarged, and covered with bumps. The

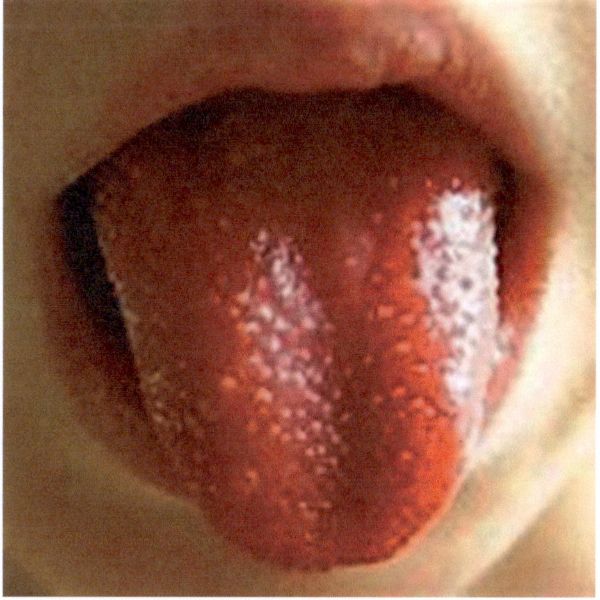

Fig. 12.5 Strawberry tongue involving the dorsal surface of the tongue

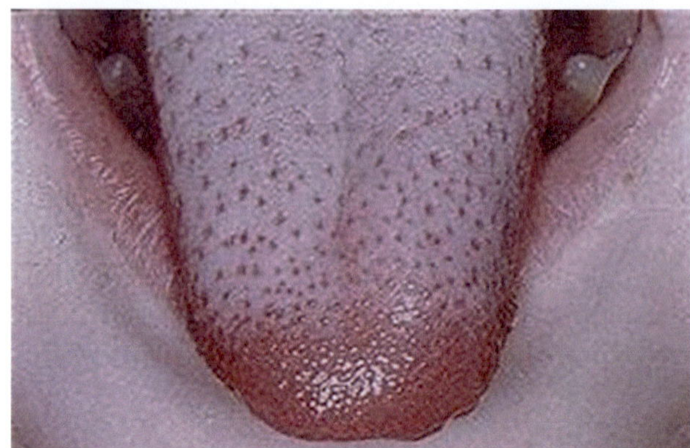

Fig. 12.6 Strawberry tongue may start and whitish and then turns red

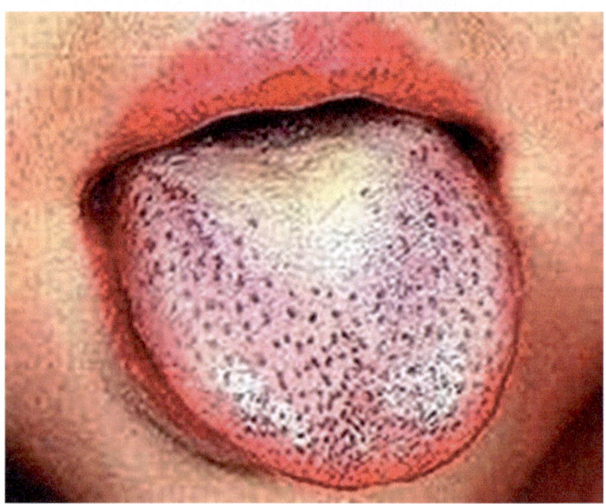

Fig. 12.7 Strawberry tongue may also show white patches

tongue may also feel irritated or painful. Other symptoms may occur in relation to the underlying condition that has caused it.

12.3.3 Etiology

Some underlying conditions that may cause strawberry tongue are explored below.

12.3.3.1 Kawasaki Disease

This disorder was first described in 1967 by Tomisaku Kawasaki in Japan [56, 57]. Kawasaki disease, also known as "mucocutaneous lymph node syndrome," is a disease in which blood vessels throughout the body become inflamed. It is a rare condition that usually affects children under the age of 5 years. It is much less common after the age of 5 and adults can be affected as well. Boys are more commonly affected than girls [55].

The cause of Kawasaki disease is exactly unknown. It may be due to an infection triggering an autoimmune response in those who are genetically predisposed. It is not contagious [55].

In addition to a strawberry tongue, the most common symptoms and signs of Kawasaki disease include high fever that lasts for more than 5 days not affected by usual medications, large lymph nodes in the neck, skin rash in the genital area, red eyes (with thick discharge in some cases) due to conjunctivitis, and erythema of the lips, palms of the hands or soles of the feet. Other symptoms include sore throat and diarrhea. Within 3 weeks of the onset of symptoms, the skin may peel from the hands and feet. Recovery then typically occurs. In some children, coronary artery aneurysms form in the heart [55, 58].

12.3.3.2 Scarlet Fever

Scarlet fever is a disease which results from bacterial infection with group A beta-hemolytic streptococcus (also known as *Streptococcus pyogenes*) [59]. It may develop when a person has strep throat (streptococcal pharyngitis) (Fig. 12.8). It most commonly affects children aged 5–15 years [59] and is transmitted by air-borne infection.

In addition to a strawberry tongue with or without white patches (Fig. 12.9), scarlet fever may cause enlarged lymph nodes (LNs), a red rash that covers most of the body and feels like *sand paper* (Fig. 12.10), bright red areas in the skin folds (particularly around the groin), a flushed face over the cheeks, high fever, sore

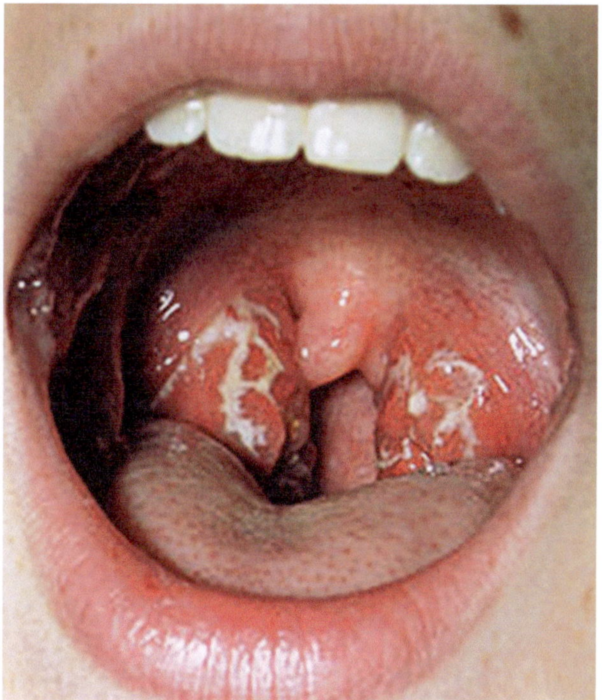

Fig. 12.8 Sore throat of a child with a positive throat culture for streptococcal pharyngitis (throat strep)

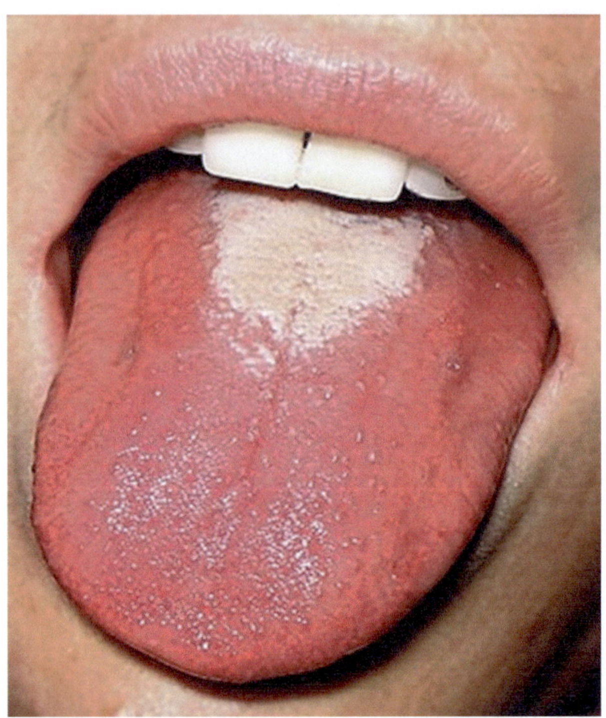

Fig. 12.9 Strawberry tongue with a white patch caused by scarlet fever

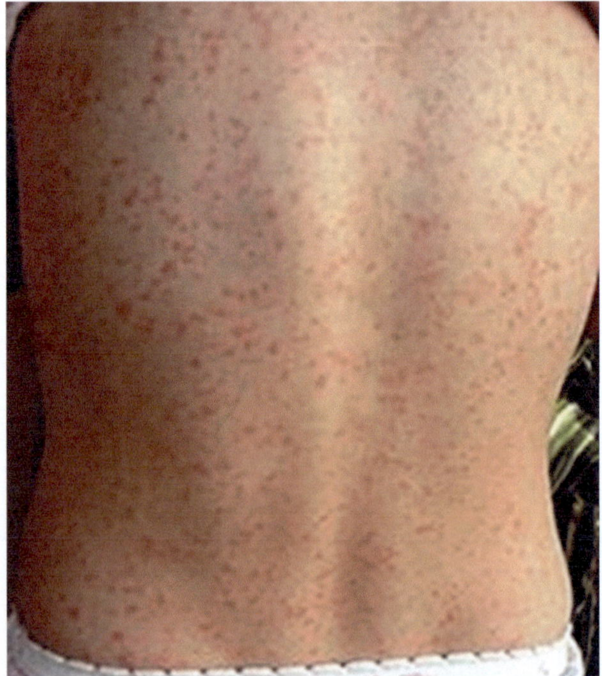

Fig. 12.10 Characteristic appearance of the skin rash on the back of a patient with of scarlet fever

throat, and headache [59]. The characteristic rash is due to the "erythrogenic toxin" [59, 60]. Diagnosis is typically confirmed by culturing the throat [59].

12.3.3.3 Food or Drug Allergy

The consumption of certain drugs, fruits, and vegetables is a common culprit in the development of strawberry tongue as part of an allergic reaction. In addition to a strawberry tongue, allergies may cause watery and itchy eyes, scratchy mouth and throat, skin rash, and difficulty in breathing (may lead to anaphylactic shock).

12.3.3.4 Vitamin B_{12} Deficiency

Vitamin B_{12} plays a key role in the functioning of the nervous system and brain, as well as the formation of the red blood cells. Vitamin B_{12} deficiency may cause a strawberry tongue. Coexistent symptoms of include easy fatigability, weakness, amnesia, vertigo, numbness or tingling, and glossitis.

12.3.3.5 Toxic Shock Syndrome

Toxic shock syndrome (TSS) is a rare complication that has been associated with using tampons and nasal gauze packing. Contrary to popular belief, simply leaving in a tampon for a long time does *not* cause TSS [61].

TSS is usually caused by infection with *Staphylococcus aureus* but can also be caused by the same bacterial species of group A *Streptococcus*, which causes scarlet fever. The synthetic, higher-absorbency tampons makes it easier for the bacterium to multiply and spread. Some of the risk factors include open wounds, surgery, and the use of a prosthetic device [61].

In addition to a strawberry tongue, TSS may cause the following symptoms: sudden high fever, hypotension, headache, confusion, sore throat, muscle aches, nausea, vomiting, and diarrhea, as well as the development of a rash that looks like a sunburn on soles of the feet and palms of the hands. This condition can be life-threatening if the patient does not seek treatment [61].

12.3.4 Complications

A swollen tongue may interfere with food ingestion and increase the risk of biting the tongue. If the conditions causing strawberry tongue are left untreated, complications may arise. These conditions include the following:

- *Kawasaki disease:* Without treatment, coronary artery aneurysms occur in up to 25% and about 1% die [62, 63]. With treatment, the risk of death is reduced to 0.17% [63].
- *Scarlet fever*: If left untreated, scarlet fever may lead to rheumatic fever (can involve the heart (rheumatic heart disease), joints (arthritis), and nervous system), renal disease (glomerulonephritis), severe otitis media, dermatitis, skin infection, and abscess formation [59]. It was a leading cause of death in children in the early twentieth century [64, 65].

- *Toxic shock syndrome (TSS):* Left untreated, TSS causes shock, multiple system/organ failure, and could be fatal.
- *Anaphylactic shock*: If a person does not receive treatment, anaphylactic shock can be fatal, typically due to circulatory and respiratory failure [66].

12.3.5 Differential Diagnosis: Glossitis

The differentiating factor between strawberry tongue and *glossitis* is that strawberry tongue results in prominent red bumps on the tongue, whereas glossitis refers to the red coloring and inflammation of the tongue, which becomes smooth (i.e., not characterized by bumps).

Similar to strawberry tongue, glossitis is often a symptom of illnesses and not a disease on its own. However, it generally occurs as a result of an underlying condition that does not have any relation to those causing strawberry tongue.

The most common conditions that cause glossitis include the following:

- Anemia (iron deficiency and pernicious forms)
- Deficiencies in vitamin B complex
- Untreated coeliac/celiac disease
- Xerostomia
- Allergic reactions
- Infections of the mouth (bacterial, viral, or fungal)
- Hormonal imbalances
- Tongue injury by burns, ill-fitting dentures, or rough teeth

Symptoms caused by glossitis may include the following:

- A red, inflamed tongue that has a smooth surface (no papillae are evident)
- A sore tongue
- Swelling of the tongue (which, although rare, when severe may block the airway)
- Difficulty in speaking, chewing, or swallowing due to discomfort and pain

12.3.6 Treatment

Treatment for strawberry tongue usually depends on the underlying cause as follows:

- *Kawasaki disease*: Salicylates help reduce artery inflammation, and supporting the immune system helps to reduce the risk of damage to the arteries. Thus, typically, initial treatment consists of high doses of aspirin and immunoglobulin administered intravenously [59]. Usually, with treatment, fever resolves within 24 h and there is a full recovery. If the coronary arteries are involved, ongoing treatment or surgery may occasionally be required [59].

- *Scarlet fever*: There is no vaccine for scarlet fever [59]. It is treated with antibiotic therapy, which prevents most complications [59]. It is normally a short-term illness and will resolve within a number of days or weeks with proper treatment.
- *Toxic shock syndrome*: This is treated with antibiotics, intravenous (IV) fluids, and stabilizing the blood pressure.
- *Allergies*: Antihistamines help to reduce the symptoms of an allergic reaction. Anaphylactic shock is typically treated with an injection of epinephrine, IV glucocorticoid, and IV antihistamine.
- *Vitamin deficiency*: Supplements, dietary changes, or possibly an injection of vitamins can help resolve any deficiency.

12.3.7 Prognosis

The outlook for a person with strawberry tongue depends on the underlying condition. Anaphylaxis and toxic shock syndrome can be immediately life-threatening, but both are very treatable with good outcome.

12.4 Yellow Tongue

12.4.1 Introduction

A wide variety of factors can cause or contribute to the development of yellow tongue, which is ordinarily a harmless condition that causes a thick, yellowish coating on the tongue. A yellow tongue tends to form when dead cells, bacteria, or discoloring particles become trapped or buildup on the tongue's surface.

Mostly, yellow tongue clears up with basic home care within a matter of days to weeks. However, on rare occasions, the condition is a symptom of a more serious health condition, usually *jaundice*.

12.4.2 Etiology

A few specific habits, conditions, and medications are known to increase the risk of developing a yellow tongue; these include the following:

12.4.2.1 Oral Hygiene Products with Oxidizing Agents

Some oral hygiene products, such as mouthwashes, rinses, and toothpaste, contain chemicals or particles that cause dry mouth, irritate the tongue, or cause its discoloration. Common compounds that are known to cause yellow tongue discoloration include peroxides, witch hazel, menthol, alcohol, thymol, and eucalyptus [67].

12.4.2.2 Poor Oral Hygiene

Teeth and tongue cleaning help reduce bacteria on the surface of the tongue, reducing the risk of developing yellow tongue [67].

12.4.2.3 Tobacco Use

Tobacco products contain compounds and toxins that can discolor skin cells or irritate them. Tobacco can cause cells to swell, increasing the chances of trapping particles and bacteria.

12.4.2.4 Mouth Breathing or Dry Mouth

Saliva naturally helps clear excess bacteria and particles from the tongue's surface. Dehydration reduces saliva production, increasing the risk of bacterial overgrowth. Mouth breathing, especially at night, increases the risk of dry mouth.

12.4.2.5 Black Hairy Tongue

Black hairy tongue is a fairly common, noncancerous condition where bacteria or fungi cause an enlarged, elongated, hair-like carpet of filiform papillae to appear on the surface of the tongue. Although the tongue most commonly appears black, it may also turn yellow, blue, or green. Most people seek treatment for the condition due to its appearance only, though others may experience nausea, gagging, halitosis, and a burning sensation in the mouth [16].

12.4.2.6 Oral Thrush

Overgrowth of the bacteria or fungi (*Candida)* can cause white patches on the tongue that eventually develop a yellow tone.

12.4.2.7 Geographic Tongue

Geographic tongue is a noncancerous condition that causes red or white patches on the top and sides of the tongue, often surrounded by a yellow border. The condition has no known cause but primarily affects children between the ages of 4 and 5 years. Patches tend to occur where skin cells are missing and occasionally are painful [68, 69].

12.4.2.8 Certain Foods

Many foods contain dyes or colorants that can stain the tongue yellow or are sticky and remain stuck to the tongue, discoloring its surface.

12.4.2.9 Certain Medications and Drugs

Several medications and drugs also contain staining particles, cause pigment discoloration, or weaken the immune system. These include diabetes and hypoglycemic drugs, antibiotics, lansoprazole (Prevacid), chlorhexidine (found in some disinfectant mouth rinses), iron salts, minocycline, bismuth subsalicylate, chemotherapy and radiotherapy, and antipsychotic medications. Some illicit drugs, such as cocaine, can also cause the tongue to discolor [70, 71].

12.4.2.10 Piercing, Tooth Extraction, or Tonsillectomy

A yellow tongue may follow a piercing, tooth extraction, or tonsillectomy as a result of papillae inflammation. Proper oral care after these procedures is important to reduce the risk of infection.

12.4.2.11 Yellow Tongue with Other Diseases [72, 73]

As mentioned, yellow tongue could be a warning sign of another disease, such as:

12.4.2.11.1 Urinary and Respiratory Tract Infections

A thick yellow coating, especially at the *back* of the tongue, could be an early warning sign of a urinary tract infection. But the same yellow coating toward the *front* is a sign of an upper respiratory infection.

12.4.2.11.2 Scarlet Fever

Scarlet fever due to bacterial infection with *Streptococcus pyogenes* (strep throat) can cause bumps on the tongue along with a yellow or white coating. Accompanying symptoms include fever, painful swallowing, and enlarged lymph nodes.

12.4.2.11.3 Jaundice

In jaundice, bilirubin builds up abnormally in tissues. Sometimes, only specific parts of the body become yellowed, such as the sclera. Other times, the entire skin may take on a yellow glow or hue. Unlike many of the causes of yellow tongue, jaundice requires immediate medical attention and often treatment as it is might be a sign of life-threatening conditions, such as liver failure.

12.4.2.11.4 Eczema and Autoimmune Conditions

Some autoimmune conditions such as eczema weaken the body's immune system, allowing otherwise harmless bacteria to overgrow on the tongue. In a 2017 study by Yu et al., out of 35 individuals with yellow tongue coating, 32 (91.4%) had acute or severe eczema. In the same study, out of 122 patients with white tongue coating, only three (2.46%) had acute eczema [73].

12.4.2.11.5 Chronic Gastritis

Several studies have confirmed that a yellow, thickened tongue coating is associated with chronic cases of gastritis, especially when caused by the bacteria *Helicobacter pylori* [72].

12.4.2.11.6 Postnasal Drainage

Postnasal drainage may cause a yellow or even white tongue, which can also cause halitosis. Excessive mucus accumulating at the back of the nose and throat is commonly caused by allergies, acid reflux, or swallowing disorders.

12.4.2.11.7 Malignancy

Yellow buildup, coating, or film on the tongue could sometimes, though quite rare, signal cancer.

12.4.2.11.8 Infectious Mononucleosis (IMN)

This viral infection—IMN—is known as the "kissing disease" as it is transmitted through the sharing of saliva. Accompanying symptoms include fatigue, fever, skin rash, headache, enlarged lymph nodes, and sore throat.

12.4.2.11.9 Human Immunodeficiency Virus (HIV)

Yellow tongue is a rare symptom of HIV but can sometimes reveal a compromised immune system. Yellow tongue could also be a sign of oral thrush—yeast infection of the mouth.

12.4.2.11.10 Yellow Under-Tongue

Common causes of a yellow under-tongue include biliary colic, alcoholic hepatitis, hepatitis A and B, IMN, gallstones, and Epstein-Barr virus (EBV).

12.4.3 Risk Factors

Though anyone can develop a yellow tongue at any age, a few factors are known to increase the likelihood of developing this condition. Risk factors for developing a yellow tongue include the following:

- Poor oral hygiene
- Tobacco and alcohol use
- Heavy consumption of coffee or black tea
- Betel nut use
- Dehydration
- Cancer
- Autoimmune conditions
- Neurological conditions
- Debilitating diseases

12.4.4 Symptoms

Yellow coating of the tongue may take different forms or shapes. The common symptoms associated with a yellow tongue may include the following:

- Bad breath (halitosis), bad taste, and dry mouth
- Additional white patches, film, or coating on the tongue or mucous membranes
- Small, raised bumps on the tongue; hairy tongue
- Pain, sore throat, and burning sensation
- Acid reflux or indigestion
- Fever

12.4.5 Complications

The only complications associated with yellow tongue are those linked to more serious underlying conditions, such as jaundice. Potential complications with *jaundice* include the following:

- Liver cirrhosis, failure, and cancer.
- Gastrointestinal inflammation, damage, and swelling.
- Fluid retention, ascites, and lower body edema.
- Splenomegaly and splenitis.
- Hepatic encephalopathy.
- In newborns, severe complications include cerebral palsy and deafness.

12.4.6 Prevention and Treatment Options

Common methods to treat and prevent yellow tongue include the following:

- Increasing frequency and thoroughness of teeth brushing or rinsing with an antibacterial or fluoride mouth rinse after meals
- Brushing the tongue gently with a soft-bristled toothbrush and daily scraping the tongue gently. Applying baking soda directly to the tongue for 60 s before rinsing off
- Increasing fluid intake and using a humidifier to reduce the chances of dry mouth
- Limiting the intake of starch or simple carbohydrate-rich foods and sugary and sticky sweets, increasing fiber intake in diet and consuming oral probiotics or yogurt
- Avoiding colored or dyed drinks, sugary drinks, alcohol, and caffeine as well as quitting smoking or using tobacco products or recreational or illicit drugs
- Using decongesting nose sprays and treating sinus infections and jaw conditions
- Avoiding unsterile needle punctures

Medications that may be used to treat yellow tongue include the following:

- Topical steroids or rinses and salicylic acid mouth rinses
- Retinoid (vitamin A)
- Antihistaminics
- Topical antifungal medications for thrush
- Topical anesthetic medications
- Antimicrobials to treat underlying infections
- Analgesics for pain

12.5 White Tongue

"White tongue" is a term used to describe any area of the tongue that has a grayish-white coating on it. The entire tongue may be coated, or the coating may appear in patches. There are a few different reasons for a white tongue, and each has a specific treatment. A white tongue is usually a harmless symptom, but, in rare cases, it can indicate a serious condition such as leukoplakia.

12.5.1 Etiology

12.5.1.1 Poor Oral Hygiene

The most common cause of a white tongue is poor oral hygiene, which causes the tongue papillae to become swollen and inflamed. Plenty of germs, debris, food particles, and dead cells can get stuck in between these papillae. This causes the tongue to appear white as the particles build up. Oral and hygiene issues that can lead to a white tongue include the following [74]:

- Dry mouth caused by mouth breathing or sleeping with the mouth open
- Not brushing or flossing the teeth correctly or cleaning the tongue
- Dehydration
- Irritation from sharp edges inside the mouth, such as teeth, braces, or dentures
- Regular alcohol consumption
- Smoking, chewing, or dipping tobacco

12.5.1.2 Leukoplakia: Oral/Tongue Cancer

Leukoplakia causes thick, white patches to form on the tongue and mouth. The exact cause of leukoplakia is unknown [75], but known risk factors include smoking, chewing tobacco, excessive alcohol, and betel nuts [76, 77]. It may also result from inflammatory conditions and chronic irritation from ill-fitting dentures. It is known to be precancerous resulting in squamous cell carcinoma (SCC) [76]. Oral and tongue cancer can also cause a white tongue.

12.5.1.3 Oral Lichen Planus (LP)

Oral lichen planus is a chronic inflammatory and immune-mediated disease condition that affects the skin, nails, hair, and mucous membranes [78]. It is characterized by polygonal, flat-topped, violaceous papules, and plaques with overlying, reticulated, fine white scale (*Wickham's striae*), commonly affecting dorsal hands, flexural wrists and forearms, trunk, anterior lower legs, and oral mucosa [78]. Oral LP causes thick, white patches to appear in the mouth and tongue among other symptoms including ulcers or painful cheeks and gums [79]. The cause is unknown, but it is thought to be the result of an autoimmune process with an unknown initial trigger.

12.5.1.4 Oral Thrush

Oral thrush, caused by fungal infection (*Candida*), is one condition that may cause an unpleasant taste and white or off-white patches in the tongue. Oral thrush can also be painful, especially during eating or drinking. The reported risk factors for developing oral thrush include the following [80]:

- Diabetes mellitus
- Extremes of age (very young or very old)
- Iron or vitamin B_{12} deficiency
- Immunocompromised patients
- Ill-fitting dentures
- Poor oral hygiene, dry mouth, or dehydration
- Smoking
- Drugs: antibiotics, chemotherapy, or corticosteroids
- Hypothyroidism

12.5.1.5 Geographic Tongue

A geographic tongue is a noncancerous condition that causes red or white patches on the top and sides of the tongue, often surrounded by a yellow border. The condition has no known cause, but primarily affects children between the ages of 4 and 5 years. Patches tend to occur where skin cells are missing and occasionally are painful [68, 69].

12.5.1.6 Syphilis

Syphilis is a sexually transmitted infection that, if untreated, can cause white patches to appear on the tongue and sores in the mouth

12.5.2 Clinical Presentation: Diagnosis

White tongue can be seen on oral examination (Fig. 12.11). It differs in its clinical presentation according to its etiology. History-taking and general physical examination are both essential to reach a sound diagnosis.

12.5.2.1 Leukoplakia

The onset is usually after the age of 30 years [76] and has been reported to occur in 8% of men above the age of 70 years [75]. Leukoplakia produces one or more firmly attached white patches in the mouth or on the tongue (on a mucous membrane) that changes with time [75, 76, 81]. The patch is usually painless and somewhat raised. Patches may also appear on the top or bottom of the mouth, the insides of the cheeks, the lower lip, or the gums.

Leukoplakia should be differentiated from fungal infection, lichen planus, and keratosis resulting from repeated minor trauma [76]. Diagnosis of leukoplakia is

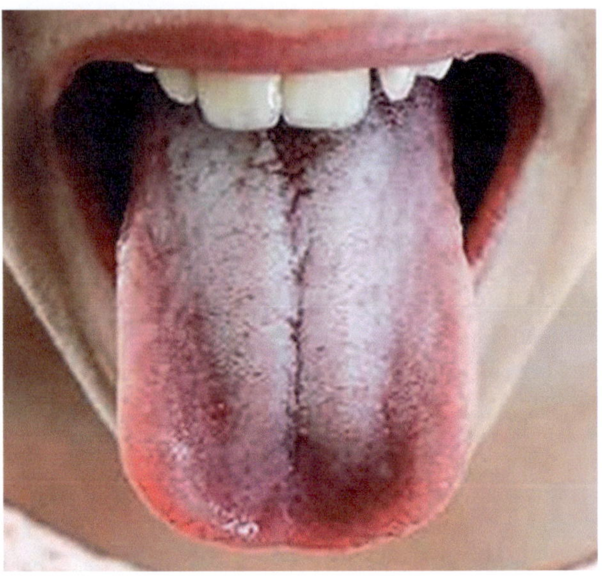

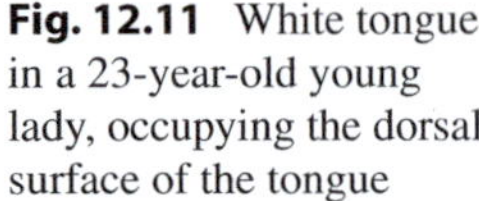

Fig. 12.11 White tongue in a 23-year-old young lady, occupying the dorsal surface of the tongue

made after exclusion of other causes and by its characteristic histological appearance on biopsy [75], which is essential as it is known to be precancerous, resulting in squamous cell carcinoma.

12.5.2.2 Oral Lichen Planus

Oral lichen planus produces white patches on the gums, tongue, or insides of the cheeks. A mild case is usually not painful; in more serious cases, the patient may have a burning sensation, painful red gums, and sore patches on the insides of the cheeks, especially when eating or drinking [79].

A full examination that includes the evaluation of the mucosal and cutaneous surfaces, including the vulva, vagina or penis, scalp, and nails, should be performed. Thorough examination may lead to the detection of extraoral manifestations of LP that provide additional support for the diagnosis or the identification of clinical findings that suggest another diagnosis [80, 81].

Tissue biopsies of oral LP help to confirm the diagnosis and are particularly of value for erythematous and erosive LP, which share features with multiple other mucosal disorders, including oral malignancy. Biopsies to confirm oral LP are less essential in patients who present with classic reticular LP, particularly in patients in whom a diagnosis of LP has already been confirmed through biopsy of an extraoral manifestation of this disorder [82, 83].

12.5.2.3 Oral Thrush

Oral thrush is marked by the following clinical features: white patches in the mouth that can be wiped away leaving behind red or even bloody surface, burning sensation of the tongue and mouth, loss of taste or unpleasant taste in the mouth, red areas inside the mouth and throat, and cracked corners on the mouth. Symptoms will continue unless the condition is treated. In severe cases that are not treated, serious infection could spread to other areas of the body.

12.5.2.4 Geographic Tongue

Geographic tongue appears on the top and sides of the tongue, and sometimes on the bottom, as wavy white lines surrounding red areas simulating the outlines of a map (and hence its name). After some weeks or months, the lines and patches may change their position or shape.

12.5.2.5 Syphilis

A small painless sore on the tongue may appear from 10 days to 3 months after exposure to infection during oral sex. If it is not treated, a condition called syphilitic leukoplakia will produce white plaques on the tongue. Other symptoms may include headache, joint pain, fever, and swollen glands. Diagnosis is established by the appropriate laboratory tests.

12.5.3 Treatment

12.5.3.1 Good Oral Hygiene

Good oral hygiene and reducing irritants in the mouth may help clear up the white patches. Practicing good oral hygiene on regular basis includes the following [80]:

- Using a soft toothbrush and a mild toothpaste that does not include sodium lauryl sulfate
- Brushing the tongue or using a tongue scraper from back to front to remove the white coating
- Using a straw to drink cold drinks
- Avoiding tongue irritants, such as alcohol, cigarettes, and food and drinks that are spicy, salty, acidic, or very hot in temperature

12.5.3.2 Other Measures

12.5.3.2.1 Probiotics

Although the evidence is not conclusive, probiotics (strains of bacteria that are good for the digestive system) are another way to influence oral symptoms such as a white tongue. They can be found in fermented foods and drinks, such as kimchi, pickles, and kombucha. Yogurt also often contains probiotics [84].

12.5.3.2.2 Baking Soda Scrub

Adding food-grade baking soda to a toothbrush and scrubbing the tongue, teeth, and gums may help reduce the bacteria (e.g., *Streptococcus*) and *Candida* that cause a white tongue.

12.5.3.2.3 Raw Garlic

Eating raw garlic (allicin) has been reported to be effective in fighting off infections caused by *Candida albicans* [85].

12.5.3.3 Specific Treatment

A white tongue caused by a certain disorder requires a specific medical treatment such as antifungal drugs for oral thrush, corticosteroids for lichen planus, and penicillin for syphilis.

- *Leukoplakia*: Avoiding alcohol and discontinuing tobacco smoking or chewing. Surgical resection is mandatory to prevent turning malignant [76].
- *Oral lichen planus*: Mouthwashes and sprays to reduce discomfort from symptoms such as burning or sore gums. It is also important to maintain good oral hygiene and avoid all kinds of irritants [79]. There is no cure for lichen planus [86], and so treatment of cutaneous and oral lichen planus is for symptomatic relief or due to cosmetic concerns [86–88]. When medical treatment is pursued, first-line treatment typically involves corticosteroids [88] and removal of any triggers [89]. Without treatment, most lesions will spontaneously resolve within 6–9 months for cutaneous lesions [88] and longer for mucosal lesions [90].
- *Oral thrush*: Topical antifungal application (e.g., gel) to the patches inside the mouth, several times/day for 1–2 weeks. Oral antifungal medications may also be prescribed [80].
- *Geographic tongue*: There are no special treatments for geographic tongue. Foods and drinks that are known to increase discomfort should be avoided. Topical applications used to treat oral thrush may provide some relief. On a long-term basis, there is no risk of this condition turning malignant.
- *Syphilis*: Penicillin.

12.5.4 Prognosis

The outlook for a white tongue is typically very good. In many cases, it is harmless, though esthetically distressing. Symptoms may not always respond to improved hygiene or lifestyle choices right away, but improved oral health is suggested for anyone with a white tongue. In rare cases, a white tongue is an indication of a serious underlying condition that requires specific treatment measures.

12.6 Green Tongue

12.6.1 Introduction

It is common to have a green tongue after eating or drinking something with green food coloring, but an unexplained color change can be a sign of an underlying issue such as an infection or overgrowth of certain germs. Symptoms of a green tongue will usually resolve after treating the underlying condition.

12.6.2 Etiology

Several conditions may cause a green tongue with the most common being oral thrush and black hairy tongue.

12.6.2.1 Previously Discussed Causes [11, 69, 91, 92]

These include oral thrush, hairy black tongue, leukoplakia, geographic tongue, and lichen planus

12.6.2.2 Oral Cancer [93]

Although it is much rarer than an oral infection, oral cancer may also cause similar symptoms. One sign of oral cancer is an open sore or lesion on the tongue that does not heal. This sore may change color depending on the oral intake or bacterial proliferation.

Oral cancer often causes other symptoms, including a growth on the tongue; persistent tongue pain; easy bleeding on the tongue or gums with no known cause; loose teeth; unexplained weight loss; colored patches on the tongue (green, white, or pinkish); numbness or tingling in the lips, chin, or neck; a persistent sore throat or jaw pain; and enlarged cervical lymph nodes.

12.6.2.3 Other Causes

Other possible causes for a green tongue include the following [67]:

- Poor dental/oral hygiene
- Certain medications including antibiotics
- Upper respiratory infection that spreads to the tongue
- Discharge from an infected tongue piercing
- Illicit drug use
- Temporary color changes caused by food coloring in candy, sweets, or oral hygiene products (mouthwashes and toothpastes)

12.6.3 Diagnosis

History-taking and oral cavity examination may suffice to reach the cause of a green tongue. A *biopsy* is often only necessary for suspicious lesions on the tongue.

12.6.4 Treatment

12.6.4.1 Treatment of the Cause

Treatment depends on the underlying cause [91–93]:

- Antibiotics for bacterial infection
- Antifungal medications (e.g., nystatin, fluconazole, or clotrimazole) for oral thrush

- Vitamin A, retinoids, or surgical resection for oral leukoplakia
- Antihistamines or corticosteroids for glossitis
- Surgery, radiation therapy, chemotherapy, and nutritional changes for oral cancer

12.6.4.2 Proper Oral Hygiene

In all cases of green tongue, proper oral hygiene is essential to support treatment efforts. This includes regular teeth and tongue brushing, daily flossing, mouth washing and rinsing, drinking plenty of water, and avoiding irritants (refer back for more details) [69].

12.6.4.3 Scraping of the Tongue

Tongue scraping may also help reduce the number of germs on the tongue and in the mouth that contribute to oral issues particularly when added to brushing and flossing [69].

References

1. Prinz H. Black tongue. Br Dent J. 1925;46:1265–74.
2. Thompson DF, Kessler TL. Drug-induced black hairy tongue. Pharmacotherapy. 2010;30:585–93.
3. Waggoner WC, Volpe AR. Lingua villosa nigra: a review of black hairy tongue. J Oral Med. 1967;22:18–21.
4. Rajendran R, Sivapathasundharam B. Shafer's textbook of oral pathology. 6th ed. Delhi: Elsevier; 2009. p. 31.
5. Avcu N, Kanli A. The prevalence of tongue lesions in 5150 Turkish dental outpatients. Oral Dis. 2003;9:188–95.
6. Motallebnejad M, Babaee N, Sakhdari S, Tavasoli M. An epidemiologic study of tongue lesions in 1901 Iranian dental outpatients. J Contemp Dent Pract. 2008;9:73–80.
7. Sarti GM, Haddy RI, Schaffer D, Kihm J. Black hairy tongue. Am Fam Physician. 1990;41(6):1751–5.
8. Neville BW, Damm DD, Allen CM, Bouquot JE. Oral & maxillofacial pathology. 2nd ed. Philadelphia: WB Saunders; 2002. p. 13–4.
9. Kullaa-Mikkonen A, Mikkonen M, Kotilainen R. Prevalence of different morphologic forms of the human tongue in young Finns. Oral Surg Oral Med Oral Pathol. 1982;53:152–6.
10. Redman RS. Prevalence of geographic tongue, fissured tongue, median rhomboid glossitis, and hairy tongue among 3,611 Minnesota school children. Oral Surg Oral Med Oral Pathol. 1970;30:390–5.
11. Nisa L, Giger R. Black hairy tongue. Am J Med. 2011;124:816–7.
12. Jahanbani J, Sandvik L, Lyberg T, Ahlfors E. Evaluation of oral mucosal lesions in 598 referred Iranian patients. Open Dent J. 2009;3:42–7.
13. Vuorenkoski L. Finland health system review. Health Syst Transit. 2008;10:1–170.
14. Poulopoulos AK, Antoniades DZ, Epivatianos A, Grivea IN, Syrogiannopoulos GA. Black hairy tongue in a 2-monthold infant. J Paediatr Child Health. 2008;44:377–9.
15. Körber A, Voshege N. Black hairy tongue in an infant. CMAJ. 2012;184:6.8.
16. Gurvits GE, Tan A. Black hairy tongue syndrome. World J Gastroenterol. 2014;20(31):10845–50.
17. Scully C. Oral and maxillofacial medicine: the basis of diagnosis and treatment. 2nd ed. Edinburgh: Churchill Livingstone; 2008. p. 349.
18. Pigatto PD, Spadari F, Meroni L, Guzzi G. Black hairy tongue associated with long-term oral erythromycin use. J Eur Acad Dermatol Venereol. 2008;22:1269–70.

19. Harada Y, Gaafar H. Black hairy tongue. A scanning electron microscopic study. J Laryngol Otol. 1977;91:91–6.
20. Manabe M, Lim HW, Winzer M, Loomis CA. Architectural organization of filiform papillae in normal and black hairy tongue epithelium: dissection of differentiation pathways in a complex human epithelium according to their patterns of keratin expression. Arch Dermatol. 1999;135:177–81.
21. Taybos G. Oral changes associated with tobacco use. Am J Med Sci. 2003;326:179–82.
22. Akay BN, Sanli H, Topcuoglu P, Zincircioğlu G, Gurgan C, Heper AO. Black hairy tongue after allogeneic stem cell transplantation: an unrecognized cutaneous presentation of graft-versus-host disease. Transplant Proc. 2010;42:4603–7.
23. Farman AG. Hairy tongue (lingua villosa). J Oral Med. 1977;32:85–91.
24. Cheshire WP. Unilateral black hairy tongue in trigeminal neuralgia. Headache. 2004;44:908–10.
25. Cawson RA, Odell EW. Cawson's essentials of oral pathology and oral medicine. 7th ed. Edinburgh: Churchill Livingstone; 2002. p. 351.
26. Refaat M, Hyle E, Malhotra R, Seidman D, Dey B. Linezolid-induced lingua villosa nigra. Am J Med. 2008;121:e1.
27. Jover-Diaz F, Cuadrado-Pastor JM, Talents-Bolos A, Martin-Gonzalez C. Black tongue associated with linezolid. Am J Ther. 2010;17:115–7.
28. Tamam L, Annagur BB. Black hairy tongue associated with olanzapine treatment: a case report. Mt Sinai J Med. 2006;73:891–4.
29. Paganini AE, Zlotlow M. Hairy tongue in patients receiving phenothiazines: preliminary report. Am J Psychiatry. 1959;116:362–3.
30. Jeong JS, Lee JY, Kim MK, Yoon TY. Black hairy tongue associated with erlotinib treatment in a patient with advanced lung cancer. Ann Dermatol. 2011;23:526–8.
31. Cohen PR. Black tongue secondary to bismuth subsalicylate: case report and review of exogenous causes of macular lingual pigmentation. J Drugs Dermatol. 2009;8(12):1132–5.
32. Maynard FP. A note on melanoglossia. Ind Med Gaz. 1897;32(10):364–5.
33. McGrath EE, Bardsley P, Basran G. Black hairy tongue: what is your call? CMAJ. 2008;178:1137–8.
34. Vañó-Galván S, Jaén P. Black hairy tongue. Cleve Clin J Med. 2008;75:847–8.
35. Katz J, Barak S, Shemer J, Langevitz P, Livneh A. Black tongue associated with minocycline therapy. Arch Dermatol. 1995;131:620.
36. Tanzi EL, Hecker MS. Minocycline-induced hyperpigmentation of the tongue. Arch Dermatol. 2000;136:427–8.
37. Westbury LW, Najera A. Minocycline-induced intraoral pharmacogenic pigmentation: case reports and review of the literature. J Periodontol. 1997;68:84–91.
38. Winzer M, Gilliar U. Hairy tongue and hairy oral leukoplakia–a differential histopathologic diagnosis. Z Hautkr. 1988;63(6):517–20.
39. Pegum JS. Urea in the treatment of black hairy tongue. Br J Dermatol. 1971;84:602.
40. Sheikh Z, Khan AS, Khan S. Lingua villosa nigra. Lancet. 2011;377:1183.
41. Ramsakal A, Mangat L. Images in clinical medicine. Lingua villosa nigra. N Engl J Med. 2007;357:2388.
42. Langtry JA, Carr MM, Steele MC, Ive FA. Topical tretinoin: a new treatment for black hairy tongue (lingua villosa nigra). Clin Exp Dermatol. 1992;17:163–4.
43. Weinstein I, Rosencrans M. Treatment of black hairy tongue with triamcinolone acetonide. Report of a case. Oral Surg Oral Med Oral Pathol. 1962;15:1071–4.
44. Yuca K, Calka O, Kiroglu AF, Akdeniz N, Cankaya H. Hairy tongue: a case report. Actaotorhinolaryngol Belg. 2004;58(4):161–3.
45. Harden SA, Sheikh A, Brown RS. Orange-yellow tongue and palate: a case report. Dent Today. 2012;31(3):78–81.
46. Hsiao C, Clukay CJ. Orangeness-peeling back the myths behind carotenemia. JAMA Dermatol. 2017;153(9):873.
47. Gangakhedkar A, Somerville R, Jelleyman T. Carotenemia and hepatomegaly in an atopic child on an exclusion diet for a food allergy. Australas J Dermatol. 2017;58(1):42–4.

48. Karthik SV, Campbell-Davidson D, Isherwood D. Carotenemia in infancy and its association with prevalent feeding practices. Pediatr Dermatol. 2006;23(6):571–3.
49. Kayhan-Tetik B, Çaylan N. Beta-carotenemia with isolated nose involvement in a child: a case report. Arch Argent Pediatr. 2019;117(5):502–4.
50. Nguyen LM, Scherr RE, Linnell JD, Ermakov IV, Gellermann W, Jahns L, et al. Evaluating the relationship between plasma and skin carotenoids and reported dietary intake in elementary school children to assess fruit and vegetable intake. Arch Biochem Biophys. 2015;572:73–80.
51. Kiuchi S, Ihara H, Koyasu M, Tani A, Hashizume N. A case of β-Carotenemia misdiagnosed as jaundice by the bilirubin oxidase method. J Nutr Sci Vitaminol. 2019;65(5):451–4.
52. Takita Y, Ichimiya M, Hamamoto Y, Muto M. A case of carotenemia associated with ingestion of nutrient supplements. J Dermatol. 2006;33(2):132–4.
53. Sale TA, Stratman E. Carotenemia associated with green bean ingestion. Pediatr Dermatol. 2004;21(6):657–9.
54. Ermakov IV, Gellermann W. Optical detection methods for carotenoids in human skin. Arch Biochem Biophys. 2015;572:101–11.
55. Kawasaki disease. PubMed Health. NHLBI health topics. 2014. Archived from the original on 11 September 2017. Retrieved 26 August 2016.
56. Lai WW, Mertens LL, Cohen MS, Geva T. Echocardiography in pediatric and congenital heart disease: from fetus to adult. 2nd ed. Hoboken: Wiley; 2017. p. 739.
57. Kawasaki T. Acute febrile mucocutaneous syndrome with lymphoid involvement with specific desquamation of the fingers and toes in children. Arerugi. 1967;16(3):178–222.
58. Dietz SM, Tacke CE, de Groot E, Kuipers IM, Hutten BA, Kuijpers TW. Extracardial vasculopathy after Kawasaki disease: a long-term follow-up study. JAHA. 2016;5:e003414.
59. CDC. Scarlet fever: a group a streptococcal infection. Atlanta: Center for Disease Control and Prevention.
60. Ralph AP, Carapetis JR. Group a streptococcal diseases and their global burden. Curr Top Microbiol Immunol. 2013;368:1–27.
61. Vostral SL. Rely and toxic shock syndrome: a technological health crisis. Yale J Biol Med. 2011;84(4):447–59.
62. Kim DS. Kawasaki disease. Yonsei Med J. 2006;47(6):759–72.
63. Merck Manual, online edition: Kawasaki Disease. 2014.
64. Smallman-Raynor M. Atlas of epidemic Britain: a twentieth century picture. Oxford: Oxford University Press; 2012. p. 48.
65. Smallman-Raynor M, Andrew C, Peter HM. World atlas of epidemic diseases. London: Hodder Education; 2004. p. 76.
66. Sampson HA, Muñoz-Furlong A, Campbell RL, Adkinson NF, Bock SA, Branum A, et al. Second symposium on the definition and management of anaphylaxis: summary report - second national institute of allergy and infectious disease/food allergy and anaphylaxis network symposium. JACI. 2006;117(2):391–7.
67. Godha S, Dasar PL, Sandesh N, Mishra P, Kumar S, Balsaraf S, et al. Impact of different oral hygiene aids for the reduction of morning bad breath among dental students: a crossover clinical trial. Clujul Med. 2016;89(4):525–33.
68. Shah N, Kariya P, Dave B, Thomas P. Geographic tongue: a case report with review of literature. Adv Hum Biol. 2016;6(3):142–4.
69. Varoni E, Decani S. Geographic tongue. New Engl J Med. 2016;374(7):670.
70. Jayakaran TG. The effect of drugs in the oral cavity - a review. J Pharm Sci Res. 2014;6(2):89–96.
71. Liao PY, Hsu PC, Chen JM, Chiang JY, Lo LC. Diabetes with pyogenic liver abscess — a perspective on tongue assessment in traditional Chinese medicine. Compl Ther Med. 2014;22(2):341–8.
72. Liu X, Sun ZM, Liu YN, Ji Q, Sui H, Zhou LH, et al. The metabonomic studies of tongue coating in H. pylori-positive chronic gastritis patients. Evid Based Complement Alternat Med. 2015;2015:804085.
73. Yu Z, Zhang H, Fu L, Lu X. Objective research on tongue manifestation of patients with eczema. Technol Health Care. 2017;25(1):143–9.

74. Matsui M, Chosa N, Shimoyama Y, Minami K, Kimura S, Kishi M. Effects of tongue cleaning on bacterial flora in tongue coating and dental plaque: A crossover study. BMC Oral Health. 2014;14(1):4. https://doi.org/10.1186/1472-6831-14-4.
75. Neville BW, Damm DD, Chi AC, Allen CM. Oral and maxillofacial pathology. 4th ed. Amsterdam: Elsevier; 2015. p. 355–8.
76. Villa A, Woo SB. Leukoplakia-A diagnostic and management algorithm. J Oral Maxillofac Surg. 2017;5(4):723–34.
77. Underner M, Perriot J, Peiffer G. Smokeless tobacco. Presse Med. 2012;41(1):3–9.
78. Gorouhi F, Davari P, Fazel N. Cutaneous and mucosal lichen planus: a comprehensive review of clinical subtypes, risk factors, diagnosis, and prognosis. TSWJ. 2014;2014:742826.
79. Burkhart N. Oral lichen planus. 2013.
80. Muzurovic S, Babajic E, Masic T, Smajic R, Selmanagic A. The relationship between oral hygiene and oral colonisation with Candida species. Mediev Archaeol. 2012;66(6):415–7.
81. Scully C, Porter S. ABC of oral health: swellings and red, white, and pigmented lesions. BMJ. 2000;321(7255):225–8.
82. Agha R, Mirowski GW. The art and science of oral examination. Dermatol Ther. 2010;23(3):209–19.
83. Eisen D. The oral mucosal punch biopsy. A report of 140 cases. Arch Dermatol. 1992;128(6):815–7.
84. Haukioja A. Probiotics and oral health. Eur J Dent. 2010;4(3):348–55.
85. Khodavandi A, Alizadeh F, Harmal NS, Sidik SM, Othman F, Sekawi Z, et al. Comparison between efficacy of allicin and fluconazole against Candida albicans in vitro and in a systemic candidiasis mouse model. FEMS Microbiol Lett. 2011;315(2):87–93.
86. Kerawala C, Newlands C. Oral and maxillofacial surgery. Oxford: Oxford University Press; 2010. p. 412–3.
87. Lodi G, Manfredi M, Mercadante V, Murphy R. Interventions for treating oral lichen planus: corticosteroid therapies. Cochrane Database Syst Rev. 2020;2:CD001168.
88. Limited. Therapeutic guidelines therapeutic guidelines. 3rd ed. North Melbourne: Therapeutic Guidelines; 2009. p. 254–5.
89. Issa Y, Brunton PA, Glenny AM, Duxbury AJ. Healing of oral lichenoid lesions after replacing amalgam restorations: a systematic review. Oral Surg. 2004;98(5):553–65.
90. Scully C, El-Kom M. Lichen planus: review and update on pathogenesis. J Oral Pathol Med. 1985;14(6):431–58.
91. Lodi G, Franchini R, Warnakulasuriya S, Varoni EM, Sardella A, Kerr AR, et al. Interventions for treating oral leukoplakia to prevent oral cancer. Cochrane Database Syst Rev. 2016;7:CD001829.
92. Thongprasom K. Oral lichen planus: challenge and management. Oral Dis. 2018;24:172–3.
93. Ribeiro IP, Barroso L, Marques F, Melo JB, Carreira IM. Early detection and personalized treatment in oral cancer: the impact of omics approaches. Mol Cytogenet. 2016;9:85.

13 Tongue Fissures

13.1 Overview

13.1.1 Definition

Tongue fissures are deep grooves on the dorsum of the tongue. They are relatively common with a prevalence ranging between 6.8% [1] and 11% [2].

13.1.2 Etiology

The cause of fissured tongue is exactly unknown, but it may be *congenital* (genetic) or *acquired* such as trauma, benign migratory glossitis, syphilis, pustular psoriasis, malnutrition, and malignancy.

13.1.3 Characteristics of Fissured Tongue

- Only the tongue is affected by the fissures.
- On the top and side of the tongue cracks, clefts, or grooves may appear.
- The tongue may be separated into small lobes or sections by a number of connected grooves.
- The depth of the grooves may vary up to 6 mm.
- They are more prominent in adults and may deepen with age.

13.1.4 Symptoms of Fissured Tongue

- Occurrence of multiple fissures and visible deep grooves in the tongue.
- The tongue may appear cracked in the middle (Fig. 13.1).
- The middle of the tongue is comparatively the most affected region.

© The Author(s), under exclusive license to Springer Nature Switzerland AG 2022

M. F. Sakr, *Tongue Lesions*, https://doi.org/10.1007/978-3-031-08198-9_13

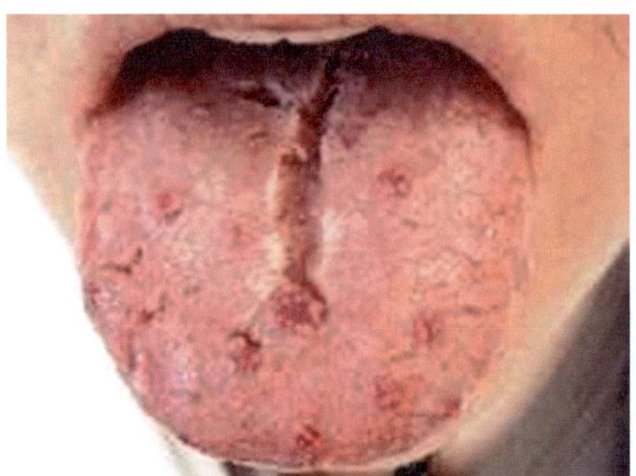

Fig. 13.1 A deep fissure on the midline of the dorsal surface of the tongue

- Different areas of the tongue may be missing the tiny pink bumps (papillae) that are normally present on the tongue. The spots missing the papillae may be smooth red with slightly raised borders.
- There may be discomfort and increasing sensitivity to substances.

13.1.5 Diagnosis

Diagnosis of fissured tongue is usually reached through routine dental checkups. It is during these sessions that the dentist is able to observe the cracks on the individual's tongue while examining his/her teeth. Usually, this condition does not require a biopsy for diagnosis.

13.1.6 Treatment of Fissured Tongue

13.1.6.1 Oral Hygiene

Maintaining proper oral hygiene is important to treat a fissured tongue. The surface of the tongue must be brushed and kept clean in order to remove food debris and avoid collection of plaque and bacteria in the fissures. This condition may also lead to tooth decay and bad breathe.

13.1.6.2 Flossing

Using a good flossing medicine could be beneficial in such situations. It cleans the mouth, and its antibiotic properties help to reduce bacteria in the mouth and reduce risk of disease, infections, and intensity of the situation.

13.1.6.3 Hydration

Drinking water helps to wash out the debris from the fissures in the tongue. It prevents the growth of bacteria in the mouth and does not allow infestation and infection. Thus, it also reduces the chances of irritation and inflammation of the tongue.

13.2 Congenital Tongue Fissures

13.2.1 Etiology

Congenital fissures may be *a genetic trait*, at least in part, with *aging* and *environmental* factors contributing to the appearance. Fissured tongue is seen in the following:

13.2.1.1 Melkersson-Rosenthal Syndrome

This is a rare neurological disorder that is transmitted to individuals genetically. It may also be due to dietary reasons or other allergens. It is characterized by the weakening of facial muscles, swelling of both or one lip (granulomatous cheilitis), swelling of the face, and a fissured tongue. These characteristics may reoccur from time to time. Facial palsy that may be permanent is another feature of this condition [3].

13.2.1.2 Down Syndrome

Down syndrome or Down's syndrome, also known as trisomy 21, is a genetic disorder caused by the presence of all or part of a third copy of chromosome 21. It is usually associated with physical growth delays, mild to moderate intellectual disability, and characteristic facial features [1]. Approximately, 80% of the people who suffer from chromosomal disorders have fissured tongue [4].

13.2.1.3 Cowden's Syndrome

Cowden's syndrome is also known as "Cowden's disease and multiple hamartoma syndrome." It is an autosomal-dominant-inherited condition characterized by hamartomas and an increased lifetime risk of breast, thyroid, uterine, and other cancers. Some patients with Cowden's syndrome develop tongue fissures [5].

13.2.2 Diagnosis and Treatment

Clinically, there is a long history of multiple fissures on the dorsum of the tongue. The mucosa looks normal. A congenital fissured tongue does not typically require treatment. Often, it does not have any symptoms.

Complications typically occur if food or other debris gets caught in the grooves. If this happens, it can cause irritation or allow bacteria to grow. The bacteria trapped in the fissures can cause *bad breath* or promote *tooth decay*. In extreme cases, *Candida albicans* may infect very deep grooves and require treatment with a topical antifungal medication.

13.3 Acquired Tongue Fissures

13.3.1 Trauma [6, 7]

13.3.1.1 Tongue Bites

The tip and sides of the tongue are closest to the teeth. While eating or talking, people may accidentally bite their tongue. These bites may also develop into sores in the future resulting in cracks or fissures that are painful to touch.

13.3.1.2 Cuts

Cuts on the tongue may occur while having food with sharp edges that can easily cut the tongue. These cuts can then develop into cracks. Eating dry foods or the presence of broken or chipped teeth in the mouth may also cause such situations.

13.3.1.3 Lacerations

Head concussions, seizures, etc. occur with excessive force. In such cases, the tongue may get caught between the teeth. They may vary in intensity. However, deep cuts may take time to heal and result in deep fissure or cracks on the tongue.

13.3.1.4 Teeth Grinding

Children having a habit of grinding their teeth while they are asleep may have fissured tongues. A mouth guard could be used in order to prevent cracks on the tip and the sides of the tongue.

13.3.2 Benign Migratory Glossitis

Benign migratory glossitis is also known as "superficial migratory glossitis," "erythema migrans," "glossitis migrans," "geographic tongue," and "wandering rash of the tongue" [8].

Although the causes behind its condition are unknown, it occurs in almost 3% of the total population. People suffering from this condition are observed to have a fissured tongue. As a result they also complain of increased sensitivity to hot or spicy food. Lesions may occur frequently. New lesions may occur as soon as the old ones begin to heal. It occurs on the erythematic area of the tongue, while the atrophy of the filiform papillae of the tongue is surrounded by white hyperkeratotic border [9].

13.3.3 Oral Psoriasis

Psoriasis is a chronic autoimmune condition that causes skin cells to grow rapidly and accumulate resulting in patches of red, scaly skin. These patches can appear anywhere on the body, including the cheeks, gums, lips and, though rare, also the tongue [10]. Fissured tongue is the most common finding in those with oral psoriasis and has been reported to occur in 6.5–20% of people with psoriasis affecting the skin [11].

Psoriasis on the tongue may be linked with an inflammatory condition affecting the sides and top of the tongue, known as "geographic tongue." More research is needed to understand this connection. Lesions on the tongue can vary in color, from white to yellowish-white to gray. The tongue may be red and inflamed, which usually occurs during an acute psoriasis flare-up.

Differential diagnosis of psoriasis of the tongue includes eczema, leukoplakia, and oral cancer. Thus, a biopsy of the tongue lesion, to rule out other possibilities and to confirm psoriasis, may be required.

In the absence of pain or difficulty in chewing or swallowing, treatment may not be necessary. Follow-up is all that is needed. Mild symptoms can be relieved by practicing good oral hygiene, anti-inflammatory drugs, and topical anesthetics. Psoriasis of the tongue can improve by treating the disease in general. Systemic medications include acitretin (Soriatane) and methotrexate (Trexall) [12]. There is no cure for psoriasis. However, treatment can help you effectively manage the disease and control its symptoms.

13.3.4 Syphilitic Tongue Fissures

Tongue fissure may be caused by syphilis, which is a sexually transmitted disease caused by the bacterium *Treponema pallidum* [13]. In secondary syphilis, a diffuse rash occurs, which frequently involves the palms of the hands and soles of the feet [14]. There may also be sores in the mouth or vagina, as well as longitudinal fissures in the tongue with areas of chronic superficial glossitis and areas of scarring [14].

Syphilis is difficult to diagnose clinically during early infection [15]. Confirmation is either via blood tests or direct visual inspection using dark field microscopy [15, 16]. Blood tests are more commonly used, as they are easier to perform [17]. They are divided into non-treponemal and treponemal tests [15]. Non-treponemal tests are used initially and include venereal disease research laboratory (VDRL) and rapid plasma reagin (RPR) tests. Because of the possibility of false positives with non-treponemal tests, confirmation is required with a treponemal test, such as treponemal pallidum particle agglutination (TPHA) or fluorescent treponemal antibody absorption test (FTA-Abs) [17]. Treponemal antibody tests usually become positive 2–5 weeks after the initial infection [15].

The first-line treatment for uncomplicated syphilis (primary or secondary stages) remains a single dose of intramuscular benzylpenicillin [17]. Doxycycline and tetracycline are alternative choices for those allergic to penicillin; however, they are not recommended during pregnancy due to the risk of birth defects [18]. Ceftriaxone, a third-generation cephalosporin antibiotic, may be as effective as penicillin-based treatment [17]. It is recommended that a treated person avoid sex until the sores are healed [19].

13.3.5 Nutritional Deficiency

13.3.5.1 Folic Acid (Vitamin B9)

Folic acid (folate) is essential for pregnant women, breastfeeding mothers, and adults during their reproductive years [20]. As humans cannot make folate, it is required in the diet, making it an essential vitamin [21]. It occurs naturally in many foods [20, 22]. The recommended adult daily intake of folate in the United States is 400 μg from foods or dietary supplements [20]. Folic acid deficiency can be caused by eating overcooked vegetables, a diet poor in fruits and vegetables, drinking too much alcohol, and Crohn's disease due to poor folate absorption. In addition to a swollen, fissured tongue and mouth sores, the patient may feel exhausted, develop gray hair, experience diarrhea, and develop peptic ulcers [20].

13.3.5.2 Biotin (B7 or B8 in France)

Biotin belongs to B vitamin family that plays a very important role in body metabolism and fat synthesis. It is also known as vitamin H [23, 24]. Most food contains this vitamin; however, various conditions can lower the absorption of biotin such as excessive consumption of alcohol, regular intake of antibiotics [23, 24], and consuming raw egg white [25]. Biotin deficiency can cause tongue fissures. Other symptoms include dry skin, hair loss, acne, dermatitis, weak nails, fatigue, gray skin, and paleness [23].

13.3.5.3 Riboflavin (Vitamin B2)

Riboflavin helps in the uptake of folate, iron, and niacin. Dietary sources include milk, cheese, liver, meat, eggs, and enriched cereal products [26, 27]. Riboflavin deficiency (ariboflavinosis) may be primary or secondary. Primary riboflavin deficiency results from inadequate intake of fortified cereals, milk, and other animal products [28]. Secondary riboflavin deficiency is most commonly caused by chronic diarrhea, malabsorption syndromes, liver disorders, hemodialysis, peritoneal dialysis, long-term use of barbiturates, and chronic alcoholism.

Under riboflavin deficiency (ariboflavinosis), people experience pallor, angular stomatitis, cheilosis, linear tongue fissures, seborrheic dermatitis, and conjunctivitis. The tongue fissures can become infected with *Candida albicans*, causing grayish-white lesions (perlèche). The tongue may appear magenta. Rarely, neovascularization and keratitis of the cornea occur, causing lacrimation and photophobia [29].

Treatment is with riboflavin supplements 5–10 mg orally once a day and other water-soluble vitamins (till recovery), or if needed, intramuscular riboflavin.

13.3.6 Malignant Tongue Fissure

Tongue fissures caused by tongue cancer are characterized with a short history, necrotic floor and hard base, infiltration of surrounding tissues, and the presence of cervical lymph node secondaries. Biopsy settles the diagnosis.

References

1. Rabiei M, Mohtashame Amiri Z, Masoodi Rad H, Niazi M, Niazi H. frequency of tongue anomalies in primary school of Lahidjan. J Guil Univ Med Sci. 2003;12(45):36–42.
2. Chernoff R. Geriatric nutrition: the health professional's handbook. Burlington: Jones & Bartlett Learning; 2006. p. 176.
3. Bakshi SS. Melkersson–Rosenthal syndrome. J Allergy Clin Immunol Pract. 2017;5(2):471–2.
4. Weijerman ME, de Winter JP. Clinical practice. The care of children with Down syndrome. Eur J Pediatr. 2010;169(12):1445–52.
5. Mester J, Eng C. Cowden syndrome: recognizing and managing a not-so-rare hereditary cancer syndrome. J Surg Oncol. 2015;111(1):125–30.
6. Das UM, Gadicherla P. Lacerated tongue injury in children. Int J Clin Pediatr Dent. 2008;1(1):39–41.
7. Bringhurst C, Herr RD, Aldous JA. Oral trauma in the emergency department. Am J Emerg Med. 1993;11(5):486–90.
8. Rajendran A, Sivapathasundharam B. Shafer's textbook of oral pathology. 7th ed. Missouri: Elsevier; 2012. p. 31–2.
9. Nandini DB, Bhavana SB, Deepak BS, Ashwini R. Paediatric geographic tongue: a case report, review and recent updates. J Clin Diagn Res. 2016;10(2):5–9.
10. Raychaudhuri SK, Maverakis E, Raychaudhuri SP. Diagnosis and classification of psoriasis. Autoimmun Rev. 2014;13(4):490–5.
11. Greenberg MS, Glick M, Ship JA. Burket's oral medicine. 11th ed. Hamilton: BC Decker; 2008. p. 103–4.
12. Rustin MH. Long-term safety of biologics in the treatment of moderate-to-severe plaque psoriasis: review of current data. Br J Dermatol. 2012;167(3):3–11.
13. Collaborators GBD. 2015 disease and injury incidence and prevalence. Lancet. 2016;388(10053):1545–602.
14. CDC. Syphilis – CDC fact sheet (detailed). 2015.
15. Eccleston K, Collins L, Higgins SP. Primary syphilis. Int J STD AIDS. 2008;19(3):145–51.
16. Ratnam S. The laboratory diagnosis of syphilis. Can J Infect Dis Med Microbiol. 2005;16(1):45–51.
17. Kent ME, Romanelli F. Reexamining syphilis: an update on epidemiology, clinical manifestations, and management. Ann Pharmacother. 2008;42(2):226–36.
18. Center for Disease Control and Prevention (CDC). Syphilis-CDC fact sheet. Atlanta: CDC; 2015.
19. CDC. Syphilis & MSM (men who have sex with men) - CDC fact sheet. Atlanta: Centers for Disease Control and Prevention (CDC); 2014.
20. Fact sheet for health professionals – folate. National Institutes of Health. 2011.
21. Pommerville JC. Alcamo's fundamentals of microbiology: body systems. Burlington: Jones & Bartlett Publishers; 2009. p. 511.

22. Micronutrient Information Center, Linus Pauling Institute, Oregon State University. 2014.
23. Biotin – fact sheet for health professionals. Office of dietary supplements. US National Institutes of Health. 2017.
24. Micronutrient Information Center, Linus Pauling Institute, Oregon State University. 2015.
25. Biotin: MedlinePlus supplements. 2013.
26. The American Society of Health-System Pharmacists. Riboflavin. Drugs.com. Bethesda: The American Society of Health-System Pharmacists; 2016.
27. US National Institutes of Health. Riboflavin: fact sheet for health professionals. Office of dietary supplements. Bethesda: US National Institutes of Health; 2018.
28. Brody T. Nutritional biochemistry. San Diego: Academic; 1999.
29. Sebrell WH, Butler RE. Riboflavin deficiency in man (ariboflavinosis). Public Health Rep. 1939;54(48):2121–31.

Ulcers of the Tongue

14

14.1 Classification

Ulcers of the tongue are classified according to their etiology into traumatic, inflammatory, dyspeptic, and malignant ulcers as shown below.

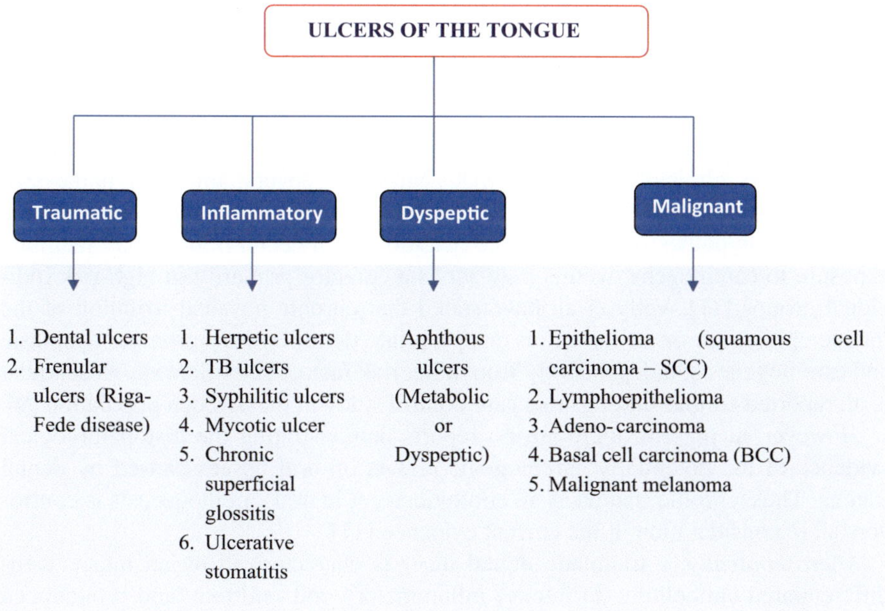

© The Author(s), under exclusive license to Springer Nature Switzerland AG 2022
M. F. Sakr, *Tongue Lesions*, https://doi.org/10.1007/978-3-031-08198-9_14

14.2 Traumatic Ulcers

Among the etiological factors of a tongue ulcer, a chronic traumatic ulcer (CTU) of mechanical nature plays an important role [1].

14.2.1 Dental Ulcers

14.2.1.1 Etiology

Prosthetic irregularities, ill-fitting dentures, metal wires, and cracked or broken teeth are the most common causes of CTU with subsequent hyperplasia and fibrosis resulting from the impact on the oral mucosa.

14.2.1.2 Location

The edges and surface of the tongue opposite a broken tooth or ill-fitting dentures, as well as the occlusal axis of the cheek mucosa, are usually the most involved sites [2, 3].

14.2.1.3 Clinical Picture and Diagnosis

It is painful, with sloping serrated *edges*, elongated shallow *floor* covered with granulation tissue, and soft or mildly indurated *base*. It heals in a few days when the cause is removed; otherwise it should be biopsied, particularly if malignancy (squamous cell carcinoma—SCC) is suspected. Lymph nodes (LNs) may be enlarged, firm, and tender.

A chronic traumatic ulcer (CTU) may be painless with a hard indurated base and raised borders, clinically simulating SCC. Moreover, several authors hypothesized a cause-and-effect relationship between repetitive dental trauma and oral carcinoma [2–10]. It is hypothesized that chronic irritation from dental trauma may facilitate exposure to carcinogens, so this may act as a cofactor primarily in high-risk individual groups [11]. Velly et al. have stated that chronic physical irritation of the tongue epithelium on action of an inappropriate dentition may promote dysplasia and carcinogenesis, independently from other risk factors [2]. Likewise, Rosenquist et al. reported similar findings in a case control study in the Sweden population [9].

However, at present, there are no reports demonstrating the histopathological evidence of the potentially carcinogenic effects on oral tissues caused by dental trauma. Thus, chronic trauma as an etiologic agent in oral carcinogenesis is controversial, in consideration of the current evidence [11].

Microscopically, a traumatic dental ulcer is characterized by an intact, well-differentiated epithelium; an intense inflammatory cell infiltrate; and pronounced eosinophilia [12]. In addition, traumatic oral ulcers are associated with an identifiable mechanical, chemical, thermal, and/or radiotherapeutic cause.

14.2.1.4 Treatment

Treatment of dental ulcers entails extraction of the ragged tooth or ill-fitting dentures (removal of the cause of tissue irritation), appropriate antibiotics, and good oral hygiene.

14.2.1.5 Prognosis

The rapid healing of dental ulcers of the tongue suggests that early dysplastic lesions may be reversible if the source of irritation can be eliminated [13].

14.2.2 Frenular Ulcers

14.2.2.1 Synonyms

A frenular ulcer is also known as "Riga-Fede disease, lesion, or syndrome," "Riga's disease," "traumatic sublingual ulceration," and "pertussis ulcer."

14.2.2.2 Definition

It is a rare condition that occurs in infants and is characterized by ulceration on the ventral surface of the tongue or on the inner surface of the lower lip (Fig. 14.1). It can be described as a sublingual traumatic ulceration [14]. Although it begins as an ulcer, it may progress to a large fibrous mass (ulcerative granuloma) with repeated trauma [15].

The lesion was first described by Antonio Riga, an Italian physician in 1881. Histological studies and additional cases were subsequently published by F. Fede in 1890 [16]. It has been subsequently known as "Riga-Fede disease."

14.2.2.3 Etiology

Traumatic ulceration on the ventral surface of the tongue is most commonly associated with natal or neonatal teeth which are present at birth or erupt in newborns during the first month of life [17, 18]. It may also occur in older infants after the eruption of primary lower incisors with repetitive tongue thrusting habits [16] or coughing (whooping cough) and in children with familial dysautonomia (insensitivity to pain) [19].

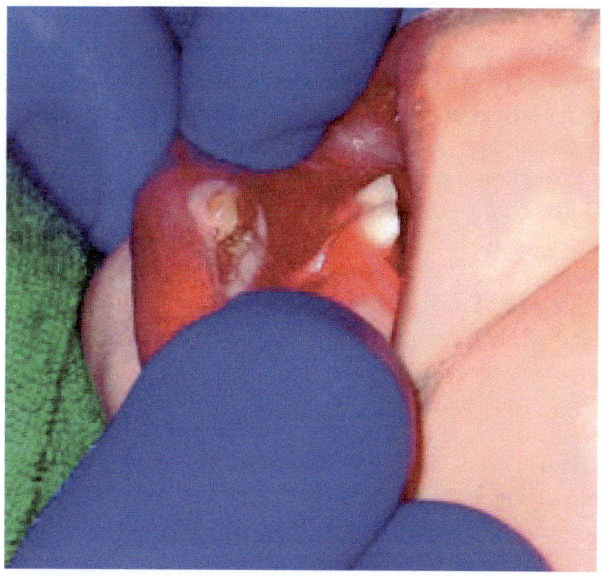

Fig. 14.1 Riga-Fede disease of the inner surface of the lower lip (traumatic ulceration)

14.2.2.4 Location

This ulcer occurs on the frenulum or on the under surface of the tongue on either side of the frenulum of children. It may also occur on the inner surface of the lower lip.

14.2.2.5 Clinical Picture

The ulcer may interfere with proper suckling and feeding and put the neonate at risk for nutritional deficiencies. In such instances, dental intervention may be required. Complications such as discomfort during feeding, laceration of the mother's breasts, deglutition, or aspiration of the teeth may occur [20].

14.2.2.6 Treatment

Treatment of Riga-Fede disease is a challenging task and has varied over the years. Early treatment consisted of excision of the lesion. Due to the erroneous diagnosis of the etiology, resolution of the lesion occurred only upon weaning of the child.

In case of mild to moderate irritation to the tongue, conservative treatment of the lesion on the ventral surface of the tongue may be performed by removing the causative agent or wear on the incisal edge of the tooth by using a polishing disc (of the Soflex type) [21]. Alternatively, a small increment of composite may be bonded to the incisal edges of the teeth [22]. Early diagnosis and intervention prevent malnutrition, and reduce discomfort for the baby and mother, making it possible to resume feeding and complete regression of the lesion [23].

Conventional therapy for Riga-Fede lesions is by the removal of the trauma and topical corticosteroid application for relief of the symptoms and healing the lesion. Within this context, *irradiation* of the soft tissues with low-level laser has been widely used, showing the potential to reduce painful sensitivity (analgesia) and accelerating the repair process in recurrent aphthous stomatitis, when compared with conventional therapies using corticosteroids [24].

However, in pediatric dentistry, *laser therapy* is not routinely used. It may be associated with conventional therapy, promoting faster improvement in the baby's nutrition. In 2017, da Silva et al. [25] reported that for the treatment of Riga-Fede disease, they used low-level laser application with a wavelength of 660 (red) emitting a power of 100 mW nm 1 J of energy, 10 seconds per point of irradiation, on the center and on the edges of the ulceration.

Irradiation was performed on the day after extraction of the tooth, for three sessions on consecutive days, and continued application of triamcinolone acetonide on the ulcerated lesion to help healing and relieve the painful symptoms, until the lesion healed. They concluded that laser therapy is a possible treatment option for Riga-Fede lesions as it reduces the healing time to 4 days, allowing the return to feeding and improvement in the pain symptoms from the first day of application [25].

Laser therapy has several advantages. These include (1) the absence of side effects, (2) being a noninvasive technique that is easily applied, and (3) one that does not generate heat in the irradiated tissue. These characteristics assure good acceptance of laser therapy by individuals, in addition to being reported to be a promising and safe therapy if performed by a qualified professional [26].

The decision about whether or not to keep the tooth in place will depend on several factors including (1) its implantation and degree of mobility, (2) interference with feeding, (3) possibility of traumatic injury to the mother's breast and ventral surface of the child's tongue, and (4) whether the tooth is supernumerary or part of the normal series [27]. Approximately, only 1–10% of natal and neonatal teeth are supernumerary [28]. Tooth extraction may be the treatment option in cases when even reduced incisal edges still contact and traumatize the tongue during suckling enough to delay healing.

14.3 Inflammatory Ulcers

14.3.1 Herpetic Ulcers (True Herpes Linguis)

14.3.1.1 Etiology

Tongue ulcers may be caused by herpes simplex virus (HSV0) [29]. The name is from Greek—ἕρπης *herpēs*—which is related to the meaning "to creep," referring to spreading blisters [30]. They are transmitted by direct contact with body fluids or lesions of an infected individual [29]. Transmission may still occur when symptoms are not present [29].

14.3.1.2 Classification of HSV

Herpes simplex virus is divided into two types [31]. However, each may cause infections in all areas [31].

- HSV-1 (orofacial herpes) causes infections primarily in the mouth, throat, face, eye, and central nervous system [31].
- HSV-2 (genital herpes) causes primarily anogenital infections [31].

14.3.1.3 Epidemiology of HSV

Worldwide rates of either HSV-1 and/or HSV-2 are between 60% and 95% in adults. HSV-1 is more common than HSV-2, with rates of both increasing as people age [31]. HSV-1 rates are between 70% and 80% in populations of low socioeconomic status and 40% to 60% in populations of higher socioeconomic status [31]. An estimated 536 million people or 16% of the population worldwide were infected with HSV-2 as of 2003 with greater rates among women and in those in the developing world [32]. Rates of infection are determined by the presence of antibodies against either viral species [33].

In the United States, 58% of the population is infected with HSV-1 [34], and 16% are infected with HSV-2. Among those who are HSV-2 seropositive, only 19% were aware they were infected [35]. During 2005–2008, the prevalence of HSV-2 was 39% in Blacks and 21% in women [36].

14.3.1.4 Site

Oral (orofacial) herpetic ulcers usually affect the tongue and angles of the mouth.

14.3.1.5 Clinical Picture

It presents with severe unilateral pain followed within a few hours by multiple blisters or vesicles small blisters in groups often called cold sores or fever blisters. These vesicles burst to become multiple, superficial, oval, small, painful ulcers.

Prodromal symptoms that occur before the appearance of herpetic lesions help differentiate HSV symptoms from the similar symptoms of other disorders, such as allergic stomatitis. When lesions do not appear inside the mouth, primary orofacial herpes is sometimes mistaken for impetigo, a bacterial infection. Common mouth ulcers (aphthous ulcer) also resemble intraoral herpes, but do not present a vesicular stage [37].

Other disorders caused by herpes simplex include herpetic whitlow when it involves the fingers [38], herpes of the eye, herpes infection of the brain [39], and neonatal herpes when it affects a newborn, among others [40].

14.3.1.6 Pathophysiology

In all cases, HSV is never removed from the body by the immune system. Following a primary infection, the virus enters the nerves at the site of primary infection, migrates to the cell body of the neuron, and becomes latent in the ganglion [41]. As a result of the primary infection, the body produces antibodies to the particular type of HSV involved, preventing a subsequent infection of that type at a different site. In HSV-1-infected individuals, seroconversion after an oral infection prevents additional HSV-1 infections such as whitlow, genital herpes, and herpes of the eye. Prior HSV-1 seroconversion seems to reduce the symptoms of a later HSV-2 infection, although HSV-2 can still be contracted.

14.3.1.7 Laboratory Tests

Until the 1980s, serological tests for antibodies to HSV were rarely useful to diagnosis and not routinely used in clinical practice [37]. The older IgM serologic assay could not differentiate between antibodies generated in response to HSV-1 or HSV-2 infection. However, a glycoprotein G-specific (IgG) HSV test introduced in the 1980s is more than 98% specific at discriminating HSV-1 from HSV-2 [42].

14.3.1.8 Differential Diagnosis

Herpetic oral ulcers should not be confused with conditions caused by other viruses in the *Herpesviridae* family such as herpes zoster, which is caused by varicella-zoster virus. The differential diagnosis includes hand, foot, and mouth disease due to similar lesions on the skin. Lymphangioma circumscriptum and dermatitis herpetiformis may also have a similar appearance.

14.3.1.9 Management

No method eradicates herpes virus from the body, but *antiviral* medications can reduce the frequency, duration, and severity of outbreaks. *Analgesics* such as ibuprofen and paracetamol (acetaminophen) can ameliorate pain and reduce fever. *Topical anesthetic* treatments such as prilocaine, lidocaine, benzocaine, or tetracaine can also relieve itching and pain [43–45].

14.3.1.9.1 Antiviral Medications

Several antiviral drugs are effective in treating herpes, including acyclovir (acyclovir), valaciclovir, famciclovir, and penciclovir. Acyclovir was the first discovered, and valaciclovir is slightly more effective than acyclovir for reducing lesion healing time [46]. Evidence supports the use of acyclovir and valaciclovir in the treatment of herpes labialis [47] as well as herpes infections in people with cancer [48]. The evidence to support the use of acyclovir in primary herpetic gingivostomatitis is weaker [49].

14.3.1.9.2 Topical Antivirals

A number of topical antivirals are effective for herpes labialis; these include acyclovir, penciclovir, and docosanol [47, 50].

14.3.1.9.3 Alternative Medicine

Evidence is insufficient to support the use of many of alternative medicine compounds such as echinacea, eleuthero, L-lysine, zinc, monolaurin bee products, and aloe vera [51]. While a number of small studies show possible benefit from *monolaurin, L-lysine, aspirin, lemon balm, topical zinc, or licorice root cream* in treatment, these preliminary studies have not been confirmed by higher-quality randomized controlled studies [52].

14.3.2 Tuberculous (TB) Ulcers

14.3.2.1 Etiology

Tuberculosis is a chronic granulomatous disease caused by various strains of mycobacteria, usually the *Mycobacterium tuberculosis* in humans [53]. *Robert Koch*, a German physician, discovered the tuberculosis bacillus in 1882 [54]. The prevalence of TB is decreasing, but it has re-emerged as an opportunistic infection in immunocompromised individuals such as transplanted patients under immunosuppression and those affected with human immunodeficiency virus (HIV) infection especially in the developed countries. However, in developing countries, it has a high prevalence rate. Although TB can affect almost every organ in the body, the lungs are the most commonly affected organ [55]. Extrapulmonary TB in the head and neck regions includes cervical lymphadenitis, TB of the larynx, TB of the tonsils, TB of the salivary glands, tubercular otitis media, and TB of the nose and nasopharynx. Tuberculosis of oral cavity is an uncommon disease with an incidence of 0.5–1.5% [56]. Oral tuberculosis may occur at any location on the oral mucous membrane, but the *tongue is most commonly affected*. Other sites include the gingiva, lips, buccal mucosa, palate, tonsils, and floor of the mouth.

Tuberculosis of the oral cavity can be primary or secondary. *Primary lesions* are uncommon, seen in younger patients, and present as single painless ulcer with regional lymph node enlargement. *The secondary lesions* are common, often associated with pulmonary disease. They usually present as single, indurated, irregular, painful ulcer covered by inflammatory exudates in patients of any age group but relatively more common in middle-aged and elderly patients [57, 58].

Oral lesions of TB may present as ulcer, diffuse fibrosis, woody tongue, nodule, fissure, tuberculoma, or granuloma [59]. Of all these oral lesions, the ulcerative form is the most common [60, 61]. It is often painful, with no caseation of the dependent lymph nodes (LNs).

Tuberculosis of the oral cavity is rare because of continuous cleaning of oral mucosa by saliva and the resistance of epithelium of the oral mucosa to the mycobacterium. The *risk factors* responsible for the development of oral TB include oral mucosal trauma, smoking, and poor oral hygiene. The breach in the mucosal integrity can predispose to the inoculation with the mycobacterium.

14.3.2.2 Site

Tuberculous ulcers usually occur at the tip and sides of the tongue, which rest against rough, sharp, or broken teeth or at the site of other irritants. Patients with oral tubercular lesions often have a history of preexisting trauma.

14.3.2.3 Clinical Picture

The patient presents with multiple, painful, *shallow* ulcers with undermined *edges* which are tender due to exposed nerve endings, yellowish *floor*, and soft *base*. The presence of pulmonary TB should point to diagnosis [62].

14.3.2.4 Diagnosis

Investigations such as chest X-ray, erythrocyte sedimentation rate (ESR), Mantoux test, and sputum for acid-fast bacillus (AFB) are mandatory in the diagnosis and the treatment of TB, especially the pulmonary TB, which is the most common form of TB that is frequently associated with various types of extrapulmonary TB. To diagnose the extrapulmonary TB, there are a number of investigations including mycobacterial stain and culture, examination of body fluid for measurement of adenosine deaminase (ADA), tissue biopsy, polymerase chain reaction (PCR), and immunological test such as tuberculin skin test. Beside these tests radio imaging is also a frequently done test.

Biopsy of ulcerated lesions of the tongue should include the deeper tissue as the superficial biopsy may lead to inconclusive diagnosis such as chronic nonspecific inflammation, mandating a repeated biopsy.

14.3.2.5 Differential Diagnosis

Although the tuberculosis of the oral cavity is rare, it should be considered in a differential diagnosis of any long-standing ulcer of the tongue. The more common differential diagnosis of such ulcerated tongue lesions includes malignant ulcer and traumatic ulcers. Similarly, a major aphthous ulcer can cause diagnostic dilemma occasionally.

Histologically, the granulomatous inflammatory reaction of tubercular ulcer may mimic other granulomatous diseases such as Wegener's granulomatosis, syphilitic ulcer, actinomycosis, mycotic infections, sarcoidosis, Crohn's disease, cat-scratch disease, foreign body reactions, tertiary syphilis, and Melkersson-Rosenthal syndrome [62, 63]. Most importantly ulcerated lesion has to be differentiated from carcinoma of the tongue because the tongue is a one of the commonest sites for malignancy of the upper gastrointestinal tract.

14.3.2.6 Treatment

The treatment of oral tuberculosis lesions is the same as the systemic TB. Currently, the most effective regimens require a combination of four drugs (isoniazid, rifampicin, pyrazinamide, and ethambutol) administered daily for the first 2 months, followed by an additional 4 months with only two drugs (isoniazid and rifampicin) [64]. The complexity of this regimen prompted the World Health Organization (WHO) to launch a new global strategy for TB control known as "directly observed therapy, short course" (DOTS) in 1997. The central component of this strategy is direct observation, by trained personnel, which both ensures patient compliance with the drug regimen and reduces the likelihood of drug resistance. However, this strategy also increases the cost of treatment and makes TB therapy more inconvenient.

Control of TB is difficult because of two primary factors: *persistence and resistance*. In spite of the fact that antibiotics are available, *M. tuberculosis* is highly persistent, possibly because the bacterium induces chronic inflammation that sequesters it within the tissues, protecting it against drug exposure [65]. Thus, drug treatment must be extended to fully destroy the bacterium and prevent relapse. Drug resistance is the result of genetic mutations that cause a heritable loss of drug susceptibility. Although resistance to a single drug does not render therapy ineffective, multidrug-resistant strains make TB much more costly and difficult to treat [65]. For this reason, the need for newer and more effective drugs that achieve multiple goals in improving TB control is imperative [66].

There are two types of resistance usually observed in the context of TB: MDR (multidrug resistant TB) and XDR (extensively drug resistant). MDR-TB is defined as *Mycobacterium tuberculosis* (*M. tuberculosis*) resistant to the most potent first-line anti-TB medications, isoniazid and rifampicin, while XDR-TB has additional multidrug resistance to the most active second-line agents, injectable drugs (aminoglycosides and/or cyclic polypeptides—capreomycin, kanamycin, and amikacin) and fluoroquinolones.

Potential new agents should reduce treatment duration, have an acceptable tolerability profile, be active against MDR/XDR TB, be of use in HIV-infected patients with TB, and be active against latent TB. Numerous novel drugs have been introduced in recent times, which promise to be a better alternative like the nitroimidazole group (PA 824, OPC 67683), diarylquinolines (TMC 207 or bedaquiline or J compound) [67], oxazolidinones (PNU-100480 and AZD5847), SQ109, phenothiazines (thioridazine), and LL3858 for the effective treatment of TB [68].

14.3.3 Syphilitic Ulcers

Syphilis is a systemic bacterial infection caused by *Treponema pallidum*. The incubation period is usually 21–30 days after contact, ranging from 10 to 90 days, according to the number and virulence of *Treponema* and the host response [69]. It is estimated that there are more than 12 million cases per year in the world [70].

According to Eyer-Silva et al. [71], the occurrence of oral lesions in syphilis would be between 12% and 15%, while Lautenschlager found oral manifestations in about one-third to one-half of patients with secondary syphilis [72].

14.3.3.1 Transmission

Syphilis is transmitted *horizontally* by sexual contact (where bacteria can enter the body through cuts or sores in the vagina, penis, anus, or mouth) and *vertically* from the mother to the baby after 14–16 weeks of gestation when *Treponema pallidum* crosses the placental barrier [73–75]. Other means of transmission have been reported, especially among health professionals. Although the genital areas are the most common site of manifestation, unusual extragenital regions were cited for the onset of cancrum, such as the oral cavity, fingers, nose, eyelids, arm, and nipple [76]. Syphilis is *not* spread through sharing eating utensils or drinking glasses.

14.3.3.2 Clinical Presentation

Signs and symptoms of syphilis vary according to the disease stage [69]. Oral manifestations are, in many cases, one of the first signs of the disease and can guide early diagnosis [70]. The lip is the most commonly involved part, followed by the tongue and tonsils [77, 78]. An important characteristic of the syphilitic oral lesion is the absence of pain; therefore, this condition must be differentiated from squamous cell carcinoma (SCC) [77].

14.3.3.2.1 First Stage: Primary Syphilis

The recent primary infection is characterized by the appearance of *chancre* or sore (self-limited nonspecific ulcer), which in oral syphilis may be inside the mouth, on the lip and commissure, or at the tip of the tongue [78].

The patient may present with painless and noninflammatory bilateral satellite adenopathy of submandibular and submental lymph nodes (LNs) [77]. Serologic tests are positive, and spirochetes are detected in the discharge obtained from the sore.

14.3.3.2.2 Second Stage: Secondary Syphilis

Secondary syphilis is associated with hematogenous dissemination of the microorganism. Clinical manifestations of the disease may be quite heterogeneous and nonspecific [77–79]. The patient may present with fever, headache, tearing, nasal secretion, pharyngitis, sore throat, weight loss, generalized arthralgia, and myalgia [78]. The disease, at this stage, is characterized by systemic involvement, generalized lymphadenopathy, and diffuse and painless, whitish/reddish, oval macules covered by a fibrinous pseudomembrane, or papular eruptions may be observed in the mucous membranes, associated or not with skin lesions [80]. This maculopapular cutaneous rash is known as *syphilitic rosette* [79].

Sometimes, in addition to the cutaneous lesions, this systemic condition can be associated to palmoplantar lesions that can affect several areas of the oral cavity [79]. It may also present a form of condyloma latum or Hutchinson's warts, characterized by nodular, firm lesions or discretely elevated mucous plaques, which may be superficially eroded or ulcerated [73].

Tongue ulcers at this stage are described as multiple, yellowish-white snail-track ulcers occurring at the sides and dorsum of the tongue.

Differential diagnosis of these ulcers is broad and varied and includes aphthous ulceration, oral ulceration associated with human immunodeficiency virus (HIV), tuberculosis (TB), lymphoma, mycosis, leishmaniasis, eosinophilic ulcer, squamous cell carcinoma (SCC), necrotizing sialometaplasia, cytomegalovirus (CMV), gonorrhea, and traumatic ulcers [21].

14.3.3.2.3 Late Stage

Late infection is represented by various signs and symptoms, such as vascular symptoms, and in the mouth, oral syphilis may eventually develop a nodular ulcerated granulomatous palatal mass [69], gummatous ulcer, or syphilitic glossitis [78]. The ulcer occurs at the midline of the dorsum of the tongue. It is painless, single, with clear-cut edges and wash-leather floor. Leukoplakia or diffuse fibrosis may also be present.

14.3.3.3 Diagnosis

Simply observing a chancre or ulcer is not enough for a diagnosis. Blood or a fluid sample from the sore is needed for further testing. There are two blood tests: non-treponemal and treponemal tests. Neither test alone is definitive, but the two tests together can confirm a diagnosis of syphilis.

A *biopsy* of tissue or fluid is sometimes used to diagnose oral syphilis. The histopathological characteristics of secondary syphilis are as variable as the lesions. Whereas the changes are often nonspecific, findings of endothelial cell swelling, perivascular infiltrates with a preponderance of plasma cells, and epidermal psoriasiform hyperplasia support the diagnosis of syphilis [81].

14.3.3.4 Treatment of Oral Syphilis

The standard treatment for most oral syphilis is the antibiotic *benzathine penicillin G* [82]. Left untreated, syphilis sores may go away spontaneously in a few weeks. However, that does not mean the infection is gone. The bacteria are still present in the body and additional symptoms are likely to appear later. What is more, untreated syphilis can cause long-term damage to your organs, such as your heart and brain. Ultimately, this damage can be fatal [83].

14.3.4 Chronic Superficial Glossitis

Chronic superficial glossitis may be associated with chronic repeated nonspecific ulcers, usually on the dorsum of the tongue. Ulcers are superficial, small, and painful. They are associated with fissures or vesicles and have a unilateral distribution.

14.3.4.1 Clinical Stages

Chronic superficial glossitis has the following clinical stages:

1. Hyperkeratosis with hypertrophy of papillae causing mild thickening of the surface and the formation of a thin milky film
2. White patches (*leukoplakia*) as if it is covered with a smooth paint
3. Red patches (*erythroplakia*) due to loss of papillae (painful—precancerous)
4. Cracks or fissures in those red patches (looks like wrinkled paint)
5. Small projections (carcinoma in situ)
6. Finally, epithelioma (squamous cell carcinoma—SCC)

14.3.4.2 Treatment

Management entails avoidance of the predisposing factors plus alkaline mouth gargles and excision of red patches. Close follow-up is indicated and biopsy of any developing lesions is highly recommended.

14.3.5 Chronic Ulcerative Stomatitis (CUS)

14.3.5.1 Definition

Tongue ulcers may occur in connection with chronic ulcerative stomatitis (CUS), which is a painful chronic ulcerative process that occurs in the mouth but can occasionally be associated with skin lesions. Chronic ulcerative stomatitis is defined as an "immune-mediated disorder characterized by oral erosions and ulcers that are usually refractory to conventional treatments" [84]. This condition was originally described by Jaremko et al. [85] and Parodi and Cardo [86].

14.3.5.2 Clinical Picture

The disease often involves middle-aged and older women with painful lesions sometimes resembling those of erosive oral lichen planus (OLP). The most affected sites are the buccal mucosa, the gingiva, and the *tongue*, but the skin is involved in 22.5% of cases.

14.3.5.3 Diagnosis

Histopathological features in CUS are nonspecific and indistinguishable from those of OLP, with the exception of the presence of a mixed infiltrate composed of lymphocytes and plasma cells. Direct immunofluorescence (DIF) analysis reveals the presence of stratified epithelium-specific antinuclear antibodies (SES-ANA) in the lower third of the epithelium. The IgG antibodies detected on DIF are directed against the $\Delta Np63\alpha$ isoform of p63 expressed in the nuclei of the epithelial basal cells.

14.3.5.4 Treatment

A distinguishing feature of chronic ulcerative stomatitis is the low response to conventional corticosteroid therapy and the good outcome with hydroxychloroquine at the dosage of 200 mg/day or higher dosages [87].

14.4 Dyspeptic (Aphthous) Ulcers

14.4.1 Introduction

The word "aphthous" originated from the Greek word "aphtha," the meaning of which is "ulcer." Aphthous stomatitis is one of most common ulcerative disease associated mainly with the oral mucosa. It was delineated in 400 BC by Hippocrates; the disease is known by lay public and professionals by several other names such as *cold sores*, *canker sores*, *recurrent aphthous stomatitis* (*RAS*), and *recurrent aphthous ulcers* (*RAU*).

14.4.2 Clinical Presentation

Aphthous stomatitis is characterized by the extremely painful, recurring, solitary, or multiple ulcers in the upper throat and oral cavity. These types of ulcers are usually small, multiple, ovoid, or round with circumscribed margin, grayish-white or yellow floor, sloping edges, soft base, and are encompassed by erythematous halo [88, 89]. Lymph nodes are *not* enlarged.

Both minor and major subtypes of aphthous stomatitis usually produce lesions on the nonkeratinized oral mucosa (i.e., the inside of the cheeks, lips, underneath the tongue, and the floor of the mouth), but less commonly major aphthous ulcers may occur in other parts of the mouth on keratinized mucosal surfaces.

This is the most prevailing oral ulcerative disorder [90]. It usually affects the tip (Fig. 14.2) and sides (Fig. 14.3) of the mouth. The pain it causes may result in difficulty in eating, speaking, and swallowing [91].

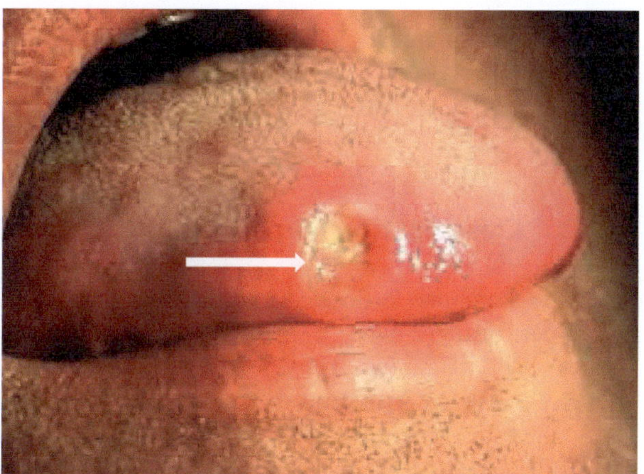

Fig. 14.2 An aphthous ulcer affecting the tip of the tongue (arrow)

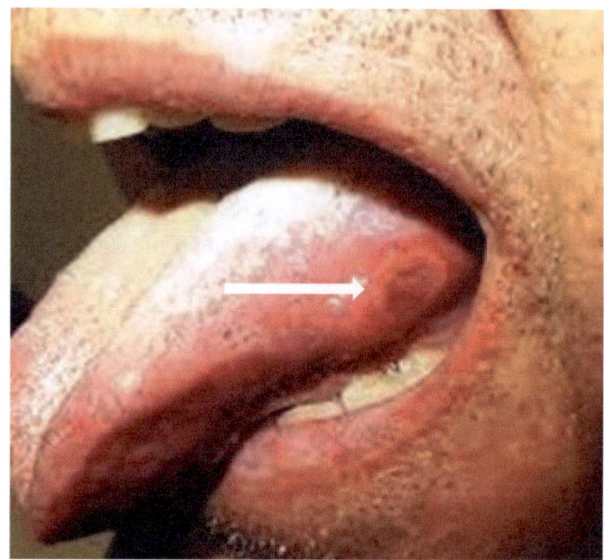

Fig. 14.3 An aphthous ulcer affecting the side of the tongue (arrow)

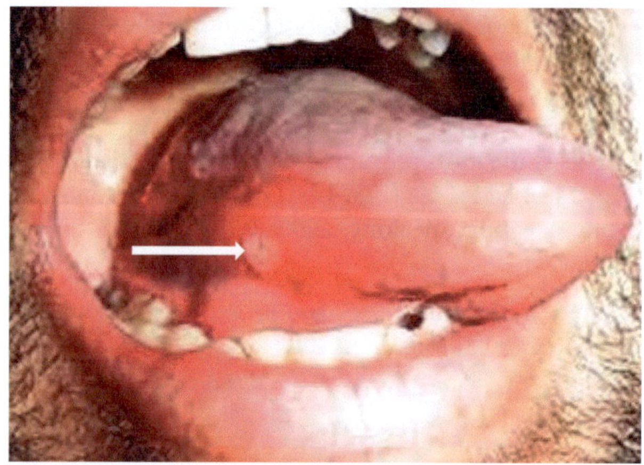

Fig. 14.4 A minor aphthous ulcer (<1 cm in size) affecting the undersurface of the side of the tongue (arrow)

14.4.3 Classification (Types of Aphthous Ulcers)

Aphthous stomatitis is divided into three varieties: minor aphthae, major aphthae, and herpetiform [92–94].

14.4.3.1 Minor Aphthae

Minor aphthae also known as "Miculiz's aphthae" is the most common variant constituting 75–85% of all recurrent aphthous stomatitis (RAS) cases. These types of ulcers are usually less than 1 cm (Fig. 14.4) and heal without scarring within 10–14 days. It is commonly found in nonkeratinized mucosal surfaces like the buccal mucosa, labial mucosa, and floor of the mouth.

14.4.3.2 Major Aphthae

Major aphthous ulcers, also known as "Sutton's disease," usually exceeds 1 cm (Fig. 14.5) in size, causes deeper ulceration, and thus leaves scar. It constitutes only 10–15% of RAS cases. These ulcers may remain for about 10–20 days or may even last for months. The usual sites are throat, lips, and soft palate, but the tongue may be also affected.

14.4.3.3 Herpetiform Aphthae

The herpetiform type is the least common variant of recurrent aphthous stomatitis (RAS) that constitutes only 7–10% of cases. Ulcer size is very small usually measuring only 2–3 mm in diameter. Herpetiform aphthous ulcers are numerous in number reaching up to approximately 100 ulcers at the same time (Fig. 14.6). These small ulcers can fuse together producing large irregular lesions that may last for 7–10 days without leaving scars.

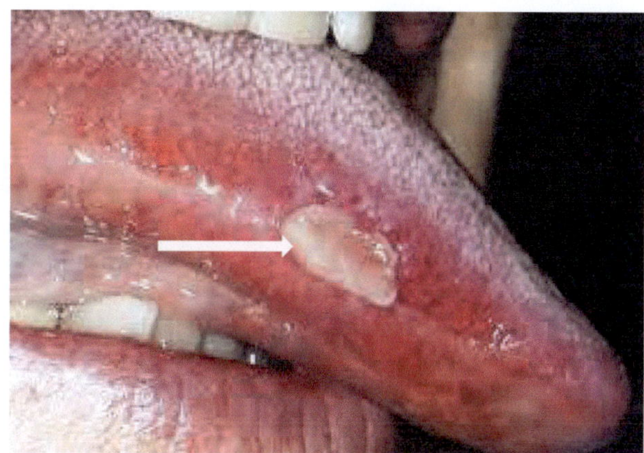

Fig. 14.5 A major aphthous ulcer (more than 1 cm in size) affecting the side of the tongue (arrow)

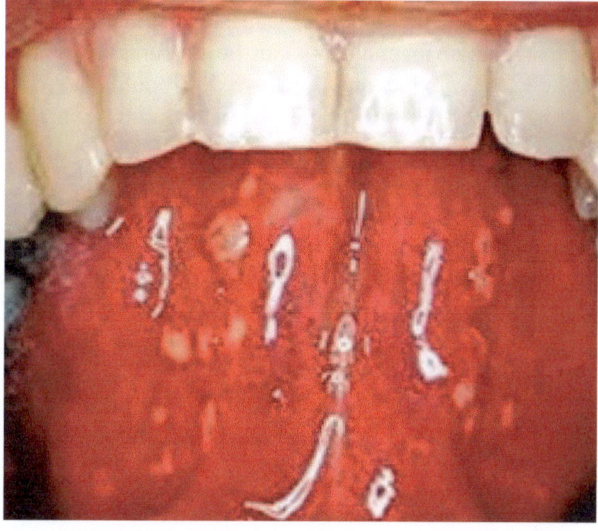

Fig. 14.6 Numerous herpetiform ulcers (recurrent) affecting the undersurface of the tongue

14.4.4 Etiology/Pathogenesis

The precise etiopathogenesis of aphthous stomatitis is not fully disclosed. The potential factors responsible for aphthous ulcers are genetic predisposition, mechanical injury, microelement and vitamin B-12 deficiencies, increased oxidative stress, food allergies, microbial factors, anxiety, hormonal defects, and systemic diseases (e.g., ulcerative colitis, celiac disease, AIDS, Crohn's disease) [95].

14.4.4.1 Genetic Predisposition

Genetic predisposition is responsible for the development of aphthous stomatitis in about 40% of patients who have a positive family history. These persons usually develop ulcers, which are of severe nature, at an earlier age [96].

14.4.4.2 Mechanical Injury

Mechanical injury resulting from local anesthetic injections, dental treatments, sharp tooth, or injury by a tooth brush may render the patient susceptible to the occurrence of recurrent aphthous ulceration [97]. Lack of adequate saliva that lubricates and protects the oral mucosa from injury and antigenic exposure may raise the risk of development of RAS [98].

14.4.4.3 Microelement and Vitamin B12 Deficiencies

Deficiencies of vitamin B12, folic acid, and iron may contribute to the development of RAS. The lack of these microelements is two times more usual in these persons as compared to controls. Contradictory detections in different investigations linking the relationship of hematinic deficiency and RAS have been elaborated because of altered genetic backgrounds and dietary habits [99].

14.4.4.4 Stress

Stress and psychological imbalance have been linked with recurrent aphthous ulcers. Patients often report increased stress with inception of aphthous ulcers. Antidepressant therapy has been suggested to reduce the incidence of aphthous ulcers. Several mechanisms can be postulated for a cause-and-effect relationship between trait anxiety and RAS. Anxiety could lead to para-functional habits including lip and cheek biting and physical trauma, which might initiate the ulcerative process in susceptible individuals [100, 101].

14.4.4.5 Food Allergies

Food containing gluten such as chocolate, coffee, almonds, cereals, peanuts, strawberries, tomatoes, cheese, and wheat flour may be responsible for the development of aphthous ulcers [102].

14.4.4.6 Microbial Factors

There is a limited consistent confirmation to support the presumption that RAS constitutes an infectious disease. In particular from investigations to examine whether there might be an association between previously suspect L-forms of streptococci and RAS or the adenoviruses, herpes simplex virus (HSV), varicella-zoster virus or cytomegalovirus (CMV), and RAS, the accessible proof indicates that none of these microorganisms appears to be directly responsible for RAS in spite of continued speculation about their feasible role.

The antiviral agent acyclovir has been reported to provide no valuable outcome in preventing or reducing episodic outburst of the condition, which weakens the suggestion of a possible viral causation for RAS. However, in a narrow subset of individuals who suffer from herpes simplex virus (HSV), the virus may serve as an antigenic "trigger" that initiates the cascade of immunological events that result in RAS. Presumably, such patients would benefit from appropriate therapeutic and prophylactic antiviral therapy, coupled with treatments specifically aimed at reducing the severity and frequency of the RAS episodes by modulating their supposedly heightened immune responses to the viral "trigger."

It must be emphasized, however, that regarding most aphthous patients, any suggestion of a causative nexus between RAS and HSV seems to represent unsubstantiated conjecture rather than proven fact [94].

14.4.4.7 Tobacco Smoking

Nonsmokers usually are more prone to RAS, and there is a lower occurrence and severity of RAS among heavy smokers as compared to moderate smokers. Few patients report an onset of RAS after cessation of smoking, while others report control on smoking reinitiation. The usage of smokeless tobacco is linked with a remarkably lower universality of RAS [103].

14.4.4.8 Immunopathogenesis

There is a rise in antibody-dependent cell cytotoxicity and higher levels of serum immunoglobulins in patients with RAS. Lymphocytes from patients with serious RAS show growing numbers of T-helper/inducer cells, decreased numbers of T-suppressor/inducer cells, and depressed responses to mitogens. Activated T lymphocytes aggregate in the periphery of RAS lesions mediated immune response. Immunohistochemical studies of lymphocyte subsets in aphthous ulcers of HIV-seronegative patients and HIV-seropositive patients have yielded similar findings, which strongly indicate that these ulcers represent a cell-mediated immunological dysfunction in which infiltrating T lymphocytes play a primary role [104].

14.4.4.9 Hormonal Defects

It appears from different studies that a minor subset of women with RAU have cyclical oral ulceration related to the onset of menstruation or luteal phase of the menstrual cycle. Complete remission during pregnancy has been reported with exacerbation occurring in the puerperium. Although 10% of women had their first episode of RAU between the ages of 50 and 59, more recent work has not uncovered an association between RAU and the menopause [105].

14.4.4.10 Drugs

Drugs such as nonsteroidal anti-inflammatory drugs (NSAIDs, e.g., diclofenac phenylacetic acid and propionic acid) can cause oral ulcers identical to those of RAU, accompanied with genital ulceration or only oral ulcers in the case of piroxicam. A relationship between beta-blockers and aphthous ulcers was also proposed. These types of ulcers commonly occur as an adverse side effect and fade away when the usage of drug is discontinued [105].

14.4.4.11 Systemic Diseases

Behcet's disease (BD) is a multisystem, chronic, relapsing vasculitis that affects nearly all organs and systems. It is associated with multiple oral and genital ulcers, arthritis, hematemesis, melena, and epigastric pain as predominant manifestations. RAS and BD have similar presenting symptoms such as oral lesions and abdominal pain [106].

Celiac disease (CD) is caused by gluten sensitivity of the small intestines. The reported CD prevalence (40%) in patients with RAS is higher than in the normal population. It is also described that RAS may be the presenting sign of the disease and may be used as a marker for the CD [107].

In *Crohn's disease*, intraoral involvement is observed in nearly 9% of cases, and oral inflammation precedes intestinal symptoms in about 60% of these patients. It is thus important to consider Crohn's disease in the differential diagnosis of subjects with intestinal symptoms and RAS [108].

14.4.5 Management and Treatment of Aphthous Stomatitis

In spite of much clinical and research studies, the root causes continue to exist, the ulcers are unavoidable, and therapy is symptomatic. There is no specific treatment for RAS, and management strategies depend on the symptoms, duration, and severity [109].

The goals of therapy are threefold: (1) controlling the ulcer pain, (2) promoting healing of the ulcer, and (3) preventing recurrence. For determination of the appropriate treatment, medical history of the patient, pain severity, frequency, and medication tolerance should be considered before commencing treatment. As there is no single treatment available which is uniformly effective in RAS, it is important to explore a spectrum of therapies to validate a definitive treatment strategy [109].

The first choice for aphthous stomatitis treatment is the "topical agents" because they are effective, safe, and not expensive. The problem with topical agents is obtaining effective drug delivery, because substances applied to mucosal surfaces are inevitably rubbed or rinsed away. Topical management may not be enough for recurring and severe ulcerations. In such cases, "systemic medications" are employed [110, 111].

14.4.6 First-Line Therapy/Topical Therapy

When there is incidence of recurrent aphthous ulcers, whether minor or major, in a limited number, closely opposed to one another and scattered on readily available oral surfaces such as the labial or vestibular mucosa or the anterior portion of the tongue, the first-line therapeutic management should be conservative topical therapy [112].

14.4.6.1 Topical Gels, Creams, and Pastes

Different gels and pastes can be employed to cover the ulcer surface and form a defensive guard against secondary infection and further mechanical irritation. A little amount of cream or gel should be applied 3–4 times a day by the patient who should stay away from drinking or eating for 30 minutes [113]. The inflammatory process that occurred with the development of aphthae may be limited by topical corticosteroids. Al-Namah et al. concluded that the novel dexamucobase was found to be equally effective in treating oral aphthous ulceration, with some advantages, as the widely used preparation Kenalog in Orabase [114]. Meng et al. indicated that amlexanox oral adhesive pellicles are as effective and safe as amlexanox oral adhesive tablets in the treatment of minor RAS for this Chinese cohort. Pellicles seem to be more comfortable to use when compared with the dosage form of tablets. Therefore in clinical practice, amlexanox oral adhesive pellicles may be a better choice for RAS patients [115].

14.4.6.2 Topical Anesthetic

Lidocaine (2%) is found to alleviate pain related to RAS, but a mixture of adrenaline (1:8000) further enhances the pain relief period, which permits the patient more time to take the meals. The patient is directed to apply 2–3 drops of it onto the surface of ulcer [116].

14.4.6.3 Topical Antimicrobials

In RAS management, the aqueous mouth rinse containing chlorhexidine gluconate provides some beneficial effects. Investigations indicate that it decreases the ulcer's duration but cannot prevent recurrence. It is generally used as 0.2% w/w (weight for weight) mouth rinse, but the 0.1% w/w mouthwash or 1% gel can also be beneficial [117].

14.4.6.4 Topical Antibiotics

The antibacterial effect of tetracycline is also known to decrease the breakdown of collagen. This can be employed in a mouth rinse form prepared by dissolving the capsule of 250 mg into 180 ml of water. The patient is advised to swish and spit four times a day for 4–5 days. Tetracycline is considered inferior to minocycline due to the additional immunomodulatory effects of minocycline. It can be used by dissolving the 100 mg tablets in 180 ml of water and asking the patient to rinse two times daily for 4–5 days. In both cases the patient should be directed to stay away from food or drink for at least 30 min [118].

14.4.6.5 Topical Corticosteroids

Topical corticosteroids are the backbone of RAS treatment. Different types of topical corticosteroids are employed that alleviate the symptoms of RAS with no suppression of adrenal function. Some of the currently available agents are designed in a new drug delivery system in the form of a protective film that is designed to attach firmly to the wet moving mucous, thereby forming a protective film over the ulcer area. It has applied in a paste form, 2–3 times a day. This leads to rapid healing and faster relief of pain. These steroids may develop local candidiasis on long-term use. Other topical corticosteroids include clobetasol propionate 0.05%, triamcinolone acetonide, and fluocinonide 0.05% [119, 120].

14.4.6.6 Topical Anti-Inflammatory Agents

Five percent amlexanox in a paste form possesses anti-inflammatory and anti-allergic properties and has been found to be efficient and clinically safe in many clinical investigations for RAS management [121].

Topical sucralfate when given at 5 ml, four times a day, was also found to be very effective in the treatment of RAS. It forms a protective barrier on the affected area by adhering to mucous membrane tissues, there by exerting a soothing effect on the lesions. It was commonly employed for the treatment of peptic ulcers [122].

14.4.6.7 Topical Analgesic/Anti-Inflammatory Spray and Rinses

Topical analgesic sprays or rinses such as benzydamine hydrochloride can be utilized to alleviate discomfort in aphthous stomatitis due to its analgesic, anti-inflammatory, antimicrobial, and anesthetic activity [123].

14.4.6.8 Topical Hyaluronic Acid

Topical application of hyaluronic acid in the form of a 0.2% gel was found to be beneficial in RAS treatment. The main function of hyaluronic acid is activation and moderation of angiogenesis, promoting re-epithelization via proliferation of basal keratinocytes and reducing collagen disposition and scarring [124].

14.4.7 Second-Line Therapy/Systemic Therapy

The outbreaks of RAS normally resolve with topical treatment, though in some cases these measures prove insufficient because of the severity of the lesions or for unknown reasons. This is when second-line therapy with systemic drugs is utilized.

14.4.7.1 Levamisole

Due to its vast immunostimulatory effects, it was recommended as a possible treatment for RAS. Levamisole at a dose of 10–15 mg/day for a period of 2–3 months helps in alleviating the pain, frequency, number, and duration of aphthous ulcers. Due to its hazardous side effects such as dyspepsia, nausea, agranulocytosis, and hyperemia, the use of this drug is limited [125].

14.4.7.2 Thalidomide

Thalidomide is one of the few drugs that are very efficacious in the management of RAS. It retards the synthesis of tumor necrosis factor alpha (TNF-α) and neutrophil function and also aids in the healing of aphthae, alleviation of pain, and delay or prevent recurrence. When it is given in standard dosing levels of 100–300 mg/day or 50 mg/day, a dose-dependent effect originates in 7–10 weeks following treatment. Due to its widely known adverse reaction-like teratogenicity and irreversible polyneuropathy, the therapy should be given only in the case of severe ulceration and confined to patients with ulceration related to HIV [126].

14.4.7.3 Pentoxifylline

Pentoxifylline is a drug that retards the synthesis of TNF-α, chemotaxis, and neutrophil function. When administered at a dosage of 400 mg, three times a day, it alleviates the level of pain and reduces the ulcer size and number during episodes of RAS. Owing to its low adverse effects and its escalating results, pentoxifylline is regarded as the primary systemic medication for RAS treatment [127].

14.4.7.4 Colchicine

Colchicine, with anti-inflammatory activity, may be of clinical benefit in the treatment of severe cases of RAS and Behcet's disease. Therefore, a therapeutic trial at least over 4–6 weeks, at a dose of 1–2 mg/day orally is recommended, which is followed by long-term therapy according to tolerability by the patient and clinical response [128].

14.4.7.5 Zinc Sulfate

Systemic *zinc* treatment causes an improvement or remission in patients with RAS. It is given systemically, at a total dose of 660 mg of zinc sulfate per day, in divided doses [129].

14.4.7.6 Azathioprine

Azathioprine has been shown to be effective in reducing the incidence, severity, and frequency of severe oral and genital aphthae when it is administered alone or in combination with other immunosuppressive drugs. It is administered at a dosage of 1–2 mg/kg/day [120].

14.4.7.7 Methotrexate

Methotrexate, an analogue of folic acid, was found to be very beneficial in severe oro-genital aphthosis when administered in a dosage of 3–6 mg/kg or 7.5–20 mg weekly [120].

14.4.7.8 Prednisone

Prednisone can be utilized in association with topical mouth rinses and gels. Systemic treatment of prednisone should be started at a dose of 1.0 mg/kg a day as a single dose in patients with severe RAU. It should be reduced after 1–2 weeks because long-term exposure to the drug carries the risk of several adverse effects such as hyperglycemia, moon faces, depression, lipodystrophy, and hypothalamic-pituitary-adrenal axis suppression. In order to provide an effective treatment, it can be given along with other immunosuppressive agents such as azathioprine to reduce the dosage of prednisone [105].

14.4.7.9 Vitamin B12

When patients suffering from RAS were treated with 1000 μg of vitamin B12, the number of ulcers, duration of outbreaks, and level of pain were remarkably reduced after 5–6 months of treatment. During the treatment of around 6 months, "no aphthous ulcers status" was obtained by 74.1% of 31 interventional group participants. It was concluded that treatment of RAS with vitamin B12 seems to be effective irrespective of their initial level of serum vitamin B12 [130].

14.4.7.10 Dapsone

Dapsone is an extensively employed drug for the treatment of leprosy. However, it had a limited success in the management of major aphthae. It is administered orally at a dosage of 100 mg in divided doses and can be increased at the rate of 50 mg/day per week to a maximum of 300 mg/day. Due to its toxic nature, it can precipitate hemolytic anemia; therefore, strict patient monitoring for methemoglobinemia, hemolysis, agranulocytosis, and anemia is required [131].

14.4.7.11 Rebamipide

Rebamipide is the first anti-ulcer drug that enhances endogenous prostaglandins in the mucosa and retards the production of oxygen-derived free radicals. In 2013, Kudur et al. [132] reported that when the drug is administered orally at a dose of 100 mg, three times daily for 7 days, it decreases the pain and number of aphthae with excellent recovery by the seventh day.

14.4.7.12 Irsogladin

When irsogladin, which is used for the treatment of peptic ulcer and gastritis, is administered orally 2–4 mg/day, it was found to decrease the ulcer numbers and prevent the recurrence of aphthous stomatitis when regularly taken [133].

14.4.7.13 Cyclosporine a (CyA)

At a dose of 3–6 mg/kg, CyA was found to be effective in about 50% of patients suffering from aphthosis. However, abrupt withdrawal of therapy may lead to a rebound phenomenon. Due to its potential severe side effects, clinical and serological observation is required [111].

14.4.7.14 Adalimumab

Adalimumab is an anti-TNF-monoclonal antibody that has been used to treat severe RAS, but in view of the risk of serious adverse effects, it should be used with extreme caution [134].

14.4.7.15 Acyclovir

Acyclovir (400 mg twice daily for 1 year) was used in a double-blind study in 25 patients with RAS without any benefit in prevention of ulcers. Alternatively, higher dosages (800 mg twice daily for 8 weeks) were used in one study of eight patients with RAS, and six experienced either total regression of existing ulcers or relief of symptoms within 2 days of therapy [135].

14.4.7.16 Montelukast

A study was carried out by Femiano et al. in which 20 participants received a daily oral dosage of 10 mg Montelukast for 1 month followed by alternate days for the second month. It was concluded that the time (in days) to resolution of the first ulcer was shorter, accompanied with a remarkable reduction in the total count of new lesions over the treatment period of 2 months [136].

14.4.7.17 Infliximab (Remicade)

Recently, it has been shown by that infliximab (Remicade), a chimeric anti-TNF antibody, is very effective in the management of refractory and recurrent oral and genital ulcers. It is usually given intravenously at a dose of 5 mg/kg body weight in different schemes (e.g., 2, 6, and 32 weeks after the first injection) [120].

14.4.7.18 Etanercept (Enbrel)

Etanercept (Enbrel) is a recombinant TNF-soluble receptor that can be used in cases of recurrent ulceration at a dose of 25 mg subcutaneously twice a week. The only adverse effect reported is mild erythema, induration, and tenderness at the injection site [137].

14.4.7.19 Clofazimine

Clofazimine is an antimicrobial drug used for the treatment of leprosy in combination with other drugs such as rifampicin and dapsone. In application to treat severe RAS, and when administered at a dose of 100 mg/day over 6 months, the emergence of new lesions was found to be inhibited by the drug during the prescribed period of treatment [138].

Table 14.1 Treatment options for aphthous stomatitis

First-line therapy	
Topical antiseptics	Chlorhexidine gluconate, triclosan
Topical/systemic anti-inflammatory/analgesics	Benzydamine hydrochloride, diclofenac
Topical anesthetic	Lidocaine, benzocaine
Topical antibiotics	Chlortetracycline, doxycycline
Topical corticosteroids	Hydrocortisone hemisuccinate, triamcinolone acetonide, betamethasone valerate, beclomethasone dipropionate, budesonide, clobetasol
Second-line therapy	
Systemic immunomodulators	Levamisole, colchicine, hydrocortisone and triamcinolone, thalidomide, dapsone, pentoxifylline, 5-amino salicylic acid, azathioprine, prostaglandin E2
Systemic antibiotics	Penicillin G potassium
Systemic corticosteroids	Prednisone

14.4.7.20 Penicillin G Potassium

Penicillin G potassium in 50 mg tablets administered four times a day for 4 days reduces the size of the ulcers and ameliorates pain [139].

First-line and second-line treatment options available for the management of aphthous stomatitis are summarized in Table 14.1 [140].

14.5 Malignant Ulcers

14.5.1 Historical Perspectives

- In 1928, *VP Blair* of St. Louis was the first to advocate surgery as the best management of oral cancers.
- *Billroth* appreciated the importance of good access and took the procedure a stage further, removing a section of the mandibular body to reach the tongue and oropharynx.
- In 1875, *Bernhard von Langenbeck* resected the ramus of the mandible in continuity with the primary tumor [141].
- In 1917, *Esser* was the first to describe an axial flap based on the temporal artery [142].
- By 1923, radiotherapy was used to treat neck metastases.
- In the 1930s, *Hayes Martin* was the first to focus on improving cure rates by treating the primary tumor with X-rays by the "Coutard method" supplemented with gold radium seeds.
- By 1950, development of bleeding control methods, antibiotics, and blood transfusion made it possible to do advanced surgeries for cancers.
- A major initiative of the 1970s and 1980s was chemotherapy for patients unfit for surgery.

14.5.2 Classification of Oral Tumors

There is no specific established system for the classification of tongue cancer; however, it is classified as part of the oral cancers. *Oral tumors* can be classified into three types based on the potential to spread to other parts of the body (1) malignant tumors, (2) precancerous conditions, and (3) benign tumors (Table 14.2).

The most common type of malignant tumors of the mouth is SCC, which is further classified based on macroscopic and microscopic features. About 5% of oral cavity cancers are rare malignant tumors that start in different types of cells in the oral cavity. These include salivary gland cancer, melanoma, bone and soft tissue sarcoma, extramedullary plasmacytoma, Hodgkin lymphoma, non-Hodgkin lymphoma (NHL), and metastatic cancer.

14.5.2.1 Malignant Tumors of the Oral Cavity

14.5.2.1.1 Squamous Cell Carcinoma (SCC)

Since the oral cavity is lined with squamous epithelium, SCC makes up to 95% of all oral cavity cancers. They are classified based on macroscopic or microscopic features as follows:

Table 14.2 Classification of oral cavity tumors

Malignant tumors (MTs)	Precancerous conditions	Benign tumors and conditions
Squamous cell carcinoma (SCC) • Classical or conventional SCC • Variants Verrucous carcinoma Basaloid SCC Papillary SCC Spindle cell carcinoma (SpCC) Acantholytic SCC Adenosquamous carcinoma Lymphoepithelial carcinoma	• Leukoplakia • Erythroplakia • Erythro-leukoplakia (speckled leukoplakia) • Proliferative verrucous leukoplakia (PVL) • Oral submucous fibrosis	*Benign tumors* • Hyperplasia • Papillomas • Pleomorphic adenoma • Soft tissue tumors Hemangioma/ lymphangioma Neurofibroma Lipoma • Benign odontogenic tumors Osteoma Ossifying fibroma
Rare MTs • Salivary gland cancer • Melanoma • Bone and soft tissue sarcomas • Extramedullary Plasmacytoma • Hodgkin lymphoma • Non-Hodgkin lymphoma • Metastatic cancer		*Benign conditions* • Candidacies • Aphthous ulcers • Recurrent herpes labialis • Erythema migrans • Hairy tongue • Lichen planus • Hyperkeratosis • Mucocele

According to Macroscopic Features

1. *Infiltrative*: Cancer is growing into the deep layers of the oral cavity.
2. *Exophytic*: Cancer is growing outward from the surface of the oral cavity.
3. *Verrucous*: Cancer has a wart-like appearance.
4. *Ulcerated*: Cancer appears as an open sore (ulcer).
5. *Flat*: Cancer appears as an abnormal area in the lining of the oral cavity.

According to Microscopic Features

1. *Classical or Conventional SCC*

   Most cancers of the oral cavity are classical (conventional) SCC. This type starts in the squamous epithelium that lines the oral cavity and occurs most often on the lower lip, tongue, and floor of the mouth.
2. *Variants of SCC*

   These variants of SCC have distinct microscopic features that make them look and behave differently from the classical SCC.

- Verrucous carcinoma
- Basaloid SCC
- Papillary SCC
- Spindle cell carcinoma (SpCC) (fusiform cell carcinoma or sarcomatoid)
- Acantholytic SCC
- Adenosquamous carcinoma

14.5.2.1.2 Rare Malignant Tumors

About 5% of oral cavity cancers are rare malignant tumors that start in different types of cells in the oral cavity. These include the following:

- Salivary gland cancer
- Melanoma
- Bone and soft tissue sarcomas
- Extramedullary plasmacytomas
- Hodgkin lymphoma
- Non-Hodgkin lymphoma
- Metastatic cancer

14.5.2.2 Precancerous Lesions of the Oral Cavity

A premalignant (precancerous) lesion is defined as a "benign, morphologically altered tissue that has a greater than normal risk of malignant transformation." The most common precancerous conditions of the oral cavity are as follows:

1. *Leukoplakia* (white patches)
2. *Erythroplakia* (red patches)
3. *Erythro-leukoplakia* (speckled leukoplakia) (mixed white and red patches)
4. *Proliferative verrucous leukoplakia* (PVL)
5. *Oral submucous fibrosis*

14.5.2.3 Benign Tumors and Conditions of the Oral Cavity

14.5.2.3.1 Benign Tumors

- Hyperplasia
- Papilloma
- Pleomorphic adenoma
- Soft tissue tumors (lymphangioma, hemangioma, neurofibroma, lipoma)
- Benign odontogenic tumors (osteoma, ossifying fibroma)

14.5.2.3.2 Benign Conditions

- Candidiasis (thrush)
- Aphthous ulcers (canker sores)
- Recurrent herpes labialis (cold sores)
- Erythema migrans (geographic tongue)
- Hairy tongue
- Lichen planus
- Frictional hyperkeratosis
- Mucocele

14.5.3 TNM Staging Classification of Oral Cavity Carcinoma

TNM classification of oral cavity carcinoma according to staging system of the American Joint Committee on Cancer is shown in Table 14.3, and stage grouping is depicted in Table 14.4 [143].

14.5.4 Epidemiology and Demographics

In the United States, cancer of the *oral cavity* represents 2% of all cancers diagnosed annually. Likewise, in Australia and Europe, the incidence of oral cavity cancer accounts for less than 5% of all cancers. In France, oral cavity cancer is the third most common cancer in males and the second most common cause of death [144].

14.5.4.1 Incidence of Tongue Cancer

In 2009, the incidence of tongue cancer was estimated to be 10,530 cases per 100,000 individuals in the United States. Approximately, 1 in 324 men and women will be diagnosed with tongue cancer in their lifetime. According to the National Cancer Institute in the year 2011, the incidence of tongue cancer was estimated to be approximately 12,060 cases per 100,000 individuals. Out of those approximately 71% ($n = 8560$) were men and 29% ($n = 3500$) were women.

14.5.4.2 Gender

Men are more commonly affected with tongue cancer than women, with a ratio of approximately 2:1 [145].

Table 14.3 TNM staging of oral cancer

TNM staging of oral cavity cancers	
Tumor	
TX	Primary tumor cannot be assessed
T0	No evidence of primary tumor
Tis	Carcinoma in situ
T1	Tumor <2 cm in greatest dimension
T2	Tumor >2 cm but not >4 cm in greatest dimension
T3	Tumor >4 cm in greatest dimension
T4 (lip)	Tumor invades through cortical bone, inferior alveolar nerve, floor of the mouth, or skin of the face (e.g., chin or nose)
T4a (oral cavity)	Tumor invades adjacent structures (e.g., through cortical bone into deep (extrinsic) muscles of the tongue (genioglossus, hyoglossus, palatoglossus, and styloglossus), maxillary sinus, or skin of the face)
T4b	Tumor invades masticator space, pterygoid plates, or skull base and/or encases internal carotid canal
Regional lymph nodes (N)	
NX	Regional lymph nodes (LNs) cannot be assessed
N0	No regional LN metastasis
N1	Metastasis in a single ipsilateral LN 3 cm or less
N2a	Metastasis in a single ipsilateral LN >3 cm but not >6 cm
N2b	Metastasis in multiple ipsilateral LNs, >6 cm
N2c	Metastasis in bilateral or contralateral LNs, none >6 cm
N3	Metastasis in a LN more than 6 cm in greatest dimension
Distant metastasis (M)	
MX	Distant metastasis cannot be assessed
cM0	No distant metastasis
cM1	Distant metastasis
pM1	Distant metastasis, microscopically confirmed

Table 14.4 Stage grouping of oral SCC

Stage	Tumor (T)	Nodes (N)	Metastases (M)
0	Tis	N0	M0
I	T1	N0	M0
II	T2	N0	M0
III	T3	N0	M0
	T1,T2,T3	N1	M0
IVA	T1, T2, or T3	N2	M0
IVB	T4a	N0, N1, or N2	M0
IVC	Any T	N3	M0
	T4b	Any N	M0
	Any T	Any N	M1

Tis carcinoma in situ

Table 14.5 Risk of tongue cancer according to age

Age at diagnosis (years)	Percent of people with tongue cancer out of all tongue cancer diagnosis (%)
<20	0.2
20–34	2.0
35–44	6.0
45–54	20.8
55–64	31
65–74	21.9
75–84	13.5
≥85	4.6

14.5.4.3 Race

There is no racial predilection to the development of tongue cancer [146].

14.5.4.4 Age

The incidence of tongue cancer increases with age; the median age at diagnosis is 61 years. Approximately, one-third of all diagnoses occurred in patients under the age of 55 years. According to the National Cancer Institute from 2004 to 2008, the age at diagnosis and percentage of people diagnosed with tongue cancer are shown in Table 14.5.

14.5.5 Etiology/Risk Factors

The main cause of tongue cancer is genetic mutations due to precancerous lesions or chronic inflammation [147].

Mutations in tumor suppressor genes have been reported in patients with cancers of the oral cavity. The most abundant carcinogens in tobacco are *nitrosamines* that can damage DNA, leading to point mutations, which lead to deregulation of tumor suppressor genes (*TP53*), which is located on chromosome 17. The other oncogenes associated with oral SCC of the tongue include *c-myc* and *erb-b1*.

Tobacco exposure causes progressive sequential histological changes to the oral mucosa. Prolonged period of exposure eventually leads to neoplastic transformation, in particular changes in the expression of *p53* mutations.

14.5.5.1 Precancerous Lesions

A premalignant (or precancerous) lesion is defined as "a benign, morphologically altered tissue that has a greater than normal risk of malignant transformation." There are several different types of premalignant lesion that occur in the mouth. These include the following:

14.5.5.1.1 Oral Leukoplakia

Leukoplakia is defined as a "white patch of mucosa that cannot be characterized clinically or pathologically as any other disease." It presents as a "white plaque on the surface of the tongue that cannot be wiped away." It is considered a premalignant condition from the chronic irritation of the mucous membranes, resulting in increased rates of epithelial and connective tissue proliferation. It usually occurs after the age of 40 years, with the peak incidence before 50 years, and is 2–3 times more common in men than in women [148]. The rate of malignant transformation of leukoplakia lesions range from less than 1% to as high as 17.5%, averaging 4.5–6%.

Leukoplakia can be divided into the following [149]:

1. *Homogenous lesions*: flat, thin, and white [150]
2. *Non-homogenous lesions*: white and red lesion

Oral leukoplakia should be confirmed by biopsy. Surgical excision should be recommended in the presence of moderate and severe epithelial *dysplasia*. In the case of using topical retinoic acid, recurrence rates are 50% after withdrawal [151].

Risk factors of malignant transformation of *leukoplakia* include the following [149]:

1. Female gender
2. Long duration of leukoplakia
3. Leukoplakia in nonsmokers
4. Location on the tongue and floor of the mouth
5. Size >200 mm
6. Nonhomogenous type
7. Presence of epithelial dysplasia

14.5.5.1.2 Oral Erythroplakia

Erythroplakia is defined as "any lesion of the oral mucosa that presents as bright red velvety plaques, which cannot be characterized clinically or pathologically as any other recognizable condition" [152]. It occurs in middle-aged and elderly patients and affects mainly the soft palate, floor of the mouth, and buccal mucosa [153]. No sex predilection is recognized in erythroplakia, and it is rarely found on the tongue compared with other sites in the oral cavity.

Tobacco and alcohol consumption are the most common risk factors for the development of oral erythroplakia. The lesion is usually <1.5 cm in diameter, but its size may range between 1 and 4 cm. Early effective treatment is mandatory as malignant transformation rates are very high.

14.5.5.1.3 Oral Erythro-Leukoplakia

Erythroplakia may occur together with leukoplakia leading to erythro-leukoplakia, which is formed of mixed white and red patches [154]. Among the oral potentially malignant disorders, erythro-leukoplakia and nodular leukoplakia exhibit the highest rate of malignant transformation(approximately, 45% of cases develop malignancy) [154–156].

14.5.5.1.4 Oral Lichen Planus

Lichen planus is a "chronic inflammatory disease, which may affect oral mucosa between other areas of body" [157]. It is characterized by remissions and recurrences and mainly occurs in females between the third and sixth decades of life. Lichen planus may occur in multifocal, papular, bullous, erosive, reticular, and atrophic forms. The atrophic and erosive patterns are associated with a burning sensation and pain and a higher risk of malignant transformation than other forms, reaching up to 10% of patients. Histologically, lesions show liquefactive necrosis of basal cells, infiltrative lymphocytes of superficial dermis, saw-tooth rete ridges, and hyperkeratosis.

14.5.5.1.5 Oral Submucous Fibrosis and Actinic Cheilitis [158]

In India, oral submucous fibrosis is very common due to betel nut chewing. This is a progressive lesion in which the opening of the mouth becomes progressively limited, and later on even normal eating becomes difficult. It occurs almost exclusively in India and Indian communities living abroad.

14.5.5.2 Risk Factors

The most potent risk factors in the development of oral cancer are alcohol intake, tobacco use, and human papillomavirus (HPV) transmitted through sexual contact. Other risk factors include history of betel quid intake, male gender, age over 55 years, ultraviolet light exposure, Fanconi anemia, dyskeratosis congenita, lichen planus, graft-versus-host disease (GVHD), immunosuppression, and mouthwash and chronic irritation from dentures.

14.5.5.2.1 Major Tongue Cancer Risk Factors

Major risk factors in the development of tongue cancer include the following [159–161]:

Tobacco Smoking

Cancer of the tongue is correlated the closest with the use of tobacco products. Approximately, 90% of patients with oral cavity cancers use tobacco products, and the relative risk of oral cavity cancers increases with the amount smoked and the duration of smoking. In smokers, the incidence of oral cavity cancers is approximately six times that of nonsmokers.

Tobacco exposure causes progressive sequential histological changes to the oral mucosa. Prolonged exposure eventually leads to neoplastic transformation. The most abundant carcinogens in tobacco are nitrosamines, which damage the DNA, leading to point mutations that result in deregulation of tumor suppressor genes (*TP53*), which is located on chromosome 17. If the tobacco exposure is discontinued, these changes may be reversible. The other oncogenes associated with oral squamous cell cancers of the tongue include *c-myc* and *erb-b1*.

There is compelling evidence supporting the benefit of head and neck cancer patients to cease smoking after treatment for their cancer. Approximately, 40% of patients who continued to smoke after definitive treatment for an oral cavity malignancy developed recurrence or developed a second head and neck malignancy. In patients who stopped smoking after treatment, only about 6% developed a recurrence.

There has been an increase in the incidence of oral cavity cancer in young adults in the recent years. The explosive use of smokeless tobacco, or snuff, in certain regions of the United States has led to increased numbers of mandibular alveolus, buccal mucosa, and tongue cancers.

Alcohol Ingestion

The correlation between alcohol consumption, particularly hard liquor, and oral cavity cancer is significant, especially in patients taking >4 consumptions/day. Nearly 75% of patients who develop oral cavity cancers consume alcohol, and cancer occurs six times more often in persons who drink alcohol than in those who do not. The role of alcohol consumption in the development of tongue cancer appears to be independent of *smoking*. The use of alcohol with smoking has a synergistic rather than cumulative effect. The risk for a person who drinks alcohol and smokes tobacco is 15 times that of an individual with neither of these habits.

Human Papillomavirus (HPV)

Infection with human papillomavirus (HPV), particularly type 16 (there are over 180 types), is a known risk factor and independent causative factor for oral cancer. The HPV has been detected in various amounts in persons with leukoplakia, oral dysplasia, and malignancy. In the subset of patients without other risk factors (tobacco and alcohol consumption), HPV (especially HPV type 16) should be considered as an etiological factor [162].

HPV-16 (along with HPV-18) is the same virus responsible for the vast majority of all cervical cancers and is the most common sexually transmitted infection in the United States. Oral cancer in this group tends to favor the tonsil and tonsillar pillars, *base of the tongue*, and the oropharynx. Recent data suggest that individuals who develop the disease from this particular cause have a significant survival advantage as the disease responds better to radiation treatments than tobacco caused disease.

Plummer-Vinson Syndrome (PVS)

Plummer-Vinson syndrome (iron deficiency anemia, achlorhydria, and mucosal atrophy of the mouth, pharynx, and esophagus) has been associated with an increased risk of tongue cancer. Studies have suggested that vitamins A and C, along with carotenoids, may be protective against epithelial cancers. Iron and riboflavin deficiencies are known to produce dysplastic changes to the oral mucosa.

Stem Cell Transplantation

After stem cell transplantation, the risk of developing oral SCC is significantly increased. Oral cancer in these patients may be more aggressive with poorer prognosis due to the continuous life-long immune suppression and chronic oral graft-versus-host disease [163].

14.5.5.2.2 Other Less Potent Risk Factors

Lifestyle: Betel Nut Intake

- Betel intake (it is an Asian evergreen climbing plant, related to pepper, which in the east is chewed as a mild stimulant).
- Chewing betel nut, pan, and areca is known to be a strong risk factor for developing oral cancer even in the absence of tobacco. It increases the rate of oral cancer 2.1 times, through a variety of genetic and related effects through local irritation of the mucous membrane cells, particularly from the areca nut and slaked lime [164]. In India where such practices are common, oral cancer represents up to 40% of all cancers, compared to just 4% in the United Kingdom.

Genetic Factors

- Fanconi anemia
- Dyskeratosis congenita
- Family history of SCC

General Factors

- Male gender
- Age over 55 year
- Ultraviolet light
- GVHD
- Immune system suppression

Unproven Risk Factors

- Alcohol-containing mouthwash
- Irritation from dentures

14.5.6 Pathogenesis

14.5.6.1 WHO Grading for Oral Cancer Dysplasia

The World Health Organization (WHO) classified oral cancer into mild, moderate, and severe dysplasia [165].

- *Mild dysplasia:* Abnormal cytological features largely confined to the lower third of the epithelium.
- *Moderate dysplasia:* The dysplastic process extends into the middle third of the epithelium.
- *Severe dysplasia:* Extension of the dysplasia into the *upper third* of the epithelium.
- *Carcinoma* in situ*:* Full thickness involvement is present in the absence of invasion.

14.5.6.2 Precancerous Conditions

The two most common types of precancerous conditions on the tongue are *leukoplakia* and *erythroplakia*. They both have the greatest potential for malignant transformation into tongue cancer (squamous cell carcinoma—SCC) [166].

14.5.6.3 Genetics

Oral SCC is the end-product of an unregulated proliferation of mucous basal cells. A single precursor cell is transformed into a clone consisting of many daughter cells with an accumulation of altered genes called *oncogenes*.

Genes involved in the pathogenesis of tongue cancer include *TP53*, which is located on chromosome 17 [147]. The carcinogens in tobacco smoke, for example, increase the prevalence and spectrum of TP53 mutations [167]. Other oncogenes associated with SCC of the tongue include *c-myc* and *erb-b1*.

More than 50% of oropharyngeal carcinomas harbor integrated HPV DNA. The E6 and E7 viral onc-proteins bind and inactivate the TP53 and retinoblastoma gene products, respectively, disengaging two of the more critical pathways involved in cell cycle regulation.

Local tumor recurrence reflects extension of genetically damaged cells beyond the clinical and microscopic boundaries of carcinoma to the margins of surgical resection [168]. Head and neck SCCs have been identified by circulating plasma or serum changes, which can be used for follow-up and screening.

14.5.7 Pathology

14.5.7.1 Gross Pathology

Squamous cell carcinoma (SCC) is the most common malignancy of the tongue. It typically has 3 main gross morphologic growth patterns, namely exophytic, ulcerative, and infiltrative. The infiltrative and ulcerative (Fig. 14.7) are the types most commonly observed on the tongue.

The macroscopic appearance of tongue cancer depends on the following:

- Duration of the lesion.
- The amount of keratinization.
- The changes in the adjoining mucosa.
- A fully developed tongue lesion appears as an exophytic bulky lesion that is gray to grayish-red and has a rough, shaggy, or papillomatous surface.

The macroscopic types (patterns or forms) of tongue cancer include the following:

- *Ulcer*: Everted edges, necrotic floor, and hard indurated base.
- *Nodular*: A nodule with an indurated base.
- *Cauliflower-like Mass*: It has a bad prognosis.
- *Fissure*: A deep, often infected fissure with surrounding induration.
- *Diffuse (woody) type*: It has the worst prognosis.

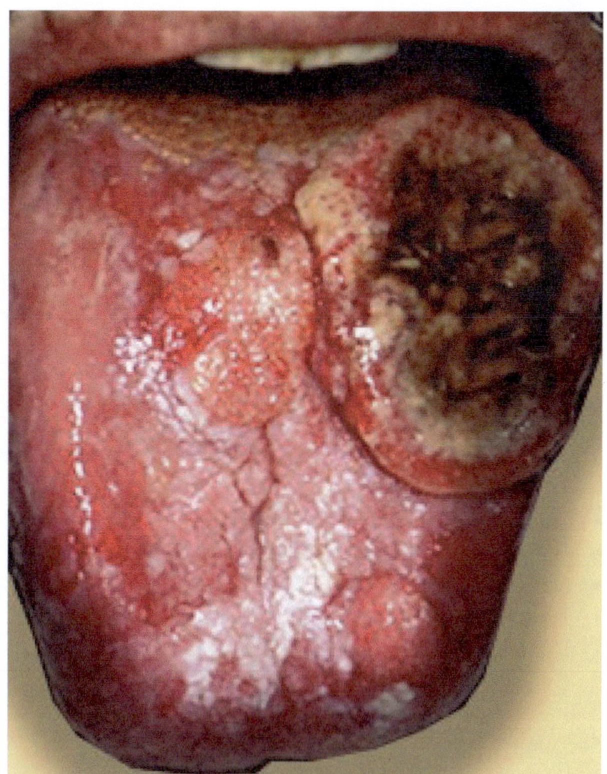

Fig. 14.7 Gross pathology of SCC of the tongue. Ulcerative lesion with everted edges and necrotic floor

14.5.7.2 Microscopic Pathology

Tongue cancer constitutes of squamous cells with rare mitoses. The surface of the lesion is covered with compressed invaginating folds of *keratin* layers. A stroma-like inflammatory reaction and a blunt pushing margin may be seen (Fig. 14.8). Squamous cell carcinoma is subdivided by the World Health Organization into the following types [169]:

1. *Keratinizing* type: It carries the worst prognosis.
2. *Undifferentiated type:* It is associated with *EBV* and has an intermediate prognosis [170].
3. *Nonkeratinizing type*: It is associated with *EBV* and has a good prognosis.

14.5.7.2.1 Microscopic Types of Tongue Cancer

Microscopic types of tongue cancer include the following:

Primary Tumor

- SCC (conventional type—variants): SCC occurs mainly in the anterior two-thirds of the tongue.
- Lympho-epithelioma: mainly in the posterior third of the tongue.

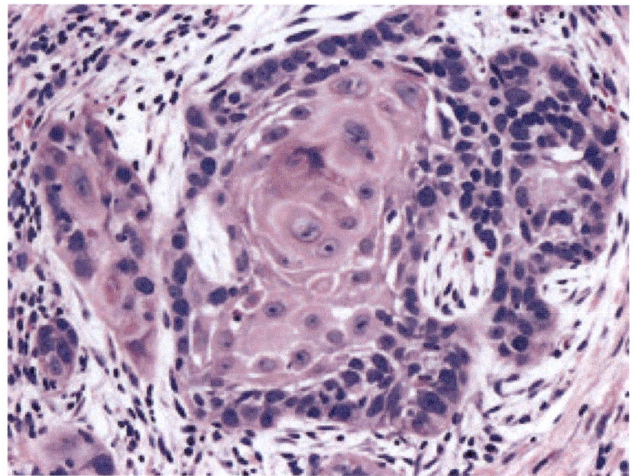

Fig. 14.8 Microscopic picture of SCC of the tongue showing the characteristic "epithelial pearls"

- Adeno-carcinoma: arising from the minor salivary glands of the tongue.
- Basal cell carcinoma (BCC).
- Melanoma (very rare).
- Hemangioendothelioma.
- Rhabdo-myosarcoma.
- Lymphoma.

Secondary Tumor

It is rare and the primary is usually a breast cancer.

14.5.7.2.2 Histopathology of SCC and Its Variants [171]

Conventional Type

Histopathologically, the most common variant is the conventional type of SCC accounting for approximately 53.7% of cases. This variety is made out of neoplastic cells with varying degrees of squamous differentiation, in which the well-differentiated ones almost resemble Malpighian cells of the normal epithelium, but they disrupt the basal membrane and invade the underlying corium under various patterns, with disorderly growth, loss of polarity, development of dyskeratosis, and formation of "epithelial pearls." There is also over unity of the nucleus/cytoplasm ratio and constant presence of typical and atypical mitoses (Fig. 14.9).

Acantholytic Subtype

The second most common histopathological subtype is "acantholytic," accounting for about 26% of patients. The growth pattern in this type is the *lobular/insular* one with the central presence of pseudo-glandular/pseudo-luminal spaces resulting from the acantholysis, delimited by polygonal neoplastic cells. Often, in these lumens, discrete, acantholytic neoplastic cells can be observed (Fig. 14.10). Tumor cells from the periphery of the tumor lobules show an obvious nuclear pleomorphism,

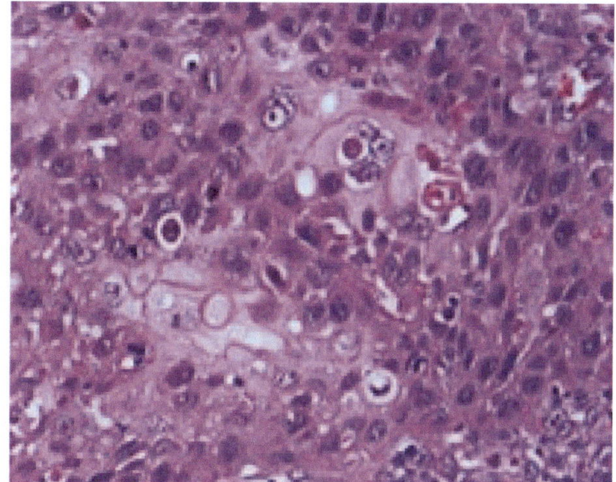

Fig. 14.9 Microscopic picture of tongue SCC (conventional type) showing malignant features of neoplastic proliferations, nuclear atypia, and atypical mitosis, H&E stain, ×400

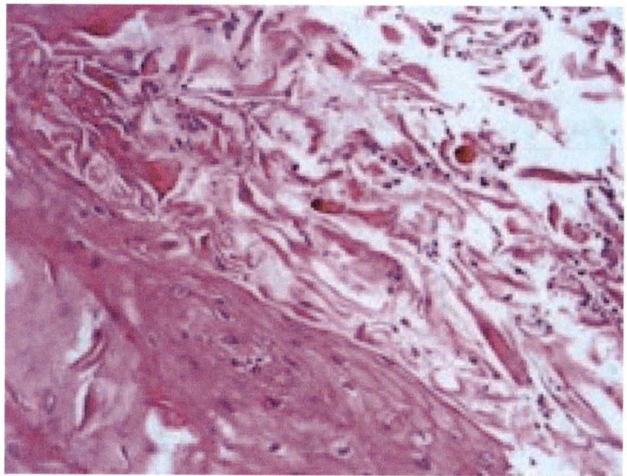

Fig. 14.10 Microscopic picture of tongue SCC (conventional type) showing the presence of acantholytic dyskeratotic cells in the neoplastic pseudolumens. H&E stain, ×200

nuclear anisochromia, dense eosinophilic cytoplasm, and frequent mitosis. Focally, keratotic pearls and areas of conventional SCC can also be highlighted.

Basaloid Subtype

The basaloid subtype of tongue SCC is rather uncommon, representing approximately 13% of cases. The growth pattern in such tumor subtype is variable with lobular/insular areas, trabecular areas, cribriform areas, and nests of neoplastic cells.

The characteristics of this subtype are the neoplastic cells from periphery of the neoplastic proliferations that present a "basaloid" morphology (cubico-cylindrical with a little cytoplasm and tachychromatic nuclei) (Fig. 14.11). Often, in the central area of tumor proliferations, comedonecrosis can be shown. Focally, conventional SCC areas in close contact with basaloid proliferations may be also observed.

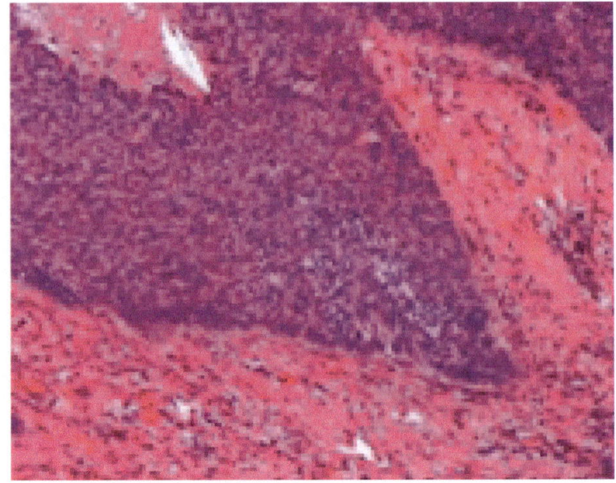

Fig. 14.11 Microscopic picture of tongue SCC (basaloid subtype) showing the presence of peripheral palisades in the neoplastic proliferations, H&E stain, ×200

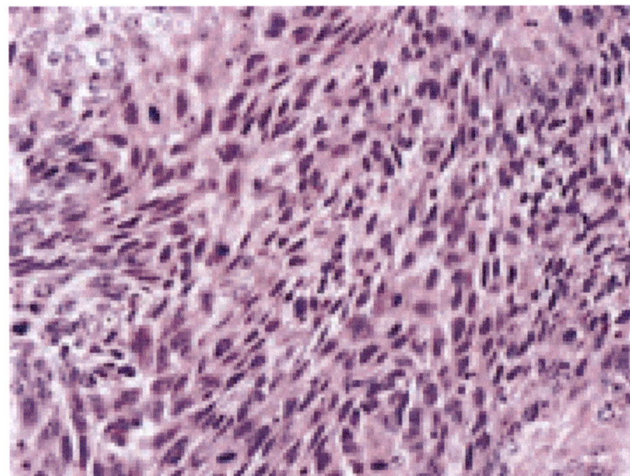

Fig. 14.12 Microscopic picture of tongue SCC (sarcomatoid subtype) showing fusiform morphology of neoplastic cells in sarcomatoid proliferation; H&E stain, x400

Spindle (Fusiform) Cell Subtype or Sarcomatoid

The sarcomatoid subtype of SCC is rare accounting for about (5.5%) of all cases. It shows a biphasic histological appearance with surface epithelium showing features of mild dysplasia to invasive carcinoma and an atypical stroma composed of fusiform cells giving a fibrosarcoma-like appearance. The *epithelial component* is usually found within the stalk or periphery of the lesion and forms a minor portion of the tumor mass. The *sarcomatous component* usually makes up the tumor bulk and consists mainly of plump spindle cells. Mixed areas of conventional SCC with malignant fusiform cell proliferation may be seen.

The sarcomatoid proliferation pattern is predominantly “fascicular” and rarely “storiform”; neoplastic cells being mixed with inflammatory cells and rarely the neoplastic cells present epithelioid morphology (Fig. 14.12).

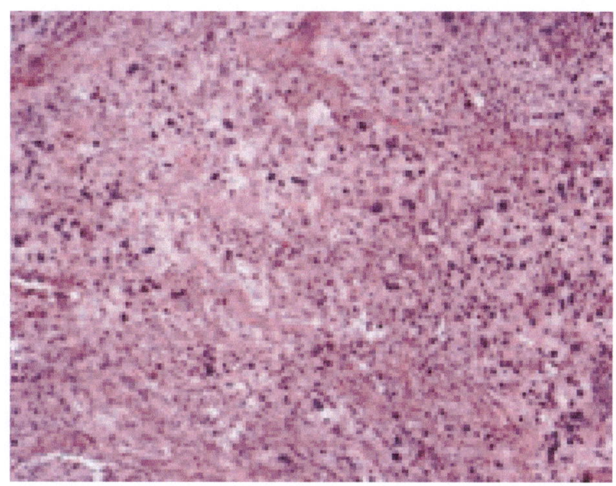

Fig. 14.13 Microscopic picture of tongue SCC showing poorly differentiated conventional tongue SCC, neoplastic cells with marked atypia and atypical mitosis, H&E stain, x100

Verrucous Subtype

The verrucous subtype is very rare, and its peculiar microscopic aspect is the broad invasion of the underlying corium that takes the form of plump papillary invaginations of thickened epithelium, with minimal atypia. The epithelium of the surface usually shows hyperparakeratosis, more evident especially at the level of the sites of invaginations. At the level of the broad neoplastic epithelial ridges that invade the corium, some cystic structure with keratin in the lumen may be seen.

Generally, tongue SCC is represented by the moderately differentiated G2 forms, followed by well-differentiated G1 forms, and lastly by the poorly differentiated G3 forms (Fig. 14.13). Brandwein-Gensler scores include most of the moderate grades, followed by the high grade, and lastly, the low grade. Regarding the pTNM stage, the most commonly diagnosed stage is stage III, closely followed by stage II and at a distance by stage IV and stage I.

14.5.8 Tumor Spread

Carcinoma of the tongue spreads *early* because of the (1) rich blood supply, (2) rich communicating lymphatics, and (3) continuous movement of the tongue.

14.5.8.1 Local (Direct) Spread

Tongue cancer can spread locally to the floor of the mouth, gums, mandible, fauces, and glottis. It can also spread to the soft palate and pharynx if it lies in the posterior third of the tongue

Tumor involving the lateral margin of tongue tends to spread in depth. The intrinsic muscles of tongue run in all directions. The floor of mouth SCC spreads superficially without invading into the mylohyoid muscle or the sublingual gland until a late stage.

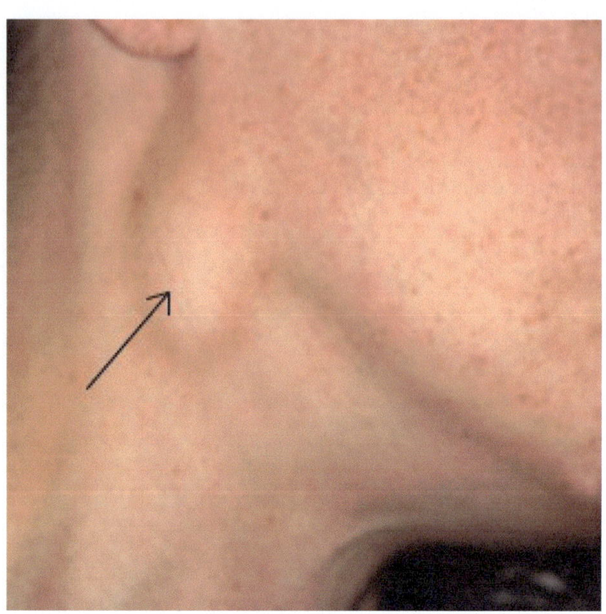

Fig. 14.14 Spread of cancer to cervical lymph nodes from tongue cancer

14.5.8.2 Lymphatic Spread

Spread to local LNs (Fig. 14.14) worsens the prognosis in oral and oropharyngeal cancer. The mechanism of spread from the primary site to lymph nodes (LNs) is almost always by *embolism*, or less commonly by *permeation.*

Levels of LNs at high risk for metastasis from oral cavity SCC are levels I, II, and III and to a lesser extent level IV.

Lymphatic spread occurs within few weeks or months as follows:

- Tip and frenulum drain into submental LNs.
- Remainder of anterior 2/3 drain into submandibular LNs.
- Posterior 1/3 drain into upper deep cervical (UDC) LNs (jugulo-digastric) and then to lower deep cervical (LDC) LNs (jugulo-omohyoid).
- Central lesions are bilaterally drained.

14.5.8.3 Hematogenous Spread

Hematogenous spread is less important than local and lymphatic spread. The best predictor of the likelihood of this spread is involvement of the cervical LNs at multiple levels. This suggests that the route of entry of tumors into the circulation is most often via the *large veins* in the neck and that hematogenous spread is in effect tertiary spread following extracapsular spread from cervical LNs. Blood spread is rare (8–17%) and late and involves mainly the lungs, liver, and bone.

14.5.9 Diagnosis of Tongue Cancer

Tongue cancers usually present late, as they are usually painless and often ignored by the patient. Eventually, the patient develops a nonhealing ulcer which demonstrates growth over time. Carcinomas of the tongue base are clinically silent until they deeply infiltrate the tongue musculature.

Due to the extensive lymphatic drainage of the tongue, nodal metastases are common at the time of diagnosis, with a neck mass being the presenting complaint. Tongue cancer often begins as a white patch (leukoplakia), small lump, or sore (ulcer) on the tongue. It is often not diagnosed until it has grown and spread to other areas of the mouth, but if diagnosed early, it can be easily treated.

As the tumor enlarges, it may cause a mass effect, which can lead to respiratory compromise when the patient presents late. If left untreated, tongue cancer can send distant metastases and can cause mortality.

14.5.9.1 History-Taking and Symptoms

Symptoms of tongue cancer may include a red or white patch on the tongue; a sore throat; an ulcer or lump on the tongue; pain when swallowing, speaking, or moving the tongue; numbness in the mouth; tongue bleeding; and pain in the ear, mouth, or tongue.

14.5.9.1.1 History-Taking

Demographic history indicates that the age of the patient is usually >50–60 years but may be as early as 20 years or as late as 70 years and that men are more affected than women with a ratio of approximately 3:1.

Initial history should evaluate the duration and rapidity of growth of the lesion, the presence of pain, loss of weight, dysphagia, odynophagia, referred otalgia, hemoptysis, neck mass, hoarseness, and articulation difficulties. The patient should also be asked about personal history of tobacco and alcohol use [172].

The initial history should also evaluate the patient's swallowing and dietary status. The majority of tongue cancer patients present with malnutrition associated with history of alcoholism or as a result of dysphagia from the enlarging tumor. The patient should also be asked about any changes in speech, which may give an indication of the location, functional impairment, and severity of the tumor extent [172].

14.5.9.1.2 Symptoms

Tongue cancer may grow to a significant size before causing symptoms. Approximately, 75% of tongue cancers, which is most often well-differentiated, occur in the mobile tongue. Cancer cells may spread easily, and the tumor becomes symptomatic only when tumor size interferes with tongue mobility.

Squamous cell carcinoma of the tongue may arise in normal epithelium, in an area of chronic glossitis, or in areas of leukoplakia (or erythroplakia). These lesions are usually >2 cm at presentation, and the lateral border of the tongue is the most common subsite of origin. When the *lateral border* of the tongue is involved, the patient may develop dysfunction of speech and swallowing. When the tumor involves the lingual nerve, pain occurs and may be referred to the ear. Tongue cancer that involves the *base of the tongue* is clinically silent until it deeply infiltrates the tongue musculature. It is usually less differentiated. Tongue cancer may extend into the oral tongue or have clinical LN metastases before the diagnosis is established [172].

Symptoms of tongue cancer may include the following [172]:

- A red or white patch on the tongue.
- An ulcer (Fig. 14.15) or lump (nodule) (Fig. 14.16) or fissure on the tongue.
- Pain in the mouth or tongue (due to infection) or referred to the corresponding ear via the chorda tympani.
- Pain on swallowing, speaking, or moving the tongue.
- Difficulty in chewing, swallowing, or speaking (disarticulation).
- Sore throat.
- Numbness in the mouth.
- Unexplained bleeding from the tongue (that is not caused by tongue biting or injury. A "SCC" of the tongue is known to "bleed on touch." Hemorrhage may be severe.
- Increased salivation, which becomes blood-stained in late cases.
- Fetor oris (foul oral odor) due to necrosis and infection.
- Ankyloglossia: limited movement with fixation (no protrusion or deviation).
- Dysarthria (diminished articulation) due to pain, salivation, and ankylosis.
- Mass in the neck (LN secondaries). It may be the first symptom especially in posterior lesions (occult primary).

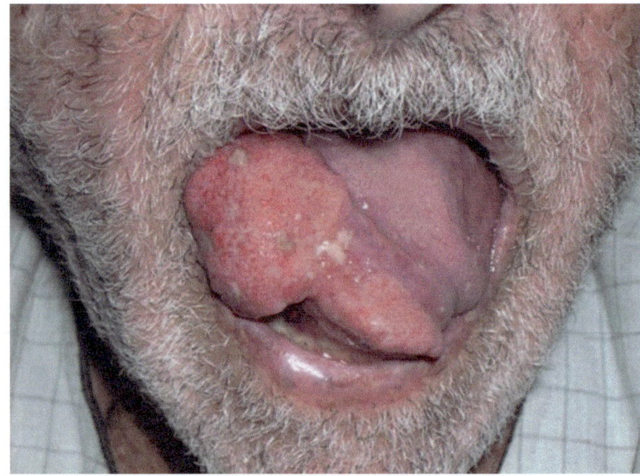

Fig. 14.15 A neglected epitheliomatous ulcer at the side of the anterior two-thirds of the tongue in a 76-year-old man. Note the large size of the ulcer, the everted edges, and the necrotic floor

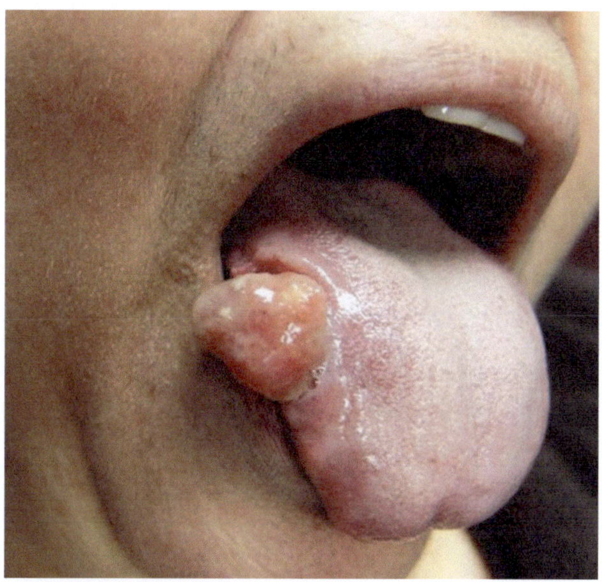

Fig. 14.16 SCC at the lateral border of the tongue presenting as a "nodule"

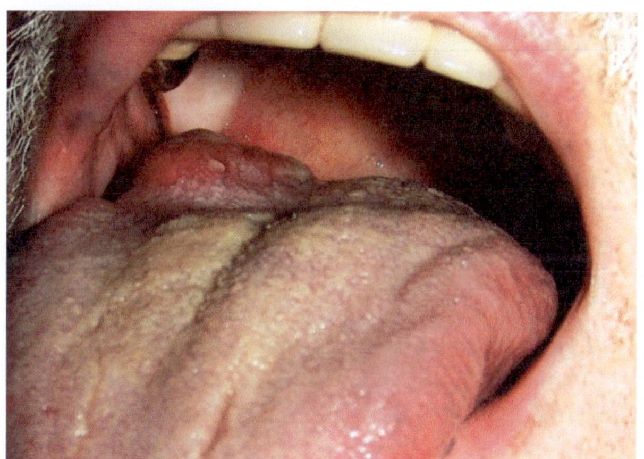

Fig. 14.17 SCC could be seen at the base of the tongue (posterior third)

- Cancer of the posterior third of the tongue (Fig. 14.17) is usually characterized by a lump in the neck (jugulo-digastric LN), dysphagia, and hoarseness due to infiltration of the epiglottis.

14.5.9.2 Physical Examination

Common physical examination findings of tongue cancer include otalgia, submandibular gland asymmetry, and cervical lymphadenopathy. During the thorough clinical examination, the physician should check the roof and floor of the mouth, the back of the throat, cervical LNs, the inside of the cheeks, the lips, and the top, sides, and underside of the tongue.

The physician should be looking for red or white patches, ulcers, or lumps. A dental evaluation is also performed, with attention to dental hygiene, integrity of the mandible, and dentition status [172].

14.5.9.2.1 Head Examination

During a complete head examination, specific attention is directed to the size, site, and the extent (infiltrating characteristics) of the lesion. The physician should also perform a thorough bimanual examination of the tumor itself, the submandibular triangles, and the surrounding floor of mouth.

Patients may present with red lesions, mixed red and white lesions, or white plaques. Extremely advanced cancers present as ulcero-proliferative growths with areas of necrosis and extension to surrounding structures, e.g., the bone. In the terminal stages, patients may present with intractable bleeding, severe anemia, and cachexia.

Cancer of the base of the tongue presents late in the course of the disease as a grossly ulcerated, painful, indurated growth [172].

Physical Examination (Epitheliomatous Ulcer)

- *Site*: Commonest site is the *anterior* two-thirds (not in the midline).
- *Edge*: Raised everted edge.
- *Floor*: Necrotic floor that bleeds easily.
- *Base*: Hard indurated.
- *Other clinical findings*: The patient has a foul smell of breath and may be limited or deviated protrusion of the tongue.
- *Regional LNs* are usually *enlarged* (hard, mobile, or fixed) ± infiltration of deeper tissues.
- *Other benign lesions* should be ruled out and *suspicious lesions* should be biopsied.

14.5.9.2.2 Neck Examination

- Submandibular gland asymmetry may be evident.
- Cervical lymphadenopathy may be bilateral [173].

14.5.9.3 Clinical Presentation of Complications

14.5.9.3.1 Terminal Events

- Secondary infection
- Aspiration pneumonia
- Asphyxia (due to edema of the glottis or compression of air passages by LNs)
- Hemorrhage from the primary tumor/ulcer or LNs due to erosion of a blood vessel, e.g., lingual artery
- Starvation and cancer cachexia
- Spread of malignancy by direct (local) infiltration and/or lymphatic or hematogenous routes.

14.5.9.3.2 Direct Surgical Complications

- Infection
- Bleeding
- Aspiration
- Wound breakdown
- Flap loss
- Fistula formation

14.5.9.3.3 Complications of Chemotherapy [174]

- Neurotoxicity: a side effect of certain classes of drugs, such as the vinca alkaloids
- Bleeding

14.5.9.3.4 Complications of Radiation Therapy [175]

- Radiation caries
- Trismus
- Osteonecrosis

14.5.9.3.5 Complications of Chemotherapy and Radiation [176]

- Oral mucositis
- Chronic dysphagia
- Anemia
- Pharyngo-cutaneous fistula
- Aspiration
- Xerostomia (dry mouth)
- Infections; viral, bacterial, and fungal that result from myelosuppression, xerostomia, and damage to the mucosa from radiotherapy or chemotherapy
- Functional disabilities such as impaired ability to swallow, eat, taste, and speak because of trismus, dry mouth, mucositis, and infection
- Nutritional compromise such as poor nutrition from eating difficulties caused by dry mouth, mucositis, dysphagia, and loss of taste
- Abnormal dental development
- Altered tooth development, craniofacial growth, or skeletal development in children secondary to high doses of chemotherapy and radiotherapy before the age of 9 years

14.5.9.4 Laboratory Investigations

A complete blood cell count is a useful general screen that helps the physician to decide if further testing is warranted. In a patient with a suspected bleeding diathesis, investigations may also include tests of prothrombin time (PT), activated partial thromboplastic time (aPTT), and international normalized ratio (INR) [177]. Wassermann reaction (WR) should also be performed if syphilis is suspected (fissure type).

14.5.9.5 Plain X-Ray

There are *no* X-ray findings associated with tongue cancer. However, an X-ray may be helpful in the evaluation of metastases to the lungs, skull, and mandible. Periapical dental films are needed for detecting minimal invasion of the mandible [178].

14.5.9.6 Computed Tomography (CT) Scan

The most commonly used modality for assessment of tongue SCC is the CT scan. Lesions typically appear more attenuating than normal tongue musculature (on the account of keratin) and enhance following contrast administration (Fig. 14.18).

Noncontrast scans of the neck may demonstrate increased attenuation of involved LNs due to keratin production by tumor deposits [179]. CT scan is better for the evaluation of bone destruction (erosion) and assessment of cartilage invasion [180].

Pathological LNs are enlarged and exhibit central necrosis. Size criteria based on measurement of minimal axial diameter are considered the most accurate and effective [181]. Pathological LNs show also loss of normal fatty hilum, increased or heterogeneous contrast enhancement, and LN clustering [182]. Sensitivity is 83% and specificity is 83% [183].

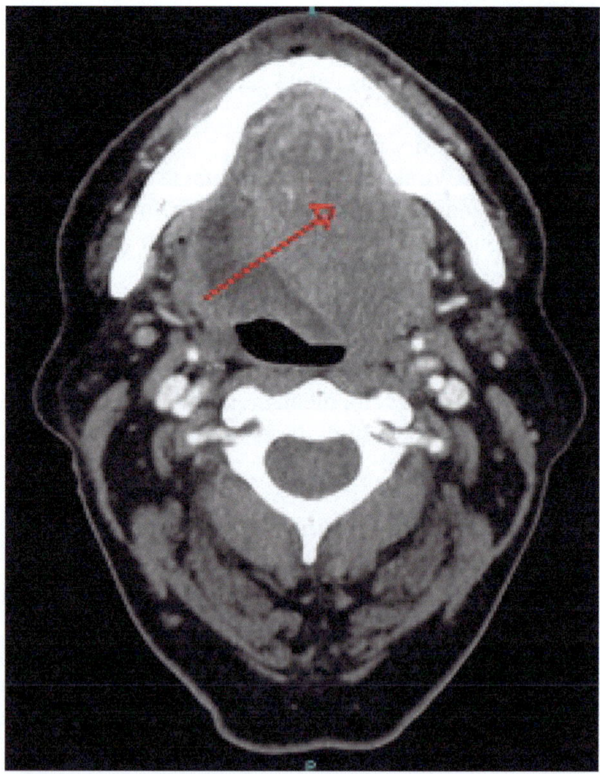

Fig. 14.18 A large squamous cell carcinoma (SCC) of the tongue as seen on CT imaging (red arrow)

14.5.9.7 Positron Emission Tomography (PET)-CT Scan

Positron emission tomography (PET) appears to be as sensitive and specific as CT and magnetic resonance imaging (MRI) in detecting primary head and neck tumors [184]. It is superior to both CT and MRI in detecting regional LN metastases, as well as distant metastases and second primary tumors [185]. False negative results of PET scan may be seen in small LNs less than 5 mm, necrotic or cystic LNs, and tumors of low metabolic activity. PET-CT is sensitive and superior for the evaluation of deep lesions.

14.5.9.8 Magnetic Resonance Imaging (MRI)

Compared to CT scan, MRI can provide more accurate definition of tumors of the tongue and is more sensitive for superficial tumors [186]. It is also better than CT scan for discriminating tumor from mucus and in detecting bone marrow invasion [187].

In addition, MRI is superior to CT scan for evaluation of perineural spread, skull base invasion, and intracranial extension of head and neck cancer. MRI can be useful for evaluation of cartilage invasion, particularly for non-ossified cartilage that can pose difficulty for CT.

MRI may also provide additional benefits compared with CT in the evaluation of the base of the tongue and parotid glands. It is the imaging modality recommended by the National Comprehensive Cancer Network (NCCN) guidelines to evaluate skull base erosion. MRI is also excellent at identifying the extent of tumor infiltration and is especially useful in patients with significant dental amalgam, which causes artifact on CT [188].

On the other hand, CT scan is better than MRI in detection of bone cortex invasion since MRI shows no bony detail [189]. Moreover, CT scanning outperforms MRI in the detection of pathological nodal metastases.

On MRI, tongue cancer is characterized by isointense to hypointense mass on T1-weighted MRI and isointense to hyperintense mass on T2-weighted MRI (Table 14.6).

In larger lesions that abut the mandible, MRI is more sensitive than CT at identifying early marrow change (low T1 signal, high T2 signal, and enhancement) but less sensitive at visualizing cortical erosion.

14.5.9.9 Ultrasonography

Ultrasonography may be performed to detect *metastases* of tongue cancer to cervical LNs and to aid in FNAC of suspicious nodes. It is possible to assess the *primary tumor* in some instances directly with a small high-frequency probe, to try and evaluate tumor thickness as shown in [190].

Table 14.6 Characteristic features of the MRI component

MRI component	Characteristic features
T1	Intermediate to low signal
T2	Intermediate to high signal
T1 contrast + gadolinium with fat saturation	Tumors enhance

14.5.9.10 Other Diagnostic Studies

14.5.9.10.1 Evaluation Under Anesthesia (EUA)

Evaluation under anesthesia is beneficial in defining involvement of the tumor surroundings by fibrosis or tumefaction. This helps in planning for the extent of surgical excision and reconstruction.

14.5.9.10.2 Tumor Biopsy

A sample of the lesion may be obtained as a part of the endoscopic evaluation of the tumor or in the clinical setting. Tumor (wedge) biopsy helps to evaluate viable tumor cells. The majority of biopsy findings reflect the presence of SCC (Fig. 14.19). However, in fewer instances, sarcoma and minor salivary gland cancer are discovered [191].

With biopsy, the pathologist will provide a tissue diagnosis (e.g., SCC) and classify the cell structure. Additional provided information can be used in staging and treatment planning, such as the mitotic rate, depth of invasion, and HPV status of the tissue.

As a general rule, a benign ulcer of the tongue that did not heal within 2 weeks must be biopsied.

14.5.9.10.3 Panendoscopy

Panendoscopy allows for the complete evaluation of the upper aerodigestive tract and helps rule out the presence of a *metachronous* tumor. With the help of panendoscopy, the mucous membrane of the upper aerodigestive tract is evaluated, and biopsy samples of any abnormal tissue areas are taken for assessment.

By performing tumor-specific endoscopy an intermediate view is obtained, whereby the anesthetized patient in a relaxed state can have the oral cavity examined with less difficulty. The tumor is staged after completing the evaluation. Panendoscopy is highly accurate for evaluation of smaller or more superficial second primary mucosal lesions [192].

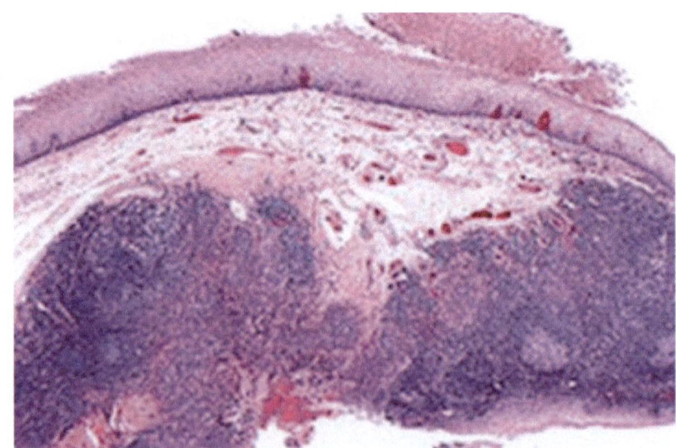

Fig. 14.19 Histopathological appearance of a poorly differentiated squamous cell carcinoma specimen. Hematoxylin-eosin stain. p16 positive, EBV negative

14.5.10 Staging

According to the TNM staging system by the American Joint Committee on Cancer, there are four stages of oral cancer based on tumor size and extension into adjacent structures (T), lymph nodes involved (N), and metastasis (M) [193, 194].

14.5.10.1 Assessment of T-Category

The following features are assessed on either CT scan or MRI [195]:

- Size of tumor and tumor thickness
- Extension across the midline
- Extension beyond the intrinsic muscles of the tongue
- Involvement of adjacent structures (neurovascular bundle and submandibular duct in the floor of the mouth—mandible)

14.5.10.2 Assessment of N-Category

Lymphatic drainage of the tongue is extensive, accounting presumably for the high rate of nodal metastases present at the time of diagnosis.

Drainage patterns depend on the location of the primary lesion:

14.5.10.2.1 Anterior Tongue

- Level Ia nodes (submental LNs)

14.5.10.2.2 Lateral Tongue

- Level Ib nodes (submandibular LNs)
- Level II nodes: upper jugulo-digasric nodes
- Level IV nodes (potentially direct drainage)

14.5.10.2.3 Posterior Tongue

- Level II nodes (upper jugulo-digasric nodes)

Significant lymphatic drainage occurs *across the midline*, and thus LNs of both sides of the neck need to be carefully examined for the presence of nodal metastases. The incidence of LN metastases correlates with tumor thickness, which is best assessed on coronal images.

14.5.10.3 Assessment of M-Category

- M1: no distant metastases
- M1: positive distant metastases

14.5.11 Differential Diagnosis

Tongue cancer must be differentiated from other malignant, benign, and nonneoplastic lesions of the oral cavity. These include lymphoma, sarcoma, metastatic

Table 14.7 Differential diagnosis of SCC of the tongue

Disease	Examples
Other malignancies	• Lymphoma • Sarcoma • Metastatic tumor • Malignant salivary gland tumors
Benign neoplasms	• Papilloma • Lipoma • Leiomyoma • Neurofibroma • Schwannoma • Granular cell tumor
Infections	• Scarlet fever • Tuberculosis • Syphilis
Metabolic	• Vitamin B deficiency • Amyloidosis • Diabetes mellitus • Hypothyroidism • Acromegaly
Immunological	• Erythema multiforme • Benign mucous membrane pemphigoid • Pemphigus
Idiopathic	• Benign migratory glossitis • Hairy tongue

tumor, malignant salivary gland tumors, tuberculosis, scarlet fever, syphilis, papilloma, lipoma, leiomyoma, neurofibroma, schwannoma, granular cell tumor, benign migratory glossitis, hairy tongue, pemphigus, erythema multiforme, mucous membrane pemphigoid, vitamin B deficiency, amyloidosis, diabetes mellitus, hypothyroidism, and acromegaly. The differential diagnosis of tongue cancer is summarized in Table 14.7.

The site, clinical presentation, and investigations of ulcers included in the differential diagnosis of tongue cancer are summarized in Tables 14.8, 14.9, 14.10, 14.11, 14.12, and 14.13.

The clinical characteristics of tongue ulcers should be accurately noticed and documented to aid in the differential diagnosis of a malignant tongue ulcer as shown in Table 14.14.

14.5.12 Prevention of Tongue Cancer

14.5.12.1 Primary Prevention

14.5.12.1.1 Screening

Tongue cancer screening is *not* a standard procedure for health assessment [212]. There is *no* effective oral cancer screening program whether general or selected

Table 14.8 Site, clinical presentation, and investigations of malignant ulcers included in the differential diagnosis

Malignant lesions	Site	Clinical presentation	Investigations
Squamous cell carcinoma (SCC)	Lateral borders	*Symptoms* • Painless ulcer or exophytic mass • History of heavy use of alcohol and tobacco *Signs* • Ulcer with rolled borders around a necrotic center • May resembles a traumatic ulcer	Biopsy CT scan
Malignant salivary gland tumor	Dorsum and ventral surface	*Symptoms* • Painless slowly growing mass *Signs* • Submucosal mass • May ulcerate in the later stages	
Metastatic tumor	Base of the tongue	*Symptoms* • Painful mass • Dysphagia • Symptoms of 1ry tumor *Signs* • Mass in tongue base • Cachexia and loss of appetite • Signs of 1ry tumor	Biopsy
Sarcoma [196]	Tongue and palate	*Symptoms* • Painless slowly growing mass • Dysphagia and weight loss *Signs* • Reddish or bluish macules that then coalesce to form purple nodules and may get ulcerated	Biopsy

(high-risk population) for oral cancer in the United States. Screening high-risk individuals in developing countries could be an effective prevention strategy to lower the stage of oral cancer at diagnosis and improve the 5-year survival [213]. Screening subjects in the subgroup who used tobacco or alcohol reduced the mortality rate from oral cancer [214].

14.5.12.1.2 Prevention

Avoiding known risk factors such as the use of *tobacco* and excessive use of *alcohol* is the best method of tongue cancer prevention [215].

The main methods for prevention are natural components such as *vitamin A*, *vitamin E*, and *beta-carotene* because they are rich in trace elements and antioxidants [216]. There is a protective effect of *diets* rich in fresh fruits and vegetables by reducing the incidence of leukoplakia [217]. Toxicity of *isotretinoin* is the main side effect, particularly in patients treated with doses higher than 2 mg/kg per day. Patients treated at the lower dose level (1 mg/kg per day) had less toxicity and did not require dose reduction [218].

Table 14.9 Site, clinical presentation, and investigations of benign tumors included in the differential diagnosis

Benign tumors	Site	Clinical presentation	Investigations
Papilloma	Dorsum and lateral borders	*Symptoms* • Painless slowly growing mass *Signs* • Warty surface or hyperkeratotic finger-like projections • Sessile or pedunculated, pink to white color	Biopsy
Lipoma [197]	Dorsum and lateral borders	*Symptoms* • Painless slowly growing mass *Signs* • Soft, sessile, and yellowish, with slippery edges	Biopsy
Leiomyoma [198]	Dorsum	*Symptoms* • Painless slowly growing mass *Signs* • Small, single or multiple, well-circumscribed mass	Biopsy
Schwannoma [199]	Dorsum and lateral borders	*Symptoms* • Painless slowly growing lesions, may be painful *Signs* • Firm, submucous mass	Biopsy
Neurofibroma [200]	Dorsum and lateral borders	*Symptoms* • Slowly growing multiple nodules • Unilateral macroglossia *Signs* • Tongue may show multiple nodules or a more diffuse involvement causing unilateral macroglossia	Biopsy
Granular cell tumor	Dorsum	*Symptoms* • Painless, firm, slowly growing nodules *Signs* • Submucosal nodules with a yellowish or pinkish color	Biopsy

14.5.12.2 Secondary Prevention

14.5.12.2.1 Follow-Up: Monitoring

Postoperative patients are monitored monthly for the first 12–18 months. In patients who undergo nonsurgical treatment, follow-up diagnostic imaging studies are recommended in the first 6 months. The aim of the regular follow-up visits is to assess nutrition, dental health, speech, swallowing function, and recurrence.

14.5.12.2.2 Natural Components

Beta-carotene and vitamin E are used as secondary chemo-protective agents [219].

Table 14.10 Site, clinical picture, and investigations of infections included in differential diagnosis

Infections	Site	Clinical Presentation	Investigations
Tuberculosis (TB) [201]	Dorsum	*Symptoms* • 1ry TB symptoms: Night fever and sweating, hemoptysis, loss of weight • Painful tongue ulcers *Signs* • Ulcer: Irregular outline, undulated borders, and yellowish-gray fibrinous floor	• Culture • Biopsy • Chest X-ray for 1ry infection • Tuberculin skin test
Scarlet fever [202]	Dorsum	*Symptoms* • Fever, malaise, headache, pharyngitis • Red skin rash • Swelling of tongue, white and red coating *Signs* • Heavy gray-white coating • Enlargement of fungiform papillae, which appear as multiple red dots • Dots disappear with time	• Throat swab culture • Rapid streptococcal antigen tests
Syphilis [203]	Dorsum	*Symptoms* • Single or multiple painless masses or ulcers according to stage • White patches (leukoplakia) • Symptoms of syphilis in 2ry and 3ry stages especially generalized LN↑ *Signs* 1ry stage • Lingual chancre (solitary, painless, slightly raised, well-demarcated ulcer) • Enlarged, painless, regional LNs 2ry stage • Mucous patches (slightly raised, grayish-white, usually surrounded by a red halo) • If scraped, it leaves a raw, bleeding surface Third stage • Gumma (a painless, elastic mass that undergoes central necrosis and ulceration) • Atrophy of the papillae • Frequently associated with leukoplakia, which may turn malignant	• Dark-field illumination to reveal the organism • Rapid plasma reagin • Venereal disease research laboratory

Table 14.11 Site, clinical picture, and investigations of metabolic disorders included in the differential diagnosis

Metabolic	Site	Clinical presentation	Investigations
Diabetes mellitus	Dorsum	*Symptoms* • Burning and dryness ± • White plaques on the dorsum due to *Candida* infection if uncontrolled *Signs* • Lingual papillary atrophy	• Throat swab • Blood glucose level • HbA1C
Hypothyroidism		*Symptoms* • Dry mouth • Difficulties in eating and speaking • Tongue swelling *Signs* • Tongue protrusion • Macroglossia	• TSH level • T3 and T4 levels
Acromegaly [204]	Generalized	*Symptoms* • Swollen tongue • Lingual indentations *Signs* • Hyperplasia of epithelium and connective tissue • Macroglossia • Spacing and labial tilting of the teeth	• Serum IGF-1 conc • Oral glucose tolerance test
Vitamin B deficiency [205]	Dorsum	*Symptoms* • Redness in tongue tip and margins • Swelling of the tongue • Indentations of the teeth • Associated neurological symptoms due to niacin and B12 deficiency *Signs* • Atrophy of both filiform and fungiform papillae	• Serum vitamin B12 and folate levels • CBC • Blood smear
Amyloidosis [206]	Lateral borders	*Symptoms* • Enlarged tongue • Decrease in lingual mobility • Difficulty in chewing, swallowing, and speaking *Signs* • Generalized induration • Yellowish nodules	• Tongue biopsy • Abdominal fat pad biopsy • S serum protein electrophoresis (SPEP)

Table 14.12 Site, clinical presentation, and investigations of immunological disorders included in the differential diagnosis

Immunological	Site	Clinical presentation	Investigations
Benign mucous membrane pemphigoid [207]	Generalized	*Symptoms* • Women over the age of 50 • Painful bullae or ulcerations *Signs* • Yellow or hemorrhagic bullae on an erythematous background • Bullae rupture leaving a fibrin-covered ulceration	• Biopsy • Indirect immunofluorescence • Autoantibodies against BP180, BP230, and laminin 332
Erythema multiforme [208]	Generalized	*Symptoms* • It occurs primarily in young men *Signs* • Small, erythematous plaque that then becomes a vesicle, quickly rupture and become confluent, shallow erosions covered by a pseudomembrane of necrotic tissue	• The cause of this disorder is an infectious disease such as herpes simplex, Coxsackievirus, or drug therapy
Pemphigus [209]	Generalized	*Signs* • Bullae rupture soon after formation to produce ulcers (pemphigus vulgaris) • Fungoid vegetations develop on the base of these ulcers (pemphigus vegetans)	• ELISA for antibodies to the BP180 NC16A • Biopsy

Table 14.13 Site, clinical presentation, and investigations of idiopathic ulcers included in the differential diagnosis

Idiopathic	Site	Clinical presentation	Investigations
Benign migratory glossitis [210]	Dorsum	*Symptoms* • Painless reddish ulcerative lesions *Signs* • Lesions appear as one or more irregularly shaped, reddish areas of depapillation surrounded by a narrow, whitish zone of regenerating papillae	
Hairy tongue [211]	Dorsum and ventral surface	*Risk factors* • Tobacco • Radiation therapy *Symptoms* • Tongue color changes *Signs* • Hypertrophy of the filiform papillae • Tongue color will vary from yellowish-white to brown or black	

Table 14.14 Clinical characteristics of different tongue ulcers

Features	Malignant	Aphthous	Frenular	Dental	Tuberculosis	Syphilis
Site	Side of the tongue	Dorsal and undersurface	Undersurface and frenulum	Side of the anterior 2/3	Tip or back of the tongue	Midline of dorsum
Number	Single	Multiple	Single	Single	Single or multiple	Single
Pain	++	+++	+	++	+	–
Teeth	Sepsis	±	±	Ragged	±	
Edges	Everted	Sloping	Sloping	Sloping	Undermined	Punched-out
Base	Indurated	Soft		Firm, granulation tissue	Soft	± Fibrotic
Floor	Tumor	Whitish			Yellow	Wash-leather
LNs	+	–	–	–	+	+

LNs lymph nodes

14.5.12.2.3 Synthetic Retinoids

Premalignant lesions have low levels of the nuclear retinoid receptors, which control normal growth and differentiation. Retinoids have antiangiogenic activity [220]. Synthetic retinoids response rates are 59–92%.

14.5.12.2.4 Nonsteroidal Anti-Inflammatory Drugs (NSAIDs)

Intake of NSAIDs prevents the development of intra-epithelial SCC, especially in the colon and rectum, due to inhibition COX-2 and diminished synthesis of prostaglandins [221].

14.5.12.2.5 Endothelial Growth Factor Receptor (EGFR) Inhibition

Endothelial growth factor receptor (EGFR) is highly expressed in SCC of the tongue, suggesting that EGFR inhibition may be effective in prevention of these tumors [222].

14.5.12.2.6 Human Papilloma Virus (HPV)-Related Oro-Pharyngeal Carcinoma Vaccine

The E6 and E7 HPV viral proteins in HPV 16 are responsible for promoting cell cycle progression and viral DNA replication in differentiated normal mucosal epithelial cells. While E6 protein binds to p53 tumor suppressor protein and induces its degradation, the E7 protein ubiquinates the retinoblastoma tumor suppressor protein. This process leads to driving the mucosal cells into S-phase and induces cellular DNA synthesis [223].

14.5.13 Treatment of Tongue Cancer

14.5.13.1 Overview

Surgical resection is the predominant treatment of tongue cancer. "Radical approach" is required in large lesions, impaired tongue mobility, deep tongue infiltration, and floor-of-mouth extension. A "partial glossectomy" with negative margins can preserve speech and swallowing for most stages I and II lesions of the oral tongue. "Total glossectomy" is required in cases where bilateral lingual arteries are involved by cancer. In these cases, postoperative radiotherapy (RT) or chemo-RT appears to improve disease control compared with surgery alone. Elective treatment of the neck in patients with stages I and II oral cavity cancer is *not* well established. Studies recommend a tumor thickness cutoff of 4 mm as a threshold for elective neck dissection.

Radiation therapy (RT) is indicated in patients with positive resection margins or bone invasion, patients with positive LNs, tumor thickness >4 mm, and those with regional recurrence. For patients who are not surgical candidates but can tolerate chemotherapy, a combined chemotherapy and RT is appropriate. If they cannot tolerate chemotherapy, RT alone is more appropriate.

Chemotherapy is used in patients who present with extensive primary lesions, with distant metastases or with poor prognosis. *Targeted therapy* may be used in combination with chemotherapy or RT. Targeted therapy drugs, such as monoclonal antibodies, interrupt the spread and growth of specific tongue cancer cells.

14.5.13.2 Radiation Therapy (RT)

14.5.13.2.1 Indications

Radiotherapy (RT) may be used for the treatment of small or superficial tongue cancers [224]. Because of the side effects of RT, younger patients are treated surgically. Surgery or RT may be chosen in older patients. Large lesions are treated with combined surgery and RT.

Indications of Adjuvant Therapy [225]

- Patients who have positive resection margins
- Patients with bone invasion
- Patients with positive LNs
- Tumor thickness >4 mm
- Patients with regional recurrence

14.5.13.2.2 Techniques of Radiation Therapy [226]

External Beam Radiotherapy (EBRT)

Depending on tumor size and location, nodal status, and the possible inclusion of interstitial implants, EBRT using a single ipsilateral portal or bilateral-opposed portals may be selected [224].

Brachytherapy

Brachytherapy may be used as a single modality or can be used following partial glossectomy. Most often brachytherapy is used after the tumor bed has been preliminarily treated with EBRT. It may result in tongue edema necessitating an elective tracheostomy [226, 227].

Orthovoltage Radiotherapy

In patients with well-defined margins and exophytic lesions, cone therapy is administered prior to EBRT therapy. An intraoral cone is placed against the tumor bed, and either electrons or orthovoltage may be given with equal control rates. For tumors <2 cm thick, RT of oral tongue cancer typically combines EBRT with an intraoral cone. Small lesions ≤10 mm and superficial lesions can be treated with either an intraoral cone or interstitial brachytherapy alone [228].

14.5.13.2.3 Treatment of Nonsurgical Candidates

For patients who are not surgical candidates but can tolerate chemotherapy, a combined *chemotherapy* and *radiotherapy* is appropriate [229]. For those patients who are not surgical candidates with poor medical condition and cannot tolerate chemotherapy, RT alone is more appropriate [230].

14.5.13.3 Chemotherapy

Chemotherapy is used in patients who present with extensive primary lesions, in patients with distant metastases, or those with poor prognosis [228]. Early tumors are *not* treated with chemotherapy because of the high success of either RT or surgery. There is no evidence to support the use of chemotherapy for early stage oral cavity cancer [231].

The factors to be considered if chemotherapy is being contemplated include the following:

- Stage of disease
- General medical status
- Potential efficacy
- Tolerance to adverse effects

14.5.13.3.1 Targeted Therapy

Targeted therapy may be used in combination with chemotherapy or radiation therapy. Targeted therapy drugs, such as monoclonal antibodies, interrupt the spread and growth of specific tongue cancer cells [231].

14.5.13.4 Surgical Treatment

The ideal surgical approach to the oral tongue tumors depends on tumor size and involvement of adjacent structures. For most small T1 and T2 lesions confined to the tongue, excision is possible with a hemiglossectomy or partial glossectomy.

Reconstruction of the tongue depends on the size of the defect. When less than one-third of the tongue has been resected, primary closure is possible [232].

Radical approach is required in the following conditions:

- Larger lesions
- Impaired tongue mobility
- Deep tongue infiltration
- Extension to the floor of the mouth

14.5.13.4.1 Surgical Approach

The tongue may be approached via a *lateral pharyngotomy*. A *partial glossectomy* with negative margins can preserve speech and swallowing for most stages I and II lesions of the oral tongue. Partial glossectomy is commonly required for advanced disease. *Total glossectomy* is required in cases where bilateral lingual arteries are involved by cancer. In these cases, postoperative RT or chemo-RT may improve disease control compared with surgery alone [233].

A *mandibulotomy* may be required for access if the mandible is free of tumor. Resection of the mandible is considered if the tumor involves or extends to the gingiva.

Free flap reconstruction is required for larger defects. Larger lesions, which cross the midline, are usually not resected due to the operation being poorly tolerated [234]. *Total laryngectomy* may also be required to prevent aspiration.

Assessing surgical resection margins can be difficult. Therefore, close deep surgical margins should be interpreted with caution, and more aggressive treatment may be indicated compared with close radial mucosal margins or close margins in other disease sites.

14.5.13.4.2 Management of the Neck

Elective treatment of the neck in patients with stages I and II oral cavity cancer is *not* well established [235]. Most reports have found that increasing tumor thickness is associated with an increased risk of occult metastases and reduced survival [236]. Studies recommend a tumor thickness cutoff of 4 mm for elective neck dissection [237]. The benefit was present in all subgroups, except for those with a primary tumor depth ≤3 mm.

An *ipsilateral selective neck dissection* is indicated for levels I to III/IV, for stage I cancers with >3 mm of invasion and for most stage II disease, except minimally invasive primary tumors. Levels IIB and IV of cervical LNs (Fig. 14.20) are dissected at the discretion of the surgeon. Patients with primary tumors close to or involving the midline should be managed with *bilateral neck dissection* [238].

Sentinel LN biopsy may be an important option between observation and neck dissection in patients with intermediate-thickness tumors [239]. This may be most applicable to patients with primary tumors <3 mm in depth with an intermediate risk of LN metastases and larger primary tumors. A negative sentinel LN biopsy may replace planned neck dissection [240].

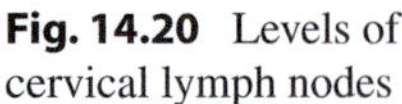

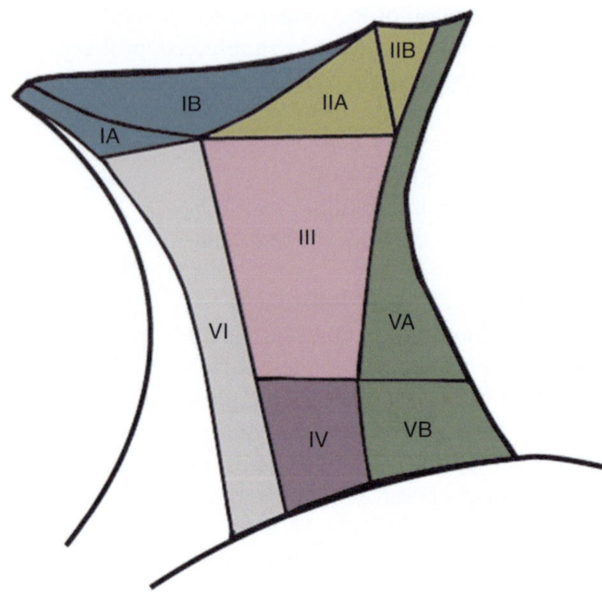

Fig. 14.20 Levels of cervical lymph nodes

Brachytherapy can be used in large lesions. The patient is then monitored post-operatively for 48 hours, during which the oncologist proceeds with the brachytherapy dosimetry and implantation of radioactive needles for periods of up to 72 h. The needles are then removed and the patient's recovery is continued in-hospital.

14.5.14 Prognosis

Prognosis of tongue cancer varies according to the extent of the tumor/ulcer at the time of diagnosis. Generally, it is regarded as "good." Neck dissection is associated with an improved prognosis. A better prognosis is provided by combination of radiotherapy (RT) and surgical treatment. The 5-year survival rate for patients with *early* oral cavity cancer is approximately 70% [241] and for those with *locally advanced* disease is about 54.7% [242].

14.5.14.1 Prognostic Factors

14.5.14.1.1 Stage of the Tumor

The later the stage, the worse the prognosis as shown by the 5-year survival rate (Table 14.15).

14.5.14.1.2 Tumor Thickness

In general, increased tumor size and thickness is significantly predictive of decreased survival and increased rate of loco-regional recurrence. Measuring tumor thickness and pattern of invasion may allow for the identification of patients with more

Table 14.15 Five-year survival rate of tongue cancer according to stage

Stage	5-year survival rate (%)
I	71
II	59
III	47
IV	37

aggressive disease. Those with tumor diameter more than 1.5 cm or tumor thickness more than 5 mm may then be considered for more aggressive adjuvant therapy and elective neck dissection regardless of stage due to increased risk for cervical LN metastasis [243–245].

Magnetic resonance imaging (MRI) is sufficiently accurate to determine tumor thickness of oral cavity SCC, although histological examination remains the standard [246–249]. Although tumor thickness reliably predicts regional nodal metastasis and decreased survival, specific treatment strategies based on tumor thickness have yet to be evaluated due to the wide range of prognostic factors related among patients with oral cavity SCC. In advanced disease (stages III and IV), tumor thickness is generally not a consideration in treatment planning as the depth usually exceeds 5 mm, and patients generally receive aggressive surgery with neoadjuvant and/or adjuvant chemo-radiotherapy.

14.5.14.1.3 Perineural Invasion

Perineural invasion is associated with increased risk local recurrence and cervical metastasis and is generally considered an independent predictor of survival for patients with oral cavity SCC [250–253].

If the presence of even small peripheral nerve involvement is pathologically confirmed, this should prompt strong consideration for a full course of postoperative RT to treat the primary tumor as outcomes related to loco-regional recurrence are poor [254, 255].

14.5.14.1.4 Positive Surgical Margins

Microscopic residual tumor resulting from positive surgical margins statistically increases local recurrence and mortality when treating SCC of the head and neck. Patients treated with surgery as the primary modality exhibit significantly improved local control rates if a negative surgical margin is obtained. Surgeons performing resections for advanced primary oral cavity SCC should strive for a minimum of 1 cm margin, with 2–3 cm margins preferred, to minimize the likelihood of positive margins. Positive surgical margins either at the primary site or within the neck after neck dissection require the use of postoperative RT to improve outcomes. The 2-year disease-free survival has been reported to improve from 33.6% to 75.6% in patients with positive surgical margins who received postoperative RT (≥62.5 Gy) [256].

14.5.14.1.5 Cervical Lymph Node Metastases

Involvement of cervical LNs is considered the single most important prognostic factor for outcome in oral cavity cancer with decreased survival and increased loco-regional recurrence. The reported 5-year survival rate of patients without and with cervical LN metastases are approximately 42% and 17.5%, respectively [257–263]. Prognosis depends on the number and size of positive LNs and the ratio of positive LNs to total number of excised LNs [264].

14.5.14.1.6 Extracapsular Extension

Advanced stage tongue SCC may present with extensive cervical nodal disease that increases the likelihood of extracapsular extension. Patients with multiple LNs exhibiting extracapsular extension generally have an extremely poor prognosis with a statistically decreased overall survival. The presence of nodal extracapsular extension is also a concern for cervical recurrence after therapy [265, 266].

14.5.14.1.7 Site of Tongue SCC

Lesions in the posterior one-third of the tongue have a worse prognosis than those in the anterior two-thirds because of (1) later diagnosis, (2) highly anaplastic nature of the tumor, and (3) early spread.

14.5.14.1.8 Other Factors

Other prognostic factors of tongue cancer associated with a poorer outcome include the following:

- *Histological grade*: Patients with high-grade tumors and with positive resection margins have bad prognosis.
- *Age of the patient*: In patients less than 40 years of age, tongue cancer has a more aggressive course [267]. The age at diagnosis of tongue cancer and the approximate percentage of deaths from tongue cancer are shown in Table 14.16.
- *Female gender.*
- *Presence of comorbidities.*
- *Lifestyle*: Patients of Southeast Asian origin with tobacco and alcohol consumption.

Table 14.16 Mortality rate of tongue cancer by age

Age at diagnosis (years)	Mortality rate of tongue cancer (%)
≤20	0.1
20–34	1.1
35–44	3.9
45–54	15.4
55–64	24.8
65–74	23.8
75–84	20.3
≥85	10.7

14.5.15 Summary: Tongue Cancer

Approximately, 25–30% of all oral cavity cancers begin in the tongue. If cancer begins in the proximal two-third of the tongue, it is described as "oral cancer," and if it begins on the distal third, it is described as "throat cancer."

More than 90% of oral cavity cancers are *squamous cell carcinomas* (SCCs); SCC of the tongue usually arises from the ventrolateral aspect of the mid and posterior tongue, probably due to adjacent pooling of carcinogens. The majority of the other lesions are of minor salivary gland origin. Non-SCCs comprise less than 3% of all lingual malignancies.

In 2009, the *incidence* of tongue cancer was estimated to be 10,530 cases per 100,000 individuals in the United States. Males are more commonly affected by tongue cancer than females. The incidence of tongue cancer increases with age. The most potent risk factor in the development of oral cancer (in general) is alcohol intake, tobacco use, and human papilloma virus (HPV) transmitted through sexual contact.

Genes involved in the pathogenesis of tongue cancer include *TP53*, *c-myc*, and *erb-b1*. On *gross pathology*, the characteristic findings of tongue cancer are the exophytic, ulcerative, and infiltrative growth patterns. Tongue cancer must be *differentiated* from other malignant lesions of the oral cavity and from few benign and nonneoplastic lesions of the oral cavity. Thus, tongue cancer must be differentiated from lymphoma, adenocarcinoma, adenoid cystic carcinoma, mucoepidermoid tumor, rhabdomyosarcoma, liposarcoma, and infections at the floor of the mouth and mandible, as well as normal adenoid tissue for lesions at the base of the tongue.

Head and neck MRI scan is *diagnostic* of tongue cancer. The predominant *therapy* is surgical resection. Adjunctive *chemotherapy*, *RT*, chemo-RT, or brachytherapy may be required. Avoiding known risk factors such as the use of tobacco and excessive use of alcohol is the best method of tongue cancer prevention.

Prognosis may vary according to the extent of the tumor at the time of diagnosis and is generally regarded as "good." Neck dissection is associated with an improved prognosis. The 5-year survival rate for patients with *early* oral cavity cancer is 70% and for those with *locally advanced* disease is 54.7%.

Causes of death from tongue cancer include cachexia, chest infection (pneumonia, Bronchiectasis, lung abscess, etc.), severe hemorrhage from erosion of blood vessels, and suffocations (usually from lesions of the posterior third of the tongue).

References

1. Bombeccari GP, Guzzi G, Pallotti F, Porrini M, Giannì AB, Spadari F. Large oral ulcer of tongue related to dental trauma. Stomatologija, Baltic Dental Maxillofac J. 2017;19:51–4.
2. Velly AM, Franco EL, Schlecht N, et al. Relationship between dental factors and upper aerodigestive tract cancer. Oral Oncol. 1998;34:284–91.
3. Kabat GC, Hebert JR, Wynder EL. Risk factors for oral cancer in women. Cancer Res. 1989;49:2803–6.
4. Gallego L, Junquera L. Oral carcinoma associated with implant-supported overdenture trauma: a casa report. Dent Traumatol. 2009;25:e3–4.

5. Piemonte ED, Lasoz JP, Brunotto M. Relationship between chronic trauma of the oral mucosa, oral potentially malignant disorders and oral cancer. J Oral Pathol Med. 2010;39:513–7.
6. Dayal, Reddy R, Anuradha Bhat K. Malignant potential of oral submucous fibrosis due to intraoral trauma. Indian J Med Sci. 2000;54:182–7.
7. Thumfart W, Weidenbecher M, Waller G, Pesch HJ. Chronic mechanical trauma in the etiology of oropharyngeal carcinoma. J Maxillofac Surg. 1978;6:217–21.
8. Marshall JR, Graham S, Haughey BP, Shedd D, O'Shea R, Brasure J, et al. Smoking, alcohol, dentition and diet in the epidemiology of oral cancer. Eur J Cancer B Oral Oncol. 1992;28B:9–15.
9. Rosenquist K. Risk factors in oral and oropharyngeal squamous cell carcinoma: a population-based case control study in southern Sweden. Swed Dent J Suppl. 2005;179:1–66.
10. Orbak R, Bayraktar C, Kavrut F, Gűndogdu C. Poor oral hygiene and dental trauma as the precipitating factors of squamous cell carcinoma. Oral Oncol Extra. 2005;41:109–13.
11. Gonçales ES, Rubira-Bullen IF, Rubira CM, Miyazawa M, Chinellato LE, Consolaro A. Eosinophilic ulcer of the oral mucosa versus squamous cell carcinoma. Quintessence Int. 2007;38:677–80.
12. Warnakulasuriya S. Causes of oral cancer-an appraisal of controversies. Br Dent J. 2009;207:471–5.
13. Neville BW, Day TA. Oral cancer and precancerous lesions. CA Cancer J Clin. 2002;52:195–215.
14. Meij EHVD, Vries TWD, Eggink HF, Visscher JG. Traumatic lingual ulceration in a newborn: Riga-Fede disease. Ital J Pediatr. 2012;38:20. https://doi.org/10.1186/1824-7288-38-20.
15. Hegde RJ. Sublingual traumatic ulceration due to neonatal teeth (Riga-Fede disease). J Indian Soc Predod Prev Dent. 2005;23:51–2.
16. Slaryton R. Treatment alternatives for sublingual traumatic ulceration (Riga-Fede disease). Fed Dent. 2000;22:413–4.
17. Goho C. Neonatal sublingual ulceration (Riga-Fede disease): reports of cases. J Dent Child. 1996;63:362–4.
18. Buchanan S, Jenkins CK. Riga-Fede syndrome: natal or neonatal teeth associated with tongue ulceration, case report. Aust Dent J. 1997;42:225–7.
19. Rakocz M, Frand M, Brand N. Familial dysautonomia with Riga-Fede disease: report of cases. ASDC J Dent Child. 1987;54:57–9.
20. Leung AKC, Robson WLM. Natal teeth: a review. J Natl Med Assoc. 2006;98(2):226–8.
21. Moreira FCL, Gonçalves IMF. Dentes natais e doença de Riga-Fede. RGO, Rev Gaúcha Odontol. 2010;58(2):257–61.
22. Baghdadi ZD. Riga-Fede disease: report of 9 cases and review. J Cl Fed Dent. 2001;25:209–13.
23. Volpato LER, Simões CAD, Simões F, Nespolo PA, Borges AH. Case report Riga-Fede disease associated with natal teeth: two different approaches in the same case. Case Rep Dent. 2015;2015:234961. https://doi.org/10.1155/2015/234961.
24. Dezan CC, Walter LRDF, Gasparoni KW, Sangiorgio JPM, Nogari B, Fernandes KBP. Sublingual traumatic ulcerative lesions caused by the eruption of primary mandibular molars: a case report. Int J Morphol. 2011;29(4):1136–8.
25. da Silva DC, de Freitas PM, Calvo AFB, Gimenez T, Zanola M, Imparato JCP. Treatment of Riga-Fede disease using laser therapy: clinical case report. Odontologia. 2017;65(1):87–91.
26. Vazzoller RMS, Fernandes RD, de Sena RMM, de Sena AM. Tratamento do herpes simplex por meio da leserterapia: relato de casos. Rev Cient ITPAC. 2016;9(1):1–11.
27. Khandelwal V, Nayak UA, Nayak PA, Bafna Y. Management of an infant having natal teeth. BMJ Case Rep. 2013:31–3. https://doi.org/10.1136/bcr-2013-010049.
28. Basavanthappa NN, Kagathur U, Basavanthappa RN, Suryaprakash ST. Natal and neonatal teeth: a retrospective study of 15 cases. Eur J Dent. 2011;5(2):168–72.
29. Genital Herpes – CDC Fact Sheet. cdc.gov. Dec 8, 2014. Archived from the original on 31 Dec 2014.
30. Beswick TSL. The origin and the use of the word herpes. Med Hist. 1962;6(3):214–32.

31. Chayavichitsilp P, Buckwalter JV, Krakowski AC, Friedlander SF. Herpes simplex. Pediatr Rev. 2009;30(4):119–29.
32. Looker KJ, Garnett GP, Schmid GP. An estimate of the global prevalence and incidence of herpes simplex virus type 2 infection. Bull WHO 2008. 2008;86(10):805–12.
33. Smith JS, Robinson NJ. Age-specific prevalence of infection with herpes simplex virus types 2 and 1: a global review. J Infect Dis. 2002;186(Suppl 1):S3–28.
34. Xu F, Fujie X, Maya RS, Benny JK, Geraldine MM, Francis KL, et al. Trends in herpes simplex virus type 1 and type 2 seroprevalence in the United States. JAMA. 2006;296(8):964–73.
35. Xu F, Sternberg MR, Gottlieb SL, Berman SM, Markowitz LE, et al. Seroprevalence of Herpes simplex virus type 2 among persons aged 14–49 years – United States, 2005–2008. MMWR. 2010;59(15):456–9.
36. CDC Study Finds U.S. Herpes Rates Remain High. Center for Disease Control and Prevention. 2010. Archived from the original on 2016.
37. Fatahzadeh M, Schwartz RA. Human herpes simplex virus infections: epidemiology, pathogenesis, symptomatology, diagnosis, and management. J Am Acad Dermatol. 2007;57(5):737–63.
38. Wu IB, Schwartz RA. Herpetic whitlow. Cutis. 2007;79(3):193–06.
39. Steiner I, Benninger F. Update on herpes virus infections of the nervous system. Current Curr Neurol Neurosci Rep. 2013;13(12):414.
40. Stephenson-Famy A, Gardella C. 2014 herpes simplex virus infection during pregnancy. Obstet Gynecol Clin N Am. 2014;41(4):601–14.
41. Gupta R, Warren T, Wald A. Genital herpes. Lancet. 2007;370(9605):2127–37.
42. Ashley RL, Militoni, Lee F, Nahmias A, Cores L. Comparison of Western blot (immunoblot) and glycoprotein G-specific immunodot enzyme assay for detecting antibodies to herpes simplex virus types 1 and 2 in human sera. J Clin Microbiol. 1988;26(4):662–7.
43. O'Mahony C, Timms MS, Ramsden RT. Local anesthetic creams. BMJ. 1988;297(6661):1468.
44. Kaminester LH, Pariser RJ, Pariser DM, Weiss JS, Shavin JS, Landsman L, et al. A double-blind, placebo-controlled study of topical tetracaine in the treatment of herpes labialis. J Am Acad Dermatol. 1999;41(6):996–1001.
45. Leung DT, Sacks SL. Current treatment options to prevent perinatal transmission of herpes simplex virus. Expert Opin Pharmacother. 2003;4(10):1809–19.
46. Chen F, Xu H, Liu J, Cui Y, Luo X, Zhou Y, et al. Efficacy and safety of nucleoside antiviral drugs for treatment of recurrent herpes labialis: a systematic review and meta-analysis. J Oral Pathol Med. 2017;46(8):561–8.
47. Chon T, Nguyen L, Elliott TC. Clinical inquiries. What are the best treatments for herpes labialis? J Fam Pract. 2007;56(7):576–8.
48. Glenny AM, Fernandez Mauleffinch LM, Pavitt S, Walsh T. Interventions for the prevention and treatment of herpes simplex virus in patients being treated for cancer. Cochrane Database Syst Rev. 2009;(1):CD006706.
49. Nasser M, Fedorowicz Z, Khoshnevisan MH, Tabarestani MS. Acyclovir for treating primary herpetic gingivostomatitis. Cochrane Database Syst Rev. 2008;(4):CD006700.
50. Treister NS, Woo SB. Topical n-docosanol for management of recurrent herpes labialis. Expert Opin Pharmacother. 2010;11(5):853–60.
51. Perfect MM, Bourne N, Ebel C, Rosenthal SL. Use of complementary and alternative medicine for the treatment of genital herpes. Herpes. 2005;12(2):38–41.
52. Beauman JG. Genital herpes: a review. Am Fam Physician. 2005;72(8):1527–34.
53. Dimitrakopoulos I, Zouloumis L, Lazaridis N, Karakasis D, Trigonidis G, Sichletidis L. Primary tuberculosis of the oral cavity. Oral Surg Oral Med Oral Pathol. 1991;72:712–5.
54. Gregory, Guptha RB. Incidence of oral manifestations in tuberculosis. J Oral Maxillofac Surg. 1980;53(2):1334–40.
55. Krawiecka E, Szponar E. Tuberculosis of the oral cavity: an uncommon but still a live issue. Postepy Dermatologii Alergologii. 2015;32(4):302–6.
56. Nalini B, Vinayak S. Tuberculosis in ear, nose, and throat practice: is presentation and diagnosis. Am J Otolaryngol Head Neck Med Surg. 2006;27(1):39–45.

57. Pekiner FN, Erseven G, Borahan MO, Gumru B. Natural barrier in primary tuberculosis inoculation: oral mucous membrane. Int J Tuberc Lung Dis. 2006;10(12):1418.
58. Mignogna MD, Muzio LL, Favia G, Ruoppo E, Sammartino G, Zarrelli C. Oral tuberculosis: a clinical evaluation of 42 cases. Oral Dis. 2000;6:25–30.
59. Dimitrakopoulos I, Zouloumis L, Lazaridis N, Karakasis D, Trigonidis G, Sichletidis L. Primary tuberculosis of the oral cavity. Oral Surg Oral Med Oral Pathol Oral Radiol. 1991;72(6):712–5.
60. Weir MR, Thornton GF. Extrapulmonary tuberculosis. Experience of a community hospital and review of the literature. Am J Med. 1985;79:467–78.
61. Iype EM, Ramdas K, Pandey M, Jayasree K, Thomas G, Sebestian P, et al. Primary tuberculosis of the tongue: report of three cases. Br J Oral Maxillofac Surg. 2001;39:402–3.
62. Gupta PP, Fotedar S, Agarwal D, Sansanwal P. Primary tuberculous glossitis in an immunocompetent patient. Hong Kong Med J. 2007;13(4):330–1.
63. Von Arx DP. Oral tuberculosis. Br Dent J. 2001;190(8):420–2.
64. Sierra C, Fortún J, Barros C, Melcon E, Condes E, Cobo J, et al. Extra-laryngeal head and neck tuberculosis. Clin Microbiol Infect. 2000;6:644–8.
65. Sacchettini JC, Rubin EJ, Freundlich JS. Drugs versus bugs: in pursuit of the persistent predator mycobacterium tuberculosis. Nat Rev Microbiol. 2008;6:41–52.
66. Spigelman MK. New tuberculosis therapeutics: a growing pipeline. J Infect Dis. 2007;196:s28–34.
67. Chan B, Khadem TM, Brown J. A review of tuberculosis: focus on bedaquiline. Am J Health Syst Pharm. 2013;70(22):1984–94.
68. van den Boogaard J, Kibiki GS, Kisanga ER, Boeree MJ, Aarnoutse RE. New drugs against tuberculosis: problems, progress and evaluation of agents in clinical development. Antimicrob Agents Chemother. 2009;53(3):849.
69. Akgoz A, Mukundan S, Lee TC. Imaging of rickettsial, spirochetal, and parasitic infections. Neuroimaging Clin N Am. 2012;22:633–57.
70. Guidelines for the treatment of Treponema pallidum (syphilis). Geneva: World Health Organization; 2016.
71. Eyer-Silva WA, Freire MAL, Horta-Araujo CA, Almeida Rosa da Silva G, Francisco da Cunha Pinto J, Raphael de Almeida Ferry F. Secondary syphilis presenting as glossodynia, plaques en Prairie Fauchée, and a split papule at the oral commissure: case report and review. Case Rep Med. 2017;19:897–8.
72. Lautenschlager S. Diagnosis of syphilis: clinical and laboratory problems. JDDG. 2006;4:1058–74.
73. Boellaard R, O'Doherty MJ, Weber WA, Mottaghy FM, Lonsdale MN, Stroobants SG. FDG PET and PET/CT: EANM procedure guidelines for tumour PET imaging: version 1.0. Eur J Nucl Med Mol Imaging. 2010;37:181–200.
74. Seibt CE, Munerato MC. Secondary syphilis in the oral cavity and the role of the dental surgeon in STD prevention, diagnosis and treatment: a case series study. Braz J Infect Dis. 2016;24:393–9.
75. France CM, Mugayar LR. Intrauterine infections: a literature review. Spec Care Dentist. 2004;24:250–3.
76. Walker GJA, Walker DG. Congenital syphilis: a continuing but neglected problem. Semin Fetal Neonatal Med. 2007;12:198–206.
77. Scheurkogel MM, Tim J, Jeurissen FJ, Quarles van Ufford HM. Gummatous syphilis of the adrenal gland. Clin Nucl Med. 2012;37:e231–3.
78. Shim HJ. Tertiary syphilis mimicking hepatic metastases of underlying primary peritoneal serous carcinoma. World J Hepatol. 2010;2:362–6.
79. Pires FR, da Silva PJ, Natal RF, Alves FA, Pinto CA, Rumayor A. Clinicopathologic features, microvessel density, and immunohistochemical expression of ICAM-1 and VEGF in 15 cases of secondary syphilis with oral manifestations. Oral Surg Oral Med Oral Pathol Oral Radiol. 2016;121:274–81.

80. Tamura S, Takimoto Y, Hoshida Y, Okada K, Yoshimura M, Uji K. A case of primary oropharyngeal and gastric syphilis mimicking oropharyngeal cancer. Endoscopy. 2008;40:235–6.
81. Willeford WG, Bachmann LH. Syphilis ascendant: a brief history and modern trends. Trop Dis Travel Med Vaccines. 2016;26:20.
82. Azulay RD. Dermatologia, vol. 10. 2nd ed. Rio de Janeiro: Guanabara Koogan; 1997. p. 190–202.
83. de Andrade R-S, de Freitas E-M, Rocha B-A, Gusmão ES, Filho M-R-M. JúniorH-M.Oral findings in secondary syphilis. Med Oral Patol Oral Cir Bucal. 2018;23(2):e138–43.
84. Qari H, Villasante C, Richert J, Rees T, Kessler H. The diagnostic challenges of separating chronic ulcerative stomatitis from oral lichen planus. Oral Surg Oral Med Oral Pathol Oral Radiol. 2015;120:622–7.
85. Jaremko WM, Beutner EH, Kumar V, Kipping H, Condry P, Zeid MY, et al. Chronic ulcerative stomatitis associated with a specific immunological marker. J Am Acad Dermatol. 1990;22:215–20.
86. Parodi A, Cardo PP. Patients with erosive lichen planus may have antibodies directed to a nuclear antigen of epithelial cells: a study on the antigen nature. J Invest Dermatol. 1990;94:689–93.
87. Azzi L, Cerati M, Lambardo M, Pellilli M, Croveri F, Maurino V, et al. Chronic ulcerative stomatitis: a comprehensive review and proposal for diagnostic criteria. Oral Dis. 2019;25(6):1465–91.
88. Preeti L, Magesh K, Rajkumar K, Karthik R. Recurrent aphthous stomatitis. J Oral Maxillofac Pathol. 2011;15:252–6.
89. Pongissawaranun W, Laohapand PP. Epidemiologic study on recurrent aphthous stomatitis in a Thai dental patient population. Community Dent Oral Epidemiol. 1991;19:52–3.
90. Shashy RG, Ridley MB. Aphthous ulcers: a difficult clinical entity. Amer J Otolaryngol. 2000;21:389–93.
91. Wadhawan R, Sharma S, Solanki G, Vaishnav R. Alternative medicine for aphthous stomatitis: a review. Int J Adv Case Rep. 2014;1:5–10.
92. Munoz-Corcuera M, Esparza-Gomez G, Gonzalez-Moles MA, BasconesMartinez A. Oral ulcers: clinical aspects. A tool for dermatologists: Part I, Acute ulcers. Clin Exp Dermatol. 2009;34:289–94.
93. Tarakji B, Gazal G, Al-Maweri SA, Azzeghaiby SN, Alaizari N. Guideline for the diagnosis and treatment of recurrent aphthous stomatitis for dental practitioners. J Int Oral Health. 2015;7:74–8.
94. Swain N, Pathak J, Poonja LS, Penkar Y. Etiological factors of recurrent aphthous stomatitis: a common perplexity. J Contemp Dent. 2012;2:96–100.
95. Slebioda Z, Szponar E, Kowalska A. Etiopathogenesis of recurrent aphthous stomatitis and the role of immunologic aspects: literature review. Arch Immunol Her Exp. 2014;62:205–15.
96. Scully C, Porter S. Oral mucosal disease: recurrent aphthous stomatitis. Br J Oral Maxillofac Surg. 2008;46:198–206.
97. Jurge S, Kuffer R, Scully C, Porter SR. Recurrent aphthous stomatitis. Oral Dis. 2006;12:1–21.
98. Ship JA, Chavez EM, Doerr PA, Henson BS, Sarmadi M. Recurrent aphthous stomatitis. Quintessence Int. 2001;31:95–112.
99. Edgar NR, Saleh D, Miller RA. Recurrent aphthous stomatitis: a review. J Clin Aesth Dermatol. 2017;10:26–36.
100. Akintoye SO, Greenberg MS. Recurrent aphthous stomatitis. Dent Clin N Am. 2005;49:31–47.
101. Shastri A, Srivastava R. Etiopathogenesis, diagnosis and recent treatment modalities for recurrent aphthous stomatitis: a review. Int J Contemp Med Res. 2015;2:1–5.
102. Scully C, Nur FL. Diagnosis and management of recurrent Aphthous stomatitis. He J Amer Dent Assoc. 2003;134:200–7.
103. Arun Kumar M, Ananthakrishnan V, Goturu J. Etiology and pathophysiology of recurrent aphthous stomatitis: a review. Int J Cur Res Rev. 2014;6:16–22.

104. Ship JA. Recurrent aphthous stomatitis: an update. Oral Surg Oral Med Oral Pathol Oral Radiol Endod. 1996;81(2):141–7.
105. Natah SS, Konttinen YT, Enattah NS, Ashammakhi N, Sharkey KA, et al. Recurrent aphthous ulcers today: a review of the growing knowledge. Int J Oral Maxillofac Surg. 2004;33:221–34.
106. Rhee SH, Kim YB, Lee ES. Comparison of Behcet's disease and recurrent aphthous ulcer according to characteristics of gastrointestinal symptoms. J Korean Med Sci. 2005;20:971–6.
107. Aydemir S, Tekin NS, Aktunç E, Numanoglu G, Ustundag Y. Celiac disease in patients having recurrent aphthous stomatitis. Turk J Gastroenterol. 2004;15:192–5.
108. Rogers RS. Recurrent aphthous stomatitis: clinical characteristics and associated systemic disorders. Semin Cut Med Surg. 1997;16:278–83.
109. Vivek V, Bindu JN. Recurrent aphthous stomatitis: current concepts in diagnosis and management. J Ind Acad Oral Med Radiol. 2011;23:232–6.
110. Guallar IB, Soriano YJ, Lozano AC. Treatment of recurrent aphthous stomatitis. A literature review. J Clin Exp Dent. 2014;6:168–74.
111. Pramod GV. Management strategies for recurrent oral aphthous ulcers. J Dent. 2013;3:352–60.
112. Eisenberg E. Diagnosis and treatment of recurrent aphthous stomatitis. Oral Maxillofacial Surg Clin N Am. 2003;15:111–22.
113. Casiglia JM. Recurrent aphthous stomatitis: etiology, diagnosis, and treatment. Gen Dent. 2002;50:157–66.
114. Al-Namah ZM, Carson R, Hanoon IA. Dexamucobase: a novel treatment for oral aphthous ulceration. Quintessence Int. 2009;40:399–404.
115. Meng W, Dong Y, Liu J, Wang Z, Zhong X, et al. A clinical evaluation of amlexanox oral adhesive pellicles in the treatment of recurrent aphthous stomatitis and comparison with amlexanox oral tablets: a randomized, placebo controlled, blinded, multicenter clinical trial. Trials. 2009;10:30.
116. Aljbab AA, Almuhaiza M, Patil SR, Alanezi K. Management of recurrent aphthous ulcers: an update. Int J Dent Oral Health. 2015;2:1–4.
117. Piccione N. Use of chlorhexidine in the therapy of some stomatological diseases. Minerva Stomatol. 1979;28:209–14.
118. Graykowski EA, Kingman A. Double-blind trial of tetracycline in recurrent aphthous ulceration. J Oral Pathol. 1978;7:376–82.
119. Pimlott SJ, Walker DM. A controlled clinical trial of the efficacy of topically applied fluocinonide in the treatment of recurrent aphthous ulceration. Br Dent J. 1983;154:174–7.
120. Altenburg A, Zouboulis CC. Current concepts in the treatment of recurrent aphthous stomatitis. Skin Herapy Lett. 2008;13:1–10.
121. Khandwala A, Van Inwegen RG, Alfano MC. 5% Amlexanox oral paste, a new treatment for recurrent minor aphthous stomatitis. Oral Surg Oral Med Oral Pathol Oral Radiol Endod. 1997;83:222–30.
122. Ricer RE. Sucralfate vs. placebo for the treatment of aphthous ulcers: a double-blinded prospective clinical trial. Fam Pract Res J. 1989;9:33–41.
123. Qnane PA, Graham GG, Ziegler JB. Pharmacology of Benzydamine. Inflammopharmacology. 1998;6:95–107.
124. Nolan A, Baillie C, Badminton J, Rudralingham M, Seymour RA. The efficacy of topical hyaluronic acid in the management of recurrent aphthous ulceration. J Oral Pathol Med. 2006;35:461–5.
125. Scheinfeld N, Rosenberg JD, Weinberg JM. Levamisole in dermatology: a review. Am J Clin Dermatol. 2004;5:97–104.
126. Genvo MF, Faure M, Hivolet J. Treatment of aphthosis with thalidomide and with colchicine. Dermatologica. 1984;168:182–8.
127. Pizarro A, Navarro A, Fonseca E, Vidaurrazaga C, Herranz P. Treatment of recurrent aphthous stomatitis with pentoxifylline. Br J Dermatol. 1995;133:659–60.
128. Puri N, Gill JK, Kaur H, Kaur N, Kaur J. Recurrent aphthous stomatitis: Herapeutic management from topicals to systemics. J Adv Med Dent Sc Res. 2015;3:165–70.

129. Bor NM, Karabiyikoglu A, Karabiyikoglu T. Treatment of recurrent aphthous stomatitis with systemic zinc sulphate. J Islam Acad Sci. 1990;3:343–7.
130. Cui RZ, Bruce AJ, Rogers RS. Recurrent aphthous stomatitis. Clin Dermatol. 2016;34:475–81.
131. Sarmadi M, Ship JA. Refractory major aphthous stomatitis managed with systemic immunosuppressants: a case report. Quintessence Int. 2004;35:39–48.
132. Kudur MH, Hulmani M. Rebamipide: a novel agent in the treatment of recurrent aphthous ulcer and Behcet's syndrome. Indian J Dermatol. 2013;58:352–4.
133. Nanke Y, Kamatani N, Okamoto T, Ogiuchi H, Kotake S. Irsogladine is effective for recurrent oral ulcers in patients with Behçet's disease: an open-label, single-Centre study. Drugs R D. 2008;9:455–9.
134. Vujevich J, Zirwas M. Treatment of severe, recalcitrant, major aphthous stomatitis with adalimumab. Cutis. 2005;76:129–32.
135. Pedersen A. Acyclovir in the prevention of severe aphthous ulcers. Arch Dermatol. 1992;128:119–20.
136. Femiano F, Buonaiuto C, Gombos F, Lanza A, Cirillo N. Pilot study on recurrent aphthous stomatitis (RAS): a randomized placebo-controlled trial for the comparative therapeutic effects of systemic prednisone and systemic montelukast in subjects unresponsive to topical therapy. Oral Surg Oral Med Oral Pathol Oral Radiol Endod. 2010;109:402–7.
137. Robinson ND. Recalcitrant, recurrent aphthous stomatitis treated with etanercept. Arch Dermatol. 2003;139:1259–62.
138. De Abreu MA, Hirata CH, Pimentel DR, Weckx LL. Treatment of recurrent aphthous stomatitis with clofazimine. Oral Surg Oral Med Oral Pathol Oral Radiol Endod. 2009;108:714–21.
139. Zhou Y, Chen Q, Meng W, Jiang L, Wang Z, et al. Evaluation of penicillin G potassium troches in the treatment of minor recurrent aphthous ulceration in a chinese cohort: a randomized, double-blinded, placebo and no-treatment-controlled, multicenter clinical trial. Oral Surg Oral Med Oral Pathol Oral Radiol Endod. 2010;109:561–6.
140. Sharma D, Garg R. Comprehensive review on aphthous stomatitis, its types, management and treatment available. J Dev Drugs. 2018;7(2):188–95.
141. Alberti PW. Panel discussion: the historical development of laryngectomy. II. The evolution of laryngology and laryngectomy in the mid-19th century. Laryngoscope. 1975;85(2):288–98.
142. Esser JF. Studies in plastic surgery of the face: i. use of skin from the neck to replace face defects. ii. Plastic operations about the mouth. iii. The epidermic inlay. Ann Surg. 1917;65(3):297–315.
143. Sobin LH. TNM classification of malignant tumours. Chichester, West Sussex, UK, Hoboken, NJ: Wiley-Blackwell; 2009.
144. Bray F, Ren JS, Masuyer E, Ferlay J. Global estimates of cancer prevalence for 27 sites in the adult population in 2008. Int J Cancer. 2013;132(5):1133–45.
145. Siegel RL, Miller KD, Jemal A. Cancer statistics. CA Cancer J Clin. 2017;67(1):7–30.
146. Gatta G, Botta L, Sánchez MJ, Anderson LA, Pierannunzio D, Licitra L, et al. Prognoses and improvement for head and neck cancers diagnosed in Europe in early 2000s: the EUROCARE-5 population-based study. Eur J Cancer. 2015;51(15):2130–43.
147. Abbas NF, Labib El-Sharkawy S, Abbas EA, Abdel Monem El-Shaer M. Immunohistochemical study of p53 and angiogenesis in benign and preneoplastic oral lesions and oral squamous cell carcinoma. Oral Surg Oral Med Oral Pathol Oral Radiol Endod. 2007;103(3):385–90.
148. Greer RO. Pathology of malignant and premalignant oral epithelial lesions. Otolaryngol Clin N Am. 2006;39(2):249–75.
149. van der Waal I. Potentially malignant disorders of the oral and oropharyngeal mucosa; present concepts of management. Oral Oncol. 2010;46(6):423–5.
150. van der Waal I. Potentially malignant disorders of the oral and oropharyngeal mucosa; terminology, classification and present concepts of management. Oral Oncol. 2009;45(4–5):317–23.
151. Gorsky M, Epstein JB. The effect of retinoids on premalignant oral lesions: focus on topical therapy. Cancer. 2002;95(6):1258–64.
152. Reichart PA, Philipsen HP. Oral erythroplakia--a review. Oral Oncol. 2005;41(6):551–61.

153. Hashibe M, Mathew B, Kuruvilla B, Thomas G, Sankaranarayanan R, Parkin DM, et al. Chewing tobacco, alcohol, and the risk of erythroplakia. Cancer Epidemiol Biomark Prev. 2000;9(7):639–45.
154. van der Waal I, Schepman KP, van der Meij EH, Smeele LE. Oral leukoplakia: a clinicopathological review. Oral Oncol. 1997;33(5):291–301.
155. Napier SS, Speight PM. Natural history of potentially malignant oral lesions and conditions: an overview of the literature. J Oral Pathol Med. 2008;37(1):1–10.
156. Lee J-J, Hung H-C, Cheng S-J, Chen Y-J, Chiang C-P, Liu B-Y, et al. Carcinoma and dysplasia in oral leukoplakias in Taiwan: prevalence and risk factors. Oral Surg Oral Med Oral Pathol Oral Radiol Endod. 2006;101(4):472–80.
157. Parashar P. Oral lichen planus. Otolaryngol Clin N Am. 2011;44(1):89–107.
158. Patrick G. Sataloff's comprehensive textbook of otolaryngology: head and neck surgery: head and neck surgery, vol. 5. New Delhi: The Health Sciences Publisher; 2016. p. 600.
159. Doherty G. Current diagnosis and treatment: surgery. New York, NY: Lange Medical Books/McGraw-Hill; 2010.
160. Som P. Head and neck imaging. St. Louis, Missori, MO: Mosby; 2003.
161. Harrison L. Head and neck cancer: a multidisciplinary approach. Philadelphia, PA: Lipppincott Williams & Wilkins; 2009.
162. Martín-Hernán F, Sánchez-Hernández JG, Cano J, Campo J, del Romero J. Oral cancer, HPV infection and evidence of sexual transmission. Medicina Oral, Patologia Oral y Cirugia Bucal. 2013;18(3):e439–44.
163. Elad S, Zadik Y, Zeevi I, Miyazaki A, de Figueiredo MA, Or R. Oral cancer in patients after hematopoietic stem-cell transplantation: long-term follow-up suggests an increased risk for recurrence. Transplantation. 2010;90(11):1243–4.
164. Mashberg A, Barsa P, Grossman ML. A study of the relationship between mouthwash use and oral and pharyngeal cancer. JADA. 1985;110(5):731–4.
165. Lee CC, Ho HC, Su YC, Yu CH, Yang CC. Modified tumor classification with inclusion of tumor characteristics improves discrimination and prediction accuracy in oral and hypopharyngeal cancer patients who underwent surgery. Medicine (Baltimore). 2015;94(27):e1114.
166. Abbey LM. Precancerous lesions of the mouth. Curr Opin Dent. 1991;1(6):773–6.
167. Stelow EB, Jo VY, Stoler MH, Mills SE. Human papillomavirus-associated squamous cell carcinoma of the upper aerodigestive tract. Am J Surg Pathol. 2010;34(7):e15–24.
168. Schlecht NF, Brandwein-Gensler M, Nuovo GJ, Li M, Dunne A, Kawachi N, et al. A comparison of clinically utilized human papillomavirus detection methods in head and neck cancer. Mod Pathol. 2011;24(10):1295–305.
169. Peterson BR, Nelson BL. Nonkeratinizing undifferentiated nasopharyngeal carcinoma. Head Neck Pathol. 2013;7(1):73–5.
170. Pathmanathan R, Prasad U, Chandrika G, Sadler R, Flynn K, Raab-Traub N. Undifferentiated, nonkeratinizing, and squamous cell carcinoma of the nasopharynx. Variants of Epstein-Barr virus-infected neoplasia. Am J Pathol. 1995;146(6):1355–67.
171. Marasescu F, Marasescu P-C, Matei M, Florescu AM, Margaritescu C, Peterscu S-M-S, Dumiterscu C. Epidemiological and histopathological aspects of tongue squamous cell carcinomas-retrospective study. Curr Health Sci J. 2018;44(3):211–24.
172. Stambuk HE, Karimi S, Lee N, Patel SG. Oral cavity and oropharynx tumors. Radiol Clin N Am. 2007;45(1):1–20.
173. Edward H. Perez and Brady's principles and practice of radiation oncology. Philadelphia, PA: Wolters Kluwer Health/Lippincott Williams & Wilkins; 2008.
174. Pauloski BR, Rademaker AW, Logemann JA, Colangelo LA. Speech and swallowing in irradiated and nonirradiated postsurgical oral cancer patients. Otolaryngol Head Neck Surg. 1998;118(5):616–24.
175. Gomez DR, Zhung JE, Gomez J, Chan K, Wu AJ, Wolden SL, et al. Intensity-modulated radiotherapy in postoperative treatment of oral cavity cancers. Int JRadiat Oncol Biol Phys. 2009;73(4):1096–103.

176. Oh HK, Chambers MS, Martin JW, Lim HJ, Park HJ. Osteoradionecrosis of the mandible: treatment outcomes and factors influencing the progress of osteoradionecrosis. J Oral Maxillofac Surg. 2009;677:1378–86.
177. Chip developed to diagnose oral cancer in ten minutes. Br Dent J. 2010;209(4):155.
178. Shaha A. Preoperative evaluation of the mandible in patients with carcinoma of the floor of mouth. Head Neck. 1991;13(5):398–402.
179. Hayashi T, Tanaka R, Taira S, Koyama J, Katsura K, Kobayashi F. Non-contrast-enhanced CT findings of high attenuation within metastatic cervical lymph nodes in patients with stage I or II tongue carcinoma during a follow-up period. AJNR Am J Neuroradiol. 2003;24(7):1330–3.
180. Kuno H, Onaya H, Iwata R, Kobayashi T, Fujii S, Hayashi R, et al. Evaluation of cartilage invasion by laryngeal and hypopharyngeal squamous cell carcinoma with dual-energy CT. Radiology. 2012;265(2):488–96.
181. van den Brekel MW, Stel HV, Castelijns JA, Nauta JJ, van der Waal I, Valk J, et al. Cervical lymph node metastasis: assessment of radiologic criteria. Radiology. 1990;177(2):379–84.
182. Curtin HD, Ishwaran H, Mancuso AA, Dalley RW, Caudry DJ, McNeil BJ. Comparison of CT and MR imaging in staging of neck metastases. Radiology. 1998;207(1):123–30.
183. Merritt RM, Williams MF, James TH, Porubsky ES. Detection of cervical metastasis. A meta-analysis comparing computed tomography with physical examination. Arch Otolaryngol Head Neck Surg. 1997;123(2):149–52.
184. Rudmik L, Lau HY, Matthews TW, Bosch JD, Kloiber R, Molnar CP, et al. Clinical utility of PET/CT in the evaluation of head and neck squamous cell carcinoma with an unknown primary: a prospective clinical trial. Head Neck. 2011;33(7):935–40.
185. Escott EJ. Role of positron emission tomography/computed tomography (PET/CT) in head and neck cancer. Radiol Clin N Am. 2013;51(5):881–93.
186. Sakata K, Hareyama M, Tamakawa M, Oouchi A, Sido M, Nagakura H, et al. Prognostic factors of nasopharynx tumors investigated by MR imaging and the value of MR imaging in the newly published TNM staging. Int J Radiat Oncol Biol Phys. 1999;43(2):273–8.
187. Rasch C, Keus R, Pameijer FA, Koops W, de Ru V, Muller S, et al. The potential impact of CT-MRI matching on tumor volume delineation in advanced head and neck cancer. Int J Radiat Oncol Biol Phys. 1997;39(4):841–8.
188. Squamous cell carcinoma of the tongue. Radiopedia. http://radiopaedia.org/articles/squamous-cell-carcinoma-of-the-tongue. Accessed on 17 Nov 2015.
189. Kuno H, Onaya H, Fujii S, Ojiri H, Otani K, Satake M. Primary staging of laryngeal and hypopharyngeal cancer: CT, MR imaging and dual-energy CT. Eur J Radiol. 2014;83(1):e23–35.
190. Lodder WL, Teertstra HJ, Tan IB, Pameijer FA, Smeele LE, van Velthuysen ML, et al. Tumour thickness in oral cancer using an intra-oral ultrasound probe. Eur Radiol. 2011;2(1):98–106.
191. Liu J, Wang XL, Liu L, Xue LY, Liu K, Huang H, et al. Application value of sentinel node biopsy in early stage oral tongue cancer with clinically negative neck. Zhonghua Zhong Liu Za Zhi. 2013;35(6):459–62.
192. Kim SY, Roh JL, Yeo NK, Kim JS, Lee JH, Choi SH, et al. Combined 18F-fluorodeoxyglucose-positron emission tomography and computed tomography as a primary screening method for detecting second primary cancers and distant metastases in patients with head and neck cancer. Ann Oncol. 2007;18(10):1698–703.
193. Anil A. Imaging in head and neck cancer: a practical approach. London San Francisco: Greenwich Medical Media; 2003. ISBN 1841100900
194. Stephen E. AJCC cancer staging manual. New York, NY: Springer; 2010. ISBN 0387884408
195. Sigal R, Zagdanski AM, Schwaab G, Bosq J, Auperin A, Laplanche A, et al. CT and MR imaging of squamous cell carcinoma of the tongue and floor of the mouth. Radiographics. 1996;16(4):787–810.
196. Anbarasi K, Sathasivasubramanian S, Kuruvilla S. Susruthan. Alveolar soft-part sarcoma of tongue. Indian J Pathol Microbiol. 2011;54(3):581–3.
197. Agarwal R, Kumar V, Kaushal A, Singh RK. Intraoral lipoma: a rare clinical entity. BMJ Case Rep. 2013;2013:bcr2012007889.

198. Baden E, Doyle JL, Lederman DA. Leiomyoma of the oral cavity: a light microscopic and immunohistochemical study with review of the literature from 1884 to 1992. Eur J Cancer B Oral Oncol. 1994;30B(1):1–7.
199. Abreu I, Roriz D, Rodrigues P, Moreira Â, Marques C, Alves FC. Schwannoma of the tongue-a common tumour in a rare location: a case report. Eur J Radiol Open. 2017;4:1–3.
200. Acampa O, Frojo M, Palomba F, Rullo R. A case of solitary neurofibroma of the tongue. Arch Stomatol (Napoli). 1990;31(4):821–5.
201. Ajay GN, Laxmikanth C, Prashanth SK. Tuberculous ulcer of tongue with oral complications of oral antituberculosis therapy. Indian J Dent Res. 2006;17(2):87–90.
202. Kutsuna S, Hayakawa K, Ohmagari N. Scarlet fever in an adult. Intern Med. 2014;53(2):167–8.
203. Abdullaev AK. Characteristics of the clinical picture of syphilis in recent years. Vestn Dermatol Venerol. 1972;46(2):61–5.
204. Anoun N, El Ouahabi H. Acromegaly features in the aging population. Pan Afr Med J. 2017;27:169.
205. Spatz R, Thimm R, Heinze HG, Ross A, König M. Changes in the clinical picture of vitamin B-12 deficiency diseases. Nervenarzt. 1976;47(3):169–72.
206. Akin RK, Baron K, Walters PJ. Amyloidosis, macroglossia, and carpal tunnel syndrome associated with myeloma. J Oral Surg. 1975;33(9):690–2.
207. Chan LS, Ahmed AR, Anhalt GJ, Bernauer W, Cooper KD, Elder MJ, et al. Diagnosis and therapy of mucous membrane pemphigoid. Results of the 1st international consensus conference. Hautarzt. 2002;53(5):371–2.
208. Farthing PM, Maragou P, Coates M, Tatnall F, Leigh IM, Williams DM. Characteristics of the oral lesions in patients with cutaneous recurrent erythema multiforme. J Oral Pathol Med. 1995;24(1):9–13.
209. Apalla Z, Sotiriou E, Lazaridou E, Manousari A, Trigoni A, Papagarifallou I, et al. Pemphigus vegetans of the tongue: a diagnostic and therapeutic challenge. Int J Dermatol. 2013;52(3):350–1.
210. Abensour M, Grosshans E. Geographic tongue or benign migratory glossitis. Ann Dermatol Venereol. 1999;126(11):849–52.
211. Gurvits GE, Tan A. Black hairy tongue syndrome. World J Gastroenterol. 2014;20(31):10845–50.
212. Sankaranarayanan R, Ramadas K, Thomas G, Muwonge R, Thara S, Mathew B, et al. Effect of screening on oral cancer mortality in Kerala, India: a cluster-randomised controlled trial. Lancet. 2005;365(9475):1927–33.
213. Santana JC, Delgado L, Miranda J, Sánchez M. Oral cancer case finding program (OCCFP). Oral Oncol. 1997;33(1):10–2.
214. Sankaranarayanan R. Health care auxiliaries in the detection and prevention of oral cancer. Oral Oncol. 1997;33(3):149–54.
215. Shin DM, Zhang H, Saba NF, Chen AY, Nannapaneni S, Amin AR, et al. Chemoprevention of head and neck cancer by simultaneous blocking of epidermal growth factor receptor and cyclooxygenase-2 signaling pathways: preclinical and clinical studies. Clin Cancer Res. 2013;19(5):1244–56.
216. Kreimer AR, Chaturvedi AK. HPV-associated oropharyngeal cancers--are they preventable? Cancer Prev Res (Phila). 2011;4(9):1346–9.
217. Stich HF, Hornby AP, Mathew B, Sankaranarayanan R, Nair MK. Response of oral leukoplakias to the administration of vitamin a. Cancer Lett. 1988;40(1):93–101.
218. Wirth LJ, Haddad RI, Lindeman NI, Zhao X, Lee JC, Joshi VA, et al. Phase I study of gefitinib plus celecoxib in recurrent or metastatic squamous cell carcinoma of the head and neck. J Clin Oncol. 2005;23(28):6976–81.
219. Bairati I, Meyer F, Gélinas M, Fortin A, Nabid A, Brochet F, et al. A randomized trial of antioxidant vitamins to prevent second primary cancers in head and neck cancer patients. J Natl Cancer Inst. 2005;97(7):481–8.

220. Soriano AF, Helfrich B, Chan DC, Heasley LE, Bunn PA, Chou TC. Synergistic effects of new chemopreventive agents and conventional cytotoxic agents against human lung cancer cell lines. Cancer Res. 1999;59(24):6178–84.
221. Lingen MW, Polverini PJ, Bouck NP. Retinoic acid and interferon alpha act synergistically as antiangiogenic and antitumor agents against human head and neck squamous cell carcinoma. Cancer Res. 1998;58(23):5551–8.
222. Klijn JG, Berns PM, Schmitz PI, Foekens JA. The clinical significance of epidermal growth factor receptor (EGF-R) in human breast cancer: a review on 5232 patients. Endocr Rev. 1992;13(1):3–17.
223. Rampias T, Sasaki C, Psyrri A. Molecular mechanisms of HPV induced carcinogenesis in head and neck. Oral Oncol. 2014;50(5):356–63.
224. Bourgier C, Coche-Déquéant B, Fournier C, Castelain B, Prévost B, Lefebvre JL, et al. Exclusive low-dose-rate brachytherapy in 279 patients with T2N0 mobile tongue carcinoma. Int J Radiat Oncol Biol Phys. 2005;63(2):434–40.
225. Ganly I, Goldstein D, Carlson DL, Patel SG, O'Sullivan B, Lee N, et al. Long-term regional control and survival in patients with "low-risk," early stage oral tongue cancer managed by partial glossectomy and neck dissection without postoperative radiation: the importance of tumor thickness. Cancer. 2013;119(6):1168–76.
226. McGregor AD, MacDonald DG. Patterns of spread of squamous cell carcinoma within the mandible. Head Neck. 1989;11(5):457–61.
227. McGregor AD, MacDonald DG. Routes of entry of squamous cell carcinoma to the mandible. Head Neck Surg. 1988;10(5):294–301.
228. Wendt CD, Peters LJ, Delclos L, Ang KK, Morrison WH, Maor MH, et al. Primary radiotherapy in the treatment of stage I and II oral tongue cancers: importance of the proportion of therapy delivered with interstitial therapy. Int J Radiat Oncol Biol Phys. 1990;18(6):1287–92.
229. Licitra L, Grandi C, Guzzo M, Mariani L, Lo Vullo S, Valvo F, et al. Primary chemotherapy in resectable oral cavity squamous cell cancer: a randomized controlled trial. J Clin Oncol. 2003;21(2):327–33.
230. Stenson KM, Kunnavakkam R, Cohen EE, Portugal LD, Blair E, Haraf DJ, et al. Chemoradiation for patients with advanced oral cavity cancer. Laryngoscope. 2010;120(1):93–9.
231. Gomez DR, Zhung JE, Gomez J, Chan K, Wu AJ, Wolden SL, et al. Intensity-modulated radiotherapy in postoperative treatment of oral cavity cancers. Int J Radiat Oncol Biol Phys. 2009;73(4):1096–103.
232. Fujita M, Hirokawa Y, Kashiwado K, Akagi Y, Kashimoto K, Kiriu H, et al. An analysis of mandibular bone complications in radiotherapy for T1 and T2 carcinoma of the oral tongue. Int J Radiat Oncol Biol Phys. 1996;342:333–9.
233. Fein DA, Mendenhall WM, Parsons JT, McCarty PJ, Stringer SP, Million RR, et al. Carcinoma of the oral tongue: a comparison of results and complications of treatment with radiotherapy and/or surgery. Head Neck. 1994;16(4):358–65.
234. Matsuura K, Hirokawa Y, Fujita M, Akagi Y, Ito K. Treatment results of stage I and II oral tongue cancer with interstitial brachytherapy: maximum tumor thickness is prognostic of nodal metastasis. Int J Radiat Oncol Biol Phys. 1998;40(3):535–9.
235. Bessell A, Glenny AM, Furness S, Clarkson JE, Oliver R, Conway DI, et al. Interventions for the treatment of oral and oropharyngeal cancers: surgical treatment. Cochrane Database Syst Rev. 2011;9:CD006205.
236. Huang SH, Hwang D, Lockwood G, Goldstein DP, O'Sullivan B. Predictive value of tumor thickness for cervical lymph-node involvement in squamous cell carcinoma of the oral cavity: a meta-analysis of reported studies. Cancer. 2009;115(7):1489–97.
237. D'Cruz AK, Vaish R, Kapre N, Dandekar M, Gupta S, Hawaldar R, et al. Elective versus therapeutic neck dissection in node-negative oral cancer. N Engl J Med. 2015;373(6):521–9.
238. Schilling C, Stoeckli SJ, Haerle SK, Broglie MA, Huber GF, Sorensen JA, et al. Sentinel European Node Trial (SENT): 3-year results of sentinel node biopsy in oral cancer. Eur J Cancer. 2015;51(18):2777–84.

239. Pedersen NJ, Jensen DH, Hedbäck N, Frendø M, Kiss K, Lelkaitis G, et al. Staging of early lymph node metastases with the sentinel lymph node technique and predictive factors in T1/T2 oral cavity cancer: a retrospective single-center study. Head Neck. 2016;38(Suppl 1):E1033–40.
240. Abdul-Razak M, Chung H, Wong E, Palme C, Veness M, Farlow D, et al. Sentinel lymph node biopsy for early oral cancers: Westmead Hospital experience. ANZ J Surg. 2017;87(1–2):65–9.
241. Luryi AL, Chen MM, Mehra S, Roman SA, Sosa JA, Judson BL. Treatment factors associated with survival in early-stage oral cavity cancer: analysis of 6830 cases from the national cancer data base. JAMA Otolaryngol Head Neck Surg. 2015;141(7):593–8.
242. Liao CT, Chang JT, Wang HM, Ng SH, Hsueh C, Lee LY, et al. Survival in squamous cell carcinoma of the oral cavity: differences between pT4 N0 and other stage IVA categories. Cancer. 2007;110(3):564–71.
243. Ichimiya Y, Fuwa N, Kamata M, Kodaira T, Furutani K, Tachibana H. Treatment results of stage I oral tongue cancer with definitive radiotherapy. Oral Oncol. 2005;41(5):520–5.
244. Jing J, Li L, He W, Sun G. Prognostic predictors of squamous cell carcinoma of the buccal mucosa with negative surgical margins. J Oral Maxillofac Surg. 2006;64(6):896–901.
245. Mücke T, Kanatas A, Ritschl LM, Koerdt S, Tannapfel A, Wolff KD, et al. Tumor thickness and risk of lymph node metastasis in patients with squamous cell carcinoma of the tongue. Oral Oncol. 2016;53:80–4.
246. Lam P, Au-Yeung KM, Cheng PW, Wei WI, Yuen AP, Trendell-Smith N. Correlating MRI and histologic tumor thickness in the assessment of oral tongue cancer. AJR Am J Roentgenol. 2004;182(3):803–8.
247. Preda L, Chiesa F, Calabrese L, Latronico A, Bruschini R, Leon ME. Relationship between histologic thickness of tongue carcinoma and thickness estimated from preoperative MRI. Eur Radiol. 2006;16(10):2242–8.
248. Kwon M, Moon H, Nam SY, Lee JH, Kim JW, Lee YS, et al. Clinical significance of three-dimensional measurement of tumour thickness on magnetic resonance imaging in patients with oral tongue squamous cell carcinoma. Eur Radiol. 2016;26(3):858–65.
249. Alsaffar HA, Goldstein DP, King EV, de Almeida JR, Brown DH, Gilbert RW, et al. Correlation between clinical and MRI assessment of depth of invasion in oral tongue squamous cell carcinoma. J Otolaryngol Head Neck Surg. 2016;45(1):61.
250. Pentenero M, Gandolfo S, Carrozzo M. Importance of tumor thickness and depth of invasion in nodal involvement and prognosis of oral squamous cell carcinoma: a review of the literature. Head Neck. 2005;27(12):1080–91.
251. Kurtz KA, Hoffman HT, Zimmerman MB, Robinson RA. Perineural and vascular invasion in oral cavity squamous carcinoma: increased incidence on re-review of slides and by using immunohistochemical enhancement. Arch Pathol Lab Med. 2005;129(3):354–9.
252. Sparano A, Weinstein G, Chalian A, Yodul M, Weber R. Multivariate predictors of occult neck metastasis in early oral tongue cancer. Otolaryngol Head Neck Surg. 2004;131(4):472–6.
253. Garzino-Demo P, Dell'Acqua A, Dalmasso P, Fasolis M, La Terra Maggiore GM, Ramieri G. Clinicopathological parameters and outcome of 245 patients operated for oral squamous cell carcinoma. J Craniomaxillofac Surg. 2006;34(6):344–50.
254. Rahima B, Shingaki S, Nagata M, Saito C. Prognostic significance of perineural invasion in oral and oropharyngeal carcinoma. Oral Surg Oral Med Oral Pathol Oral Radiol Endod. 2004;97(4):423–31.
255. McMahon J, O'Brien CJ, Pathak I, Hamill R, McNeil E, Hammersley N. Influence of condition of surgical margins on local recurrence and disease-specific survival in oral and oropharyngeal cancer. Br J Oral Maxillofac Surg. 2003;41(4):224–31.
256. Smeele LE, Leemans CR, Langendijk JA, Tiwari R, Slotman BJ, van Der Waal I. Positive surgical margins in neck dissection specimens in patients with head and neck squamous cell carcinoma and the effect of radiotherapy. Head Neck. 2000;22(6):559–63.
257. Carvalho AL, Singh B, Spiro RH, Kowalski LP, Shah JP. Cancer of the oral cavity: a comparison between institutions in a developing and a developed nation. Head Neck. 2004;26(1):31–8.

258. Sheahan P, O'Keane C, Sheahan JN, O'Dwyer TP. Predictors of survival in early oral cancer. Otolaryngol Head Neck Surg. 2003;129(5):571–6.
259. Tankere F, Camproux A, Barry B, Guedon C, Depondt J, Gehanno P. Prognostic value of lymph node involvement in oral cancers: a study of 137 cases. Laryngoscope. 2000;110(12):2061–5.
260. Duvvuri U, Simental AA Jr, D'Angelo G, Johnson JT, Ferris RL, Gooding W. Elective neck dissection and survival in patients with squamous cell carcinoma of the oral cavity and oropharynx. Laryngoscope. 2004;114(12):2228–34.
261. Zbaren P, Nuyens M, Caversaccio M, Stauffer E. Elective neck dissection for carcinomas of the oral cavity: occult metastases, neck recurrences, and adjuvant treatment of pathologically positive necks. Am J Surg. 2006;191(6):756–60.
262. De Vicente JC, Recio OR, Pendas SL, Lopez-Arranz JS. Oral squamous cell carcinoma of the mandibular region: a survival study. Head Neck. 2001;23(7):536–43.
263. Carvalho AL, Ikeda MK, Magrin J, Kowalski LP. Trends of 37.oral and oropharyngeal cancer survival over five decades in 3267 patients treated in a single institution. Oral Oncol. 2004;40(1):71–6.
264. Gross ND, Patel SG, Carvalho AL, Chu PY, Kowalski LP, Boyle JO, et al. Nomogram for deciding adjuvant treatment after surgery for oral cavity squamous cell carcinoma. Head Neck. 2008;30(10):1352–60.
265. Fagan JJ, Collins B, Barnes L, D'Amico F, Myers EN, Johnson JT. Perineural invasion in squamous cell carcinoma of the head and neck. Arch Otolaryngol Head Neck Surg. 1998;124(6):637–40.
266. Diaz EM Jr, Holsinger FC, Zuniga ER, Roberts DB, Sorensen DM. Squamous cell carcinoma of the buccal mucosa: one institution's experience with 119 previously untreated patients. Head Neck. 2003;25(4):267–73.
267. Truitt TO, Gleich LL, Huntress GP, Gluckman JL. Surgical management of hard palate malignancies. Otolaryngol Head Neck Surg. 1999;121(5):548–52.

15 Glossectomy

15.1 Introduction

The term "glossectomy" is used to describe a variety of surgical procedures for the resection of tongue tumors. In 1978, *Péri* described four types of transoral glossectomy for noncancer-related diseases of the tongue to reduce tongue volume [1]. Later on, other attempts were made to classify macroglossia-related surgery [2] and tongue cancer-related surgery [3].

A thorough review of literature to define surgical removal of tongue cancers identified the following expressions: glossectomy, partial glossectomy, hemiglossectomy, subtotal glossectomy, transoral glossectomy, total glossectomy, cuneiform glossectomy, and compartmental glossectomy. The lack of a clear anatomical and functional definition of the various glossectomies reported in the literature leads to much confusion and misunderstanding.

In the last century, the majority of the early- and intermediate-staged tongue cancers were treated by a partial glossectomy with a safety margin of about 0.5–1 cm [4]. At the beginning of this century, the more frequent approach was a wide resection with larger free macroscopic margins (1.5–2 cm) [5]. Today, we can better plan how to perform tongue tumor excision owing to the improved knowledge of the manner of tumor spread [6–12], the improved imaging techniques [13, 14], and the new eighth edition American Joint Committee on Cancer (AJCC) TNM staging system [15–17]. Surgical treatment of tongue cancers should thus be planned according to these clinical, pathological, and imaging findings. From a functional point of view, the effect of tongue resection on muscle function should be addressed [18, 19]. Early stages can usually be approached via the transoral route as the affected tissue is limited to the tongue mucosa or intrinsic muscles and, thus, can be radically excised without necessitating extraoral access. When, however, the tumor affects one or more extrinsic muscles, which have extra-lingual insertions, it is necessary to perform an en bloc combined transoral and lateral cervical approach to remove the muscles in toto from their insertions [19–23].

© The Author(s), under exclusive license to Springer Nature Switzerland AG 2022

M. F. Sakr, *Tongue Lesions*, https://doi.org/10.1007/978-3-031-08198-9_15

15.2 Indications and Contraindications

15.2.1 Indications

Glossectomy is commonly performed for the extirpation of *malignant* and *precancerous* (or "potentially malignant") oral cavity lesions. Other indications include the following [24, 25]:

1 Excisional or incisional biopsy of tongue lesions of undetermined etiology
2 Benign neoplasms of the tongue
3 Obstructive sleep apnea
4 Macroglossia

15.2.2 Contraindications

Other than *medical comorbidities* that may preclude the patient from undergoing surgery, the principal contraindication is an *unresectable disease* in the case of malignancies. This includes the following:

1 Metastatic disease
2 Extensive or total carotid artery encasement
3 Skull base extension
4 Invasion into the paraspinal musculature

15.3 Classification of Glossectomy

While there are many classifications for glossectomy, it is commonly classified by the laterality and the proportion (volume) of the tongue removed [24, 25].

15.3.1 Classification of Glossectomy by Laterality

1 Right
2 Left
3 Midline

15.3.2 Classification of Glossectomy by Resected Volume

Glossectomy is classified according to the volume (percentage) of the tongue resected into the following categories:

1. Partial glossectomy (less than one-half of the tongue)
2. Hemiglossectomy (half of the tongue)

3. Near-total glossectomy (more than half, but less than a total glossectomy)
4. Total glossectomy (whole tongue excision)

15.3.3 Recently Proposed Classification

Recently, Ansari et al. (2019) developed a classification of glossectomies that clearly highlights what structures are involved and therefore which type of glossectomy is indicated for achieving a complete removal with minimal functional impact. This classification includes five types of glossectomy (I–V) as follows [24]:

15.3.3.1 Type I Glossectomy (Mucosectomy)

15.3.3.1.1 Definition

Mucosectomy means incision of the mucosa in healthy tissue with appropriate safety margins (1.0–1.5 cm), depending on whether or not the lesion is well-defined. The mucosa and submucosa are included up to the intrinsic muscle fibers of the tongue. The deep resection margin should include a thin layer of the intrinsic muscles because of a possible invasion of the submucosa (Fig. 15.1). Generally, the wound is left to heal by secondary intention, although the defect may be partially closed primarily or covered with a skin graft.

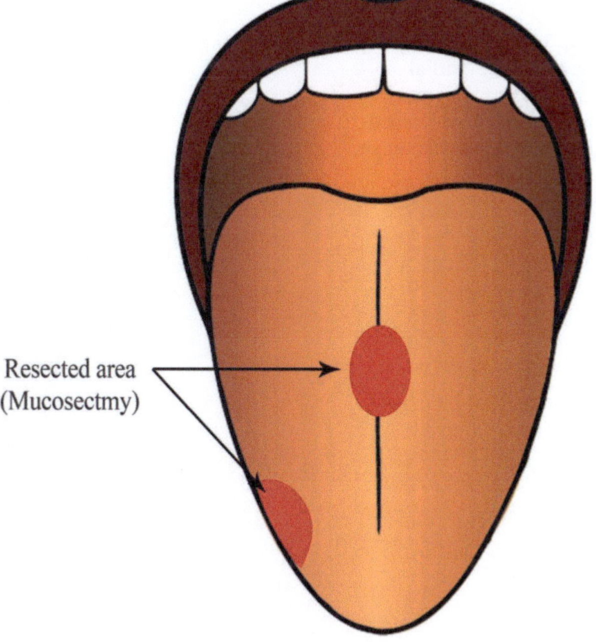

Fig. 15.1 Type I glossectomy (mucosectomy). Note the red-colored resected areas in the midline and at the lateral border of the tongue

15.3.3.1.2 Indications

Precancerous, superficial suspicious lesions, limited to the epithelium of the tongue without previous biopsy, are the indications of mucosectomy. The aim of surgery in this case is to excise the whole lesion with adequate margins up to the healthy tissue with both diagnostic and curative intent.

15.3.3.2 Type II Glossectomy (Partial Glossectomy)

15.3.3.2.1 Definition

Partial glossectomy includes the lesion and adjacent normal mucosa, submucosa, and the intrinsic muscles up to the surface of the extrinsic muscles (when the directions of the muscle fibers change), with appropriate safety margins of approximately 1.5 cm.

The resection is usually diamond-shaped on the surface, while more deeply it is shaped like a truncated cone with the intrinsic muscles as the apex (Fig. 15.2). The terminal branches of the lingual artery should be ligated, and the lingual nerve is usually preserved. Closure may be partial or total with the objective of avoiding bleeding, postoperative edema, and retracted scars.

15.3.3.2.2 Indications

Indications of partial glossectomy include lesions infiltrating the submucosa and superficially into the intrinsic, but *not* extrinsic, muscles or infiltration <10 mm deep [15].

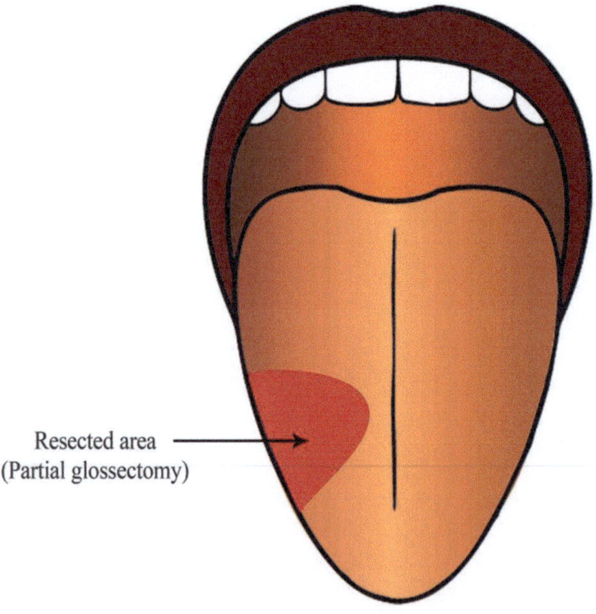

Fig. 15.2 Type II glossectomy (partial glossectomy). Note the red-colored cone-shaped resected area of the tongue

15.3.3.3 Type IIIa Glossectomy (Hemiglossectomy)

15.3.3.3.1 Definition

The resected specimen in this type includes the mucosa, submucosa, and intrinsic and extrinsic muscles ipsilateral to the lesion. The mucosa is resected up to healthy tissue with appropriate safety margins of at least 1.5 cm. The lingual artery must be ligated and removed en bloc with the lingual and hypoglossal nerves in the specimen of the primary tumor and cervical lymph nodes (LNs). The base of the ipsilateral tongue is preserved. The tip of the tongue may or may not be preserved (Fig. 15.3).

15.3.3.3.2 Indications

Indications of this type of glossectomy (IIIa) are lesions infiltrating the intrinsic and, minimally, the extrinsic muscles or infiltration >10 mm, but confined within the ipsilateral tongue [15].

15.3.3.4 Type IIIb Glossectomy (Compartmental Hemiglossectomy)

15.3.3.4.1 Definition

The specimen of compartmental hemiglossectomy includes the mucosa, submucosa, intrinsic and extrinsic muscles ipsilateral to the lesion, genioglossus, hyoglossus and styloglossus muscles, and the inferior portion of the palatoglossus muscle. Medially, the midline raphe is included in the resection (Fig. 15.4).

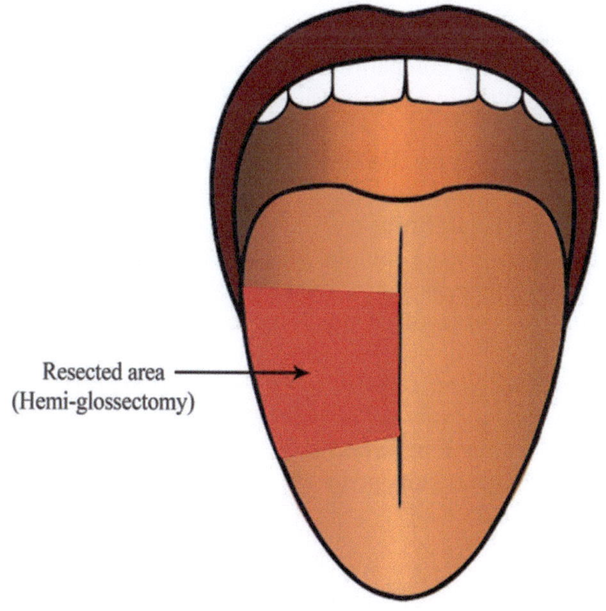

Fig. 15.3 Type IIIa glossectomy (hemiglossectomy). Note the red-colored resected area of the tongue restricted to the ipsilateral side of the lesion. The base of the ipsilateral tongue is preserved and so is the contralateral half of the tongue

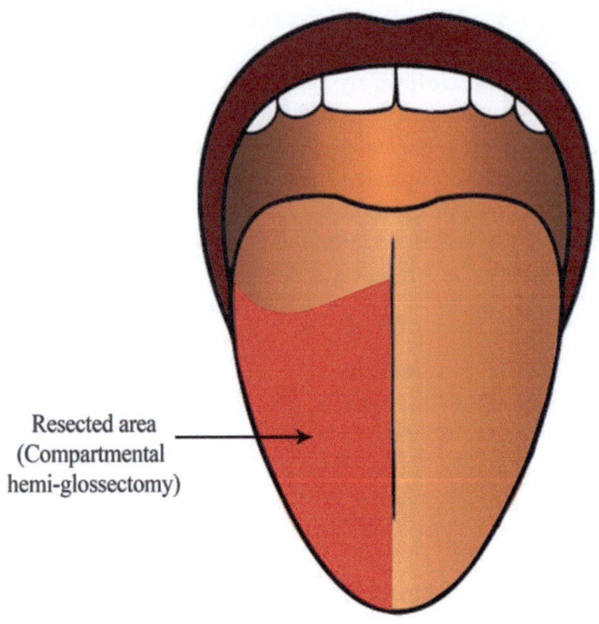

Fig. 15.4 Type IIIb glossectomy (compartmental hemiglossectomy). Note the red-colored resected area of the tongue restricted to the ipsilateral side of the lesion. Medially, the midline raphe is included in the resection

The lingual nerve is resected as far cranially as possible. The hypoglossal nerve is removed after the ansa; the lingual artery and vein are ligated in proximity to the horn of the hyoid bone and removed en bloc with the specimen and cervical lymph nodes.

15.3.3.4.2 Indications

Indications of compartmental hemiglossectomy include lesions massively infiltrating the intrinsic and extrinsic muscles but still confined to the ipsilateral tongue.

15.3.3.5 Type IVa Glossectomy (Subtotal Glossectomy)

15.3.3.5.1 Definition

This is an anterior subtotal glossectomy with preservation of both sides of the base of the tongue, posterior hyoglossus muscle, and hypoglossal and lingual nerves, from the less involved side (Fig. 15.5).

15.3.3.5.2 Indications

Indications of subtotal glossectomy include lesions that arise in the anterior portion of the mobile tongue and exceed the hemilingual area of origin involving the contralateral genioglossus muscle, but limited to the mobile tongue.

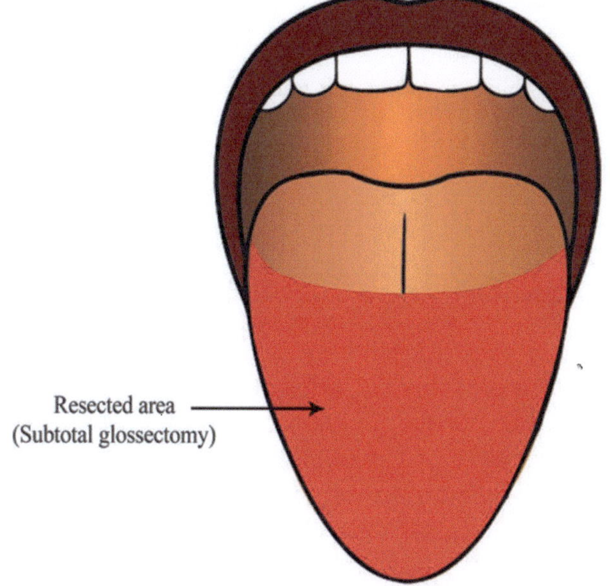

Fig. 15.5 Type IVa glossectomy (subtotal glossectomy). Note the red-colored resected area with preservation of both sides of the base of the tongue

15.3.3.6 Type IVb Glossectomy (Near-Total Glossectomy)

15.3.3.6.1 Definition

Type IVb glossectomy (near-total glossectomy) is similar to type IVa glossectomy (subtotal glossectomy) but with extension to the ipsilateral base of the tongue. The following contralateral structures are preserved: hyoglossus and styloglossus muscles, hypoglossal and lingual nerves, and lingual artery (functional unit of the base of the tongue) (Fig. 15.6).

15.3.3.6.2 Indications

Near-total glossectomy is indicated for massive lesions that exceed the border of the hemilingual area of origin, infiltrating the ipsilateral base of the tongue, and the contralateral genioglossus muscle.

15.3.3.7 Type V Glossectomy (Total Glossectomy)

15.3.3.7.1 Definition

Total glossectomy entails excision of all of the mobile tongue and the base of the tongue, which is transected at the level of the vallecula. The specimen includes intrinsic and extrinsic muscles, both lingual arteries, hypoglossal, lingual nerves, and the floor of the mouth (Fig. 15.7).

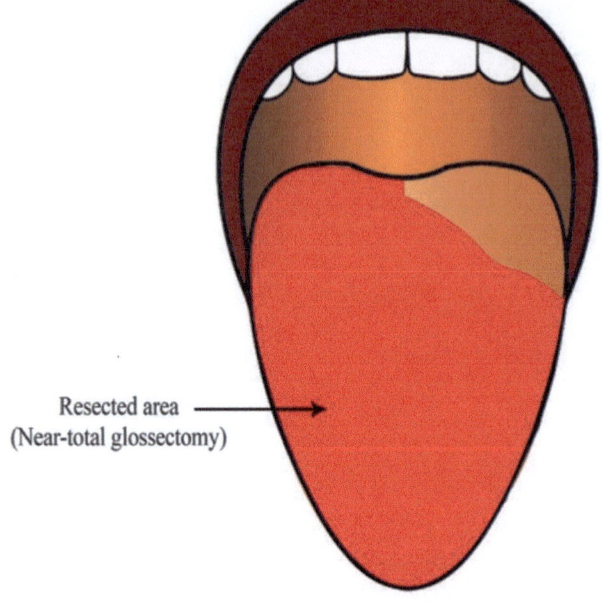

Fig. 15.6 Type IVb glossectomy (near-total glossectomy). Note the red-colored resected area with extension to the ipsilateral base of the tongue

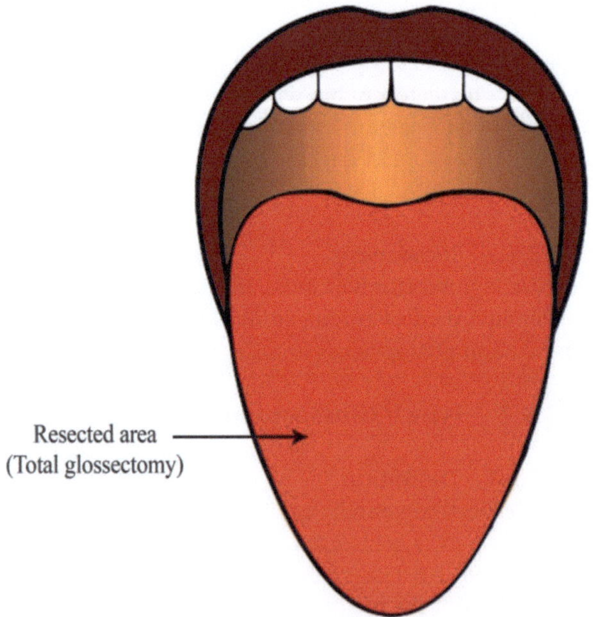

Fig. 15.7 Type V glossectomy (total glossectomy). Note the red-colored resected area including all of the mobile tongue and the base of the tongue

15.3.3.7.2 Indications

Total glossectomy is indicated for massive infiltrating lesions such as those of the anterior ventral surface of the tongue, dorsum of the tongue, or the tongue base, which bilaterally involve the genioglossus, hyoglossus, and styloglossus with impairment of the mobility of the tongue.

15.3.3.8 Impact of Glossectomy Classification on Neck Dissection

The extent of tongue resection (type of glossectomy) is a reflection of the three-dimensional extent of the primary tumor, and thus would entail the need for elective neck dissection based on the rising risk of occult metastases in the clinically negative neck.

Type I glossectomy should *not* require prophylactic neck dissection. In *type II glossectomy*, supra-omohyoid neck dissection should be carried out based on the probability of occult metastases and according to the institutional and international guidelines. From the *type III glossectomy onward*, the dissection of the neck should be done as an en bloc procedure. In the *type IV* and *V glossectomies*, the en bloc resection should be performed with *bilateral* neck dissection.

15.4 Surgical Preparation

Surgery is the recommended primary treatment for oral tongue cancer. If there are no contraindications to surgery, the NCCN guidelines favor surgery over radiation for oral cavity cancers. Understanding the limitations and advantages of various approaches to glossectomy can help facilitate resection and allow appropriate counseling of patients on the expected perioperative and postoperative course.

15.4.1 Equipment

Equipment used to optimize exposure of the tongue is the key to achieving a successful oncological resection. Equipment should include the following [26]:

- Adequate lighting is important in the oral cavity. A headlight is recommended to allow additional light into the oral cavity.
- Mouth gags, bite blocks, and lip retractors are essential to free the hands of the surgeons.
- Mouth gags can be used in conjunction with a bite block or cheek/lip retractor.
- Traction sutures (e.g., 2.0 or 3.0 silk) or locking fine-tipped forceps can help deliver the tongue out of the mouth for additional exposure.
- For mucosal and muscle cuts, electrocautery can provide hemostasis. However, excessive cautery can affect margin interpretation. Cold dissection can be done with bipolar cautery for hemostasis. The CO_2 laser offers the advantage over cautery of limiting collateral tissue damage and preserving margin interpretation but offers limited hemostasis by itself.

- If mandibulotomy or mandibulectomy is planned, bone cutting instruments will be needed; as well as a mandibular plating set to reconstruct the jaw after glossectomy is completed.

15.4.2 Personnel

The essential personnel that need to be available for this procedure include the experienced primary head and neck surgeon, one or two surgical assistants, a scrub nurse, a circulating/operating room nurse, a surgical technologist, and an anesthesiologist. To secure the airway of the patients, airway management should be discussed with the anesthesiologist prior to starting the procedure.

15.4.3 Preoperative Assessment

Preparation begins with the preoperative assessment of the tumor and the formulation of an airway plan. This starts with a comprehensive history and physical examination.

15.4.3.1 History-Taking

A comprehensive clinical history should be obtained at the initial clinical consult and should include the following:

- *Prior oncological treatments*, including the status of other cancers, prior surgeries, chemotherapy, and history of head and neck radiation
- *Other head and neck procedures*, including prior neck surgeries/procedures, vascular surgeries, trauma reconstructions, and airway procedures
- *Conditions that may affect wound healing*, including prior head and neck radiation, malnutrition, hypothyroidism, chronic steroid use, autoimmune conditions, and smoking
- *Peripheral vascular disease* if tissue transfer is planned
- *Airway conditions*, including a history of difficult intubations, subglottic stenosis, prior intubations, and history of tracheostomy, as these will affect the airway plan

15.4.3.2 Physical Examination

Physical examination should be performed during preoperative consultation to evaluate transoral exposure, as well as visual inspection and palpation of the tumor to delineate its clinical characteristics.

Transoral exposure is assessed by asking the patient to open the mouth. Patients with a good opening and a favorable tumor location may need the transoral approach alone. If the patient has severe trismus, the transoral approach will be impossible; a lip-split mandibulotomy will generally be needed for these patients. Edentulous patients are advantageous for glossectomy; as exposure is superior, there is no risk of damaging their teeth, and the flap inset may be performed without the need for circum-dental sutures in patients who may otherwise have poor dentition and periodontal hygiene.

Tumor inspection provides an accurate assessment of the size, location, depth, and anticipated mucosal margins. The surgeon must predict nearby structures that need to be recruited into the composite specimen for microscopically cancer-negative margins, including the floor of the mouth, base of the tongue, contralateral tongue, pharynx, soft palate, retromolar trigone, maxilla, buccal mucosa, hyoid bone, mandible, and even the larynx.

Manual palpation of the tongue is equally important to assess the submucosal extent of the tumor and to evaluate for fixation to surrounding structures. Superficial ulcers may give the appearance of a T1 or T2 tumor, but palpation may reveal a T3 tumor with submucosal extension crossing the midline. This may alter the approach from a transoral partial glossectomy to a mandibulotomy with subtotal glossectomy and soft tissue reconstruction.

Palpation of tumors involving the middle one-third of the tongue may necessitate resection of the tongue base, retromolar trigone, or soft palate to obtain adequate margins. Palpation is also important in cases of tumor extending along the floor of the mouth, as it may suggest mandibular invasion requiring segmental mandibulectomy and osseous reconstruction. Patients in severe pain may be difficult to examine in the office. Because in-office assessment may be confounded by patient discomfort, it is important to repeat a rigorous physical examination under anesthesia at the beginning of the procedure.

15.4.3.3 Laryngoscopy and Imaging

Preoperative flexible laryngoscopy and imaging are powerful adjuncts in evaluating tumor extension and the airway. If flexible laryngoscopy and/or imaging demonstrates tumor extension into the pharynx or larynx, the transoral approach alone will be insufficient. Assessment of airway landmarks with flexible laryngoscopy may predict potential intubation difficulties and help formulate a plan to safely secure the airway.

15.4.4 Securing the Airway

In cases of early-stage oral tongue cancer, there are rarely obstacles to securing the airway. Such patients can be nasally intubated to avoid obstruction of the operative field by the endotracheal tube. With more advanced-stage cancer, the patient may demonstrate findings that portend a difficult airway, such as trismus, tongue fixation, or mass obstruction of the airway. A good total or partial view of laryngeal landmarks may lend itself well to intubation via video-assisted laryngoscopy or awake fiberoptic nasal or oral intubation depending on the surgical plan. With effacement of laryngeal landmarks and increased laryngeal obstruction, an awake-tracheostomy may be indicated in order to secure the airway. Having an airway plan is essential in preparing for a glossectomy procedure.

Patients with severe trismus are difficult to examine preoperatively as previously discussed; they will need a more sophisticated airway plan. Awake nasal fiberoptic intubation may be recommended if good airway landmarks are present. Awake tracheostomy may be preferred if airway landmarks are effaced or if the surgeon feels it is the safest option.

15.4.5 Examination Under Anesthesia (EUA)

Once the airway is secured, an examination under anesthesia (EUA) should be performed. Once again, feasibility of the transoral exposure, visual examination, and palpation of the tumor should be repeated as the planned glossectomy approach may change depending on the findings, including tumor progression in the interval. Patients that were previously difficult to examine in the office due to trismus or severe pain may provide a different surgical assessment when under anesthesia. Direct laryngoscopy at the beginning of the procedure may also be performed to assess for tumor extent.

15.4.6 Draping

The patient is prepped and draped based on the overall planned surgery. Transoral glossectomy without neck dissection is often considered a *clean-contaminated* procedure. If a neck dissection and reconstruction is to be performed, the patient can be prepped and draped once for a *sterile* procedure, whether or not there is anticipated contamination by a connection between the oral cavity and the neck. If a transoral glossectomy is performed with a neck dissection without connecting to the neck, some surgeons may perform the glossectomy in a nonsterile fashion first. After the primary tumor is resected and negative margins confirmed, the patient may then be prepped and draped for the neck dissection for a sterile procedure. It is surgeon preference. Likewise, the administration and choice of antibiotics are at the discretion of the surgeon.

15.5 Surgical Approach

Oncological resection should include at least a 2-cm margin from the macroscopic border of the malignant lesion. Nearly all tongue lesions can be accessed via the combined oral and cervical approaches [27].

Glossectomy can be done via a few different approaches depending on what part and how much of the tongue needs to be excised and what associated procedures might be required. These approaches include the following:

1. Transoral approach
   (a) Transoral conventional approach
   (b) Transoral robotic-assisted surgery (TORS)
   (c) Transoral laser microsurgery (TLM) or transoral laser surgery (TOLS)
2. Lip-splitting mandibulotomy (mandibular swing)
3. Trans-cervical pull-through approach combined with a pharyngotomy

- **Transoral Conventional Approach**
  Conceptually, transoral conventional glossectomy is the simplest; it means the removal of the tongue tissue through the mouth. It requires the least steps, and in the appropriate case, it is the "easiest" approach. It does, however, have limited posterior access and exposure. Because the overwhelming majority of glossectomies are done for cancer, adequate access and exposure are mandatory for achieving a microscopically margin-negative resection.
- **Transoral Robotic-Assisted Surgery (TORS)**
  Transoral robotic-assisted surgery (TORS) represents a good tool for staging and treating neoplasms of the base of the tongue (BOT). The procedure is safe and can radically remove selected T1-T2 oropharyngeal tumors of the tongue base with good functional outcomes and without adverse effects and also allow the possibility to deintensify adjuvant treatments [28].

  One advantage of TORS is that it allows a clear and wide view of the surgical field and good 3D visualization of structures, enabling access to the tumor via a smaller approach than the external one. Another advantage is the use of miniaturized tools. This allows mimicking standard surgical instruments and arm movements, with tremor filtration. In addition, it permits a frontal view and reaches "blind corners" of the pharyngo-laryngeal complex, not perpendicularly positioned to the visual line due to the possibility to use a 30° telescope [29].
- **Transoral Laser Surgery (TOLS)/Transoral Laser Microsurgery (TLM)**
  The transoral laser approach is ideal for T1 and T2 malignant tumors of the tongue, exophytic T3 malignant disease, or benign tumors with limited extension into surrounding tissues. The main advantages of this approach are its minimal invasiveness, the ability to keep the pharyngeal musculature and neural innervation intact, the decreased tracheostomy tube and gastrostomy tube dependence postoperatively [30], the ability to keep the mandible intact, and the ease with which surgeons can proceed to the open approaches when necessary.
- **Lip-Split Mandibulotomy Approach (Mandibular Swing)**
  The lip-split mandibulotomy gives the widest exposure, but it is the most time-consuming and carries more risk of complications. In the lip-split mandibulotomy, a sagittal osteotomy is performed to splay open or swing the mandible open to allow inferior displacement of the tongue for a transoral transcervical expo-

sure of the posterior tongue and pharynx. It requires mandible reconstruction after ablation is completed. If the lip-split with mandible osteotomy is performed, then complications from this procedure may be decreased by combining the paramedian approach (including stair step) with rigid fixation of the osteotomy with titanium plates/screws.

- **Trans-Cervical Pull-Through Approach**
  Glossectomy via the trans-cervical pull-through is a technique that releases the tongue into the neck through the floor of the mouth by opening the sublingual and submental compartments. It provides inferior displacement of the tongue for improved visualization of the posterior tongue. This approach is simpler than the lip-split mandibulotomy approach because of the intact mandible and unnecessary mandibular reconstruction.

15.5.1 How to Choose the Appropriate Approach

The most effective approach is the one that best facilitates a microscopically margin-negative resection. The "easiest" approach may not always be the fastest one; it may be the approach that requires the most additional steps for exposure with the highest risks of complication. The overall impression of weighing the risks and benefits of each approach will help determine the most effective approach.

Choosing the appropriate approach for glossectomy depends on several factors, including the size, depth, and location of the ablation. Other surgical factors include also the presence of cervical LN metastases, the need for reconstruction, presence of trismus, and prior head and neck irradiation.

Size In general, *smaller and shallower*, Tis, T1, and T2, tumors lend themselves well to transoral resection alone. Larger tumors or tumors with significant depth, such as large T2 to T4a, are better addressed by either trans-cervical pull-through or lip-split mandibulotomy because of the improved access. T4b disease is unresectable, and surgery is usually contraindicated.

Site The location of the tumor is equally important in deciding the optimal surgical approach. The more anterior the ablation is, the more amenable it is to transoral resection. As more of the posterior tongue gets involved, exposure becomes a limiting factor.

Size and site It is important to consider both the size and location of the ablation. For example, a larger tumor (T3) of the tongue tip or anterior half of the tongue may be amenable to resection by a transoral approach only. In contrast, a shallow, 3-cm T2 tumor of the posterior middle-third of the tongue that extends onto the base of the tongue (BOT) may be difficult to remove by a transoral approach alone and may be assisted by a trans-cervical pull-through. The base of tongue (BOT) is a three-dimensional anatomical region within the upper aerodigestive tract that is intricately involved in respiration, articulation, and deglutition. Circumvallate papillae form the anterior anatomical and embryological boundary, thus separating the pharyngeal BOT from the oral tongue [31]. The BOT is further defined laterally by the glosso-palatine sulci and posteriorly or inferiorly by the vallecula and pharyngo-epiglottic folds.

Neck dissection is almost always considered in glossectomy due to the high rate of cervical LN metastases. In cases involving resection of the floor of the mouth, combined with submandibular triangle (level IB) nodal dissection, reconstruction may be required to recreate the floor and separate the neck from the oral cavity to prevent fistula. *Reconstruction* may also be indicated to recreate form and function to a certain degree if a sufficient amount of tongue is resected. Both reconstruction and neck dissection require trans-cervical approaches. It may be advantageous to perform an extended procedure if the neck is to be opened. The tumor might extend into the mandible and other neck compartments, such as the sublingual space, submental space, or other deep spaces in the neck, and may benefit from the exposure afforded by an extended approach.

Severe trismus is an obstacle to transoral glossectomy. If the jaw cannot be opened even with the administration of paralytics, lip-split mandibulotomy or trans-cervical pull-through may be indicated. Trans-cervical pull-through requires transoral mucosal cuts that might not be possible in very severe trismus cases. In patients with *prior head and neck radiation*, lip-split mandibulotomy carries the risk of osteoradionecrosis. If feasible, cervical pull-through may be favored over the mandibulotomy due to the theoretical risk of osteoradionecrosis.

15.6 Surgical Technique

15.6.1 Transoral Conventional Glossectomy

In the appropriately selected patient, transoral glossectomy can provide excellent oncological clearance with the lowest risk of morbidity.

15.6.1.1 Indications and Contraindications

Transoral conventional glossectomy is indicated in T1/T2 tumors and anterior or shallow tongue tumors. However, this approach provides the poorest exposure to the posterior tongue and therefore is contraindicated in tumors or lesions of the base of the tongue (BOT). It may be necessary to convert the transoral approach to a lip-split mandibulotomy or cervical pull-through if the exposure is suboptimal for cancer extirpation.

15.6.1.2 Operative Technique

Under general anesthesia, with the patient in the supine position, self-retaining retractors and mouth gags are used to obtain transoral exposure and free the hands of the surgeon and their assistants. There are a variety of mouth gags that can be

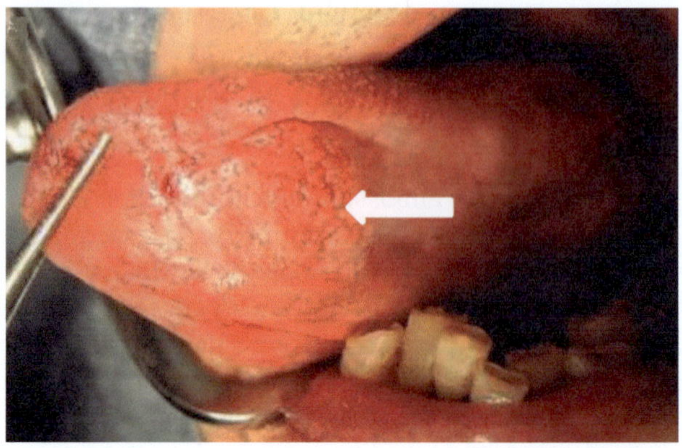

Fig. 15.8 Traction of the tip of the tongue to facilitate exposure and dissection of the lesion (arrow)

used. Commonly used are the Molt, Fergusson, and Jennings mouth gags. Mouth gags may be used in conjunction with a cheek or lip retractor to allow more light into the operative field. Traction on the tongue facilitates the resection. This can be accomplished by placing traction sutures or a fine-point ratcheting (locking) forceps on the tongue. Handling the tongue with a non-locking, toothed forceps may be difficult due to the bulk and fluidity of the tongue (Fig. 15.8).

Owing to the high vascularity of the tongue, mucosal and muscle incisions can be made with cautery, laser, ultrasonic, or thermal scalpel. Monopolar cautery provides excellent hemostasis. Because the tongue is highly vascular, excessive cautery can muddle margin analysis of malignant and premalignant margins. In patients where monopolar cautery is not advised, such as patients with cochlear implants or defibrillators, a combination of cold steel and bipolar cautery can be used. The CO_2 laser may also be utilized for its advantage in margin interpretation due to its limited collateral tissue damage.

The surgical technique combines visual and haptic feedback. Manually handling the specimen helps gauge tumor depth and improves the likelihood of a negative deep muscle margin. Once exposure and traction are obtained, 1–2 cm mucosal margin incisions are made down to the muscle. The anterior cuts are generally made first because the more anterior margins are the easiest to gauge. Making posterior cuts early, if feasible, may be considered because blood trickling from the front of the mouth may obscure the posterior cuts.

Placement of a second traction suture on the specimen adds another vector of counter traction (Fig. 15.9). With the specimen in hand, muscular incisions are made to recruit normal tissue onto the deep margin. Good hemostasis and adequate margins are of vast importance during the muscular dissection. Ventral margins may extend onto the floor of the mouth, and contents of the sublingual compartment may need to be recruited into the specimen for a cancer-free deep margin. As the specimen is being excised, there is usually improved mobility of the specimen. Forward traction on both the tongue and specimen facilitates the posterior mucosal cuts, which should also be made with at least 1 cm margins in the case of cancer. The deep tongue muscle dissection can be joined by the posterior mucosal cuts to deliver

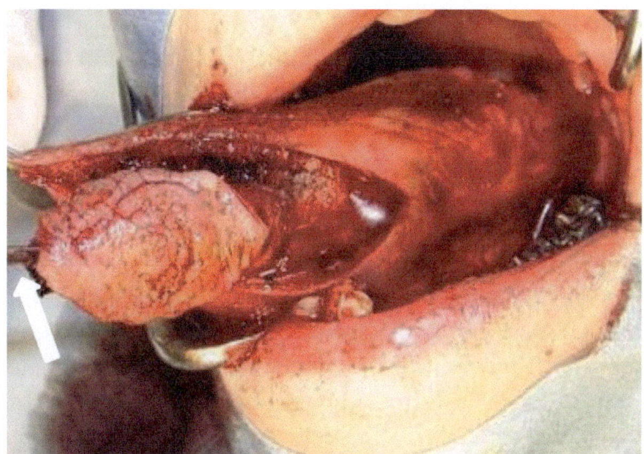

Fig. 15.9 Traction of the lesion (arrow) to facilitate its dissection from the normal tongue tissue

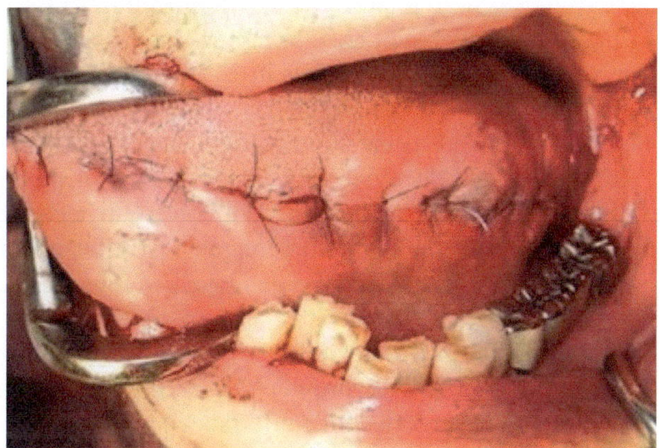

Fig. 15.10 Primary closure of the defect for reconstruction of the tongue

an en bloc specimen. Mucosal and deep muscle margins are sent for intraoperative histological margin analysis.

Depending on the amount of the tongue removed, the tongue can be closed primarily (Fig. 15.10), left to heal by secondary intention, or reconstructed.

15.6.2 Glossectomy via Transoral Robotic-Assisted Surgery (TORS)

Transoral robotic surgery (TORS) is a modern surgical technique used to treat tumors of the mouth and throat via direct access through the mouth. In "TORS," the surgeon uses a surgical robot to view and access structures in the oral cavity (mouth) and pharynx (back of the throat) without any incisions through the neck, chin, or lip that are necessary in traditional, nonrobotic approaches. Current "TORS" procedures include hemiglossectomy and other procedures such as radical tonsillectomy, resection of palate and base of skull tumors, and resection of tumors above and involving the larynx [32].

15.6.2.1 History

The use of TORS started in animal models in 2003. It was first applied in humans in 2005 for vallecula cyst [33]. In 2006, O'Malley and colleagues published the first three cases of tumor of the base of the tongue excised by TORS [34]. They demonstrated that the da Vinci robot provided excellent visualization and enabled transoral removal of the tumor while preserving key structures and nerves. In addition, they showed that it further allowed a complete resection with negative surgical margins and without complications.

Over the following several years, numerous studies demonstrated the efficacy and safety of the TORS technique [29, 34–41]. These studies proved the efficacy of the TORS procedures for cancer cure, without the potentially disastrous complications of the established otolaryngological techniques of open surgical resection and conventional endoscopic surgery. TORS resulted in cancer cure with less operating time, blood loss, and complication frequency. In light of this data, the FDA approved the da Vinci system to perform TORS procedures in 2009 [42, 43].

In 2013, Mercante et al. [28] reported a global time of TORS of 95 min for the resection of tongue base lesions in 13 consecutive patients. The mean hospital stay was 9 days ranging from 3 to 30 days in a patient submitted to excision of the tongue base and extended to the supraglottis. Thaler and colleagues, at the University of Pennsylvania, conducted a research that was published in 2016, on the applications of the TORS approach to patients with obstructive sleep apnea. They reported that a multilevel approach, including tongue resection and uvulopalatopharyngoplasty, increased airway space and oxygen levels in most cases [44].

15.6.2.2 Indications

The procedure of TORS provides an excellent alternative to chemoradiation and traditional open surgeries for some cancers of the mouth, throat, larynx, and base of the skull. Chemotherapy and radiation therapy are associated with long-term, potentially harmful toxicities, and open surgeries are highly invasive and prone to serious complications and extended hospital stays. TORS avoids these issues by avoiding the external incisions and reducing surgical time, both of which are associated with increased blood loss and infection [34].

One of the most common tumors arising in the base of the tongue (BOT) is squamous cell carcinoma (SCC); however, the differential diagnosis is broad and includes lymphoma, infections such as tuberculosis, granular cell tumors, salivary gland tumors (both benign and malignant), rhabdomyosarcoma, and metastatic disease [45]. In addition, benign processes such as ectopic lingual thyroid [46], ectopic gastric mucosa [47], and schwannomas must be considered. Surgery as a primary modality is an effective treatment for many of these benign and malignant processes. Numerous studies have repeatedly shown TORS to be both safe and effective in treating malignant and benign tumors of the head and neck [48, 49].

15.6.2.3 Operative Technique

To begin a "TORS" procedure, the patient is anesthetized in the supine position. A retractor is used to open the mouth to create room for the robotic camera and surgical instruments. The da Vinci patient-side cart is then brought to the bedside, and the robotic instruments and camera are guided into the patient's mouth. Once the operation begins, the surgeon sits at the surgeon's console and views the patient's throat through a three-dimensional view finder. As the surgeon manipulates the instrument controls, the robotic instruments move deep inside the patient's mouth and the operation performed. Resection of tissue and suturing are accomplished with the advantages of the surgical robot at the back of the pharynx. Variations in the TORS technique are due to the location of the cancer or obstruction and to the surgeon's preference.

15.6.2.4 Outcome of TORS as a Cancer Treatment

To date, the largest study of TORS as a cancer treatment included data from 410 patients. This study demonstrated 91.8% 2-year locoregional control of the cancer and 94.5% 2-year disease-specific survival. These numbers are similar to those of other head and neck cancer treatment options [48]. A separate study of 62 patients reported that 69% resumed oral intake prior to discharge and 83% within 2 weeks [50].

15.6.2.5 Complications

Many studies have evaluated TORS patient outcomes and have found complications in 10–25% of cases. Most of these are minor, including dehydration, tooth injury, bleeding, dysphagia, dysgeusia, and uncontrolled pain. Fewer patients develop major complications, which include hemorrhage, deep venous thrombosis, pneumonia, pulmonary embolism, or death [42, 51, 52].

15.6.2.6 Current Challenges

Despite being a relatively novel procedure, the application of TORS has increased in recent years as a consequence of advances in technology and surgical techniques. However, many obstacles have slowed the propagation of TORS. Firstly, the cost of instrumentation has a significant impact on the justification of its use in some cases, as well as the accessibility to the robotic system, as it is often shared with more than one surgical specialty [53]. Equally, the lack of dedicated equipment for head and neck surgery can hinder the progress from traditional to robotic surgery. Finally, the use of a robotic approach can cause prolongation of surgical time, especially with the setup and the docking phase of surgery, although data has shown that its impact is minimal on the total operation time and that with experience it can be reduced significantly [54]. However, at the moment, robotic surgery is widely used, and its application in head and neck oncological field is widely documented and described, though its impact on the treatment of benign tumors and functional disorders has not yet been clearly defined.

15.6.3 Transoral Laser Surgery (TOLS)/Transoral Laser Microsurgery (TLM)

Transoral CO_2 laser microsurgery (TLM) was originally introduced by Strong and Jako for the treatment of small laryngeal lesions [55]. It was developed further by Steiner et al. [56, 57] and Canis et al. [58–61] to be used for the treatment of small and large tumors in multiple regions of the upper aerodigestive tract including the base of the tongue (BOT).

15.6.3.1 Indications

Transoral laser microsurgery is a form of minimally invasive surgery used to remove small- and medium-sized tumors through the mouth. It can be selectively used for larger tumors. Transoral laser microsurgery allows surgeons to remove tumors from the larynx and oropharynx with no external incisions and is especially applied to human papilloma virus (HPV)-mediated oropharynx malignancy (tonsils, base of the tongue). It also allows access to tumors that are not reachable with robotic surgery and is significantly conserving of normal tissue.

15.6.3.2 Contraindications

For functional or technical reasons, contraindications of TLM include (1) extensive spread with involvement of the Eustachian tube or invasion of the carotid sheath; (2) insufficient tumor was accessed, for example, when there is extensive vertebral fixation or trismus; (3) multiple primary synchronous malignant tumors; (4) N3 neck disease; (5) simultaneous distant metastases; and (6) recurrent disease of oropharyngeal malignancies. It is noteworthy that "age" is not a contraindication to surgery with curative intent [62].

15.6.3.3 Operative Technique [56, 63, 64]

A microscope helps the surgeon clearly view the deep and perimeter margins of the tumor, ensuring complete clearance of the tumor and minimizing the amount of normal tissue removed or damaged during surgery. TLM is performed with a CO_2 laser in a continuous super-pulse mode. The CO_2 laser is used for removing the tumor with high precision so that the pathologist can evaluate the margin status at the edge of the surgical specimen. The laser leaves a particularly "light" surgical foot print in the patient's throat tissues. This technique helps give the patient as much speech and swallowing function as possible after surgery [65–69].

TLM involves a step-by-step resection with cutting through the tumor, if necessary, allowing the surgeon to inspect the boundary between normal and abnormal tissue under magnification more accurately compared to conventional surgery. Thus, the surgeon preserves as much healthy tissue as possible and inspects the depth of tumor invasion intraoperatively.

Optimal visualization is achieved using different tongue depressors, retractors, or closed and distending laryngo-pharyngoscopes. Protrusion of the tongue base into the line of vision can be prevented by using a distending pharyngoscope with lateral wings. Furthermore, the differentiation between tumor and healthy tissue is possible by evaluating the lasers' cutting characteristics (e.g., carbonization) under microscopic magnification.

An appropriate resection margin of at least 5–10 mm can be maintained to ensure R0 resection status by frozen section analysis. Evaluation of frozen sections required particular attention at the tongue base, since the lingual tonsil tissue makes intraoperative differentiation between tumor and healthy tissue more difficult. Here, not only tumor tissue but also normal tissue will show increased carbonization as a result of the high tissue density, lymphatic tissue, and fibrosis. One advantage of TLM is that it can be easily repeated if inadequate resection margins are found postoperatively [70].

If the patient has extended local disease (cT3-4a), the tumor infiltration depth exceeds 3 mm, or if preoperative imaging reveals suspicious lymph nodes (LNs), a neck dissection (ND) is performed. In cN0 cases, it is done as a selective ND including levels II–IV. In cN+ cases, a selective ND with levels II–IV is performed. Bilateral NDs are carried out if imaging reveals suspicious LNs bilaterally or the primary tumor had an advanced stage with midline localization.

15.6.3.4 Complications

One advantage of TLM is the low complication rate. Weiss et al. [62] conducted research on 368 patients (249 men (80.4%) and 72 women (19.6%)) who underwent elective TLM for SCC of the oropharynx at the Department of Otorhinolaryngology, Head and Neck Surgery, University Medical Center Göttingen, between October 1986 and October 2015. Eighty-nine patients (24%) had their lesion at the base of the tongue (BOT). They reported that the most common complication was postoperative bleeding, which occurred in 11% ($n = 42$) of their series. The majority of cases of postoperative hemorrhage are usually managed by transoral electrocautery or clipping [62, 68, 71, 72]. Large tumors (T3-T4) have a significant higher risk for complications [73] reaching up to 65.9% [62].

15.6.4 Glossectomy via Lip-Split Mandibulotomy

The lip-split mandibulotomy (mandibular swing) combines the transoral glossectomy technique with a sagittal mandibular osteotomy. While the transoral glossectomy can be thought of as a "bird's eye" view of the tumor, the mandibulotomy provides a more "head-on" view of the depth of the tumor. It provides excellent access to the sublingual and submental compartments, as well as the supra-hyoid tongue musculature. It also allows inferior displacement of the tongue for a wide view of the posterior tongue and pharynx. Though this approach offers the best overall exposure of the tongue, it requires additional steps that increase the risk of complications.

15.6.4.1 Indications and Contraindications

This approach is *indicated* in patients with (1) severe trismus, (2) complicated anatomy, (3) deeply invasive tumors, and (4) tumors that are intimately related to the carotid vasculature. Lip-split mandibulotomy allows the surgeon to appreciate the extent of the tumor by palpation and visualization, allows excellent access to the head and neck vasculature for control of bleeding, and allows the surgeon wide access to the surgical defect for placement of reconstructive flaps.

Although most patients recover without significant cosmetic deformity, this procedure is largely *contraindicated* in patients who are concerned with cosmetic outcome. In addition, mandibulotomy is not recommended for those patients with poor wound healing owing to risk of wound breakdown, infection, and mandibular nonunion. These clinical conditions can include uncontrolled diabetes mellites, a history of radiation therapy, or immunosuppression. In addition, this procedure should be reserved for cases that need wide exposure, and therefore, it is not suitable for small BOT lesions that are accessible through less-invasive techniques [74].

15.6.4.2 Operative Technique [74]

In order to ensure adequate ventilation of the patient both intraoperatively and postoperatively and to allow unencumbered visualization and access to the surgical field, a *tracheotomy* is performed at the beginning of the operation. A 3-cm horizontal incision is made just inferior to the cricoid cartilage. Dissection is carried down to the strap muscles. The paired muscles are divided in the midline and retracted laterally. The thyroid isthmus is exposed and either retracted superiorly or divided and suture ligated.

An inferiorly based flap (Björk flap) of the second or third tracheal ring is created and sutured to the overlaying skin. The previously placed endotracheal tube is removed, and a reinforced endotracheal tube is placed into the tracheotomy site and secured, and further ventilation is carried out through this tube.

The technique requires trans-cervical mandibular exposure and a trans-facial lip-split. As neck dissection is usually performed with this procedure, the neck dissection incision can be extended superiorly from the midline to the lip. A mucosal lip incision is made approximately 1 cm anterior to the gingiva to provide a cuff of tissue sufficient for closure. The incision is extended along the mucosal lip in the sagittal plane between the central incisors for a median mandibulotomy (or between the lateral incisor and the canine for a paramedian mandibulotomy). It is extended anteriorly toward the cutaneous lip, through the vermillion border. The labial artery is usually encountered in the process and is clipped or cauterized. Though the incision can be extended along the midline through the chin (Fig. 15.11), it is preferable to place the incision along the semicircular contour of the chin subunit (Fig. 15.12). Muscular cuts are made through the orbicularis oris, mentalis, and the lip depressors, onto the periosteum of the mandible.

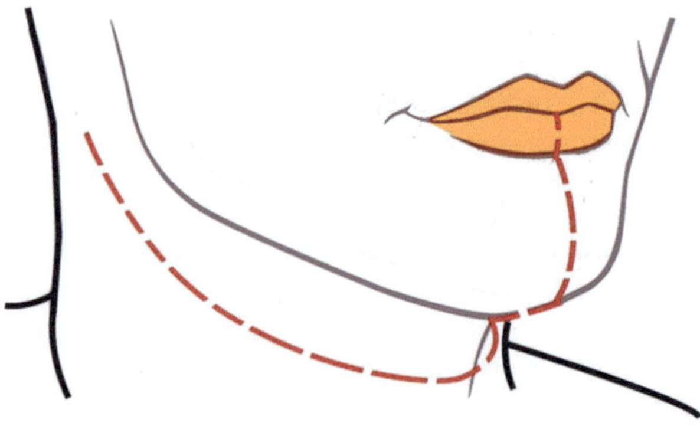

Fig. 15.11 The labial incision is extended along the midline through the chin

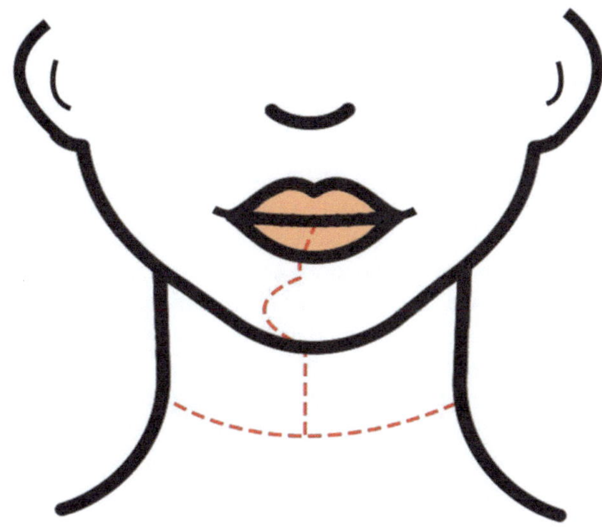

Fig. 15.12 Incision placed along the semicircular contour of the chin subunit (better cosmetically than extending the incision from the midline of the chin)

Gingival cuts are then made. Management of the central incisors is at the surgeon's discretion. If not extracted, the roots are at risk of exposure or being dislodged from their periodontal ligament during the sagittal osteotomy. A 15-blade is best for making the gingival cuts between the central incisors. It preserves the most mucosa and does not transmit unintended heat damage that could occur with monopolar cautery. It is often the case, especially in radiated tissue, that monopolar cautery use at this step ablates the gingival tissue, leaving a tissue gap, and increases the risk of a salivary fistula.

Ipsilateral or bilateral neck dissection is then performed, as indicated, before proceeding to mandibulotomy. Dissection of level I lymph nodes of the neck on the side of the tumor and skeletonization of the digastric muscle, mylohyoid muscle, lingual and hypoglossal nerves, and lingual artery on this side facilitate the mandibulotomy approach. The ipsilateral lingual artery is ligated in the neck. It is imperative to preserve the contralateral lingual artery and hypoglossal nerve if the patient is to maintain speech and swallowing function postoperatively.

The flaps over the mandible are then elevated in the subperiosteal plane to expose the bone. Subperiosteal dissection need only to provide enough exposure to place a fixation plate across the osteotomy.

In cases of prior head and neck irradiation, a conservative periosteal elevation is best to reduce the risk of osteonecrosis of the jaw. If exposure beyond the canines is needed, care should be taken to avoid damage to the mental nerve as it exits the mental foramen. At this point, it is advisable to place a reconstruction plate on the inferior border of the mandible while it is in continuity. The plate is contoured, and the drill holes and screws are placed. The plate is then removed, oriented, and stored with the screws until the mandible needs to be fixated. Sagittal osteotomy is then performed. The mandible is splayed open, and the mylohyoid muscle between the mandibular segments can be appreciated. If the muscle is involved with tumor, it should be excised to a negative margin. Myotomy of the mylohyoid completely releases the mandible segments from one another, further improving exposure. The oncological advantages of this approach are apparent at this step of the procedure; the ability to appreciate the depth of the tumor and a tremendous transoral/trans-cervical exposure.

Glossectomy can be performed with the ability to not only pull the tongue anteriorly out of the mouth but to also pull the specimen inferiorly into the neck to view the posterior cuts. The margins should be sent for intraoperative histological analysis. Tumors that extend along the floor of the mouth may be adherent to the mandible as shown by physical examination and imaging. Instead of a midline mandibulotomy, segmental mandibulectomy of the involved bone by the trans-cervical approach is another technique for completing the primary resection. Subplatysmal flaps are elevated beyond the mandible. The marginal mandibular branch of the facial nerve is identified and safely retracted. The soft tissue over planned osteotomies is ablated down to the cortical bone. Bone cuts are made, and the released bone can be retracted to provide additional exposure and an additional traction vector for combined transoral/trans-cervical resection of the primary tumor.

Glossectomies warranting mandibulotomy/mandibulectomy will usually require soft tissue and mandibular reconstruction. Soft tissue is reconstructed with either a loco-regional flap or free tissue transfer. Resected bone is reconstructed with a free bone graft or vascularized osseous-free tissue transfer. Reduction and internal fixation can be made with mandibular plates or lag screws. Closure is completed by closing the entire soft tissue defect in a watertight fashion with resorbable mattress sutures, fixing the mandible, and closing the lip wound meticulously with mucosal, muscle, and skin stitches. The neck wounds are closed over suction drains.

15.6.4.3 Complications

Mandibulotomy commonly involves perioperative edema and prolonged healing time that can delay return to speech and swallowing for several weeks. Complications of mandibulotomy include cosmetic defects of the skin of the neck, lip, and chin. These can be minimized with meticulous closure technique, careful approximation of the orbicularis muscle and vermillion–cutaneous junction, and appropriate choice of sutures. Patients are frequently worried about the cosmesis of the procedure, but cosmetic results are commonly acceptable. Malocclusion, loss of dentition, and mastication problems can occur. The incidence of these can be minimized with careful operative planning, execution, and careful plating of the mandibulotomy defect [74].

Mandibulotomy coupled with postoperative radiotherapy can result in malunion of the mandibulotomy site, hardware exposure, and osteonecrosis around the mandibulotomy site. These are the most troublesome complications of mandibulotomy that can occur years after the procedure, and sometimes require hardware removal or replacement, or even mandibular vascularized reconstruction. Because these bony complications can be difficult to repair, some surgeons avoid the approach. A compromise that will allow adequate exposure without sacrificing the mandible is the "trans-cervical pull-through" technique [74].

15.6.5 Glossectomy via Trans-Cervical Pull-Through with Visor Incision

Though mandibulotomy provides excellent exposure, the added steps of the lip-split, osteotomy, and mandibular fixation compound risks of postoperative complications. Head and neck cancer patients with hypothyroidism, diabetes mellites, or previous irradiation experience have an increased risk of fistula formation, wound dehiscence, and delayed wound healing. Mandibular osteoradionecrosis is another risk in previously irradiated head and neck patients.

Glossectomy via trans-cervical pull-through is an alternative resection technique to transoral glossectomy and the lip-split mandibulotomy. It is a combined transoral/trans-cervical technique, whereby the tongue, floor of the mouth, and the sublingual compartment are released through the submental and submandibular compartments into the neck. Compared to transoral glossectomy alone, this approach provides better exposure for a posterior resection. Transoral glossectomy can be converted to a pull-through without adding a significant length of time to the procedure. The exposure is not as wide as the lip-split mandibulotomy. It does not require a mandibular osteotomy and thus avoids the added procedure time for mandibular reconstruction and its associated complications. Flap inset requires thoughtful and disciplined closure to reduce the risk of a postoperative fistula.

15.6.5.1 Indications and Contraindications

The pull-through technique is *indicated* for large tumors of the BOT when the surgeon needs wide exposure but does not want to split the mandible or lip. The visor incision can be cosmetically preferable to the lip-split incision and may be preferable in younger patients or patients with high cosmetic demands who require extensive BOT surgery. Partial pull-through can be performed for unilateral resections, whereas bilateral pull-through can be performed for larger tumors that cross the midline or when total glossectomy is to be performed. The technique is *contraindicated* in smaller tumors when transoral resection will suffice or when the patient is not tolerant of tracheostomy placement.

15.6.5.2 Operative Technique [74]

As in the mandibulotomy approach, the procedure is initiated with tracheostomy, followed by a bilateral horizontal mid neck incision, ideally placed in a horizontal neck rhytid (Fig. 15.13). It is carried through skin and subcutaneous tissues and platysma muscle, and flaps are raised superiorly and inferiorly in a subplatysmal plane to expose the entire neck.

The superior flap is raised in the subplatysmal plane up to the submandibular level. The marginal mandibular branch of the facial nerve is identified bilaterally, released inferiorly, and retracted superior to the mandibular border in order to avoid injury during the resection. The facial arteries and veins are divided beneath the mandibular notches, and the mental nerve is divided if this step is part of the planned resection. The flaps are then raised deep to the marginal nerves and superior vessels above the mandibular border. Care should be taken to avoid undue tension of or

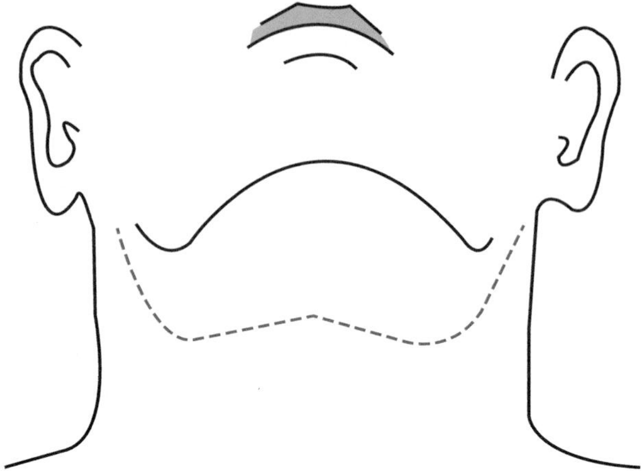

Fig. 15.13 The neck incision is carried out in a mid-neck crease from mastoid tip to mastoid tip

injury to the mental nerve on the contralateral side during elevation of the flap. The flap is secured in a superior position.

Neck dissection is then carried out as appropriate. The mylohyoid and digastric muscles are released from the mandible, followed by the genioglossus muscles. Intra-oral mucosal cuts are then performed transorally with cautery along the lingual surface of the mandible, taking care to preserve a mucosal cuff of the tissues along the inner surface of the mandible to allow for closure. Continuing the cuts up to the retromolar trigone and into the tonsillar fossa and pharynx allows for enough mobility of the tongue so that it can be dropped beneath the mandible and visualized in the neck. The surgeon can then proceed with tumor removal by making cautery cuts through the tongue mucosa, intrinsic muscles, and extrinsic muscles, as necessary. The tumor should be kept in view and be available for palpation during extirpation to prevent violation. As with other tongue resections, generous margins of normal tissue (1–1.5 cm) confirmed by frozen-section pathology ensure complete tumor extirpation.

After tumor removal, closure begins by first thoroughly irrigating the tongue surface and neck and ensuring hemostasis. A nasogastric feeding tube should be placed and the tongue returned to its native position. A watertight closure of the mucosal edges by meticulous placement of resorbable vertical mattress sutures (e.g., 3-0 Vicryl) is performed. This is essential to avoid an orocutaneous fistulae and subsequent infection at the surgical site. Care must be taken during closure to avoid injury to the vascular pedicle which may be traversing the defect. The mouth is then irrigated with inspection of the neck to assess for leak, and any leaks are repaired either with transoral or trans-cervical placement of sutures. Closure with a soft tissue flap may be necessary, depending on the extent of resection. The genioglossus and mylohyoid muscles may be reapproximated, and then the neck is closed over suction drains (e.g., Jackson-Pratt drains) brought out through stab incisions in the skin. If a vascularized flap has been used for reconstruction, the drains must be placed as so as to not overlay the vascular pedicle of the flap.

The neck is closed in layers. The platysma muscle and deep dermis are closed with resorbable interrupted sutures in a buried fashion. The skin is closed with a fine (e.g., 5/0) running resorbable or non-resorbable suture [74].

15.6.5.3 Complications

The tongue pull-through technique can be associated with *fistula formation*. However, this can be prevented with meticulous preservation of mucosal tissue, atraumatic and meticulous technique of resection, and careful closure. In patients who have been previously treated, are malnourished, or have severe comorbidities, delayed healing, and mandible, *exposure* can occur, requiring soft tissue-vascularized flaps for reconstruction. *Dysarthria and dysphagia* can also occur. Preservation of one lingual artery and one hypoglossal nerve is essential, and preservation of both hypoglossal nerves and lingual arteries is preferable, to maximize speech and swallowing function. However, oncological resection should never be compromised for this purpose. *Ranulas* can also occur after this procedure but can be minimized by removal of the sublingual glands and submandibular glands ipsilateral to the tumor and more extensive surgical resection [74].

15.7 Complications/Risks of Glossectomy

The risks for glossectomy include those pertinent to most surgical head and neck procedures, including pain, bleeding, infection, healing disorders, injury to nearby structures, and the need for future procedures. Risks of *general anesthesia*, including cardiopulmonary event, stroke, and death, though remote, must also be considered and discussed with the patient. Discussion about *procedure-specific risks* to speech and swallow function is essential in counseling patients. Varying degrees of dysarthria and difficulties with speech or are almost guaranteed with every glossectomy. The long-term functional outcomes may also vary [75].

The smaller the region of the removed tongue, the lesser the chance of many of these complications to be encountered especially difficulty with speaking and swallowing. The location of the tongue lesion is also of vast importance. Complications associated with transoral resection of the "base of the tongue" (BOT) lesions can be divided into minor and major categories. *Minor complications* include altered taste, chipped teeth, odynophagia, trismus, dysphagia, and otalgia. Occurrence of such complications may be minimized by taking care to preserve uninvolved neurovascular structures and choosing instruments that decrease injury to adjacent normal tissue. *Major complications* include postoperative intraoral hemorrhage, hematoma, airway compromise, urgent or emergent tracheostomy, and aspiration pneumonia. The risk of *perioperative death* is rarely reported in current series and may be minimized by appropriately selecting surgical patients [30, 36, 76].

15.7.1 Bleeding/Hematoma

Although rare, the occurrence of life-threatening oropharyngeal hemorrhage in the postoperative period has been reported. Identifying and ligating the ipsilateral facial and lingual arteries during neck dissection are recommended to decrease this risk. In addition, taking care to identify and properly clip the dorsal lingual artery transorally is important and often required for large tongue resections. If bleeding after the procedure is severe, surgical intervention for hemostasis is required. However, some mild bleeding or small hematomas can be observed [74].

The development of hematomas may be avoided by meticulous hemostasis; however, even the most careful surgeon may experience this complication. Recommended management involves returning to the operating room for evacuation of the blood clot and hemostasis, although bleeding vessels are rarely found.

15.7.2 Infection

Because the tongue has a very good blood supply, infections of the tongue are quite rare. Still, as with any surgical procedure, there is always a risk of an infection after the surgery, particularly if glossectomy is associated with additional procedures that might connect the mouth with the neck. This might require antibiotics and/or drainage of the infection.

15.7.3 Dysarthria (Difficult Speech) and Dysphagia

The extent that a patient's speech or swallowing is affected will depend on how much and what part of the tongue is removed. Dysarthria and dysphagia are secondary to the loss of intrinsic and extrinsic muscles that shape and position the tongue. Even with shallow partial glossectomy, patients may experience some degree of dysarthria secondary to postoperative changes to their tongue. Flaps used to reconstruct the tongue do not have volitional movement, and thus postoperative tongue function is influenced by the residual tongue musculature and bulk [77]. Changes in speech and swallowing may also be secondary to the *sequelae of healing*. In cases of primary closure, tongue tethering may occur and limit the freedom of movement. Even in cases of healing by secondary intention, tongue tethering can occur from unanticipated annealing of open surfaces to one another.

Careful attention to the location of the hypoglossal nerve during surgery is critical to preserve the function of the remainder of the tongue in order to optimize speech and swallowing outcomes. Rehabilitation and speech therapy may play a role in optimizing post-glossectomy functional outcomes [78].

15.7.4 Alteration of Tongue Sensation

An altered sensation of the tongue is another inevitable complication. Patients may experience neuropathic or phantom sensation from the soft tissue resection. Sensory changes can also be secondary to lingual nerve trauma during glossectomy or neck dissection. In cases where there is more significant tongue resection, sensory changes are more secondary to loss of the sensory input and from the sacrifice of the lingual nerve. In reconstructive cases with regional flaps or free tissue transfer, the reconstructive substrate is commonly non-sensate, and if the tissue used contains muscle, the muscle cannot be used in any meaningful way to restore motor function. Some institutions perform reinnervated free flap reconstructions, which provide sensation, with the exception of taste sensation taste [79]. In cases where the tongue base is resected and reconstructed, the altered sensation combined with the loss of functional tongue muscle can result in aspiration, making the patient dependent on tube feeds.

Patients commonly ask about altered taste. It is a myth that the tongue has specific topography concerning taste. All five taste senses are represented throughout the tongue. Higher acuity taste is facilitated by olfaction via retrograde airflow to the nasal cavity, which should be unaffected by glossectomy.

15.7.5 Aspiration

Aspiration occurs when a patient breathes a foreign substance, often saliva and/or food and drinks, into their airway. Having saliva and/or food and drink pass into the lungs can lead to pneumonia. Patients with large resections and reconstructions are at higher risk for this problem. Patients who develop a cough associated with eating or drinking should be suspected of having aspiration, which should be evaluated with a modified barium swallow. If this problem is identified and cannot be overcome with therapy, then a feeding tube may need to be placed through the nose or directly into the stomach.

15.7.6 Urgent or Emergent Tracheostomy

Unplanned tracheostomy can be limited by carefully examining the patient after surgical resection and performing planned tracheostomy or delaying extubation to allow abatement of the associated edema. One of the reported benefits of transoral resection of BOT tumors is the low tracheostomy and gastrostomy tube dependence rates reported in the literature [30, 80].

15.7.7 Salivary (Oro-cutaneous) Fistula

Salivary fistula means the "leakage of saliva from the mouth or pharynx into the neck." It occurs when the oral cavity is continuous with the deep neck space. It tends to occur between the floor of the mouth and the submandibular triangle. The loss of the submandibular gland and the vascularized fascia creates a direct communication between the oral cavity and the neck through the floor of the mouth. It can also happen at the site of the sagittal-split osteotomy. The chances of this complication increase if a patient has had previous treatment including radiation and/or chemotherapy, both of which impair the healing process.

In the setting of primary surgery, these wounds tend to heal or can be assisted with some local tissue rearrangement. However, salvage surgery after radiation is prevalent and leaves the operative bed with altered vascularity and impaired healing [81]. Vascularized tissue transfers have become the standard and greatly decrease the risk of fistula, even in the setting of prior radiation.

Although persistent fistula is rare, prompt recognition and management by placing a feeding tube, eliminating oral intake, and performing local wound cares can prevent acute complications and long-term functional debility [82].

15.7.8 Osteoradionecrosis

For patients undergoing lip-split mandibulotomy, there are increased risks specific to the osteotomy performed, including osteoradionecrosis of the mandible, malocclusion, and hardware complications. Osteoradionecrosis is a radiation injury resulting in the devitalized bone. If the patient develops osteoradionecrosis, they may require secondary resection and reconstruction.

15.7.9 Positive Margins

Another risk with surgery is positive margins and recurrences. Positive margins can make wound closure impossible as the reconstruction might not heal to cancer on the inset margins. The risk of salivary fistula and chronic, nonhealing wounds is almost certain in that scenario. Persistent cancer should always be on the differential in a chronic, nonhealing wound.

Even if surgery results in a microscopically negative margin resection and the wound heals, surveillance should still be complicated. In cases of transoral glossectomy without reconstruction, scar tissue from primary and secondary closure may make it difficult to survey for local recurrences, which may result in future procedures coupled with anxiety for the patient and uncertainty for the oncologists shriveling the patient.

15.7.10 Recurrence

Advanced tongue SCCs are at a significantly higher risk of developing loco-regional recurrence [83]. Patients with recurrent disease are candidates for salvage therapy by surgery, additional chemotherapy, and RT depending on the primary therapy administered. There is some evidence that surgical salvage may offer a slight outcome advantage compared to other modalities such as RT and chemotherapy. Despite the type of salvage therapy, survival outcomes in this patient population are somewhat dismal and have been reported to range between approximately 15 and 35% at 5 years [84]. Patients should be cautiously counseled regarding the morbidity of salvage therapy and the limited chance for cure prior to initiating salvage therapy for recurrent advanced stage oral cavity SCC.

References

1. Péri G. Technique of glossectomy (author's transl). Rev Stomatol Chir Maxillofac. 1978;79:335–7.
2. Balaji SM. Reduction glossectomy for large tongues. Ann Maxillofac Surg. 2013;3:167–72.
3. Sigal R, Zagdanski AM, Schwaab G, Bosq J, Auperin A, Laplanche A, et al. CT and MR imaging of squamous cell carcinoma of the tongue and floor of the mouth. Radiographics. 1996;16:787–810.
4. Royster HP, Lehr HB, Raventos A, Demuth WE. Management of patients with squamous cell carcinoma of the tongue. Ann Surg. 1961;154:563–72.
5. Calabrese L, Tagliabue M, Maffini F, Massaro MA, Santoro L. From wide excision to a compartmental approach in tongue tumors: what is going on? Curr Opin Otolaryngol Head Neck Surg. 2013;21:112–7.
6. Yuen PW, Lam KY, Chan AC, Wei WI, Lam LK. Clinicopathological analysis of local spread of carcinoma of the tongue. Am J Surg. 1998;175:242–4.
7. Jardim JF, Francisco AL, Gondak R, Damascena A, Kowalski LP. Prognostic impact of perineural invasion and lymphovascular invasion in advanced stage oral squamous cell carcinoma. Int J Oral Maxillofac Surg. 2015;44:23–8.
8. Zanoni DK, Migliacci JC, Xu B, Katabi N, et al. A proposal to redefine close surgical margins in squamous cell carcinoma of the oral tongue. JAMA Otolaryngol Head Neck Surg. 2017;143:555–60.
9. Bradley PJ, MacLennan K, Brakenhoff RH, Leemans CR. Status of primary tumour surgical margins in squamous head and neck cancer: prognostic implications. Curr Opin Otolaryngol Head Neck Surg. 2007;15:74–81.
10. Piazza C, Montalto N, Paderno A, Taglietti V, Nicolai P. Is it time to incorporate 'depth of infiltration' in the T staging of oral tongue and floor of mouth cancer? Curr Opin Otolaryngol Head Neck Surg. 2014;22:81–9.
11. Junn JC, Baugnon KL, Lacayo EA, Hudgins PA, Patel MR, Magliocca KR, et al. CT accuracy of extrinsic tongue muscle invasion in oral cavity cancer. AJNR Am J Neuroradiol. 2017;38:364–70.
12. Prince S, Bailey BM. Squamous carcinoma of the tongue: review. Br J Oral Maxillofac Surg. 1999;37:164–74.
13. Goel V, Parihar PS, Parihar A, Goel AK, Waghani K, Gupta R, et al. Accuracy of MRI in prediction of tumour thickness and nodal stage in Oral tongue and gingivobuccal cancer with clinical correlation and staging. J Clin Diagn Res. 2016;10:TC01–5.
14. Alsaffar HA, Goldstein DP, King EV, de Almeida JR, Brown DH, Gilbert RW, et al. Correlation between clinical and MRI assessment of depth of invasion in oral tongue squamous cell carcinoma. J Otolaryngol Head Neck Surg. 2016;45:61–5.
15. Amin MB, Edge SB, Greene FL, Byrd DR, Brookland RK, Washington MK, et al., editors. AJCC cancer staging manual. 8th ed. New York, NY: Springer; 2017.
16. Murthy SP, Thankappan K, Jayasankaran SC, Milind K, Prasad C, Balasubramnian D, et al. Deep extrinsic muscle involvement is a Fallacy in the American Joint Committee on Cancer's Seventh Edition of Tumor Staging of Oral Cavity Cancers. J Oral Maxillofac Surg. 2018;76:206–12.

17. Glastonbury CM, Mukherji SK, O'Sullivan B, Lydiatt WM. Setting the stage for 2018: how the changes in the American joint committee on cancer/Union for International Cancer Control cancer staging manual eighth edition impact radiologists. AJNR Am J Neuroradiol. 2017;38:2231–7.
18. Calabrese L, Giugliano G, Bruschini R, Ansarin M, Navach V, Grosso R, et al. Compartmental surgery in tongue tumours: description of a new surgical technique. Acta Otorhinolaryngol Ital. 2009;29:259–64.
19. Calabrese L, Bruschini R, Giugliano G, Ostuni A, Maffini F, Massaro MA, et al. Compartmental tongue surgery: long term oncologic results in the treatment of tongue cancer. Oral Oncol. 2011;47:174–9.
20. Sessions DG, Spector GJ, Lenox J, Haughey B, Chao C, Marks J. Analysis of treatment results for oral tongue cancer. Laryngoscope. 2002;112:616–25.
21. Omura K. Current status of oral cancer treatment strategies: surgical treatments for oral squamous cell carcinoma. Int J Clin Oncol. 2014;19:423–30.
22. Haddadin KJ, Soutar DS, Webster MH, Robertson AG, Oliver RJ, MacDonald DG. Natural history and patterns of recurrence of tongue tumours. Br J Plast Surg. 2000;53:279–85.
23. Pimenta Amaral TM, Da Silva Freire AR, Carvalho AL, Pinto CA, Kowalski LP. Predictive factors of occult metastasis and prognosis of clinical stages I and II squamous cell carcinoma of the tongue and floor of the mouth. Oral Oncol. 2004;40:780–6.
24. Ansari M, Bruschini R, Navach V, Giugliano G, Calabrese L, Chiesa F, Medina JE, Kowalski LP, Shah JP. Classification of glossectomies: proposal for tongue cancer resections. Head Neck. 2019;41(3):821–7.
25. Mannelli G, Arcuri F, Agostini T, Innocenti M, Raffaini M, Spinelli G. Classification of tongue cancer resection and treatment algorithm. J Surg Oncol. 2018;117(5):1092–9.
26. Suter VG, Altermatt HJ, Sendi P, Mettraux G, Bornstein MM. CO2 and diode laser for excisional biopsies of oral mucosal lesions. A pilot study evaluating clinical and histopathological parameters. Schweiz Monatsschr Zahnmed. 2010;120(8):664–71.
27. Myers LL, Sumer BD, Truelson JM, Ahn C, Leach JL. Resection and free tissue reconstruction of locally advanced oral cancer: avoidance of lip split. Microsurgery. 2011;31(5):347–52.
28. Mercante Ruscito P, Pellini R, Cristalli G, Spriano G. Trans-oral robotic surgery (TORS) for tongue base tumours. Acta Otorhinolaryngol Ital. 2013;33(4):230–5.
29. Weinstein GS, O'Malley BV, Hockstein NG. Transoral robotic surgery: supraglottic laryngectomy in canine model. Laryngoscope. 2005;115:1315–9.
30. Moore EJ, Olsen KD, Kasperbauer JL. Transoral robotic surgery for oropharyngeal squamous cell carcinoma: a prospective study of feasibility and functional outcomes. Laryngoscope. 2009;119:2156–64.
31. Moore EJ, Janus J, Kasperbauer J. Transoral robotic surgery of the oropharynx: clinical and anatomical considerations. Clin Anat. 2012;25:135–41.
32. Kwong FN, Puvanendran M, Paleri V. Transoral robotic surgery in head neck cancer management. B-ENT. 2015;11:7–13.
33. McLeod IK, Melder PC. DaVinci Robot assisted excision of a vallecular cyst: a case report. Ear Nose Throat J. 2005;84:170–2.
34. O'Malley BV, Weinstein GS, Sneyder W, et al. Tronsoral robotic surgery (TORS) for base of the tongue neoplasm. Laryngoscope. 2006;115:1465–72.
35. Hockstein NG, Weinstein GS, O'Malley Bert W Jr. Maintenance of hemostasis in transoral robotic surgery. ORL J Otorhinolaryngol Relat Spec. 2005;67(4):220–4.
36. O'Malley BW Jr, Weinstein GS, Hockstein NG. Transoral robotic surgery (TORS): glottic microsurgery in a canine model. J Voice. 2006;20(2):263–8.
37. Hockstein NG, O'Malley BW Jr, Weinstein GS. Assessment of intraoperative safety in transoral robotic surgery. Laryngoscope. 2006;116(2):165–8.
38. Weinstein GS, O'Malley BW Jr, Snyder W, Eric S, Quon H. Transoral robotic surgery: radical tonsillectomy. Arch Otolaryngol Head Neck Surg. 2007;133(12):1220–6.
39. O'Malley BW Jr, Weinstein GS. Robotic skull base surgery: preclinical investigations to human clinical application. Arch Otolaryngol Head Neck Surg. 2007;133(12):1215–9.

40. Solares CA, Strome M. Transoral robot-assisted CO2 laser supraglottic laryngectomy: experimental and clinical data. Laryngoscope. 2007;117(5):817–20.
41. Weinstein GS, O'Malley BW Jr, Snyder W, Hockstein NG. Transoral robotic surgery: supraglottic partial laryngectomy. Ann Otol Rhinol Laryngol. 2007;116(1):19–23.
42. Justin GA, Chang ET, Camacho M, Brietzke SE. Transoral robotic surgery for obstructive sleep apnea: a systematic review and meta-analysis. Otolaryngol Head Neck Surg. 2016;154(5):835–46.
43. Vicini C, Dallan I, Canzi P, Frassineti S, La Pietra MG, Montevecchi F. Transoral robotic tongue base resection in obstructive sleep apnoea-hypopnoea syndrome: a preliminary report. ORL J Otorhinolaryngol Relat Spec. 2016;72(1):22–7.
44. Thaler ER, Rassekh CH, Lee JM, Weinstein GS, O'Malley BW Jr. Outcomes for multilevel surgery for sleep apnea: obstructive sleep apnea, transoral robotic surgery, and uvulopalatopharyngoplasty. Laryngoscope. 2016;126(1):266–9.
45. Kim SH, Han MH, Park SW, Chang KH. Radiologic-pathologic correlation of unusual lingual masses: part II: Benign and malignant tumors. Korean J Radiol. 2001;2:42–51.
46. Van Abel KM, Carlson ML, Boettcher NL, Boettcher NL, Hafner JW, Moore EJ. Management algorithm for ectopic lingual thyroid including TORS thyroidectomy. Presented as a poster at the Combined Otolaryngology Society Meeting in Chicago, IL, April 2011; 2011.
47. Van Abel KM, Carlson ML, Narendra S. Hypopharyngeal gastric choristoma in an infant resulting in airway obstruction. Arch Otolaryngol Head Neck Surg. 2011;137:947–51.
48. Byrd JK, Ferris RL. Is there a role for robotic surgery in the treatment of head and neck cancer? Curr Treat Options in Oncol. 2016;17(6):1–12.
49. Weinstein GS, O'Malley BW Jr, Desai SC, Quon H. Transoral robotic surgery: does the ends justify the means? Curr Opin Otolaryngol Head Neck Surg. 2009;17(2):126–31.
50. Iseli TA, Kulbersh BD, Iseli CE, Carroll WR, Rosenthal, Eben L, Magnuson JS. Functional outcomes after transoral robotic surgery for head and neck cancer. Otolaryngol Head Neck Surg. 2009;141(2):166–71.
51. Glazer TA, Hoff PT, Spector ME. Transoral robotic surgery for obstructive sleep apnea: perioperative management and postoperative complications. JAMA Otolaryngol Head Neck Surg. 2014;140(12):1207–12.
52. Chia SH, Gross ND, Richmon JD. Surgeon experience and complications with transoral robotic surgery (TORS). Otolaryngol Head Neck Surg. 2013;149(6):885–92.
53. Chen AY. A shifting paradigm for patients with head and neck cancer: transoral robotic surgery (TORS). Head Neck. 2010;24:1030–2.
54. Iranmanesh P, Morel P, Wagner OJ, Inan I, Pugin F, Hagen ME. Set-up and docking of the da Vinci surgical system: prospective analysis of initial experience. Int J Med Robot Comput Assist Surg. 2010;6:57–60.
55. Strong MS, Jako GJ. Laser surgery in the larynx. Early clinical experience with continuous CO_2 laser. Ann Otol Rhinol Laryngol. 1972;81(6):791–8.
56. Steiner W. Experience in endoscopic laser surgery of malignant tumours of the upper aerodigestive tract. Adv Otorhinolaryngol. 1988;39:135–44.
57. Steiner W, Ambrosch P, Hess CF, Kron M. Organ preservation by transoral laser microsurgery in piriform sinus carcinoma. Otolaryngol Head Neck Surg. 2001;124(1):58–67.
58. Canis M, Ihler F, Wolff HA, Christiansen H, Matthias C, Steiner W. Oncologic and functional results after transoral laser microsurgery of tongue base carcinoma. Eur Arch Otorhinolaryngol. 2013;270(3):1075–83.
59. Canis M, Martin A, Ihler F, et al. Transoral laser microsurgery in treatment of pT2 and pT3 glottic laryngeal squamous cell carcinoma—results of 391 patients. Head Neck. 2014;36(6):859–66.
60. Canis M, Ihler F, Martin A, Matthias C, Steiner W. Transoral laser microsurgery for T1a glottic cancer: review of 404 cases. Head Neck. 2014;37(6):889–95.
61. Canis M, Ihler F, Martin A, Wolff HA, Matthias C, Steiner W. Organ preservation in T4a laryngeal cancer: is transoral laser microsurgery an option? Eur Arch Otorhinolaryngol. 2013;270(10):2719–27.

62. Weiss BG, Ihler F, Anczyvkowski MZ, Berlich M, Kitz J, Steiner W, Canis M, Jakob M. Transoral laser microsurgery for treatment of oropharyngeal cancer in 368 patients. Head Neck. 2019;41:3144–58.
63. Steiner W, Ambrosch P. Endoscopic laser surgery of the upper aerodigestive tract with special emphasis on cancer surgery. Stuttgart: Thieme; 2000. p. 147.
64. David SWH, Bruce H, Manuel B-S. Transoral laser microsurgery for cancer of the upper aerodigestive tract. Tuttlingen: Endo-Press; 2013.
65. Karni R, Haughey B. Transoral laser microsurgery: a new approach for unknown primaries of the head and neck. Laryngoscope. 2011;121(6):1194–201.
66. Rich J, Liu J, Haughey B. Swallowing function after transoral laser microsurgery (TLM) ± adjuvant therapy for advanced stage oropharyngeal cancer. Laryngoscope. 2011;121(11):2381–90.
67. Haughey BH, Hinni ML, Salassa JR, Grant DG, Rich JT, Milov S, Lewis JS Jr, Krishan M. Transoral laser microsurgery as primary treatment of advanced stage oropharynx cancer: a United States multicenter study. Head Neck. 2011;33(12):1683–94.
68. Rich JT, Milov S, Lewis JS Jr, Thorstad WL, Adkins DR, Haughey BH. Transoral laser microsurgery (TLM) ± adjuvant therapy for advanced stage oropharyngeal cancer: outcomes and prognostic factors. Laryngoscope. 2009;119(9):1709–19.
69. Hinni M, Salassa J, Grant D, Pearson B, Hayden R, Martin A, Christiansen H, Haughey B, Nussenbaum B, Steiner W. Transoral laser microsurgery for advanced laryngeal cancer. Arch Otolaryngol Head Neck Surg. 2007;133(12):1198–204.
70. Jackel MC, Ambrosch P, Martin A, Steiner W. Impact of re-resection for inadequate margins on the prognosis of upper aerodigestive tract cancer treated by laser microsurgery. Laryngoscope. 2007;117(2):350–6.
71. Karatzanis AD, Psychogios G, Waldfahrer F, Zenk J, Velegrakis GA, Iro H. Surgical management of T1 oropharyngeal carcinoma. Head Neck. 2012;34(9):1277–82.
72. Iro H, Mantsopoulos K, Zenk J, Waldfahrer F, Psychogios G. Results of transoral laser resection in T1-2 oropharyngeal, hypopharyngeal and laryngeal carcinomas. Laryngo-Rhino-Otologie. 2011;90(8):481–5.
73. Bernal-Sprekelsen M, Dazert S, Sudhoff H, Blanch JL, Vilaseca I. Complications of transoral laser surgery for malignant tumors of the larynx and hypopharynx. Laryngo-Rhino-Otologie. 2009;88(1):28–34.
74. Van Abel KM, Moore EJ. Surgical management of the base of tongue. Oper Tech Otolaryngol. 2013;24:74–85.
75. Vincent A, Kohlert S, Lee TS, Inman J, Ducic Y. Free-flap reconstruction of the tongue. Semin Plast Surg. 2019;33(1):38–45.
76. Henstrom DK, Moore EJ, Olsen KD, et al. Transoral resection for squamous cell carcinoma of the base of the tongue. Arch Otolaryngol Head Neck Surg. 2009;135:1231–8.
77. Lam L, Samman N. Speech and swallowing following tongue cancer surgery and free flap reconstruction--a systematic review. Oral Oncol. 2013;49(6):507–24.
78. Hutcheson KA, Lewin JS. Functional assessment and rehabilitation: how to maximize outcomes. Otolaryngol Clin N Am. 2013;46(4):657–70.
79. Biglioli F, Liviero F, Frigerio A, Rezzonico A, Brusati R. Function of the sensate free forearm flap after partial glossectomy. J Craniomaxillofac Surg. 2006;34(6):332–9.
80. Laccourreye O, Hans S, Ménard M, et al. Transoral lateral oropharyngectomy for squamous cell carcinoma of the tonsillar region: II. An analysis of the incidence, related variables, and consequences of local recurrence. Arch Otolaryngol Head Neck Surg. 2005;131:592–9.
81. Paderno A, Piazza C, Bresciani L, Vella R, Nicolai P. Microvascular head and neck reconstruction after (chemo)radiation: facts and prejudices. Curr Opin Otolaryngol Head Neck Surg. 2016;24(2):83–90.
82. Moore EJ, Olsen KD, Martin EJ. Concurrent neck dissection and transoral robotic surgery. Laryngoscope. 2011;121:541–4.
83. Lin YC, Hsiao JR, Tsai ST. Salvage surgery as the primary treatment for recurrent oral squamous cell carcinoma. Oral Oncol. 2004;40(2):183–1839.
84. Chone CT, Silva AR, Crespo AN, Schlupp WR. Regional tumor recurrence after supraomohyoid neck dissection. Arch Otolaryngol Head Neck Surg. 2003;129(1):54–8.

Surgical Management of the Neck 16

16.1 Overview

In 1906, *George W. Crile* of the Cleveland Clinic described the radical neck dissection (RND) encompassing removal of all the lymph nodes (LNs) on one side of the neck and including removal of the spinal accessory nerve (SAN), internal jugular vein (IJV), and sternocleidomastoid (SCM) muscle. In 1957, *Hayes Martin* described routine use of the RND for control of neck metastases. Later, in 1967, *Oscar Suarez* and *E. Bocca* described a more conservative operation which preserves the SAN, IJV, and SCM, and in the last three decades, further procedures have been described to selectively remove the involved regional LN groups.

Treatment of the neck (neck dissection) should always be considered when treating squamous cell carcinoma (SCC) of the tongue due to the risk of cervical lymph node (LN) metastases, even in the clinically negative (cN0) neck. *Clinically N0 necks* have been observed to harbor occult metastases at a rate of 20% [1]. Tumor thickness is also associated with cervical LN metastases [2–4]. Studies recommend a tumor thickness cutoff of 4 mm for elective neck dissection [5]. Thus, the nodal disease burden is a predictor for increased mortality, and elective neck dissection has been shown to offer a survival advantage with higher disease-free survival over therapeutic neck dissection [5, 6].

It is generally accepted that routine surgical dissection of the *node-positive neck* is required for advanced stage oral cavity SCC [7, 8]. Tongue SCC has an extremely high rate (60–80%) of clinically evident and occult cervical LN metastasis to levels I–III, with a moderate risk of level IV involvement [9, 10]. Occasionally, LNs in levels III and IV can harbor metastases *without* level I or II disease and can be considered an indication of aggressive management [11]. Neck dissection is therefore strongly recommended as it provides more accurate nodal staging and can also be therapeutic for decreasing tumor burden.

© The Author(s), under exclusive license to Springer Nature Switzerland AG 2022

M. F. Sakr, *Tongue Lesions*, https://doi.org/10.1007/978-3-031-08198-9_16

Surgical management of the *ipsilateral* neck in tongue SCC consists of the modified radical neck dissection (MRND) including levels I, II, III, and IV with preservation of the SAN, IJV, and SCM muscle [12, 13]. This is indicated for stage I cancers with >3 mm of invasion and for most stage II disease except minimally invasive primary tumors. Both T3 or T4 lesions and those lesions approaching the midline require *bilateral* MRND due to the risk of contralateral LN metastasis [14]. The risk of level V cervical LN metastasis in tongue SCC is extremely low, and therefore the utility of level V dissection in such cases may be questionable [15–17].

Sentinel LN biopsy may be an important option between observation and neck dissection in patients with intermediate-thickness tumors [18]. This may be most applicable to patients with primary tumors <3 mm in depth with an intermediate risk of LN metastases and larger primary tumors. A negative sentinel LN biopsy may replace planned neck dissection [19].

In addition to surgical management, adjunctive radiotherapy (RT) is warranted for increased regional control of disease in the presence of cervical metastasis. Zhu et al. [20] who performed with the Surveillance, Epidemiology, and End Results (SEER) database in a study of 9474 tongue cancer patients who received either surgery alone (n = 6715) or surgery and RT (n = 2759) reported that the latter group had a better prognosis in terms of survival [20]. Likewise, Maochang et al. [21] have reported a 5-year survival rate of 31.03% among patients receiving surgery only but as high as 68.08% among patients receiving combined treatment. Local recurrence has also been previously reported to be significantly reduced in patients who receive both surgery and RT as compared to surgery alone [22].

16.2 Relevant Anatomy

The lymphatic drainage of the mucosal surfaces and other tissues of the head and neck is directed to the lymph nodes (LNs) located within the fibroadipose tissue that lies between the investing (superficial) layer of the deep fascia superficially and the visceral and prevertebral layers underneath. In this space, these LNs tend to be aggregated around certain neural (SAN) and vascular (IJV and transverse cervical artery) structures [23].

The nomenclature of cervical LN regions (levels and sublevels) in popular use today comes from the Memorial Sloan Kettering Cancer Center. This classification was used to describe the patterns of metastatic dissemination observed in more than 1000 patients who were treated at the center with radical neck dissection (RND). Lymph nodes in the neck are identified by Roman numerals and grouped into levels I–VI, corresponding with the submandibular and submental nodes (level I); upper, middle, and lower jugular nodes (levels II, III, IV, respectively); posterior triangle nodes (level V); and anterior compartment nodes (level VI) (Fig. 16.1). A further level VII to denote LN groups in the superior mediastinum (from the suprasternal notch superiorly to the innominate artery inferiorly) is *no longer used.*

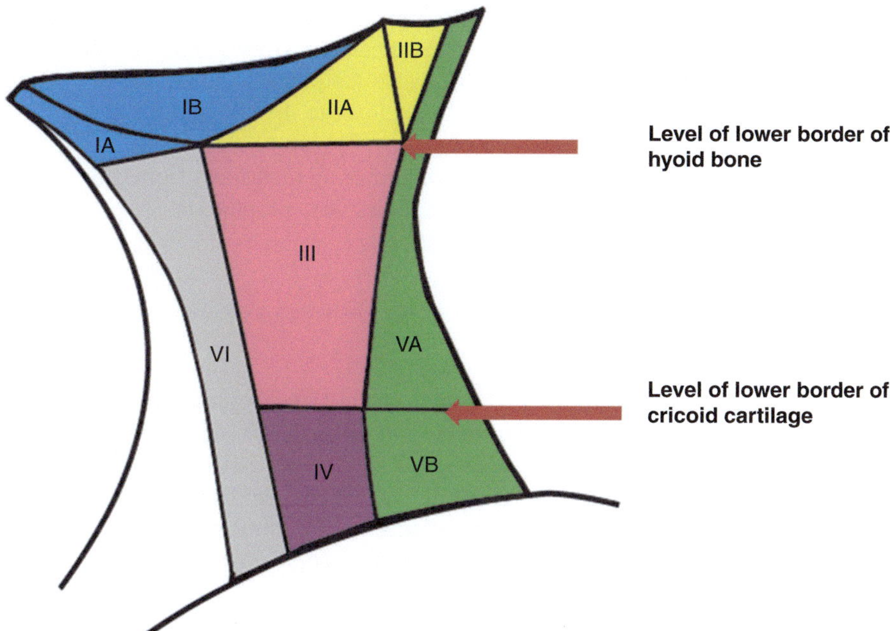

Fig. 16.1 The six levels of lymph nodes in the neck (I–VI) with sublevels

16.2.1 Level I

Level I may be divided into level Ia, which refers to the nodes in the *submental triangle* (bound by the anterior bellies of the digastric muscles and the hyoid bone), and Ib, which refers to the *submandibular triangle* nodes formed by the anterior and posterior bellies of the digastric and body of the mandible.

The nodes of level Ia are at greatest risk of harboring metastasis from cancers that arise from the floor of the mouth, anterior tongue, anterior mandibular alveolar ridge, and lower lip, while the nodes of level Ib often receive metastasis from cancers of the oral cavity, anterior nasal cavity, soft tissue structures of the midface, and submandibular gland.

16.2.2 Level II

Level II nodes are related to the upper third of the IJV, extending from the skull base superiorly to the inferior border of the hyoid bone (clinical landmark) or carotid bifurcation (surgical landmark) inferiorly. The posterior border of level II is the posterior border of the sternocleidomastoid (SCM) muscle, while the anterior border of level II has been defined as the stylohyoid muscle. However, the 2008 classification revision proposed that the vertical plane marked by the posterior edge of the submandibular gland be used as an alternative to the stylohyoid muscle boundary [24]. This region includes the upper jugular and jugulo-digastric nodes and the upper posterior cervical LNs. The spinal accessory nerve (SAN), which travels obliquely across this region, is used as a landmark to subdivide this group into IIa, the part that lies anteroinferiorly and closer to the IJV and IIb, the portion above and behind the nerve.

The nodes in level II are at greatest risk of harboring metastasis from cancers that arise from the *oral cavity*, nasal cavity, nasopharynx, oropharynx, hypopharynx, larynx, and parotid gland.

16.2.3 Level III

Level III nodes are related to the lower third of the IJV. They are located between the inferior border of the hyoid bone (or carotid bifurcation) superiorly and a horizontal plane defined by the inferior border of the cricoid cartilage inferiorly. The sternohyoid muscle marks the anterior limit of level III, and the posterior border of the SCM muscle is the posterior border. Level III most commonly receives metastasis from cancers that originate in the *oral cavity*, nasopharynx, oropharynx, hypopharynx, and larynx.

16.2.4 Level IV

This refers to the group of nodes related to the lower third of the IJV. These nodes are located between the inferior border of the cricoid cartilage superiorly and the clavicle inferiorly, and, similar to level III, the anterior boundary is the sternohyoid muscle, and the posterior border is the posterior border of the SCM muscle. The nodes of level IV commonly harbor metastasis from cancer that originates in the larynx, hypopharynx, thyroid [25], and cervical esophagus.

A literature review by Weisz Shabtay and Ronen reported that in patients with clinically negative neck (cN0) oral tongue squamous cell carcinoma (SCC), level IV involvement was found in just 16 out of 498 patients (3.2%), with the incidence of skip metastases (metastases that bypassed levels I–III and spread directly to level IV), also being low. Therefore, the investigators recommended that patients with cN0 oral tongue squamous cell carcinoma undergo elective neck dissection of levels I-III [26].

16.2.5 Level V

This refers to the LNs located in the posterior triangle of the neck. These include the spinal accessory, transverse cervical, and supraclavicular group of nodes. Level V is bound anteriorly by the posterior border of the SCM muscle and posteriorly by the anterior border of the trapezius muscle. Level V extends from the apex of the convergence of the SCM and trapezius muscle superiorly to the clavicle inferiorly. This level is subdivided by an imaginary plane defined by the inferior border of the cricoid cartilage into level Va superior to that plane and Vb inferior to it.

Level Va contains the nodes associated with the SAN, and level Vb contains the transverse cervical and supraclavicular nodes. The posterior triangle nodes are at greatest risk for harboring metastasis from cancers that arise in the nasopharynx, oropharynx, and skin of the posterior scalp and neck.

16.2.6 Level VI

Level VI nodes refer to LNs of the anterior (or central) compartment of the neck. Defined by the carotid arteries (medial border of carotid sheath) laterally, the hyoid bone superiorly, and the suprasternal notch inferiorly, it is rich in lymphatics that drain the thyroid gland, subglottic larynx, cervical trachea, hypopharynx, and cervical esophagus. Lymph nodes in this compartment are located in the tracheoesophageal groove (paratracheal nodes), in front of the trachea (pre-tracheal nodes), around the thyroid gland (para-thyroidal nodes), and on the cricothyroid membrane (precricoid or Delphian node). Lymph nodes in the central compartment are *not* routinely excised in radical neck dissection; most commonly, they are removed during surgery for thyroid, laryngeal, and hypopharyngeal cancer.

16.3 Classification of Neck Dissection

The operation of radical neck dissection (RND) dates back to 1906 when *George Crile* described the classical RND. This was subsequently popularized by *Hayes Martin* and still remains the gold standard by which other operations are judged. This operation removes the LN-bearing areas of the neck along with the SCM, IJV, and SAN muscle. The inevitable morbidity to which this led fueled an interest in more conservative approaches, and during the 1980s and 1990s, a number of less radical procedures have been popularized based on the staging of the disease at presentation. Modified radical neck dissection (MRND) differs from the classical RND in that it aims at the preservation of different structures: IJV, SAN, and SCM muscle [27].

The following are the four major types and subtypes of neck dissections (NDs) proposed by the American Academy of Otolaryngology/Head and Neck Surgery [28].

16.3.1 Radical Neck Dissection (RND)

This procedure is an en bloc clearance of all fibrofatty tissue from one side of the neck, including the LNs from levels I–V (and LNs surrounding the tail of the parotid gland) and the SAN, IJV, and SCM muscle. Radical neck dissection does *not* include the removal of the postauricular, suboccipital, peri-facial, buccinator, retropharyngeal, or central compartment LNs.

Previously used for neck disease of any stage, from microscopic to bulky nodal disease, this procedure is now limited to (1) patients with advanced neck disease, (2) recurrent disease after chemoradiation, or (3) gross extracapsular spread to the SAN, IJV, and SCM muscle.

16.3.2 Modified Radical Neck Dissection (MRND)

This operation involves excision of the same LN-bearing tissues from one side of the neck as is done in a RND (levels I–V) with the preservation of one or more non-lymphatic structure including the SAN, IJV, or SCM. The MRND is analogous to the "functional neck dissection" described by *Bocca*; however, they differ in that Bocca originally did *not* remove the submandibular gland.

- *Type I:* preservation of the SAN
- *Type II:* preservation of the SAN and IJV
- *Type III:* preservation of the SAN, IJV, and SCM muscle

The structure or structures preserved should be specifically indicated in the name of the procedure (e.g., modified radical neck dissection with preservation of accessory nerve and internal jugular vein) [29].

Modified radical neck dissection (MRND) is indicated for clinically palpable metastatic neck disease. Conversion to RND becomes necessary upon gross involvement of the SAN, IJV, and SCM muscle, although involvement of all three is unusual, except in very advanced (N3) disease.

The term "comprehensive neck dissection" is frequently mentioned in the literature. This term refers to any type of neck dissection (ND) that involves the removal of LNs from levels I–V and corresponds, therefore, to RND and MRND, according to the Academy's classification.

16.3.3 Selective Neck Dissection (SND)

This term refers to a type of neck dissection in which one or more lymph node groups normally removed in a radical neck dissection are preserved. The 1991 classification schema classified SND into the following four categories or subtypes:

- *Supra-omohyoid ND*: removal of levels I–III (Fig. 16.2)
- *Lateral ND:* removal of levels II–IV (Fig. 16.3)
- *Posterolateral ND:* removal of levels II–V, suboccipital and postauricular LNs (Fig. 16.4)
- *Anterior compartment ND:* removal of level VI (Fig. 16.5)

Because of the increased use of selective neck dissection and the increased selectivity with which lymph node groups are removed, the Committee for Head and Neck Surgery and Oncology revised the classification of selective neck dissection in 2002. Because the

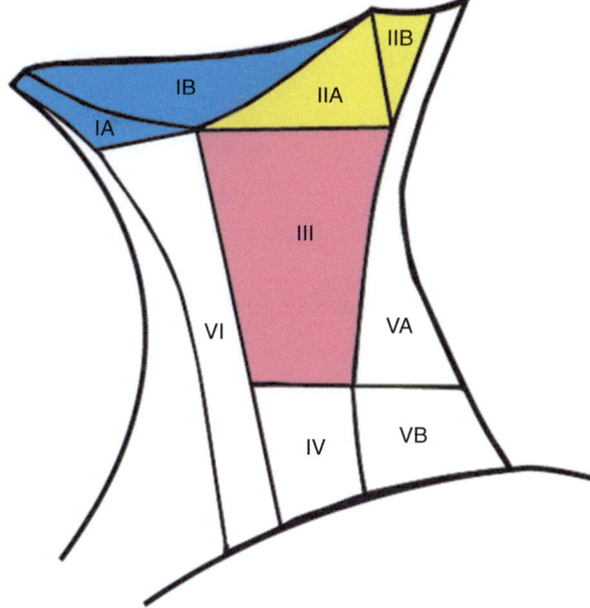

Fig. 16.2 Selective neck dissection (SND), levels I–III (supra-omohyoid ND)

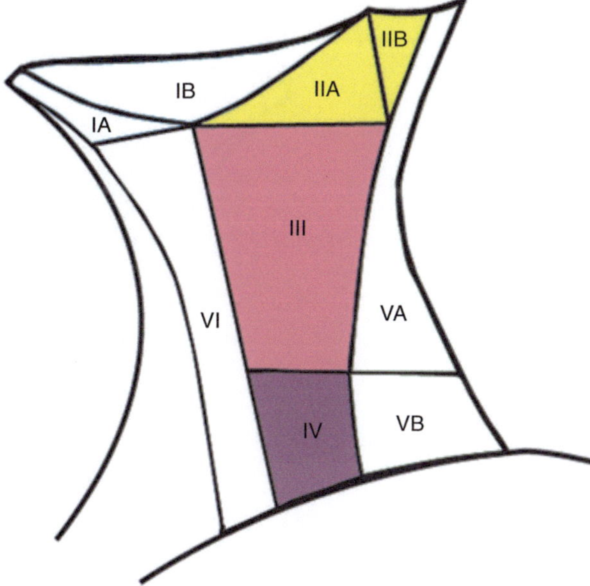

Fig. 16.3 Selective neck dissection (SND), levels II–IV (lateral ND)

1991 classification did not provide an accurate description of procedures in which the surgeon preserves certain sublevels, the 2002 classification excludes the above listed "named" selective neck dissections (SNDs). In the 2002 classification, selective neck dissections are described with respect to the lymph node levels excised. For example, a supra-omohyoid neck dissection is described as a selective neck dissection (I–III).

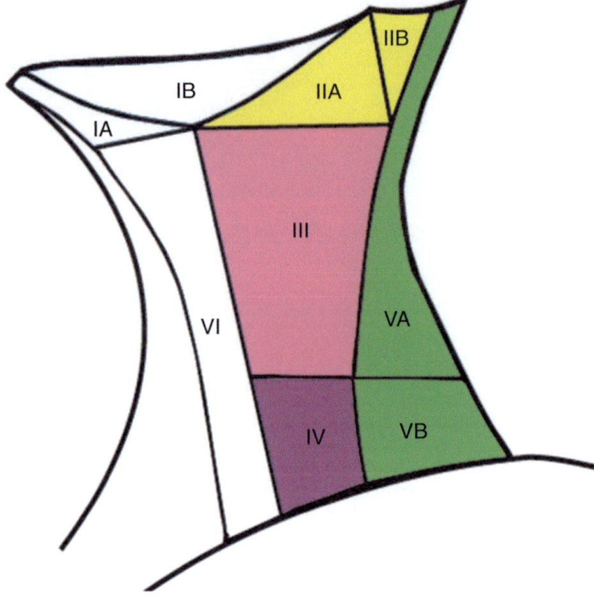

Fig. 16.4 Selective neck dissection (SND), levels II–V (posterolateral ND)

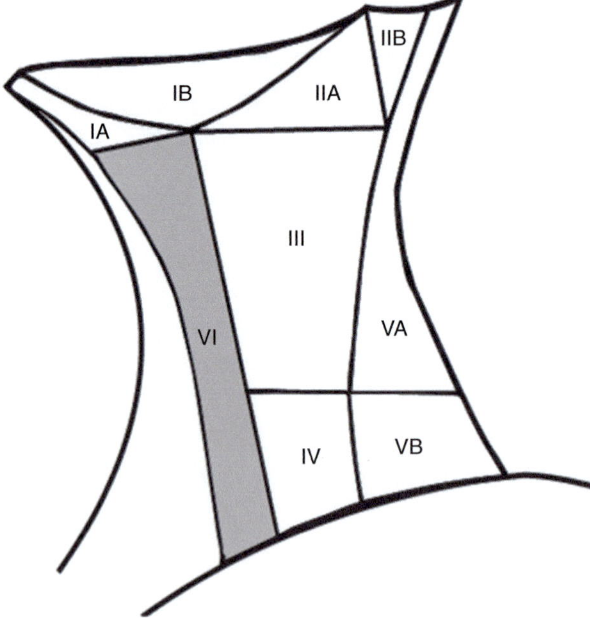

Fig. 16.5 Selective neck dissection (SND), level VI (anterior or central compartment ND)

A retrospective study by Barzan et al. [30] indicated that SND can be safely and effectively performed as primary and salvage surgery. The report involved 827 patients with primary head and neck tumors who underwent SND, with just 22 of 40 neck cancer recurrences later arising on the dissected side of the neck. The incidence of recurrence was approximately the same after primary and salvage surgery (4.4% and 5.2%, respectively) [30].

The United Kingdom (UK) National Multidisciplinary Guidelines from 2016 on the management of neck metastases in head and neck cancer included the following recommendations with regard to SND [31]:

- SND is as effective as MRND for controlling regional disease in N0 necks for all primary sites.
- SND alone is adequate treatment for pN1 neck disease without adverse histological features.

The UK National Multidisciplinary Guidelines from 2016 regarding *recurrent* head and neck cancer included the following recommendations [32]:

- Elective SND is considered in patients with recurrent primaries with N0 necks, especially in advanced cases.
- SND (with preservation of nodal levels, especially level V, that are not involved by disease) in patients with nodal (N+) recurrence appears to be as effective as MRND.

16.3.3.1 SND for Oral Cavity Cancer

Selective removal of the levels I, II, and III LNs is the *procedure of choice* for management of N0 and N1 diseases that originate from cancers of the oral cavity. However, because of the lymphatic drainage of the *oral tongue*, some authorities advocate SND (I–IV) for cancers that originate from this subsite. The operation includes resection of soft tissues in the submental triangle, along with the submandibular triangle contents, including the submandibular gland and the fibrofatty tissue along the IJV from the skull base to the omohyoid muscle (or clavicle). The dissected contents include the fascia that covers the medial aspect of the SCM muscle; the muscle itself is laterally retracted and preserved. These neck contents are peeled off from the IJV and from around the SAN, sparing these structures.

16.3.3.2 SND for Oropharyngeal, Hypopharyngeal, and Laryngeal Cancer

SND (II–IV) is the *procedure of choice* in the elective treatment of neck disease in patients with cancers that originate in the oropharynx, hypopharynx, or larynx [33]. The SAN and SCM muscle and IJV are spared in this operation, while the LNs are removed from the skull base superiorly to the clavicle inferiorly and from the cutaneous branches of the cervical plexus at the posterior border of the SCM muscle posteriorly to the sternothyroid muscle anteriorly. If the jugular chain nodes above the SAN nerve were preserved, the procedure would be named SND (IIa, III, IV).

16.3.4 Extended Neck Dissection

In cases of advanced neck disease, certain lymphatic or non-lymphatic structures not routinely included in the aforementioned NDs may have to be removed. Extended neck dissection is the term used to describe these procedures. Retropharyngeal LNs, the hypoglossal nerve, portions of the prevertebral musculature, or the carotid artery are some of the structures that may occasionally have to be excised to obtain negative margins. All additional lymphatic and non-lymphatic structures removed should be identified in parentheses.

In a recent study of extended neck dissection on 72 patients with human papillomavirus (HPV)-related oropharyngeal squamous cell carcinoma (SCC), Zenga et al. [34] reported that advanced T classification, a pathologic node number of five or more, and no employment of adjuvant radiotherapy were associated with a reduced disease-free survival rate [34].

16.4 Neck Dissection: Indications and Contraindications

16.4.1 Indications

The indications of various types of neck dissection (ND) are as follows:

- *RND:* Bulky nodal disease in the neck with extensive soft tissue involvement due to extracapsular spread [35].
- *MRND-I (preservation of SAN):* Bulky nodal disease with extracapsular spread involving the SCM and IJV, but not the SAN.
- *MRND-II (preservation of SAN and INJV):* Bulky nodal disease with SCM involvement but sparing the IJ or SAN.
- *MRND-III:* Metastatic disease with limited extracapsular spread and the IJV, SCM, and SAN can all be dissected free [24, 36].
- *SND I–III (supra-omohyoid ND):* N0 neck for primary SCC or malignant melanoma where the primary site is anterior to the ear or is located in the lower eyelid.
- *SND II–IV (lateral ND):* N0 neck for SCC of the lateral tongue, oral cavity, anterior floor of mouth, or for N1 disease in these primary sites [37] or any N-stage neck without significant extracapsular spread for SCC of the larynx and hypopharynx, for differentiated thyroid carcinoma, or for melanoma with a positive sentinel LN that drains to these nodal basins.

- *SND II–V (posterolateral ND):* Any N-stage neck cutaneous melanoma with high-risk features or melanoma with a positive sentinel LN where the primary site is posterior to the ear [13].
- *SND VI (central ND):* Clinically apparent disease (cN1a) in papillary thyroid carcinoma (therapeutic). It is debatable in clinically node-negative (cN0) neck.

16.4.2 Contraindications

16.4.2.1 Absolute Contraindications

There are no absolute contraindications to neck dissection beyond those that make a patient unfit for general anesthesia and resection, with one exception: unresectable disease (fixed neck mass in the deep neck muscles, prevertebral fascia, and/or skull base involvement).

16.4.2.2 Relative Contraindications [38, 39]

- Severe cardiopulmonary disease, chronic obstructive pulmonary disease (COPD) with poor functional status
- Preoperative imaging showing deep infiltration of the tumor in the prevertebral space, scalene muscles, levator scapula muscle, phrenic nerve, and brachial plexus
- Uncontrollable primary tumor
- Distant metastatic disease
- Tumor encasement of the carotid artery (many authors view this as "unresectable disease," as resection and grafting does not confer a survival or local control advantage, even if it is technically possible) [40]

16.5 Neck Dissection: Operative Technique

16.5.1 Preparation

There are no specific preoperative preparatory requirements for patients undergoing ND other than planning of the incisions for neck dissection, particularly if the primary tumor is undergoing resection simultaneously. Preparation of the neck dissection incisions must also take into consideration any reconstructive effort required to repair the surgical defect created after the excision of the primary tumor.

16.5.2 Anesthesia and Position

General endotracheal anesthesia is essential for performing ND, and the use of paralytic agents should be discussed between the surgeon and anesthetist. The patient is placed in the supine position with the head elevated to 30°. The neck is hyperextended with the use of a shoulder roll and rotated to the opposite side [41].

16.5.3 Incision

There are many historical incisions including the Latyshevsky and Freund, Mac Fee, Crile, Kocher, Schobinger, and Hockey stick, but in modern head and neck surgery, the operation is performed via a single incision placed in an existing neck skin crease midway down the neck. Trifurcate incisions were popular in the past and can still be used in the case of bulky posterior neck disease, but care should be taken to not place the trifurcation over the carotid artery [42, 43].

16.5.4 Raising Skin Flaps

The skin incision is deepened through the subcutaneous tissue and then through the platysma muscle. The posterior flap is then raised in the subplatysmal plane by applying traction to the flap with skin hooks and countertraction of the deeper soft tissues. The flap is elevated up to the anterior border of the trapezius muscle.

16.5.5 Identifying Marginal Mandibular Nerve

Careful identification of the marginal mandibular branch of the facial nerve is crucial. Avoidance of paralytics is advocated at this point in the operation by some surgeons. Posteriorly, the greater auricular nerve (GAN) and the external jugular vein (EJV) overlying the SCM come into view as elevation of the flap is continued. The GAN and EJV should be identified carefully and preserved. Dissection with electrocautery is not advisable as it may cause temporary damage to the nerve. This nerve lies just anterior to the submandibular fascia and superficial to the posterior facial vein. The vein is ligated, and its upper stump retracted cephalad, protecting the marginal branch of the facial nerve (Hayes-Martin maneuver). Alternately, the facial vein and marginal mandibular nerves can be skeletonized and preserved individually.

16.5.6 Dissection

16.5.6.1 Superior Dissection

The fibrous fatty tissue of the submental triangle is dissected off the anterior bellies of the digastric muscles and the mylohyoid. The fascia is then dissected off the anterior belly of the digastric muscle, and the specimen is retracted posteriorly, removing the fibrous fatty tissue containing LNs lateral to the mylohyoid muscle. When dissection reaches the posterior border of the mylohyoid, this is retracted anteriorly, exposing the facial artery, lingual nerve, and the submandibular gland (Fig. 16.6).

Finally, the facial artery is ligated as it crosses forward, under the posterior belly of the digastric muscle. Alternately, the facial artery and vein can be dissected through the substance of the submandibular gland to increase the length of these vessels available for microvascular anastomosis or if a submental flap is planned.

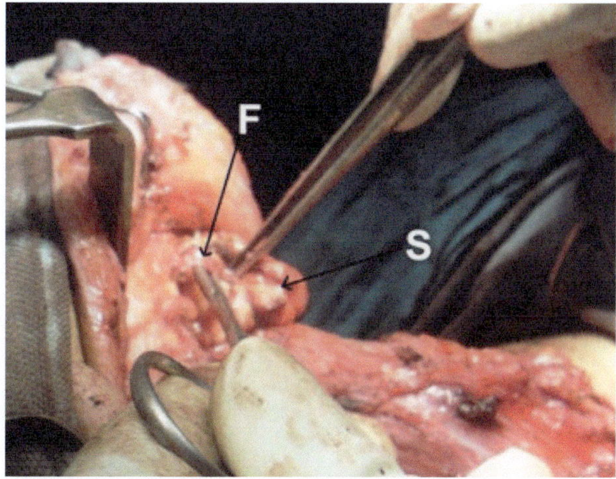

Fig. 16.6 Superior dissection exposing the facial artery (F) and submandibular gland (S)

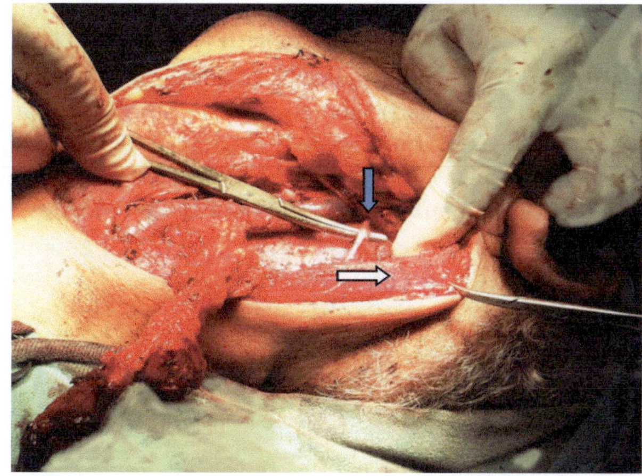

Fig. 16.7 Superior dissection exposing the internal jugular vein (IJV) (blue arrow) and spinal accessory nerve (SAN) (white arrow)

The tail of the parotid gland is elevated off of the sternocleidomastoid (SCM) muscle and deep structures, and the SCM muscle is then incised close to its insertion in the mastoid process (the SCM is preserved in MRND). The fibro-fatty tissue medial to the muscle is incised, exposing the splenius capitis and the levator scapulae muscles. Otherwise, incising the fascia below the digastric muscle and gentle inferior traction of the specimen allows identification of the hypoglossal nerve, the upper end of the IJV and the SAN. At this point in the dissection, the IJV and SAN are identified and preserved, reflecting the LN-bearing tissue inferiorly with the surgical specimen (Fig. 16.7).

16.5.6.2 Inferior Dissection

Dissection is continued posteriorly and inferiorly along the anterior border of the trapezius muscle. The SAN and the transverse cervical vessels are divided as they cross the anterior and the border of the trapezius muscle (the SAN is preserved in MRND). During this step of the operation, it is important to preserve the branches

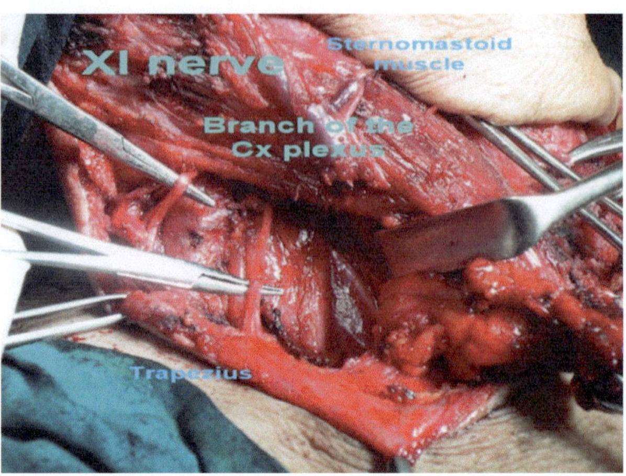

Fig. 16.8 Inferior dissection showing retraction of the sternocleidomastoid muscle (SCM) and trapezius muscle and exposing the spinal accessory nerve (SAN) (under the straight forceps) and branch of the cervical plexus (under the curved forceps)

of the cervical plexus that innervate the levator scapulae muscle, unless the extent of the disease in the neck precludes it (Fig. 16.8). The SCM muscle and the superficial layer of the deep cervical fascia are incised above the superior border of the clavicle (the SCM is preserved in MRND). The omohyoid muscle is divided, and the EJV can either be preserved or divided, depending upon the vascular needs of the reconstructive surgeon. The fibro-fatty tissue in this region is then gently pushed in an upward direction, exposing the brachial plexus, the scalenus anterior muscle, and the phrenic nerve. Posteriorly, dissection is continued to join the previous dissection along the anterior border of the trapezius.

16.5.6.3 Medial Dissection

Dissection is continued medially to expose the vagus nerve, the common carotid artery (CCA), and the IJV. Inferiorly, the phrenic nerve is identified and protected by not violating the deep fascia of the floor of the neck overlying the brachial plexus and muscles (Fig. 16.9). The surgeon must remain very vigilant on the left side to be able to identify thoracic duct, which arches downward and forward from behind the CCA to open into the IJV, the subclavian vein, or the angle formed by the junction of these two vessels (Fig. 16.10). The duct is located anterior or superficial to the anterior scalene muscle and the phrenic nerve. The thoracic duct may have multiple connections at its upper end, and at the base of the neck, it usually receives a jugular, a subclavian, and perhaps other minor lymphatic trunks, which must be individually ligated or clipped to avoid leakage.

The IJV can almost always be spared (*in MRND*) with meticulous technique (Fig. 16.11), but if resection is necessary (in RND), it is important to obtain circumferential control of the vessel proximally and distally with vessel loops before cross-clamping and dividing it. If the tumor mass is located low in the jugulo-digastric region or the mid-jugular region, the IJV is first ligated and divided superiorly. Dissection is then continued in an inferior direction, separating the specimen from the vagus nerve, the carotid artery, and the superior thyroid vessels. If instead, the

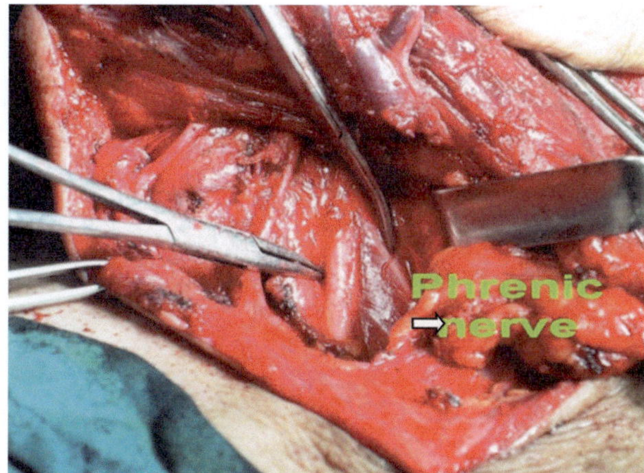

Fig. 16.9 Medial dissection showing the phrenic nerve (white arrow) without violating the deep fascia of the floor of the neck overlying the brachial plexus and muscles

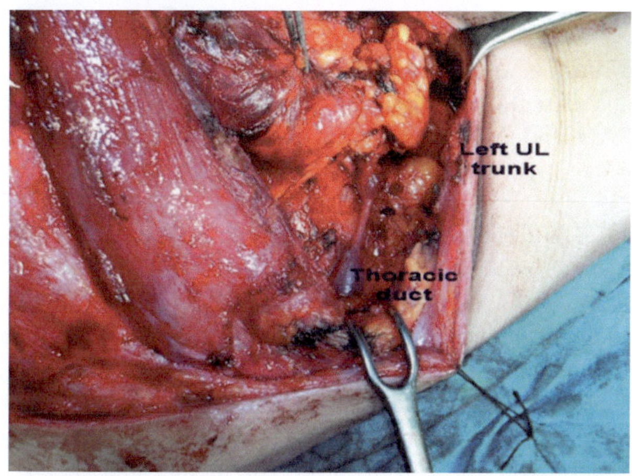

Fig. 16.10 Medial dissection showing the thoracic duct on the left side of the neck. The duct arches downward and forward from behind the common carotid artery (CCA) to open into the internal jugular vein (IJV), the subclavian vein, or the angle formed by the junction of these two vessels

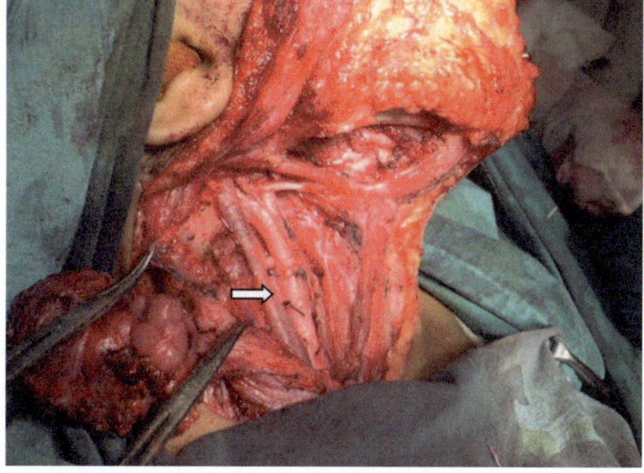

Fig. 16.11 The internal jugular vein (IJV) (white arrow) is dissected and spared in modified radical neck dissection (MRND)

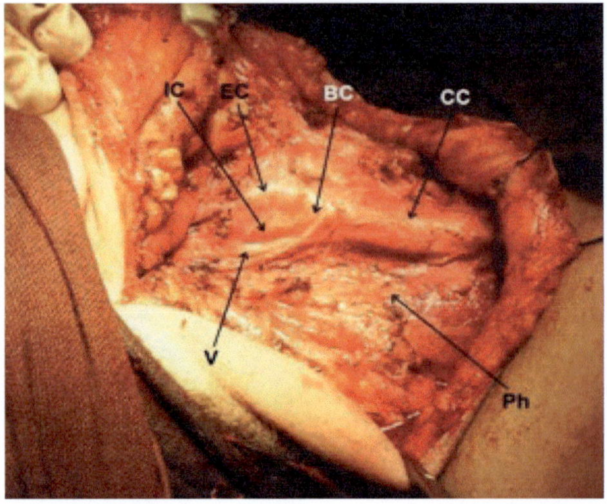

Fig. 16.12 Right neck side after RND, showing the common carotid artery (CC), carotid bifurcation (BC), external carotid artery (EC), internal carotid artery (IC), vagus nerve (V), and phrenic nerve (Ph). SCM, IJV, and SAN have been excised

disease is located high in the jugulo-digastric region, the IJV is divided inferiorly, and dissection is continued in a superior direction along the CCA. In RND, the IJV, SAN, and SCM muscles are excised with the LN specimen (Fig. 16.12).

16.5.7 Closure

Incision closure is in three layers: The first layer approximates the platysma anteriorly and the subcutaneous tissue laterally, and the second layer approximates the subcuticular layer. The skin can then be closed with sutures, staples, or dermal glue. One or two suction drains should be placed in the most dependent areas (the lateral gutter and inferior aspect near the thoracic inlet). The drain(s) should not rest immediately over the carotid artery or in the area of the thoracic duct, or atop any named nerve.

16.6 Complications of Neck Dissection

As with any surgical procedure, ND is associated with several potential complications that can be prevented by a careful preoperative assessment, meticulous surgical technique, high-quality postoperative care, and appropriate rehabilitation. Although many of these complications are rare in the hands of an experienced surgeon, some are nonetheless unavoidable.

All the possible integrity of the cranial nerves should be maintained unless it compromises tumor resection. Modified procedures should be used to reduce the adverse effects of the classical RND operation and yet preserve its effectiveness in oncological terms. A protocol-driven approach and a vigilant and proactive emphasis in the entire perioperative period can help minimize the complications.

16.6.1 Nerve Complications

Several nerves in the neck are at risk of being damaged during neck dissection. These nerves may be transected or suffer a neuropraxia during surgery.

16.6.1.1 Spinal Accessory Nerve (SAN)

The most notable sequelae observed in patients who underwent an ND are related to sacrifice or damage of the SAN. The resulting denervation of the trapezius muscle causes destabilization of the scapula with progressive flaring at the vertebral border, drooping, and lateral and anterior rotation (*shoulder syndrome*). The loss of trapezius function decreases the patient's ability to abduct the shoulder above 90°. These physical changes result in a syndrome of pain, weakness, and deformity of the shoulder girdle commonly associated with the RND [44, 45].

16.6.1.2 Marginal Mandibular Nerve (MMN)

The incidence of MMN palsy in ND is high. Despite being a recognized complication of ND surgery, there are limited data regarding rates of MMN palsy or correlation with levels of nodal clearance. Injury to the MMN often occurs during dissection of either the submental triangle or the facial group of LNs, resulting in altered function of the lip depressors. Preoperatively, the patient should be alerted to the incidence of MMN palsy, especially if level I is to be included in the dissection [46].

16.6.1.3 Phrenic Nerve

Phrenic nerve paralysis leads to ipsilateral hemidiaphragm elevation ± mediastinal shift on chest X-ray and may contribute to postoperative pulmonary complications [47]. Dugena et al. [48] reviewed the clinical records of 100 consecutive patients who underwent a neck dissection for oral cancer and reported 9% (9/100) had a radiological evidence of postoperative unilateral phrenic nerve injury. Depending on the degree of the injury, recovery may be spontaneous [48].

16.6.1.4 Sensory Branches of the Cervical Roots

Sensory branches of the cervical roots provide sensation to the skin of the neck and shoulder. As the skin flaps are elevated in sub-platysmal plane, several branches of the cervical plexus are immediately encountered overlying the SCM muscle. Sacrifice of these branches will results in a sensory deficit that extends from pinna to the chest wall below the clavicle. Most of this sensory deficit will spontaneously resolve postoperatively over a period of few months [49].

16.6.1.5 Greater Auricular Nerve

Sacrifice of this nerve during neck dissection (ND) leads to a sensory deficit of the auricle that usually diminishes with time [50].

16.6.1.6 Lingual Nerve

Level I LN dissection incorporating submandibular gland excision puts the lingual nerve at risk for injury. Clinically, injury results in loss of taste from ipsilateral anterior two third of the tongue and hypoesthesia or paresthesia of the hemi-tongue resulting in difficulty in speech and deglutition [46].

16.6.1.7 Vagus Nerve

The vagus nerve can be damaged during ligation of the IJV. High vagus nerve injuries result in significant dysphonia from ipsilateral vocal cord (VC) paralysis and dysphagia with pooling of secretions from pharyngeal paralysis and loss of sensation in the larynx, which causes a breathy voice, an inefficient cough, and a subjective sense of dyspnea. The loss of more distal vagal innervations has little clinical effect [46].

16.6.1.8 Hypoglossal Nerve

The hypoglossal nerve is susceptible to injury during dissection of levels I–II LNs. Hypoglossal nerve injury result in ipsilateral tongue weakness, deviation of the tongue to the affected side, and difficulty with speech and swallowing [51].

16.6.1.9 Sympathetic Trunk

Disruption of the sympathetic chain may also result from neck dissection, following dissection of the carotid sheath, leading to *Horner's syndrome*. However, this should be avoided by careful dissection and recognition of the sympathetic chain.

16.6.2 Wound Complications

The incidence of wound infection after surgery of the neck without entry into the aerodigestive tract is very low. Wound infection is a contributing factor to dehiscence and flap skin loss. Skin flaps should be elevated in the sub-platysmal plane in order to maximize their blood supply. Flap elevation superficial to the platysma adds to the problems of skin loss [52, 53]. Wound infection may manifest as a cellulitis with erythema, warmth, or induration of the cervical skin flaps, abscess formation from an infected seroma or hematoma, or fistula [54]. Fluid collection under the skin flaps can be prevented by using suction drainage. Seroma may be drained using a wide-bore needle and applying pressure dressing to the area.

16.6.3 Air Leak

Air leak may result from incomplete closure of the surgical incision or the presence of an improperly secured drain, which becomes displaced, exposing drain vents. Air leaks can, however, be associated with more serious consequences such as communication with a tracheotomy site. In addition to air, contaminated secretions may leak into the wound bed resulting in fistulous tracts and wound infections. Early identification of the site of leak may be difficult, and correcting the leak may require revision of the wound closure in the operating room.

16.6.4 Vascular Complications

16.6.4.1 Intraoperative Bleeding

Intraoperative bleeding can result from a series of small veins that are either present in the posterior triangle near the SAN or near the lower end of the trapezius muscle, or even in the region of the mylohyoid muscle. Injury to the transverse cervical artery with subsequent retraction of the artery behind the clavicle can lead to great difficulty in managing any hemorrhage. Similarly, trauma to the IJV may lead to severe intraoperative bleeding that may be difficult to control. As such, it is necessary that one should carry out any dissection with extreme care, so as to prevent any uncontrollable intraoperative bleeding or the formation of a hematoma.

16.6.4.2 Hematoma

Hematoma occurs in approximately 1% of neck dissections. Hematomas are avoided by careful hemostasis, application of pressure dressing, and continuous suction drainage [54]. Should a large hematoma be encountered, the patient should be taken back to the operating room as soon as possible for evacuation as it would compromise the take of any flap.

16.6.4.3 Internal Jugular Vein (IJV) Complications

The IJV has several large tributaries that enter anterosuperiorly. If it is to be spared, care must be taken to ligate these branches. Narrowing of the vein probably contributes to postoperative thrombosis and occlusion that are reported in 15% of preserved IJVs. If the IJV is to be ligated during ND, it should first be thoroughly exposed, with the position of the vagus and hypoglossal nerves being noted [24].

Although rare, the possibility of an air embolus following injury to the IJV should be borne in mind. The IJV can sometimes be torn by the inappropriate use of artery forceps below the SCM in an attempt to mobilize the muscle prior to dissection. In such a case, no attempt should be made to clamp the hole with an artery forceps or use diathermy, as this would only make the hole bigger. If a tear occurs prior to the division of the vein, pressure is applied over the vein, the operative table is tilted head down, and the area above and below the tear is securely ligated.

16.6.4.4 Carotid Artery Complications (Rupture/Blowout)

The most feared and often lethal complication after neck dissection is exposure and rupture of the carotid artery. Acute postoperative carotid artery rupture or *blow out* occurs in 3–4% of RND and is associated with a mortality rate of 50%. It is usually the culmination of several factors: (1) improper incision used in an irradiated neck, (2) damage or stripping of the adventitial layer of the carotid sheath, and (3) the involvement of the carotid artery by tumor itself. With proper design of skin incisions, the carotid seldom becomes exposed in the absence of a salivary fistula. If the carotid becomes exposed, it should be covered promptly with well-vascularized tissue. Tumor invasion of the carotid artery is a relatively uncommon event of advanced aggressive disease or revision surgery for a recurrent neck mass [46].

Carotid artery rupture can be prevented in patients who have had previous irradiation to the neck by protecting the carotid arteries with a muscle flap (usually the levator scapulae muscle), by not stripping the adventitia of the carotid sheath unless absolutely necessary and by keeping the vessel walls moist during operation. In the case of rupture, local pressure is applied to the area, the airway is protected with a cuffed tracheostomy tube, and the blood pressure is maintained with IV fluids. The patient should be taken to the operating room, with each end of the carotid artery exposed and tied off at healthy tissue using a transfixing stitch. *Neurological sequelae* due to ligation include contralateral hemiplegia, hemi-anesthesia, aphasia, and optic nerve atrophy.

16.6.4.5 Chylous Fistula

The key to the treatment of a chyle fistula is prevention, which demands knowledge of the relevant anatomy bearing in mind that up to 50% of patients exhibit more than one termination of the thoracic duct. Whereas intraoperative identification can be aided by placing the patient in the Trendelenburg position or adopting a forced Valsalva maneuver, postoperative leaks are usually identified when feeding is commenced. The reported incidence of postoperative chylous fistula varies between 1% and 2.5%. Management depends on the time of onset of the fistula, on the amount of chyle drainage in 24 h, and the presence or absence of accumulation of chyle under the skin flaps.

If a chylous leak is detected intraoperatively, every effort must be made to find the source and suture the opening. Accumulation of chyle affects flap survival, increases the risk of neck infections, and leads to emaciation of the patient. Chyle in a fasting patient is a clear-yellowish fluid as compared to the traditional milky white fluid. If a fistula is suspected postoperatively, the patient should begin IV feeding. The patient's head is kept elevated and a pressure dressing applied. Electrolytes and serum proteins should be monitored daily. The use of total parenteral nutrition feeds has largely obviated the need for re-exploration of the neck. However, when the daily output of chyle exceeds 600 mL in a day or 200–300 mL/day for 3 days, especially when the chyle fistula becomes apparent immediately after surgery, conservative closed wound management is unlikely to succeed; these are indications for surgical exploration [46].

16.6.5 Cardiac Arrhythmias

Cardiac arrhythmias can also occur during neck surgery. Manipulation of the carotid bulb during dissection of the IJV can lead to the arrhythmias that can be life-threatening. Gentle and careful handling of the carotid bulb can reduce the incidence of such irregular rhythms. The use of lidocaine injected into the adventitia surrounding the carotid bulb may reduce the risk of arrhythmias.

16.6.6 Facial/Cerebral Edema

Synchronous bilateral RND in which both IJVs are ligated may result in a (1) facial and/or cerebral edema due to inadequate venous drainage, (2) blindness, and (3) hypoxia. This typically resolves with time as collateral circulation is established. Facial edema appears more commonly in those patients with a history of previous radiation therapy (RT).

Facial edema may be prevented by preserving at least one external jugular vein when bilateral neck dissection is performed. Cerebral edema may lead to increased intracranial pressure, which may also be associated with syndrome of inappropriate antidiuretic hormone. If ligation of both IJVs is anticipated, intraoperative and perioperative fluid administration should be closely monitored.

16.6.7 Late Complications

Late complications following neck dissection tend to be less severe but may considerably affect the quality of life of the patient. The formation of a *neuroma* may considerably affect the day-to-day life of the patient. In such cases, it is important to ascertain that any lump in the neck is not a sign of recurrent disease. Similarly, *chronic shoulder pain* may impair the daily activities of the patient. Competent physiotherapy may help to improve the patient's condition.

References

1. Weiss MH, Harrison LB, Isaacs RS. Use of decision analysis in planning a management strategy for the stage N0 neck. Arch Otolaryngol Head Neck Surg. 1994;120(7):699–702.
2. Huang SH, Hwang D, Lockwood G, Goldstein DP, O'Sullivan B. Predictive value of tumor thickness for cervical lymph-node involvement in squamous cell carcinoma of the oral cavity: a meta-analysis of reported studies. Cancer. 2009;115(7):1489–97.
3. Jerjes W, Upile T, Petrie A, Riskalla A, Hamdoon Z, Vourvachis M, Karavidas K, Jay A, Sandison A, Thomas GJ, Kalavrezos N, Hopper C. Clinicopathological parameters, recurrence, locoregional and distant metastasis in 115 T1-T2 oral squamous cell carcinoma patients. Head Neck Oncol. 2010;20:2–9.
4. Tam S, Amit M, Zafereo M, Bell D, Weber RS. Depth of invasion as a predictor of nodal disease and survival in patients with oral tongue squamous cell carcinoma. Head Neck. 2019;41(1):177–84.
5. D'Cruz AK, Vaish R, Kapre N, Dandekar M, Gupta S, Hawaldar R, Agarwal JP, Pantvaidya G, Chaukar D, Deshmukh A, Kane S, Arya S, Ghosh-Laskar S, Chaturvedi P, Pai P, Nair S, Nair D, Badwe R. Head and Neck Disease Management Group. Elective versus therapeutic neck dissection in node-negative oral cancer. N Engl J Med. 2015;373(6):521–9.
6. Ho AS, Kim S, Tighiouart M, Gudino C, Mita A, Scher KS, Laury A, Prasad R, Shiao SL, Van Eyk JE, Zumsteg ZS. Metastatic lymph node burden and survival in oral cavity cancer. J Clin Oncol. 2017;35(31):3601–9.
7. Umeda M, Nishimatsu N, Teranobu O, Shimada K. Criteria for diagnosing lymph node metastasis from squamous cell carcinoma of the oral cavity: a study of the relationship

between computed tomographic and histologic findings and outcome. J Oral Maxillofac Surg. 1998;56(5):585–95.
8. Shah JP, Singh B. Keynote comment: why the lack of progress for oral cancer? Lancet Oncol. 2006;7(5):356–7.
9. Antoniades K, Lazaridis N, Vahtsevanos K, Hadjipetrou L, Antoniades V, Karakasis D. Treatment of squamous cell carcinoma of the anterior faucial pillar-retromolar trigone. Oral Oncol. 2003;39(7):680–6.
10. O'Brien CJ, Traynor SJ, McNeil E, McMahon JD, Chaplin JM. The use of clinical criteria alone in the management of the clinically negative neck among patients with squamous cell carcinoma of the oral cavity and oropharynx. Arch Otolaryngol Head Neck Surg. 2000;126(3):360–5.
11. Byers RM, Weber RS, Andrews T, McGill D, Kare R, Wolf P. Frequency and therapeutic implications of "skip metastases" in the neck from squamous carcinoma of the oral tongue. Head Neck. 1997;19(1):14–9.
12. Ambrosch P, Kron M, Pradier O, Steiner W. Efficacy of selective neck dissection: a review of 503 cases of elective and therapeutic treatment of the neck in squamous cell carcinoma of the upper aerodigestive tract. Otolaryngol Head Neck Surg. 2001;124(2):180–7.
13. Brazilian Head and Neck Cancer Study Group. Results of a prospective trial on elective modified radical classical versus supraomohyoid neck dissection in the management of oral squamous carcinoma. Am J Surg. 1998;176(5):422–7.
14. Koo BS, Lim YC, Lee JS, Choi EC. Management of contralateral N0 neck in oral cavity squamous cell carcinoma. Head Neck. 2006;28(10):896–901.
15. Schliephake H. Prognostic relevance of molecular markers of oral cancer--a review. Int J Oral Maxillofac Surg. 2003;32(3):233–45.
16. Hamoir M, Shah JP, Desuter G, Gregoire V, Ledeghen S, Plouin-Gaudon I. Prevalence of lymph nodes in the apex of level V: a plea against the necessity to dissect the apex of level V in mucosal head and neck cancer. Head Neck. 2005;27(11):963–9.
17. Brennan PA, Hoffman GR, Mackenzie N, Ethunandan M, Boote DJ, Mellor TK. Recurrent nodal metastases in the posterior triangle: implications for treatment of the atypical tumour. Br J Oral Maxillofac Surg. 2006;44(2):83–6.
18. Pedersen NJ, Jensen DH, Hedbäck N, Frendø M, Kiss K, Lelkaitis G, et al. Staging of early lymph node metastases with the sentinel lymph node technique and predictive factors in T1/T2 oral cavity cancer: a retrospective single-center study. Head Neck. 2016;38(Suppl 1):E1033–40.
19. Abdul-Razak M, Chung H, Wong E, Palme C, Veness M, Farlow D, et al. Sentinel lymph node biopsy for early oral cancers: Westmead Hospital experience. ANZ J Surg. 2017;87(1–2):65–9.
20. Zhu Y, Zhou C, He Q. Radiation therapy's efficacy on tongue cancer: a population-based survival analysis. Onco Targets Ther. 2018;11:7271–6.
21. Maochang Y, Luo YX, Zhou RJ. The curative effect of the comprehensive treatment of tongue cancer. Oral Med. 1991;11(2):79–81.
22. Cunningham MJ, Johnson JT, Myers EN, Schramm VL, Thearle PB. Cervical lymph node metastasis after local excision of early squamous cell carcinoma of the oral cavity. Am J Surg. 1986;152(4):361–6.
23. Akutsu Y, Matsubara H. The significance of lymph node status as a prognostic factor for esophageal cancer. Surg Today. 2011;41:1190–5.
24. Robbins KT, Shaha AR, Medina JE, Califano JA, Wolf GT, Ferlito A, et al. Consensus statement on the classification and terminology of neck dissection. Arch Otolaryngol Head Neck Surg. 2008;134(5):536–8.
25. McAlister ED, Goldstein DP, Rotstein LE. Redefining classification of central neck dissection in differentiated thyroid cancer. Head Neck. 2014;36(2):286–90.
26. Weisz Shabtay N, Ronen O. Level IV neck dissection as an elective treatment for oral tongue carcinoma-a systematic review and meta-analysis. Oral Surg Oral Med Oral Pathol Oral Radiol. 2020;130(4):363–72.

27. Watkinson JC, Gaze MN, Wilson JA. Metastatic neck disease. In: Watkinson JC, Gaze MN, Wilson JA, editors. Stell&Maran's head & neck surgery. 4th ed. Oxford: Butterworth Heinemann; 2000. p. 201–32.
28. Bocca E. Conservative neck dissection. Laryngoscope. 1975;85:1511–5.
29. Dua A, Desai SS. Utility of internal jugular vein reconstruction in modified radical neck dissection. Vascular. 2013;22(2):81–4.
30. Barzan L, Talamini R, Franchin G, et al. Effectiveness of selective neck dissection in head and neck cancer: the experience of two Italian centers. Laryngoscope. 2015;125(8):1849–55.
31. Paleri V, Urbano TG, Mehanna H, et al. Management of neck metastases in head and neck cancer: United Kingdom national multidisciplinary guidelines. J Laryngol Otol. 2016;130(S2):S161–9.
32. Mehanna H, Kong A, Ahmed SK. Recurrent head and neck cancer: United Kingdom national multidisciplinary guidelines. J Laryngol Otol. 2016;130(S2):S181–90.
33. Amit M, Hilly O, Leider-Trejo L, Popovtzer A, Gutfeld O, Shvero J, et al. The role of elective neck dissection in patients undergoing salvage laryngectomy. Head Neck. 2012;35(10):1392–6.
34. Zenga J, Pipkorn P, Graboyes EM, Martin EJ, Rich JT, Moore EJ, et al. Oncologic outcomes of extended neck dissections in human papillomavirus-related oropharyngeal squamous cell carcinoma. Head Neck. 2018;40(5):955–62.
35. Martin H, Del Valle B, Ehrlich H, Cahan WG. Neck dissection. Cancer. 1951;4(3):441–99.
36. Pugazhendi SK, Thangaswamy V, Venkatasetty A, Thambiah L. The functional neck dissection for lymph node neck metastasis in oral carcinoma. J Pharm Bioallied Sci. 2012;4(Suppl 2):S245–7.
37. Brazilian Head and Neck Cancer Study Group. End results of a prospective trial on elective lateral neck dissection vs type III modified radical neck dissection in the management of supraglottic and transglottic carcinomas. Head Neck. 1999;21(8):694–702.
38. Lydiatt DD, Karrer FW, Lydiatt WM, Johnson PJ. The evaluation, indications, and contraindications of selective neck dissections. Nebr Med J. 1994;79(5):140–4.
39. Byers RM. Neck dissection: concepts, controversies, and technique. Semin Surg Oncol. 1991;7(1):9–13.
40. Krol E, Brandt CT, Blakeslee-Carter J, Ahanchi SS, Dexter DJ, Karakla D, Panneton JM. Vascular interventions in head and neck cancer patients as a marker of poor survival. J Vasc Surg. 2019;69(1):181–9.
41. Hemmat SM, Wang SJ, Ryan WR. Neck dissection technique commonality and variance: a survey on neck dissection technique preferences among head and neck oncologic surgeons in the American Head and Neck Society. Int Arch Otorhinolaryngol. 2017;21(1):8–16.
42. Shaw HJ. A modification of the MacFee incisions for neck dissection. J Laryngol Otol. 1988;102(12):1124–6.
43. Chintamani. Ten commandments of safe and optimum neck dissections for cancer. Indian J Surg. 2015;77(2):85–91.
44. Dedivitis RA, Guimarães AV, Pfuetzenreiter EG, Castro MA. Neck dissection complications. Braz J Otorhinolaryngol. 2011;77(1):65–9.
45. Kerawala CJ, Heliotos M. Prevention of complications in neck dissection. Head Neck Oncol. 2009;1:35.
46. Russel WD, Ibanez ML. Thyroid carcinoma. Cancer. 1963;2:1425–9.
47. McGregor GI, Luoma A, Jackson SM. Lymph node metastases from well-differentiated thyroid cancer. A clinical review. Am J Surg. 1985;149(5):610–2.
48. Dugena O, Islam S, Hayter J. The rate of phrenic nerve injury following neck dissection for head and neck cancer and its impact on the length of hospital stay. Int J Oral Maxillofac Surg. 2017;4(S1):283.
49. Marchetta FC, Sako K, Matsuura H. Modified neck dissection for carcinoma of the thyroid gland. Am J Surg. 1970;20(2):87–93.
50. Noguchi S, Murakami N. The value of lymph-node dissection in patients with differentiated thyroid cancer. Surg Clin N Am. 1987;67(2):251–61.

51. Machens A, Holzhausen HJ, Dralle H. Skip metastases in thyroid cancer leaping the central lymph node compartment. Arch Surg. 2004;139(1):43–5.
52. Haagensen CD, Feind CR, Herter FP, Slanetz CA, Weinberg JA. The lymphatics in cancer. Philadelphia, PA: WB Saunders; 1972. p. 231–52.
53. Robbins KT, Clayman G, Levine P. Neck dissection classification update. Arch Otolaryngol. 2002;128(7):751–8.
54. Woolner LB, Beahrs OH, Black BM, McConahey WM, Keating FR. Thyroid carcinoma: general considerations and follow-up data on 1181 cases. In: Young S, Inman DR, editors. Thyroid neoplasia. London: Academic Press; 1968. p. 71–9.

Reconstruction After Glossectomy

17

17.1 Introduction

The oral tongue is the most common site of oral cavity malignancy and presents a significant reconstructive challenge due to its highly specialized function [1]. The oral tongue has a lot of functions in speech and articulation, as well as mastication, oral hygiene, and the oral phase of swallowing [2]. The oropharyngeal tongue is important for the pharyngeal phase of swallowing and prevention of aspiration. Normal swallowing begins with containing the food bolus within the oral cavity. Greater volumes of tongue resection are associated with reduction in swallowing function [3–5] since the lack of adequate tongue bulk leads to premature spillage into the pharynx [6]. Thus, the defect left by resecting malignant tumors dramatically affects speech, mastication, swallowing, and general quality of life. A variety of options are available to the head and neck surgeon for reconstruction.

Traditionally, tongue reconstruction has been defined by the quantity and location of the tongue defect. The amount of tissue missing is defined by the ablative procedure that has led to the defect (i.e., partial glossectomy, hemiglossectomy, subtotal glossectomy, total glossectomy, and total glossectomy with resection of adjacent tissues). The location of the defect is generally described as the oral tongue or base of the tongue (BOT). The ideal tongue reconstructive method closes large ablative defects in a watertight fashion that separates the oral cavity from the neck, avoids tethering tongue scars that limit tongue mobility, restores the innate functions of speech and swallowing by providing sufficient tissue volume, and provides an acceptable aesthetic result [7].

At present, no reconstructive options offer complete restoration of the form and function of the tongue. Regional and free flap options vary by the amount of bulk provided, mobility afforded, technical difficulty, operative time, and functional outcomes. Of paramount importance is the coordination of multidisciplinary reconstructive and rehabilitative teams.

© The Author(s), under exclusive license to Springer Nature Switzerland AG 2022

M. F. Sakr, *Tongue Lesions*, https://doi.org/10.1007/978-3-031-08198-9_17

17.2 Defects: Etiology and Classification

Tongue defects are commonly a result of oncological resection, but severe trauma can also lead to extensive defects. The site of most tongue malignancies is the lateral border of the anterior two-thirds of the tongue [1]. Malignancies occur with equal frequency on the left and right sides of the tongue, and approximately 75% of patients have unilateral disease that does not cross the midline [8]. Oncological margins of 1.5–2 cm are recommended for squamous cell carcinomas (SCC), the most common malignancy encountered. Therefore, even small cancers can lead to relatively large surgical defects.

In general, a partial glossectomy involves resection of less than one-third of the tongue, hemiglossectomy involves resection of one-third to half of the tongue, subtotal glossectomy involves resection of half to three-fourths of the tongue, and total glossectomy involves resection of the entire tongue. Although glossectomy refers specifically to the tongue, yet any of these resections can also involve resection of the floor of the mouth, soft palate, oropharynx, hypopharynx, mandible, or any other adjacent structures given the size and location of a malignancy.

Several authors reported that the greater the degree (volume) of tongue resection, the greater the impairment of swallowing after reconstruction [3, 9]. Similarly, larger tongue defects are associated with worse tongue mobility [10]. Some authors relied more on the location of the malignancy and hence classified surgical defects slightly differently, as involving the (1) oral tongue only, (2) base-of-tongue only, or (3) oral and base-of-tongue. Such classification has more specific prognostic and reconstructive implications.

17.3 Reconstruction Options

17.3.1 Goals of Reconstruction

The goal of tongue reconstruction is to restore function, primarily speech and swallowing, to as close to normal as possible, with an acceptable aesthetic result. When deciding between reconstructive options of the tongue, the most important considerations are (1) the size and site of the tongue defect, (2) availability of neck donor vessels, (3) involvement of the floor of the mouth, and (4) presence of concurrent mandible bony defect and/or concurrent oropharyngeal defect [10]. The radial forearm free flap (RFFF) and anterolateral thigh free flap (ALTFF) are the two most commonly used flaps to reconstruct the tongue [7].

Typically, small defects (less than one-fourth of the tongue) are amenable to healing by secondary intention, primary closure, or reconstruction with a skin graft [8] with excellent functional outcomes. Larger defects such as subtotal glossectomy, total glossectomy, or those involving the floor of the mouth require reconstruction that includes vascularized tissue replacement (free or pedicled flaps) to adequately restore bulk and prevent tethering scars and ankyloglossia [8].

17.3.2 Overview

In addition to tissue reconstruction, many patients may also require other procedures such as tracheostomy due to significant airway swelling immediately following the surgery and placement of a gastrostomy tube (G-tube) or a temporary nasogastric (NG) tube feeding to facilitate adequate postoperative nutrition.

In the case of a concurrent, full-thickness mandible bony defect with a tongue defect, in which the plan is to restore mandible continuity at the same time as tongue reconstruction, a bony free flap is likely required such as the scapula flap, fibula flap, or iliac flap.

In the case of a concurrent sizable oropharyngeal or hypopharyngeal mucosal defect, there can be dangerous communication into the neck and great vessels from the oral cavity and pharynx. In these situations, sealing off the oral cavity can prevent salivary exposure in the neck and minimize the risk of carotid blowout and fistula formation. This can be achieved by local tissue advancement or a submental island flap for smaller defects. For larger pharyngeal defects, however, transfer of bulky autologous tissue is often more ideal for better restoration of swallowing function [11].

Microvascular free-flap reconstruction necessitates that the patient has available donor vessels in the neck. If no such neck vessels are available, a pectoralis flap or a pedicled latissimus dorsi (LD) flap may be a useful option. A regional composite pectoralis flap with an osteocutaneous component from the rib has also been described. Alternatively, a vein graft can be used to reach vessels in the contralateral neck or to connect to the internal mammary vessels as the free flap donor vessels [11].

17.3.2.1 Regional Flaps

Many regional flaps have been described for tongue reconstruction, and many are still employed when free tissue transfer is contraindicated. The infrahyoid fasciomyocutaneous flap, infrahyoid myofascial flap, trapezius island myocutaneous flap, pedicled submental island flap, pedicled latissimus dorsi flap, and pectoralis major myocutaneous flap (PMMF) are examples of regional flaps that can be used to reconstruct the tongue [7, 8, 12]. Advantages of regional flaps include shorter operative times, strong reliability, and ability to harvest without a second surgical team. They can also be used as a salvage option after failed free tissue transfer [8].

The adequacy of regional flaps depends on the size of the tongue defect and the donor site's tissue bulk. In obese patients, there will be much more soft tissue available for reconstruction than thin patients. Smaller regional flaps such as submental island flap can be useful for reconstructing a small tongue defect, whereas larger regional flaps such as a pectoralis myocutaneous flap are preferred for larger defects, especially in patients with poor neck donor vessels. Even large regional flaps, however, such as a pectoralis flap or a pedicled latissimus flap, may *not* be useful for total glossectomy defect reconstruction if the donor flap lacks sufficient tissue bulk [11].

Regional flaps can be contraindicated in the case of extensive neck disease or prior neck surgery as, often, the pedicle supplying flaps has already been compromised or will be sacrificed during oncological resection [8].

17.3.2.1.1 Pectoralis Major Myocutaneous Flap/Myofacial Flap

The pectoralis flap is considered the "workhorse" of oral cavity reconstruction. It is a fan-shaped musculocutaneous flap based on the thoracoacromial artery. The *pectoral branch* of the thoracoacromial artery, which runs in the fat on the underside of the muscle, is the primary blood supply. The course of the pectoral branch artery corresponds to the line drawn from the midpoint of the clavicle continuing to the medial portion of the acromion to xyphoid line. Sacrifice of the lateral thoracic artery (secondary blood supply) is usually required to gain necessary length. The superior thoracic artery also supplies the pectoralis major but is usually divided when the flap is raised.

Advantages

Advantages of the pectoralis flap include (1) its ease of harvest as a one-stage reconstruction, (2) no need for changing the patient's position intraoperatively, (3) primary donor site closure, and (4) large skin territory (island) that can be used for defects involving two epithelial surfaces. In addition, the muscular part covers neck structures protecting the carotid artery, especially in patients who have undergone radiation therapy.

Disadvantages

Some surgeons consider the major *disadvantage* of the pectoralis flap is its bulky size, which leads to postoperative contour deformities, particularly in patients who are overweight. Other disadvantages that have been reported include the following:

1. The flap can conceal recurrences, making follow-up in the neck area more complicated.
2. In women, the flap might include breast tissue, which may lead to breast asymmetry.
3. In males, hirsute chest skin is placed intraorally.
4. The flap causes loss of pectoralis muscle function in arm adduction and/or rotation.

Indications

The pectoralis major myocutaneous flap and the myofascial flap variation are utilized in a large variety of head and neck reconstructive procedures that can include coverage of mucosal and/or cutaneous defects. The extent of coverage and the reach of the flap are dependent on the anatomy of the patient, modifications of the standard techniques of elevation, and inset. The upper limits are generally considered the zygomatic arch area externally and the superior tonsillar pole internally—patient body habitus may either limit extension short of these landmarks or permit extension beyond. The myofascial flap variation carries no skin paddle and is utilized primarily to close small mucosal defects, to protect major vascular structures and to support primary mucosal closure in a patient at increased risk of wound breakdown (prior radiation, diabetic, weight loss).

Contraindications

Contraindications of the pectoralis flap include (1) a defect that is too large or outside the potential reach of the reconstructive tissue; (2) very obese patients will have a difficult-to-handle and possibly nonviable skin paddle; (3) patients with prior chest wall trauma and/or prior chest wall surgery (mastectomy, breast implants, subclavian lines, cardiac pacemaker, etc.) who may have absent, scarred, or poorly vascularized pectoralis major muscle; (4) if removal of the muscle will affect the strength of the shoulder and arm, affecting the ability of the patient to work or participate in recreational activities; and (5) congenital absence of pectoralis muscle (Poland's syndrome).

Technique

The size and location of the skin paddle over the pectoralis major (PM) muscle are designed. Initial incision is made from the lateral edge of the designed skin paddle toward the anterior axillary line. Usually this incision is above the nipple in the male and below the breast in the female patient. The incision is carried down to the PM muscle. This allows for identification of the medial and inferior extents of the muscle, after which the design of the skin paddle can be moved inferiorly or superiorly so as to rest above the muscle tissue.

The inferior, medial, and lateral incisions are made through the muscle and fascia of the PM muscle and down to the chest wall. The superior skin flap incision is made down to the muscle fibers of the PM muscle. The skin paddle should be temporarily secured to the fascia of the muscle with 3-0 Vicryl suture.

A skin/fascia tunnel is created under the superficial PM muscle fascia, preserving the perforators to the overlying deltopectoral flap; the tunnel must extend from the superior flap incision, over the clavicle, and into the neck. The muscle flap is then elevated off the chest wall beneath the deep PM muscle fascia. Care should be taken in controlling the bleeding from the chest wall perforators at the muscular attachments to the chest. Vessel retraction into the chest can lead to hemothorax.

As the muscle is elevated from inferiorly to superiorly, the pedicle should be identified by visualization and palpation on the deep surface of the muscle. As the muscle fibers are cut along the sternal attachments, care should be taken *not* to cut the internal mammary perforators (adjacent to the sternum), which supply the deltopectoral flap. The pedicle should be in view while transecting the lateral muscle attachments.

The lateral thoracic artery is usually cut to increase the length and rotation and should be tied to prevent late bleeding and/or hematoma. Care is taken not to rotate, kink, or compress proximal flap. Increased length can also be gained by division of the clavicular portion of the PM muscle above the pedicle by debulking the muscle fibers over the proximal pedicle and by splitting and removing the middle one-third of the clavicle (this is rarely necessary and increases the risk of vessel kinking and flap failure).

Excessive fat between the muscle and skin can lead to skin paddle loss without muscle loss. When securing the flap in place, muscle fascia should be secured, independent of the skin paddle.

Closure Mobilization of the surrounding tissue of the chest should allow for primary closure in almost all cases. Split thickness skin grafts should be used, if primary closure is not possible. The neck and chest are drained with suction drains, two in each location. The drains must not cross the pedicle.

Postoperative care/flap monitoring No tracheotomy ties, gown ties, or pressure on the pedicle in the neck or over the clavicle should be applied. The flap is monitored by observation of color and needle-prick bleeding. Poor flap appearance may be improved with the use of dextran, steroids, and/or hyperbaric oxygen. Pressure points and excessive torque should be assessed and improved if possible with changes in the head and arm positions or neck suture removal. Flap failure is most likely to occur at the superior aspect of the flap/mucosa closure.

17.3.2.1.2 Platysma Flap

The platysma muscle itself lies superficial to the muscular fascial sheath of the neck. Blood vessels from the muscle to the overlying skin are not true musculocutaneous perforators, and the muscle does not have a true axial blood supply. The muscle and overlying skin receive blood from a variety of sources including the submental artery, branches of the proximal facial artery, postauricular artery, occipital artery, terminal cutaneous branches of the superior thyroid artery, superficial cervical artery, and transverse cervical artery.

The platysma flap is a reliable, thin myocutaneous regional flap. When it is used for intraoral and lower facial reconstruction, the most important blood supply to the flap are the *submental branch of the facial artery* and the *superior thyroid artery*. Reconstruction of the floor of the mouth and buccal mucosa is achievable for defects of up to 5 cm.

Indications

The platysma flap may be used to close defects on the lower face, buccal mucosa, and floor of the mouth (Fig. 17.1). In selected cases, the flap will extend to the oropharynx; however, depending on the body habitus of the patient, closure of defects in the oropharynx may require excessive tension on the flap. The flap is ideally suited for reconstruction of deep chin and low anterior cheek defects in patients not requiring neck dissection. The color match is good with facial skin. When used to resurface these areas, a dual blood supply including the submental and superior thyroid arteries may be preserved (see pertinent anatomy section).

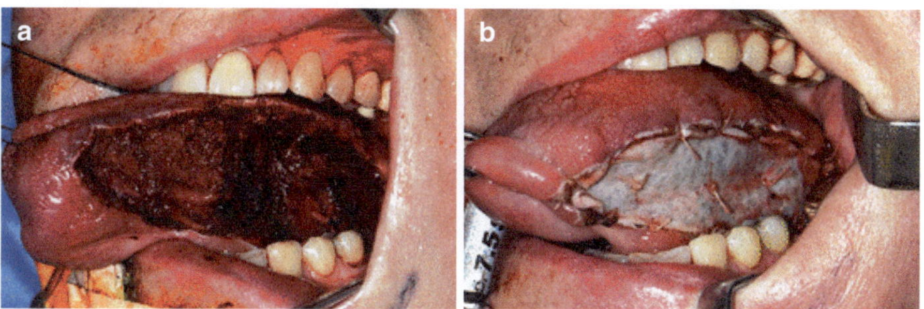

Fig. 17.1 Tongue and floor of mouth defect (**a**) covered with platysma flap (**b**)

Contraindications

Contraindications of the platysma flap include the following: (1) prior radiotherapy to the neck, which will significantly compromise the viability of the flap; (2) neck dissection that interrupts the main blood supply to the flap, i.e., submental branch of the facial artery and a cutaneous branch of the superior thyroid artery (relative contraindication); (3) the need for tissue bulk as the flap is relatively thin; (4) defects larger than 5 × 7 cm; (5) patients with extremely thin skin and a poorly developed platysma muscle; and (6) if the sternocleidomastoid (SCM) muscle will be removed as a part of the planned neck surgery.

Potential Complications

Potential complications of the platysma flap includes (1) flap failure and loss of the cutaneous paddle. Despite apparent preservation of the blood supply, if a neck dissection is performed, the risk of skin necrosis is significant. If the continuity of the facial artery between its origin and the submental branch is disrupted, the blood supply will be tenuous; (2) injury to the mandibular branch of the facial nerve and (3) distortion of the contour of the jaw line will occur to some degree with the use of this flap, and patients should be aware of that.

Technique

The terminal cutaneous blood vessels to the platysma may be delicate. The surgeon's use of loupe magnification during elevation of the flap is useful. The anticipated skin paddle should be outlined in the lower lateral neck. The lower margin of this skin paddle should not extend below the clavicle.

The method of flap elevation varies according to the indication for flap use. If an intraoral defect is to be closed, a large platysma skin flap may be raised with the inferior margin of the skin paddle defining the most distal extent. The upper skin paddle incision is not made until after it is determined that the paddle will cover the defect. The skin overlying the platysma is elevated in a plane above the muscle, just into the subcutaneous tissue. The muscle fibers should retain some connective tissue covering. The inferior margin of the muscle is divided distal to the skin paddle.

The muscle and skin paddle are mobilized toward the defect by elevation of the platysma in an inferior-to-superior direction. The plane of elevation should include the fascia of the SCM, as well as the anterior and external jugular veins. Inclusion of these veins that are left intact superiorly adds to venous drainage of the flap. By elevation of the fascia of the SCM from lateral to medial, the superior thyroid contribution should be left intact. This will create a rotation point for the flap that is relatively low, and additional length can be obtained by bringing the fascia overlying the strap muscles up with the anterior jugular veins.

The muscle may be detached along its posterior and posterosuperior margins. Mobilization of the flap may require division of the superior thyroid contribution. In such a case, every effort should be made to keep the base of the flap as wide as possible.

Closure The neck skin is closed in two layers. Mobilization of the upper chest skin will facilitate closure of the skin paddle donor site. Two 10-mm fully perforated suction drains are placed. One should lie parallel to the sternocleidomastoid in the groove anterior to it, and the other should lie posterior to it.

Postoperative care Tension on the flap is minimized if the patient's head is turned toward the donor side. This should be reinforced in the postoperative orders and accomplished with pillows or sandbags. Drains are removed when the output is less than 30 mL/day.

17.3.2.2 Free Tissue Transfer

Free tissue transfer has become the mainstay of reconstruction of large tongue defects. Free flap reconstruction of intraoral defects was first introduced in 1983 with the radial forearm free flap (RFFF) [1], and it has since expanded to include a multitude of flap types and techniques with the goal of optimizing postoperative function.

In addition to the RFFF, multiple sources of autologous tissue have been investigated, and commonly used flaps include the anterolateral thigh, rectus abdominis, and latissimus dorsi. Other less commonly used free flap options include tensor fascia lata, gracilis, scapula, iliac crest, and fibula [7, 13]. In selecting free tissue for tongue reconstruction, surgeons should consider the defect size, the need to reconstruct surrounding structures in addition to the tongue (such as bone or oropharyngeal/hypopharyngeal mucosa), donor site morbidity, potential for flap reinnervation and the reinnervation site, and whether simultaneous flap harvest and oncological resection are desirable. In general, immediate reconstruction at the time of tumor extirpation leads to optimal functional results [7]. Since many oncological patients will need postoperative radiation therapy, it is important to overcorrect the volume defect, as one can expect significant volume loss over time following radiation therapy. Failure of free flaps ranges from 0% to 15% in the immediate postoperative period [14].

17.3.2.2.1 Radial Forearm Free Flap (RFFF)

The radial forearm free flap (RFFF) is one of the most widely used microvascular free flaps in reconstructive surgery of the head and neck. The RFFF is currently preferred for reconstruction of defects involving the tongue, intraoral soft tissue, oropharynx, soft palate, hypopharynx, cervical esophagus, and selected cutaneous defects. This flap is now also being used in the reconstruction of extended hemilaryngeal defects. The RFFF is used primarily as a fascio-cutaneous flap but can also be used as a fascial flap. It is based on the *radial artery and its fascio-cutaneous branches*. The radial artery provides nutrient inflow to the flap via perforating vessels that pierce the antebrachial fascia as they course toward the subcutaneous fat and skin. The radial artery is easily palpable in the distal forearm, and its course can be marked by following the pulse proximally. Veins accompany the radial artery, and the subcutaneous cephalic vein is at the radial most edge of the forearm. This large vein can be incorporated into the flap distally or left behind to use for radial artery reconstruction after flap harvest [15].

Advantages

The RFFF has many advantages that include (1) relative ease of harvest with very consistent anatomy, (2) feasible harvesting simultaneously with oral ablation, (3) potential reinnervation through the coaptation of the lateral antebrachial cutaneous nerve to the lingual or inferior alveolar nerves [13], (4) being thin and pliable, (5) feasible harvesting with additional adipose tissue to increase its bulk, (6) availability of a long pedicle, and (7) availability of larger caliber vessels to allow easier microvascular anastomosis [8].

Disadvantages

On the other hand, the RFFF may have some disadvantages; it can leave an obvious scar on the wrist and rarely can lead to hand numbness and weakness. In the literature, partial skin graft loss has been observed at rates between 19% and 53%, donor site flexor tendon exposure was reported in 13–33% of cases, and reduction of patients' grip or pinch strength in 16–100% [1]. In addition, with RFFF harvest, there is a potential to disrupt the primary arterial supply to the hand if the patient has an unusual hand circulation pattern. Thus, preoperative assessment with *Allen's test* is imperative to avoid hand ischemia [1].

Indications

The RFFF typically provides less tissue than other free flap sources, even when extra forearm flap is harvested; therefore, it may ultimately have insufficient bulk for the reconstruction of subtotal or total glossectomy defects. In general, for tongue reconstruction, the RFFF is preferred for smaller than hemiglossectomy defects.

Contraindications

The major contraindications to the use of the RFFF are inadequate collateral blood flow to the hand via the ulnar artery, certain identifiable radial artery anomalies, and prior surgical or traumatic injury to the radial artery. The nondominant arm should be used if possible; however, functional deficit following flap harvest is minimal.

Potential Complications

The most frequent complication is incomplete healing of the skin graft placed to cover the donor site. Other potential complications include stiffness or weakness of the hand, numbness in the distribution of the superficial branch of the radial nerve, and cold intolerance of the hand.

Technique

The donor arm is placed on an operating arm board abducting the shoulder at 90° to the patient. A padded tourniquet is used proximally before prepping and draping. The size of the flap is determined and marked on the forearm, often with a template from the defect or estimate of the defect size. Because the flap can be folded, creative designs can be used in the harvest to reconstruct three-dimensional defects.

The traditional flap outline has the radial most aspect over the radial artery (Fig. 17.2). The flap can extend ulnar ward to the less hair-bearing part of the forearm as desired. If a *tendon graft* is needed, the palmaris longus (PL) is included in the flap. If the *bone* is needed, a portion of the distal radius (leaving dorsal and radial cortices) can be used. The defect can be prone to fracture, and this must be considered in postoperative mobilization or as a possible indication for prophylactic plating.

The distal aspect of the flap is raised first. Dissection proceeds deep to the antebrachial fascia, elevating the fascia with the flap. Paratendon is left on the flexor carpi radialis (FCR) tendon and PL, if the latter is to be left behind. The PL is often harvested with the flap, since it is expendable and can be used in the area of reconstruction as needed.

The radial artery and vena comitans are ligated and divided distally. The flap can then be raised from the distal aspect. As the dissection proceeds proximally, the pedicle travels under the brachioradialis tendon and muscle, necessitating retraction of this unit. Care is taken to avoid injuring the dorsal branch of the radial nerve, which exits into the distal forearm from underneath the brachioradialis muscle. The cephalic vein or a cutaneous vein can be taken with the flap. If the radial artery is to be reconstructed by a second team, the cephalic vein can be reversed and used for the reconstruction. The defect left by the flap can be primarily closed if small but is usually closed by harvesting a 0.018-inch skin graft to cover the donor defect.

The radial skin edge should be advanced to cover the exposed radial nerve; advancement of the ulnar skin edge should be avoided because the ulnar artery may be injured. The proximal arm is closed over a 10-mm fully perforated suction drain. The skin graft is sutured in place with 4-0 chromic suture, and a bolster of Adaptic dressing material and sterile foam is applied. The arm is wrapped in sterile Webril, and a volar plaster splint that places the wrist in approximately 45° of extension is

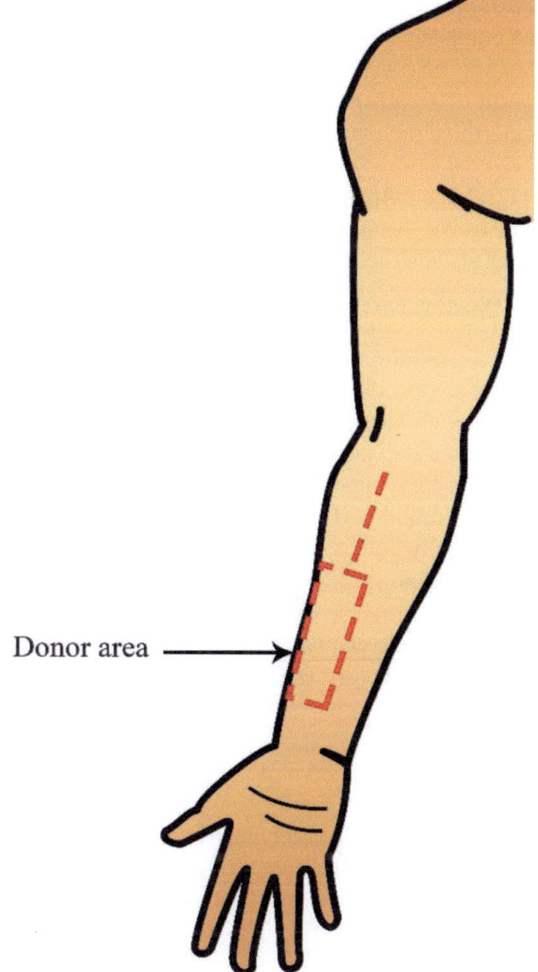

Fig. 17.2 The course of the radial pulse is determined, and the flap is outlined over the radial artery. The position of the flap can be changed depending on the needs of the recipient area. Consideration should be given to the location of the cephalic vein if that is to be used for venous drainage

placed. The splint is secured with a sterile ace wrap. A second option is using the Wound Vac system for closure. The fingers are kept free.

Complex flap design The radial forearm donor area is thin and vascular enough to allow very esoteric flap designs, with separate skin islands that allow flap folding and shaping to reconstruct complex defects.

Flap variations (1) *Radial forearm fascia flap* in which the deep fascia is harvested without skin paddle, creating a thin fascia only flap, and (2) *radial forearm osteocutaneous flap* in which a segment of the radius is harvested with the flap. It must be a unicortical block of volar radius and no wider than 1.5 cm. The radius is prone to fracture if a segment of radius is harvested.

Postoperative care The patient is allowed to use the donor hand as tolerated, with an emphasis on elevation to minimize edema and promote wound and/or skin graft healing. If donor bone is taken with the flap, stressing the radius with more than 10 lb of weight should be avoided for at least 6 weeks. Radiographs can help to determine the extent of bone healing.

17.3.2.2.2 Anterolateral Thigh Free Flap (ALTFF)

The use of the anterolateral thigh free flap (ALTFF) is now widespread for head and neck reconstruction. It is a versatile fascio-cutaneous flap based on the *descending branch of the lateral femoral circumflex artery*.

This descending branch travels deep within the space between the rectus femoris muscle and the vastus lateralis muscle (on the surface of the vastus intermedius)—often deep in the septal plane—and on occasion enters the substance of the vastus lateralis muscle as it travels distally. The septal plane can be used to identify the artery and flap perforator blood supply. This artery gives off either musculocutaneous or septocutaneous perforator vessels. Several authors have reported that the most common perforators are musculocutaneous [15–23]. A satisfactory perforator is generally found within 3 cm of the midpoint of a line connecting the anterior superior iliac spine with the superolateral border of the patella. More than half of perforators traverse the substance of the vastus lateralis muscle.

The pedicle can be as long as 7 or 8 cm. Depending on the point of ligation, the artery size can vary from 1 to 3 mm, with the major draining vein running slightly larger. Usually two veins accompany the artery and then merge into one at the profunda femoral vein junction. The flap can be innervated by a major branch of the lateral cutaneous nerve of the thigh, which enters the flap at the superior aspect, and can be traced proximally to provide length. Portions of the vastus lateralis muscle can be harvested with the flap if necessary. The position of the nerve to vastus lateralis is variable with respect to the vascular pedicle, and the nerve cannot always be left intact during harvest. It is likely that nerve division will result in morbidity.

Advantages

The ALTFF provides a tremendously versatile soft tissue flap. In selected patients, the skin paddle is as thin and pliable as in an RFFF. This flap has the advantages of (1) having the dense fascia lata on its deep surface (supra-fascial harvest is possible), (2) low or minimal long-term donor site morbidity though some patients may experience temporary leg weakness with some knee instability after flap harvest, (3) providing a significant bulk, (4) and the possibility of primary closure of the donor site with flaps up to 8 cm wide. In addition, contouring of the flap can be eased by insertion of the vascular pedicle into the midportion of the skin paddle.

Disadvantages

The anatomy of the ALTFF is less consistent than the RFFF, leading to a more difficult harvest in some cases. Furthermore, its pedicle is typically shorter than that of an RFFF [8]. However, by designing the skin flap more distally (closer to the knee), one can increase the harvested pedicle length. The most common flap-specific complication is marginal necrosis of the inset ALTFF, but total flap failure is rare [1, 24]. Some authors have suggested that the bulkiness of an ALTFF leads to less mobility of the neotongue [24]. In a comparison of tongue defects reconstructed with RFFF versus ALTFF, de Vicente et al. reported no significant differences in postoperative speech intelligibility, tongue mobility, or deglutition and concluded that because the ALTFF has less donor morbidity, it is a superior choice to the RFFF for tongue reconstruction [1].

Indications

Given that ALTFF is typically a much larger flap than RFFF, ALTFF is generally only used for larger glossectomy defects (typically larger than half of the tongue) [1].

Contraindications

The major contraindication for the ALTFF is *obesity*, which can result in unacceptable flap bulk. In addition, transmuscular perforator dissection is often required. Severe peripheral vascular disease may rarely render the flap pedicle critical to leg perfusion, making harvest unwise.

Potential Complications

Postoperative hernia is the most common complication. It is avoided by judicious harvest of the area of rectus fascia encompassing the cutaneous perforators and meticulous closure of the anterior rectus sheath. Patients may have a postoperative ileus due to manipulation of the bowel.

Technique [16, 18, 19]

The axis of the surface of the septum between the rectus femoris and the vastus lateralis is marked by a line connecting the anterior superior iliac spine and the lateral patella. This line is divided into thirds for purposes of outlining the flap. The width of the flap can reach up to 8 cm to allow primary closure (Fig. 17.3).

The junction of the proximal and middle third is often the site of a perforator that pierces the tensor fascia lata (TFL). This point can be incorporated in the flap to keep the TFL perforator as a "lifeboat" in the rare circumstance when the distal perforators are of poor quality or injured during dissection. The junction of the middle and distal third is marked and is also incorporated into the flap. The flap design can be adjusted depending on findings of a Doppler exam.

The anterior flap is elevated first, noting any vessels perforating the substance of the rectus femoris. Vessels approaching or near the septum are preserved until the posterior flap is elevated and the nourishing vessels to the flap have been identified with certainty.

The posterior flap is elevated toward the septum, again checking for major perforating vessels, this time through the vastus lateralis. Here the lower perforator can be seen to travel through the vastus. It should be dissected toward the descending branch of the LCFA. The septum is identified and any septal perforators are noted. If they are present and large in size, they can be used to perfuse the flap.

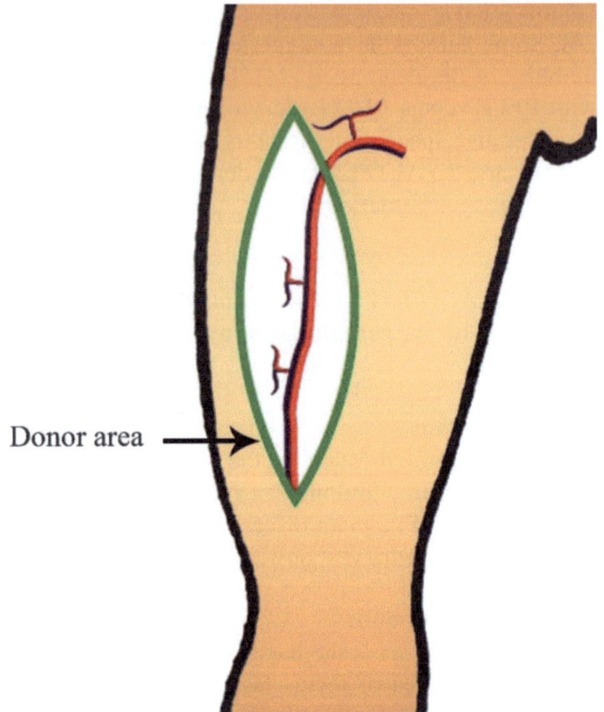

Fig. 17.3 The maximum width of the flap is judged with a pinch test. Donor sites that cannot be primarily closed (more than 8 cm) are skin grafted

If one or two good-quality perforators are visualized in the septum, then the anterior elevation can continue until the septum is isolated both medially and laterally. If the blood supply is entirely septal, the descending branch of the lateral femoral circumflex artery is found at the base of the septum between the rectus femoris and vastus lateralis and traced proximally (Fig. 17.4). When a flap perfuses from a transmuscular perforator, then this perforator is traced through the muscle to the descending branch. The size of the perforator will determine whether an additional vessel is needed. Vessels can be temporarily clamped with microvascular clamps to determine inflow dominance. The entire flap can then be isolated on the dominant perforator(s) and the descending branch of the lateral circumflex femoral vessels.

For *closure*, skin and subcutaneous tissue flaps are elevated medially and laterally at a level superficial to the fascia. These flaps are closed with interrupted suture and the skin is then approximated. Although light circumferential pressure can be applied to the thigh postoperatively, a closed suction drain is usually inserted.

Flap variations (1) *Anterolateral thigh adipofascial flap* in which the flap is harvested without the skin paddle. A thin layer of fat below Scarpa fascia is preserved with the deep fascia to create a thin fat and fascial flap (Fig. 17.5) and (2) *anterolateral thigh fascial flap* in which the muscular fascia and pedicle are harvested, and

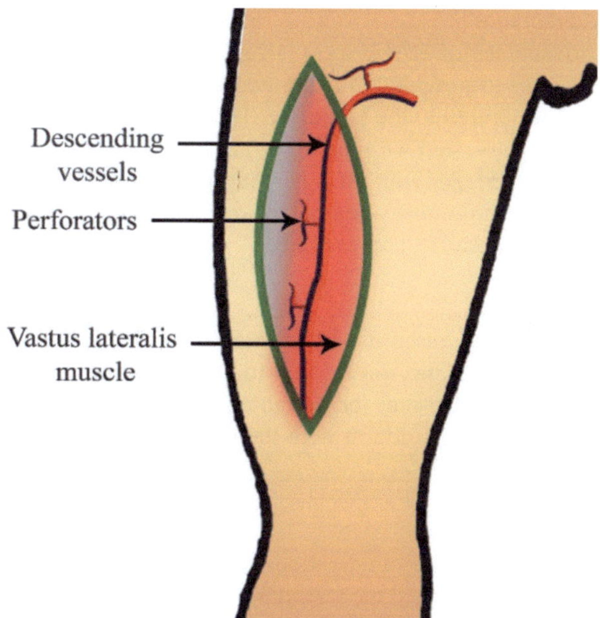

Fig. 17.4 The perforators usually travel through the muscle and must be dissected free. A bipolar cautery can be used

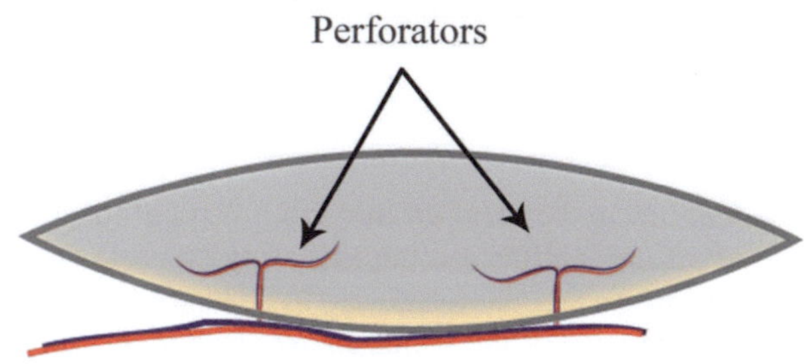

Fig. 17.5 Anterolateral thigh adipofascial flap. The flap can be harvested with just fascia and a small amount of overlying fat to create a thin fascial flap

no skin or fat is removed. Depending on the type of ALT free flap needed, the volume and thickness of the flap is tailored to the individual extent of the defect.

Postoperative care Seroma is rarely formed but can be a nuisance postoperatively. The patient is allowed to ambulate as soon as clinically indicated for the flap reconstruction. The drain is usually pulled before discharge.

17.3.2.2.3 Rectus Abdominis Free Flap (RAFF)

The rectus abdominis free flap (RAFF) has also been commonly employed for tongue reconstruction. It is a muscle flap (up to 30 cm long) that can be harvested with skin and fascia, based on the *deep inferior epigastric artery and vein*, which are long, large-diameter vessels that are ideal for microvascular anastomoses. The pedicle length depends on muscle entry and amount of intramuscular dissection performed. Approximately, 5–7 cm can be obtained easily.

Advantages

Advantages of RAFF are (1) its long vascular pedicle, (2) its ability (similar to ALTFF) to provide bulk as a neotongue, and (3) its tendinous inscriptions, which can be sutured to the mandible. The RAFF can also provide thin, pliable tissue and can be harvested with the 10th, 11th, and 12th intercostal nerves, allowing reinnervation [25]. As with all other flap reconstruction, the RAFF should be harvested larger than the measured defect size to allow for expected atrophy during the postoperative healing process [25].

Indications

With the increased use of the RFFF for intraoral and pharyngeal reconstruction, the RAFF has been relegated to a second-line choice for reconstruction of these areas. The flap may be advantageous for cases in which a large tongue defect requires reconstruction with the need for more bulk than is available through the forearm flap.

Contraindications

Flap-specific contraindications include previous abdominal or hernia surgery that may have disrupted the vascular pedicle and previous vascular surgery involving the vessels for atherosclerotic disease. Thus, this flap should be avoided in patients with a history of large umbilical or paraumbilical hernias. Although the flap may be harvested in relatively heavy patients, *extreme obesity* is a contraindication to harvest of this flap, particularly if a skin paddle is required.

Technique

The muscle can be exposed through a vertical (or lower transverse) incision. It is placed off the midline, on the axis of the muscle. The total length of the incision depends on the amount of muscle to be harvested. The subcutaneous fat is divided down to the level of the rectus sheath. Perforators are ligated and divided (cautery of the perforators may find the surgeon chasing them into the muscle and damaging the muscle).

The rectus sheath is divided longitudinally and care must be taken at the inscriptions. The fascia is elevated medially and laterally, while gentle retraction is performed with Aliss clamps. The inscriptions are tightly adherent and must be released off the muscle without damaging the muscle fibers. At the lateral inferior muscle, the thin fascial layer over the deep fat is divided, and the muscle is gently retracted medially. The deep inferior epigastric artery and its accompanying veins are identified. They can be traced down to their origin (Fig. 17.6).

The origin of the muscle near the pubis is isolated by encircling the muscle with the index finger. The muscle is then divided with cautery while protecting the pedicle. The superior muscle is likewise encircled and divided to isolate the rectus on the pedicle. The superior epigastric vessels must be securely ligated or cauterized to stop bleeding from the superior retracting muscle edge (Fig. 17.7).

Following flap harvest, meticulous hemostasis is obtained. If a large dead space is created above the fascia, as is the case in the transverse incision or often when

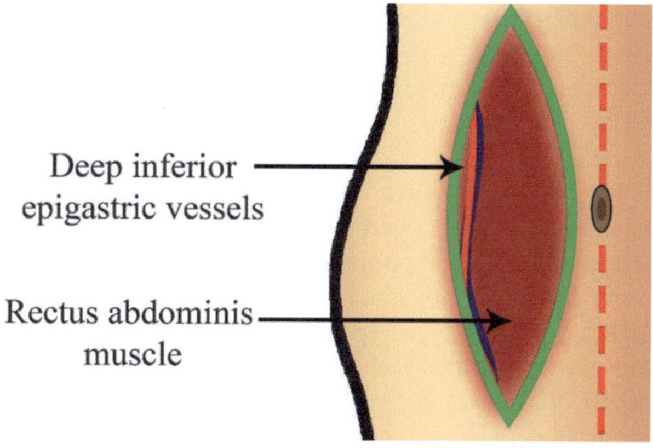

Fig. 17.6 At the lateral inferior muscle, the deep inferior epigastric artery and its accompanying veins are identified with gentle muscle medial retraction

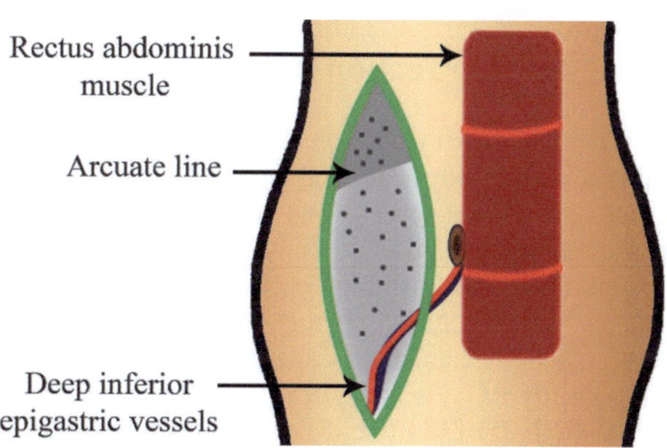

Fig. 17.7 The rectus muscle is divided superiorly and inferiorly to isolate it on the pedicle

skin paddles are harvested, then the wound should be drained. The anterior rectus sheath is closed with 0-0 nonabsorbable suture. The skin is closed with subcutaneous sutures of 2-0 Vicryl over a 10-mm fully perforated suction drain brought in inferiorly. The skin is closed with staples, and an abdominal binder is applied.

Postoperative care The suction drains are removed when drainage is less than 10 mL/8-h shift. The patient wears the abdominal binder for 2 weeks and is instructed against any heavy lifting for 6 weeks.

17.3.2.3 Reinnervation

Many studies have investigated whether reinnervation of an autologous free tissue transfer allows better outcomes. In the case of tongue reconstruction, harvested nerves can be coapted to the lingual or inferior alveolar nerves. Other recipient nerves described include the cervical plexus, hypoglossal nerve (CN-XII), and posterior auricular nerve [13]. Biglioli et al. [26] reported that reinnervated flaps show improved two-point discrimination compared with their nonreinnervated counterparts but no return of taste function [26]. More recently, Baas and colleagues [13] found that RFFF and ALTFF have been shown to regain better sensation than other flap types [13]. Furthermore, some authors suggested that a sensate ALTFF significantly improves swallowing compared with an insensate ALTFF [27, 28]. Others have also found that sensate free flaps used to reconstruct subtotal or total oral glossectomy defects lead to significantly improved speech and swallow [29–31].

The majority of reinnervated free flaps have the goal of *sensory* improvement, but the tongue has also been reconstructed with the goal of *motor* (muscular) reinnervation and improved movement of the neotongue [32]. Studies have demonstrated that, in large part, neotongues demonstrate no autologous motion, but rather move based on movements of surrounding muscles of the pharynx [33]. In 2000, Yoleri and Mavioğlu reported a case of tongue reconstruction using the gracilis muscle and obturator nerve, a flap often employed for facial reanimation. In their report, the neotongue regained some autologous movement; however, the patient unfortunately passed away before long-term evaluation could be completed [32].

17.4 Reconstruction Outcomes

In general, patients with high motivation, good family support, and regular follow-up with both a physician and a speech-language therapist develop better speech quality, swallowing ability, and overall quality of life after free flap reconstruction of the tongue [33, 34].

The QOL and functional performances are usually investigated by giving the patient validated questionnaires that include (1) the European Organization for Research and Treatment of Cancer (EORTC) Quality of Life Questionnaire Core 30 (QLQ-C30) [35]; (2) the EORTC Quality of Life Questionnaire-Head and Neck 35 (QLQ-H&N35) [36, 37]; (3) the MD Anderson Dysphagia Inventory (MDADI) [38]; and (4) the Performance Status Scale for Head and Neck (PSS-HN) [39].

The EORTC QLQ-C30 is designed to evaluate the QOL of cancer patients in general. Its 30 questions are divided into five functioning scales (physical, role, cognitivity, emotional, and social), 3 symptom scales (fatigue, pain, nausea, and vomiting), a scale for global health status and QoL, and six single-item scales (dyspnea, loss of appetite, insomnia, constipation and diarrhea, financial difficulties). Answers may vary among 1– 4, except for 29th and 30th questions, which vary between 1 and 7.

The EORTC QLQ-H&N35 is made up of 35 questions specifically investigating head and neck cancer patients' QOL. It consists of seven symptom scales (pain, swallowing, sense, speech, social eating, social contact, and sexuality); six symptom items (teeth issues, mouth opening, dry mouth, sticky saliva, coughing, and feeling ill), and five yes/no items (painkiller intake, nutritional supplements, feeding tube, weight loss, and weight gain). Thirty questions are structured as QLQ-C30, and the last five have a yes/no answer.

All scores from EORTC QLQ questionnaires must be converted to a 0–100 scale. High values for functioning or global QOL scales mean a high-functioning performance and QOL, respectively; in contrast, a higher score for symptom scale or single item denotes a higher level of disease burden.

The MDADI specifically focuses on consequences of dysphagia in everyday life of H&N cancer patients after treatment. The answer to any of the 20 questions may vary among "totally agree" to "totally disagree." A score from 1 to 5 is attributed to each question.

A part of one question is analyzing the global QOL related to swallowing; others are subdivided into three sets: physical, functional, and emotional. The final scores are converted to a 0–100 scale, where 0 means "no functioning" while 100 "extremely functioning."

The PSS-HN evaluates performance in areas of functioning most likely affected by head and neck cancer and its treatment: normalcy of diet, eating in public, and understandability of speech. Each subscale is rated from 0 to 100, with higher scores indicating better performance.

17.4.1 Speech Outcomes

17.4.1.1 Intelligibility

Free-flap reconstruction of the tongue often allows for intelligible speech production after surgery. In a series by Chien et al. [24], 13 (89%) of 15 patients with subtotal or total glossectomy defects that were reconstructed with RFFF or ALTFF went on to develop intelligible speech [24]. Similarly, in a series by Liao et al. [25], 100% of patients after RAFF for partial glossectomy defects retained intelligible speech [25]. Malignancies of the tongue often impair speech preoperatively due to bulkiness of the tumor and associated pain. In 2013, Dziegielewski et al. reported that preoperative speech intelligibility in their patient population was 78% [34]. At 1 year postoperatively, sentence intelligibility in their population dropped to 66%, whereas single-word intelligibility was 44%. They noted that patients who could attend more than 80% of speech therapy sessions, both before and after surgery, had higher scores overall [34].

Matsui et al. [40] compared speech outcomes among 126 patients who underwent RFFF, PMMF, or RAFF reconstruction of the anterior tongue. They found that overall intelligibility was not different among the three groups; however, RFFF patients performed significantly better than those using PMMF or RAFF in some articulatory sites for plosives [40]. A confounding factor in this study is that RFFF was generally used for smaller glossectomy defects, whereas PMMF and RAFF were used more for larger defects. Thus, improved function after RFFF may simply reflect the smaller defect being reconstructed. Furthermore, PMMF can sometimes lead to tongue tethering; the pedicle can only be mobilized so much before risking flap compromise, and this, in turn, can limit the final flap position and, subsequently, tongue movement.

Lam and Samman [2] and Manrique et al. [33] conducted systematic reviews of patients who underwent free flap reconstruction after glossectomy. They reported that patients undergoing anterior tongue resection with free flap reconstruction had an average preoperative *single-word intelligibility* of 90% across all studies. Intelligibility dropped to 69% at 1 month postoperatively, but it recovered to 79% at 6 months. *Sentence intelligibility* for patients undergoing anterior tongue resection and reconstruction was 77% at 1 month after surgery, improving to 91% at 6 months. Speech outcomes were better for patients undergoing base-of-tongue (BOT) resection and reconstruction; sentence intelligibility remained higher than 90% before and after surgery, but single-word intelligibility declined from 95% in the preoperative setting to 77–82% postoperatively. Finally, outcomes were worst for patients undergoing concurrent anterior and BOT resection with reconstruction. Intelligibility was reported at "good" in 29% of patients 10 months after reconstruction, "acceptable" in 53% of patients, and "poor" in 18%. Of note, essentially all patients undergoing anterior and BOT resection will also likely undergo adjuvant radiotherapy (RT) or adjuvant chemoradiotherapy, both of which may lead to undesirable tissue contracture and fat atrophy affecting tongue function [2, 33].

17.4.1.2 Factors Affecting Speech

Most studies on speech after free flap tongue reconstruction report either acoustic or perceptual evaluations of speech, and there is a wide variability in how studies measure speech quality both before and after reconstruction [2]. Intelligibility has been reported to be positively correlated with the volume and degree of protuberance of the neotongue. A positive relationship has also been reported between tongue mobility and both subjective and objective speech evaluations [33]. Multiple studies reported that larger tumors (T3/T4), resections including the tongue tip, and postoperative RT have a significantly negative affect on speech [2, 33, 41]. Furthermore, Manrique et al. demonstrated that patients who have floor-of-mouth resections have poorer postoperative speech [33]. Studies vary greatly on the type of free tissue used for reconstruction. When considering the literature as a whole, there is no definitive evidence suggesting that one type of flap leads to superior speech outcomes compared with another. There is also no definitive evidence to suggest that a reinnervated flap has better speech [33].

17.4.2 Swallowing Outcomes

In general, patients who regularly attend appointments with a trained speech-language pathologist, both before and after surgery, develop better swallowing function. Free flap reconstruction of the tongue often allows for resumption of an oral diet without the need for permanent reliance on a G-tube; however, large resections are associated with poorer swallowing ability after free flap reconstruction [2, 33]. The rates of G-*tube dependence* range from 3% to 17% [42, 43]. In a cohort of 20 patients, none were G-tube dependent after free flap reconstruction of the BOT, and only 5% developed aspiration events [44]. This is similar to a 3% aspiration rate in heterogeneous group of primary and secondary closures [45].

17.4.2.1 Objective Evaluation of Swallowing

Instrumental evaluation of swallowing is accomplished by (1) "videofluoroscopic study of swallowing" (VFSS) [46] (also known as modified barium swallow—MBS) and (2) "fiberoptic endoscopic evaluation of swallowing" (FEES) [47], which is usually repeated three times for each bolus (thick, semiliquid, and liquid). A "dysphagia score" such as that described by Dakkak and Bennett [48] and the penetration-aspiration scale (PAS) such as the eight-point PAS described by Rosenbek et al. [49] are used to score the VFFS and FEES, respectively.

17.4.2.2 Recovery Time

Many studies have compared flaps based on postoperative swallowing achieved; however, no significant benefit of any particular flap over other types has ever consistently been demonstrated [7]. Many patients with tongue cancers have some difficulty with swallowing preoperatively, but they should expect worse swallowing immediately after surgery that gradually improves with time. In general, the greater the amount of tongue resected, the poorer the postoperative swallow ability patients achieve [7].

In one study, preoperative liquid laryngeal penetration was estimated to be 50%, but long-term follow-up after anterior tongue resection and free flap reconstruction showed that liquid penetration rates had improved to 40%, whereas 0% demonstrated penetration with pudding or solids [2]. Swallow ability has been shown to improve after surgery often over the course of months, with patients achieving their best possible post-reconstructive swallow ability by around 1 year after surgery. Patients have been found to regain mobility of the tongue immediately at 4–6 months after surgery, with subsequent improvement in swallowing ability [50]. In a series by Brown et al. of 15 patients who underwent resection of 50–75% of the anterior tongue and RFFF reconstruction, there was no significant difference in the ability to swallow liquids or tongue mobility at 6 and 12 months postoperatively. Furthermore, Lam and Samma [2] reported on swallowing with videofluoroscopic swallow studies (VFSSs) and found that patients had a return to preoperative swallow parameters by 1 year postoperatively, regardless of the flap type.

17.4.2.3 Postoperative Diet

While studies consistently demonstrate that many patients resume an oral diet, the type of oral diet and the number of patients who are not permanently reliant on enteral feeding methods vary greatly. In a series by Chien et al. [24], 12 of 15 patients reconstructed with an ALTFF achieved an oral diet; three patients had persistent aspiration [24]. Rates of requiring a G-tube at 6 months postoperatively range in the literature from 0% to 87%, whereas rates at more than 1 year postoperatively range from 0% to 75% [34]. In a series by Dziegielewski et al. preoperative videofluoroscopic swallow studies (VFSSs) were compared with those performed 1 year after ALTFF reconstruction of the tongue. The authors found that there was no difference in rates of aspiration or penetration, but there was a significant increase in bolus transit times after surgery [34]. In another study by Hartl et al. two of nine patients had clinical evidence of aspiration at a 15-month follow-up, whereas one patient required enteral feeding [7].

Recent systematic reviews have reported on studies comparing patients with oral tongue resection and reconstruction, BOT resection and reconstruction, and combined oral and BOT resection and reconstruction [2, 33]. For the first group, studies have demonstrated that swallow parameters measured on VFSSs have returned to baseline by 1 year after reconstruction, regardless of flap type. Furthermore, clinical swallowing evaluations after oral tongue reconstruction showed that approximately 75% of patients achieve an unrestricted oral diet by 6 months after surgery. For patients undergoing BOT resection and free flap reconstruction, no one had preoperative aspiration; however, 14% of the patients demonstrate aspiration at a 1-year follow-up [2, 33]. Despite the high aspiration rate, 97% of patients were able to safely consume a thickened oral diet; 3% had persistent G-tube dependence. Finally, for patients undergoing combined oral and BOT resection and free flap reconstruction, 82% achieved an oral diet by 1 year, and nearly all achieved some form of an oral diet by 2 years postoperatively.

17.4.2.4 Factors Affecting Postoperative Swallow

Several studies showed that patients who undergo postoperative RT have worse long-term swallow outcomes than those who do not [2, 33, 41]. It is theorized that radiation causes increased shrinkage of tissue, leading to decreased bulk of the oropharyngeal tongue and, thus, poor swallowing function [41]. Other factors such as flap type and whether the flap was reinnervated did not significantly affect swallowing outcomes [2, 33, 41]. Overall, the literature demonstrates diverse findings when comparing patient-reported outcomes and clinical tests of dysphagia, pointing to the need to use both approaches when measuring outcomes [51, 52].

17.4.3 Quality-of-Life (QOL) Outcomes

Surgical treatment of squamous cell carcinoma (SCC) of the oral cavity has a high impact on patients' quality of life (QOL), as it variably affects their ability to speak and swallow and their social activities [53]. Evaluating QOL in cancer patients is increasingly important, not only for policymakers in public health but also for healthcare providers and patients themselves [54].

Many studies have evaluated QOL after free flap reconstruction of the tongue [33, 34, 38]. Overall QOL measured by the "EORTC H&N35" has been shown to be similar when measured before and 1 year after tongue resection and free flap reconstruction [34]. As expected, QOL scores worsened in the immediate postoperative period [34]. Hartl et al. found that resection of the BOT was specifically and significantly associated with worse swallowing function, worse QOL, and patient depression [7]. A review by Manrique et al. found that among patients undergoing subtotal glossectomy or total glossectomy without laryngectomy, 90% achieved decannulation, often within the first 2 weeks after surgery with subsequently improved QOL [33]. Patients with high motivation, good family support, and regular follow-up (both with a physician and a speech-language pathologist) have reported better EORTC H&N35 scores, whereas those patients with persistent postoperative pain and those who underwent adjuvant chemotherapy reported worse scores, reflecting a poorer QOL [33].

A case control retrospective study was conducted by Gabriele et al. [54] on 14 patients who underwent partial glossectomy for SCC of the mobile tongue at the Department of Otorhinolaryngology Head and Neck Surgery of the University Hospital of Modena, Italy, between October 2016 and February 2017. Patients were divided into two groups: group A (case group) that included seven patients whose surgical defect after tongue resection was reconstructed by a microvascular free flap (either RFFF or ALT) and group B (control group) that included seven patients who were closed primarily or by secondary healing. Their results revealed similar QOL and functional outcomes in both groups, with a slight tendency to better speech performance in the reconstructive group.

17.5 Reconstruction: Management Plan

In 2019, Vincent et al. [11] suggested that when reconstructing a tongue defect, one should always overcorrect the tissue volume, as the flap will shrink significantly with RT and flap tissue atrophy. In the initial reconstruction, they aim to place sufficient flap bulk so that the neotongue can touch the palate as long as it will not lead to excessive flap compression. Overtime, one can expect around 50% volume loss, especially if the patients undergo RT afterward.

In patients who have persistent dysarthria and dysphagia despite initial free flap tongue reconstruction, one must determine if the neotongue is tethered, and if so, releasing the scar may be considered with subsequent placement of a skin graft to minimize tethering. More commonly, however, dysarthria and dysphagia are the result of insufficient volume of the neotongue. In these cases, placement of a second flap may be considered in a delayed fashion to provide additional tongue bulk [11].

Rihani et al. [55] treated 11 patients after total glossectomy with secondary tongue augmentation through an onlay free flap (RFFF or RAFF) and reported that 63% had improved swallowing and 45.4% achieved G-tube independence [55]. All patients noted improved speech and achieved tracheostomy decannulation.

Considering all the factors described previously, Vincent et al. [11] proposed the following management plan for reconstruction after extirpation surgery for patients with defects involving the tongue only with or without the floor of the mouth, patient with concurrent tongue and mandible defects, and those with concurrent tongue and oro- or hypopharyngeal defects.

17.5.1 For Defects Involving the Tongue Only ± Floor of the Mouth

17.5.1.1 Reconstruction After Partial Glossectomy

For defects involving the tongue only, one should consider if there is a floor-of-mouth defect or not, as primary closure of defects involving the floor of the mouth are at a high risk for developing ankyloglossia and significant tongue tethering. For patients who undergo a partial glossectomy in which less than one-third of the

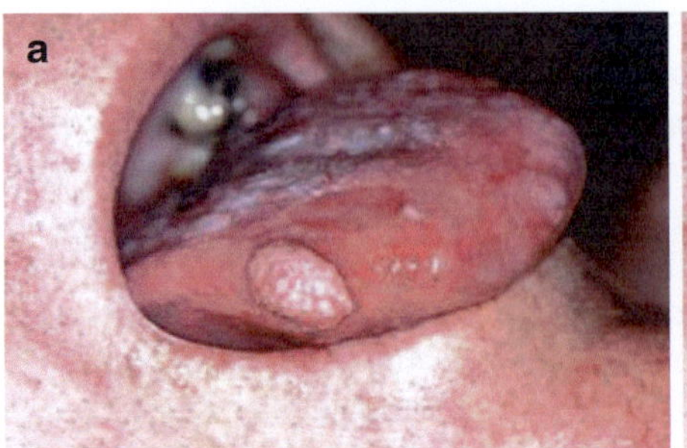

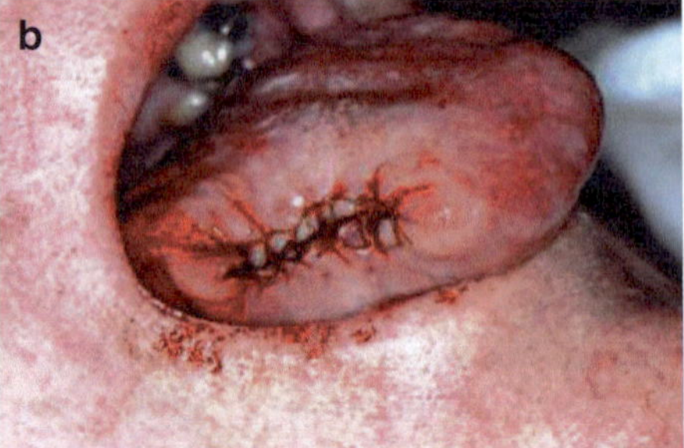

Fig. 17.8 (**a**) Small (T1N0) SCC at the right lateral border of the tongue. (**b**) Direct primary closure of the defect after partial glossectomy

tongue is removed without floor-of-mouth involvement, conservative reconstruction is appropriate to include healing by secondary intention, primary closure (Fig. 17.8), or coverage with a skin graft. Patients in this category often do not require other procedures at the time of surgery, though careful airway observation should be considered postoperatively. *Reconstruction after partial glossectomy* for small lesions have shown better results with *primary closure* than local or free flap coverage regarding oral transit times and swallowing efficiency [56]. These patients often have minimal loss of speech and swallowing function [57–59].

For patients who undergo a partial glossectomy with floor-of-mouth involvement, one may consider smaller loco-regional flaps such as a submental island flap. This will minimize the risk of tongue tethering to the floor of the mouth and optimize tongue mobility. However, a submental island flap cannot be used if the flap pedicle is resected during neck dissection for oncological reasons.

An option for reconstruction after partial glossectomy includes also microvascular flaps such as the RFFF. Overcorrection should be considered as significant flap volume loss is expected postoperatively.

17.5.1.2 Reconstruction After Hemiglossectomy

For defects approaching one-third to half of the tongue, after hemiglossectomy, an RFFF is an ideal thin pliable flap for enhanced neotongue mobility with the possibility of reinnervation (Fig. 17.9). A tracheostomy should be considered in this group of patients as one can expect significant flap swelling immediately following the surgery that may linger for several weeks. If the surgeon decides not to perform a tracheostomy, careful airway observation is of paramount importance. In some cases, a temporary NG-tube is also helpful for these patients. If the patient requires postoperative radiation therapy, concurrent placement of a G-tube feed may be helpful to transition through the radiation-related mucositis.

17.5.1.3 Reconstruction After Subtotal, Near Total, or Total Glossectomy

For patients undergoing BOT resections and *subtotal*, *near total*, or *total glossectomy* (larger than half of the tongue), RAFF and ALTFF are ideal. Significant *advantages* include (1) the ability to select the donor site that matches requirements

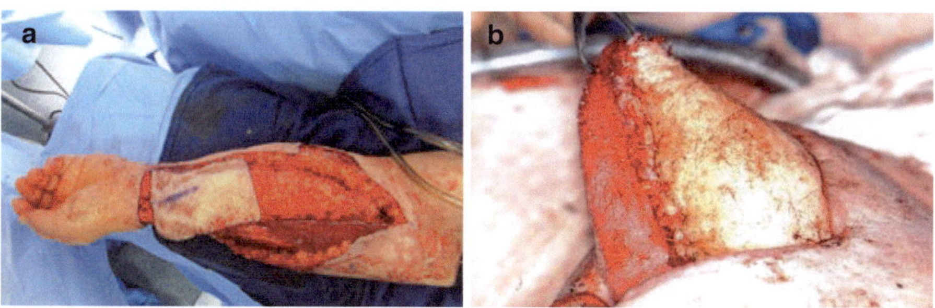

Fig. 17.9 Radial forearm free flap (RFFF) (**a**) for tongue reconstruction after hemiglossectomy (**b**)

of the defect, (2) large quantities of tissue availability including skin and fascia with the possibility of sensory/motor restoration with micro-neurorrhaphy, and (3) the ability to provide donor tissue that has not been subjected to radiation, thus offering superior vascularity and healing potential.

In this patient population, the surgeon's goal is to restore as much tongue volume as possible and to initially overcorrect the volume of the defect. It is imperative that the volume loss is overcorrected, as one can expect flap muscle atrophy and radiation-related tissue atrophy. These patients should get concurrent tracheostomy with consideration of G-tube placement, as they are likely to have significant airway swelling postoperatively and have a prolonged recovery of swallow function. Regional (pedicled) flap reconstruction of the tongue using the platysma flap or pectoralis flap is preferred when free flaps are significantly contraindicated or after a free flap failure.

When performing a total glossectomy for advanced tongue cancers, a tongue "pull though" from the oral cavity into the neck can be used. This allows for complete visualization of the macroscopic borders of the cancer. This technique is contraindicated in tumors extending to the periosteum of the lingual mandible surface. Total glossectomy defects benefit from reconstruction with the RAFF or the ALTFF due to the need for large bulk, difficult to achieve with the RFFF [60–62].

17.5.2 For Concurrent Tongue and Mandible Defects

When there are concurrent tongue and full-thickness bony mandible defects, the surgeon should first decide if the mandible continuity is to be restored and then select either a scapula flap or fibula flap based on (1) the size of the skin paddle needed for the reconstruction and (2) the length of the bone needed for the mandible reconstruction. A fibular flap can be combined with a pectoralis flap if there is a sizable tongue defect (subtotal glossectomy) for which the fibula skin paddle will not be adequate. Alternatively, a scapula flap provides significant soft tissue bulk that can easily reconstruct a subtotal glossectomy defect, but it is limited by the mandible bone defect length.

17.5.3 For Concurrent Tongue and Oropharyngeal or Hypopharyngeal Defects

If there is a concurrent oropharyngeal or hypopharyngeal defect, coverage of great vessels and the cervical spine is imperative along with the tongue reconstruction. Smaller tongue and pharyngeal mucosal defects are amenable to RFFF reconstruction. However, a larger mucosal defect will require a larger flap, such as the PMMF, ALTFF, or RAFF.

17.6 How to Improve Outcomes

Glossectomy is most commonly performed for the treatment of malignant and premalignant tongue lesions. Malignant lesions of the tongue, like other parts of the head and neck, usually require multimodality treatment that utilizes the expertise of a range of professionals, including otolaryngologists, medical oncologists, radiation oncologists, radiologists, surgical pathologists, oral surgeons, speech-language pathologists, dieticians, nurses, and pharmacists [63]. As such, all facets of the procedure, including patient selection, preoperative evaluation, type of glossectomy and surgical approach, postoperative care, and functional rehabilitation, must be performed in a multidisciplinary fashion to optimize treatment, individualized patient outcomes, and team efficiency [64–68].

17.6.1 Preoperative Measures

Preoperatively, a comprehensive clinical evaluation of the patient proposed for glossectomy must be performed by the primary surgeon, facilitated with imaging and fiberoptic examinations as necessary. Appropriate consultation referrals in anticipation of adjuvant therapy that may be required after the procedure should be made preoperatively to prevent subsequent delays in treatment. Ideally, the patient is evaluated as part of a multispecialty tumor board. Preoperative evaluation by internal medicine, cardiology, pulmonology, and/or anesthesia experts must be performed to allow identification and control of comorbidities that may significantly impact surgical safety and outcome.

17.6.2 Intraoperative Measures

During the glossectomy procedure, adequate and efficient communication between the surgeon, anesthesiologist, pathologist, and nurse is critical for ensuring a successful surgical outcome, including a margin-negative resection with adequate reconstruction as indicated so as to improve survival prognosis and transition to the next phase of care.

17.6.3 Postoperative Measures

Postoperatively, the management of the glossectomy patient will also require a variety of expertise. Pain control will be optimized with the help of pharmacists. Monitoring of the wound and reconstructive flaps will be performed by the surgical team, including specialist nurses conversant with monitoring for reconstructive tissue viability, wound infections, and other common postoperative complications. As most patients will require dietary modifications after glossectomy, dietitians will be necessary for providing appropriate oral or enteral feeding recommendations based on evaluations from the speech-language pathologists. Speech and swallowing rehabilitation through the help of the speech-language pathologists will also be required to optimize patients' quality of life and early reintegration into their preexisting lifestyle.

Thus, the need for an interprofessional approach to the preoperative, operative, and postoperative management of glossectomy patients cannot be overemphasized. It is important that professionals involved in the care of glossectomy patients be aware of the collective roles they play in the management of these patients and the need to strategically be on par with each other to improve patient outcomes.

17.6.4 Surveillance/Follow-Up

Regardless of the extent of treatment for tongue SCC, patients require close clinical surveillance. Wound care, complications, or morbidity resulting from therapy may require more frequent clinical appointments. Current practice guidelines from the American Head and Neck Society regarding the clinical surveillance of patients who have been treated for advanced oral cavity/oropharyngeal SCC are outlined below [69]:

- First-year posttreatment: 1–3 month interval
- Second-year posttreatment: 2–4 month interval
- Third-year posttreatment: 3–6 month interval
- Fourth and fifth years: 4–6 month interval
- After 5 years: Every 12 months

Physical examination including fiberoptic laryngoscopy should be performed at each visit to assess the response to therapy and monitor for recurrent and/or second malignancies.

Computed tomography (CT) scan or magnetic resonance imaging (MRI) may be obtained as clinically indicated to investigate for occult malignancy and to monitor the neck for cervical metastasis. Positron emission tomography (PET) is an excellent surveillance instrument as it represents a functional imaging modality, rather than a static imaging modality as in the case of CT scan or MRI. It has been shown to be highly effective in detecting loco-regional recurrence and distant metastases after multimodality therapy of head and neck SCC and is currently recommended by many investigators [70–72].

17.7 Summary

Autologous free flap reconstruction of the tongue allows for good speech, swallowing, and QOL outcomes in the majority of patients. There are many flap options available to surgeons, and no particular flap has consistently been demonstrated to be superior to others. Careful selection of flap reconstruction based on the tongue defect site and size, donor site flap bulk, and the presence of concurrent subunit defects is critical for successful reconstruction. Overcorrection of tissue volume defect is of paramount importance for successful postoperative speech and swallowing functions. Reinnervation of a flap has demonstrated mixed results in the literature in terms of speech and swallowing outcomes. Postoperative RT negatively affects both speech and swallowing ability. Motivated patients with good family support who comply with regular follow-up perform better and report better QOL overall. In general, there is a need for standardization of measurements, both objective and subjective, of speech, swallowing, and QOL outcomes in the patient population to allow for improved future studies.

References

1. de Vicente JC, de Villalaín L, Torre A, Peña I. Microvascular free tissue transfer for tongue reconstruction after hemiglossectomy: a functional assessment of radial forearm versus anterolateral thigh flap. J Oral Maxillofac Surg. 2008;66(11):2270–5.
2. Lam L, Samman N. Speech and swallowing following tongue cancer surgery and free flap reconstruction--a systematic review. Oral Oncol. 2013;49(06):507–24.
3. Nicoletti G, Soutar DS, Jackson MS, Wrench AA, Robertson G. Chewing and swallowing after surgical treatment for oral cancer: functional evaluation in 196 selected cases. Plast Reconstr Surg. 2004;114(2):329–38.
4. Kazi R, Johnson C, Prasad V, De Cordova J, Venkitaraman R, Nutting CM, et al. Quality of life outcome measures following partial glossectomy: assessment using the UW-QOL scale. J Cancer Res Ther. 2008;4(3):116–20.
5. Malone JP, Stephens JA, Grecula JC, Rhoades CA, Ghaheri BA, Schuller DE. Disease control, survival, and functional outcome after multimodal treatment for advanced-stage tongue base cancer. Head Neck. 2004;26(7):561–72.
6. Hsiao HT, Leu YS, Chang SH, Lee JT. Swallowing function in patients who underwent hemiglossectomy: comparison of primary closure and free radial forearm flap reconstruction with videofluoroscopy. Ann Plast Surg. 2003;50(5):450–5.
7. Hartl DM, Dauchy S, Escande C, Bretagne E, Janot F, Kolb F. Quality of life after free-flap tongue reconstruction. J Laryngol Otol. 2009;123(05):550–4.
8. Bokhari WA, Wang SJ. Tongue reconstruction: recent advances. Curr Opin Otolaryngol Head Neck Surg. 2007;15(04):202–7.
9. Diz Dios P, Fernández Feijoo J, Castro Ferreiro M, Alvarez J. Functional consequences of partial glossectomy. J Oral Maxillofac Surg. 1994;52(01):12–4.
10. Hara I, Gellrich NC, Düker J, Schon R, Nilius M, Fakler O, et al. Evaluation of swallowing function after intraoral soft tissue reconstruction with microvascular free flaps. Int J Oral Maxillofac Surg. 2003;32(06):593–9.

11. Vincent A, Kohlert S, Lee TS, Inman J, Ducic Y. Free-flap reconstruction of the tongue. Semin Plast Surg. 2019;33(1):38–45.
12. Hanna TC, Lubek JE. The hybrid submental flap for tongue reconstruction. J Oral Maxillofac Surg. 2015;73(09):18760–9.
13. Baas M, Duraku LS, Corten EML, Mureau AM. A systematic review on the sensory reinnervation of free flaps for tongue reconstruction: does improved sensibility imply functional benefits? J Plast Reconstr Aesthet Surg. 2015;68(08):1025–35.
14. Engel H, Huang JJ, Lin CY, Lam W, Kao HK, Gazyakan E. A strategic approach for tongue reconstruction to achieve predictable and improved functional and aesthetic outcomes. Plast Reconstr Surg. 2010;126(6):1967–77.
15. Wang X, Yan G, Zhang G, Li J, Liu J, Zhang Y. Functional tongue reconstruction with the anterolateral thigh flap. World J Surg Oncol. 2013;11:303–7.
16. Nasajpour H, Steele MH. Anterolateral thigh free flap for "head-to-toe" reconstruction. Ann Plast Surg. 2011;66:530–3.
17. Lee JC, Hugo SH, Christy MR, Wise MW, Rodriguez ED. Anterolateral thigh flap for trauma reconstruction. Ann Plast Surg. 2011;64:164–8.
18. Chen HC, Tang YB. Anterolateral thigh flap: an ideal soft tissue flap. Clin Plast Surg. 2003;30:383–401.
19. Sharabi SE, Hatef DA, Koshy JC, Jain A, Cole PD, Hollier LH. Is primary thinning of the anterolateral thigh flap recommended? Ann Plast Surg. 2010;65:555–9.
20. Ichinose A, Terashi H, Nakahara M. Do multiple venous anastomoses reduce risk of thrombosis in free-flap transfer? Efficacy of dual anastomoses of separate venous systems. Ann Plast Surg. 2004;52:61–3.
21. Boca R, Kuo YR, Hsieh CH, Huang EY, Jeng SF. A reliable parameter for primary closure of free anterolateral thigh donor site. Plast Reconstr Surg. 2010;126:1558–10.
22. di Candia MD, Lie K, Kumiponjera D, Simcock J, Cormack GC, Malata CM. Versatility of the anterolateral thigh free flap: the four seasons flap. Eplasty. 2012;12:e21–4.
23. Xu ZF, Dai W, Zhang EJ. Perforator-based chimeric anterolateral thigh flap for head and neck reconstruction after en bloc resection. Shanghai Kou Qiang Yi Xue. 2012;21:107–12.
24. Chien CY, Su CY, Hwang CF, Chuang HC, Jeng SF, Chen YC. Ablation of advanced tongue or base of tongue cancer and reconstruction with free flap: functional outcomes. Eur J Surg Oncol. 2006;32(03):353–7.
25. Liao G, Su Y, Zhang J, Hou J, Chen Y, Li M. Reconstruction of the tongue with reinnervated rectus abdominis musculoperitoneal flaps after hemiglossectomy. J Laryngol Otol. 2006;120(03):205–13.
26. Biglioli F, Liviero F, Frigerio A, Rezzonico A, Brusati R. Function of the sensate free forearm flap after partial glossectomy. J Craniomaxillofac Surg. 2006;34(06):332–9.
27. Yu P, Robb GL. Reconstruction for total and near-total glossectomy defects. Clin Plast Surg. 2005;32(3):411–9.
28. Yu P. Reinnervated anterolateral thigh flap for tongue reconstruction. Head Neck. 2004;26(12):1038–44.
29. Longo B, Pagnoni M, Ferri G, Morello R, Santanelli F. The mushroom-shaped anterolateral thigh perforator flap for subtotal tongue reconstruction. Plast Reconstr Surg. 2013;132(3):656–65.
30. Chang EI, Yu P, Skoracki RJ, Liu J, Hanasono MM. Comprehensive analysis of functional outcomes and survival after microvascular reconstruction of glossectomy defects. Ann Surg Oncol. 2015;22(09):3061–9.
31. Ozkan O, Ozkan O, Derin AT, Bektas G, Cinpolat A, Duymaz A, et al. True functional reconstruction of total or subtotal glossectomy defects using a chimeric anterolateral thigh flap with both sensorial and motor innervation. Ann Plast Surg. 2015;74(05):557–64.
32. Yoleri L, Mavioğlu H. Total tongue reconstruction with free functional gracilis muscle transplantation: a technical note and review of the literature. Ann Plast Surg. 2000;45(2):181–6.
33. Manrique OJ, Leland HA, Langevin CJ, Wong A, Carey JN, Ciudad P, et al. Optimizing outcomes following total and subtotal tongue reconstruction: a systematic review of the contemporary literature. J Reconstr Microsurg. 2017;33(2):103–11.

34. Dziegielewski PT, Ho ML, Rieger J, Singh P, Langille M, Harris JR, et al. Total glossectomy with laryngeal preservation and free flap reconstruction: objective functional outcomes and systematic review of the literature. Laryngoscope. 2013;123(1):140–5.
35. Aaronson NK, Ahmedzai S, Bergman B, Bullinger M, Cull A, Duez NJ, et al. The European organization for research and treatment of cancer QLQ-C30: a quality-of-life instrument for use in international clinical trials in oncology. J Natl Cancer Inst. 1993;85:365–76.
36. Bjordal K, Hammerlid E, Ahlner-Elmqvist M, de Graeff A, Boysen M, Evensen JF, et al. Quality of life in head and neck cancer patients: validation of the European organization for research and treatment of cancer quality of life questionnaire-H&N35. J Clin Oncol. 1999;17:1008–19.
37. Jansen F, Snyder CF, Leemans CR, Verdonck-de Leeuw IM. Identifying cutoff scores for the EORTC QLQ-C30 and the head and neck cancer–specific module EORTC QLQ-H&N35 representing unmet supportive care needs in patients with head and neck cancer. Head Neck. 2016;38(Suppl 1):E1493–500.
38. Chen AY, Frankowski R, Bishop-Leone J, Hebert T, Leyk S, Lewin J, et al. The development and validation of a dysphagia-specific quality-of-life questionnaire for patients with head and neck cancer: the MD Anderson dysphagia inventory. Arch Otolaryngol Head Neck Surg. 2001;127:870–6.
39. List MA, D'Antonio LL, Cella DF, Siston A, Mumby P, Haraf D, et al. The performance status scale for head and neck cancer patients and the functional assessment of cancer therapy-head and neck scale: a study of utility and validity. Cancer. 1996;77:2294–301.
40. Matsui Y, Shirota T, Yamashita Y, Ohno K. Analyses of speech intelligibility in patients after glossectomy and reconstruction with fasciocutaneous/myocutaneous flaps. Int J Oral Maxillofac Surg. 2009;38(04):339–45.
41. Shin YS, Koh YW, Kim SH, Jeong JH, Ahn S, Hong HJ, et al. Radiotherapy deteriorates postoperative functional outcome after partial glossectomy with free flap reconstruction. J Oral Maxillofac Surg. 2012;70(01):216–20.
42. Khariwala SS, Vivek PP, Lorenz RR, Esclamado RM, Wood B, Strome M, et al. Swallowing outcomes after microvascular head and neck reconstruction: a prospective review of 191 cases. Laryngoscope. 2007;117(8):1359–63.
43. Rieger JM, Zalmanowitz JG, Li SY, Sytsanko A, Harris J, Williams D. Functional outcomes after surgical reconstruction of the base of tongue using the radial forearm free flap in patients with oropharyngeal carcinoma. Head Neck. 2007;29(11):1024–32.
44. O'Connell DA, Rieger J, Harris JR, Dziegielewski P, Zalmanowitz J, Sytsanko A. Swallowing function in patients with base of tongue cancers treated with primary surgery and reconstructed with a modified radial forearm free flap. Arch Otolaryngol Head Neck Surg. 2008;134(8):857–8564.
45. Pauloski BR, Logemann JA, Rademaker AW, McConnel FM, Stein D, Beery Q. Speech and swallowing function after oral and oropharyngeal resections: one-year follow-up. Head Neck. 1994;16(4):313–22.
46. Martin-Harris B, Jones B. The videofluorographic swallowing study. Phys Med Rehabil Clin N Am. 2008;19:769–85.
47. Colodny N. Interjudge and intrajudge reliabilities in fiberoptic endoscopic evaluation of swallowing (Fees®) using the penetration–aspiration scale: a replication study. Dysphagia. 2002;17:308–15.
48. Dakkak M, Bennett JR. A new dysphagia score with objective validation. J Clin Gastroenterol. 1992;14:99–100.
49. Rosenbek JC, Robbins JA, Roecker EB, Coyle JL, Wood JL. A penetration-aspiration scale. Dysphagia. 1996;11:93–9.
50. Brown L, Rieger JM, Harris J, Seikaly H. A longitudinal study of functional outcomes after surgical resection and microvascular reconstruction for oral cancer: tongue mobility and swallowing function. J Oral Maxillofac Surg. 2010;68(11):2690–700.
51. Namin AW, Varvares MA. Functional outcomes of sensate versus insensate free flap reconstruction in oral and oropharyngeal reconstruction: a systematic review. Head Neck. 2016;38(11):1717–21.

52. Pedersen A, Wilson J, McColl E, Carding P, Patterson J. Swallowing outcome measures in head and neck cancer--how do they compare? Oral Oncol. 2016;52:104–8.
53. So WK, Chan RJ, Chan DN, Hughes BMG, Chair SY, Choi KC, et al. Quality-of-life among head and neck cancer survivors at one year after treatment–a systematic review. Eur J Cancer. 2012;48:2391–408.
54. Gabriele M, Michael G, Giulia M, Alessandro S, Andrea M, Daniele M, Livio P. Quality of life, swallowing and speech outcomes after oncological treatment for mobile tongue carcinoma. Eur J Plast Surg. 2020;43:247–56.
55. Rihani J, Lee T, Ducic Y. Secondary onlay free flap reconstruction of glossectomy defects following initial successful flap restoration. Otolaryngol Head Neck Surg. 2013;149(02):232–4.
56. McConnel FM, Pauloski BR, Logemann JA, Rademaker AW, Colangelo L, Shedd D. Functional results of primary closure vs flaps in oropharyngeal reconstruction: a prospective study of speech and swallowing. Arch Otolaryngol Head Neck Surg. 1998;124(6):625–30.
57. Urken ML, Moscoso JF, Lawson W, Biller HF. A systematic approach to functional reconstruction of the oral cavity following partial and total glossectomy. Arch Otolaryngol Head Neck Surg. 1994;120(6):589–601.
58. Michiwaki Y, Ohno K, Imai S, Yamashita Y, Suzuki N, Yoshida H. Functional effects of intraoral reconstruction with a free radial forearm flap. J Craniomaxillofac Surg. 1990;18(4):164–8.
59. McConnel FM, Cerenko D, Mendelsohn MS. Manofluorographic analysis of swallowing. Otolaryngol Clin N Am. 1988;21(4):625–35.
60. Pigno MA, Funk JJ. Prosthetic management of a total glossectomy defect after free flap reconstruction in an edentulous patient: a clinical report. J Prosthet Dent. 2003;89(2):119–22.
61. Huang CH, Chen HC, Huang YL, Mardini S, Feng GM. Comparison of the radial forearm flap and the thinned anterolateral thigh cutaneous flap for reconstruction of tongue defects: an evaluation of donor-site morbidity. Plast Reconstr Surg. 2004;114(7):1704–10.
62. Mazarro A, de Pablo A, Puiggròs C, Velasco MM, Saez M, Pamias J, et al. Indications, reconstructive techniques, and results for total glossectomy. Head Neck. 2016;38:E2004–10.
63. Gibson MK, Forastiere AA. Multidisciplinary approaches in the management of advanced head and neck tumors: state of the art. Curr Opin Oncol. 2004;16(3):220–4.
64. Brunner M, Gore SM, Read RL, Alexander A, Mehta A, Elliot M, Milross C, Boyer M, Clark JR. Head and neck multidisciplinary team meetings: effect on patient management. Head Neck. 2015;37(7):1046–50.
65. Wheless SA, McKinney KA, Zanation AM. A prospective study of the clinical impact of a multidisciplinary head and neck tumor board. Otolaryngol Head Neck Surg. 2010;143(5):650–4.
66. Patil RD, Meinzen-Derr JK, Hendricks BL, Patil YJ. Improving access and timeliness of care for veterans with head and neck squamous cell carcinoma: a multidisciplinary team's approach. Laryngoscope. 2016;126(3):627–31.
67. Wang YH, Kung PT, Tsai WC, Tai CJ, Liu SA, Tsai MH. Effects of multidisciplinary care on the survival of patients with oral cavity cancer in Taiwan. Oral Oncol. 2012;48(9):803–10.
68. Shellenberger TD, Weber RS. Multidisciplinary team planning for patients with head and neck cancer. Oral Maxillofac Surg Clin North Am. 2018;30(4):435–44.
69. American Head and Neck Society. Practice guidelines: oral cavity squamous cell carcinoma, T1-N0 and T2-N0. Los Angeles, CA: AHNS; n.d.. http://www.headandneckcancer.org/clinicalresources/docs/oralcavity.php. Accessed 2011.
70. Gourin CG, Williams HT, Seabolt WN, Herdman AV, Howington JW, Terris DJ. Utility of positron emission tomography-computed tomography in identification of residual nodal disease after chemoradiation for advanced head and neck cancer. Laryngoscope. 2006;116(5):705–10.
71. Menda Y, Graham MM. Update on 18F-fluorodeoxyglucose/positron emission tomography and positron emission tomography/computed tomography imaging of squamous head and neck cancers. Semin Nucl Med. 2005;35(4):214–9.
72. Weymuller EA, Yueh B, Deleyiannis FW, Kuntz AL, Alsarraf R, Coltrera MD. Quality of life in patients with head and neck cancer: lessons learned from 549 prospectively evaluated patients. Arch Otolaryngol Head Neck Surg. 2000;126(3):329–36.

18 Tongue Replantation After Trauma

18.1 Overview

The tongue has important roles in deglutition, speech, airway protection, taste, and sexual function, and its amputation has very serious deleterious effects. Fortunately, tongue amputation is a rare event, but replantation, which is considered the best way to reestablish oral function, is a technical challenge making attempts at tongue replantation also rare, possibly because of the friable nature of the tongue vasculature. In fact, only five *successful* tongue replants of complete amputations [1–5] and two of partial amputations [6, 7] are reported in the literature. One *unsuccessful* tongue replant for complete amputation has also been reported in the literature [8]. Case reports in the literature vary regarding the mechanism of injury, size of the amputated tongue, technical details, ischemia time, use of leeches and vein grafts, anticoagulative therapy, and outcome. On the other hand, the delayed microvascular reconstruction with heterotopic grafts using rectus abdominis, latissimus dorsi, and serratus anterior muscles have been described with poor functional results [6, 8, 9].

Successful tongue replantation is based on multiple factors that include (1) the timely evaluation and reperfusion of the amputated part typically in a two-team approach. One team prepares the recipient vessels and possible vein graft, and the second team works under the microscope preparing the amputated part. This entails maintaining the amputated part on ice, flushing the amputating part with a heparinized solution, and performing the anastomoses between the amputated part and the vein grafts, (2) meticulous micro- or supermicrosurgical technique, (3) postoperative leech therapy, (4) sedation and paralysis during the immediate postoperative period, and (5) early antipsychotic pharmacological treatment as indicated.

With venous compromise, the resultant massive swelling can itself predispose to obstruction of the oropharynx with potential threat to the respiratory tract. Prompt recognition with rapid *nasotracheal* intubation or surgical airway management must be immediately attempted [1, 8, 10, 11]. Orotracheal intubation with direct laryngoscopy is an ill-advised choice in lesions located in the base of the tongue due

© The Author(s), under exclusive license to Springer Nature Switzerland AG 2022
M. F. Sakr, *Tongue Lesions*, https://doi.org/10.1007/978-3-031-08198-9_18

to the possibility of clot dislodgment with life-threatening risks of aspiration and iatrogenic injury to the respiratory tract with the inability to visualize the laryngeal aditus.

18.2 Tongue Replantation: Animal Model

18.2.1 Introduction

Although the human tongue is not a vital organ, it adds greatly to the utility of one's everyday life and may be a vital organ in sustaining the will to live in many people. Unfortunately, the tongue can frequently be the site of traumatic injury, neurological disease, or cancer, any of which can result in the loss of the tongue and its related functions. Patients who undergo a total glossectomy are ordinarily dependent on a tracheotomy and gastrostomy tube. Although reconstructive modalities for the complete loss of the tongue have been improving, the approaches remain poor to fair at best. The latest techniques that utilize free tissue transfers with motorized segments may provide some ability to swallow and some degree of speech, but rarely to the point of the individual functioning normally [12, 13].

The morbidity associated with a glossectomy, even if coupled with the best of the current reconstructive procedures, is frequently high enough to persuade patients to refuse surgical treatment. This occurs with some regularity in treatable oral cancer patients, who elect not to have surgery, even if this decision means that their life expectancy may be shortened. The prospect of losing functionality of their tongue seems excessively life-altering to these patients. In an effort to explore the surgical feasibility of a tongue transplant and to determine the similarity of an animal model with human techniques, Day and colleagues [14] performed an autograft replantation of a tongue in a canine subject as the dog's neck, tongue, and oral anatomy represent an excellent animal model for tongue reconstruction [14]. The only previously published replantation of the tongue was reported by Buntic and Bunke in 1998 and involved the reattachment of the anterior portion of a human tongue after physical trauma that resulted in complete amputation of this part [1]. Day et al. reported the first successful *total excision* and replantation of the tongue in either a human or animal model [14].

18.2.2 Surgical Technique [14]

The tongue auto-replantation was performed on a 23-kg adult mongrel dog. After surgical preparation, which included a topical injection of 1% lidocaine with epinephrine at the points of incision, a tracheotomy was performed to protect the airway. General endotracheal anesthesia was provided throughout the procedure, and cardiorespiratory monitoring was carried out.

18.2.2.1 Resection

The neck and tongue musculature and vasculature were exposed, utilizing a transverse apron incision. Hemostasis was maintained with the use of monopolar and bipolar electrocautery. The platysma muscles were elevated bilaterally in a subplatysmal fashion to expose the anterior and external jugular veins (EJVs), which were divided and ligated. The lingual vein tributaries of the EJVs were located overlying the strap muscles and mylohyoid muscles, and approximately 5 cm of the veins were dissected free. Connecting the right and left lingual veins was a communicating vein, which also drained from the midline superior to the hyoid bone. Dissection was continued up the submental triangle where the fascia was removed to expose the digastric muscle along with the body and symphysis of the mandible. The lingual nerve was isolated deep to the digastric muscle at the anterior half of the mandible. The thick hypoglossal nerve was also isolated, running alongside the lingual artery. Both the hypoglossal nerve and lingual artery entered the tongue musculature just superior to the hyoid bone. Approximately 3 cm of the lingual artery was dissected free from its takeoff point on the external carotid artery (ECA) to the point it entered the base of the tongue.

The tongue was released from the oral cavity in a pull-through fashion and was resected from the mandible bilaterally, leaving a 1-cm periosteal cuff. At this time, the tongue was reflected down into the neck, and the remainder of the resection was then performed along the pharyngeal wall anterior to the tonsillar pillar and into the base of the tongue region. The lingual nerve was separated, along with the stylopharyngeus, styloglossus, and superior constrictor muscles. After careful retraction of the hypoglossal nerve, lingual nerve, artery, and vein, the tongue was separated from the superior aspect of the hyoid bone, thereby completely freeing the tongue musculature. Readings of 100% and 98% O_2 saturation were obtained for the left and right sides of the tongue, respectively, verifying good perfusion of the musculature. The vessels were then clamped and separated, and the tongue was removed from the dog and placed in an iced saline bath on the back table for 1 h.

18.2.2.2 Replantation

The *lingual vessels* in the neck and on the tongue were cleaned of the adventitia in preparation for reanastomosis. The tongue was replaced into the oral cavity and oropharyngeal regions and secured with 2-0 silk sutures. The right lingual artery and vein were reanastomosed using a microvascular technique with 9-0 interrupted nylon sutures. The *hypoglossal and lingual nerves* were reanastomosed to confirm the application of this technique without nerve grafting. Blood flow through the reanastomosed vessels was tested utilizing Doppler analysis. Perfusion through the tongue was monitored by utilizing a pulse oximeter sensor on the anterior portion of the replanted tongue, which registered O_2 saturation at 98%. The *tongue musculature* was attached to the periosteum of the mandible and the hyoid bone utilizing 3-0 Vicryl suture.

18.2.2.3 Closure

The surgical procedure was concluded by utilizing 3-0 Vicryl and silk sutures to close the skin. A suture was used to secure the apex of the mandible to the skin overlaying the sternum, in order to prevent hyperextension of the neck and stretching of the reanastomosed vessels. The dog remained under anesthesia and was monitored for 16 h after surgery and was then sacrificed.

18.2.3 Clinical Implications

The anatomy of the canine tongue provides an excellent model for the human tongue due to relatively similar anatomy. The canine tongue receives the majority of its arterial supply from the lingual branch of the ECA. Unlike humans, the primary venous return for the canine head is through the lingual branch of the EJV with the internal jugular vein (IJV) playing a very minor role [15]. The hypoglossal nerve provides the motor function to the canine tongue musculature via a similar course through the upper neck. The lingual nerve is identified slightly more cranial underlying the mandible in the upper neck of the canine than in the human. This experiment demonstrated the surgical feasibility of revascularization of the tongue. The canine anatomy of the oral cavity, oropharynx, tongue, and neck provided an adequate model for experiments of this nature. The same techniques employed in this experiment may be adopted eventually for human tongue transplants and could provide an alternative to free flap procedures.

18.3 Tongue Replantation in Humans

Amputation of the tongue presents in an ominous fashion, with pain, inability to articulate, and intraoral massive bleeding that might jeopardize the patient's life in few minutes due to the difficulty to control hemorrhage, shock, and direct threat to the airway.

Tongue amputation may be complete or partial (incomplete). A complete amputation means "complete separation of a tongue fragment regardless of the axis of the injury" (Fig. 18.1), unlike a partial amputation in which the fragment distal to the laceration remains attached from bands of soft tissue [7]. Fortunately, complete traumatic amputation of the tongue is very exceptional owing to its intraoral position generally providing protection. However, tongue amputations, whether partial or complete, can be found in patients with oral self-mutilation with neurological conditions such as encephalitis [16], seizures [17], schizophrenia [4], Lesch-Nyhan syndrome [18], or as a result of maxillofacial trauma with tongue bite [7].

In the case of "small" amputated tongue measuring less than 2.5 cm, "supermicrosurgery" with reimplantation has been reported with microvascular anastomosis in injured vessels smaller than 0.8 mm with good results instead of simple closure of the lingual stump [3].

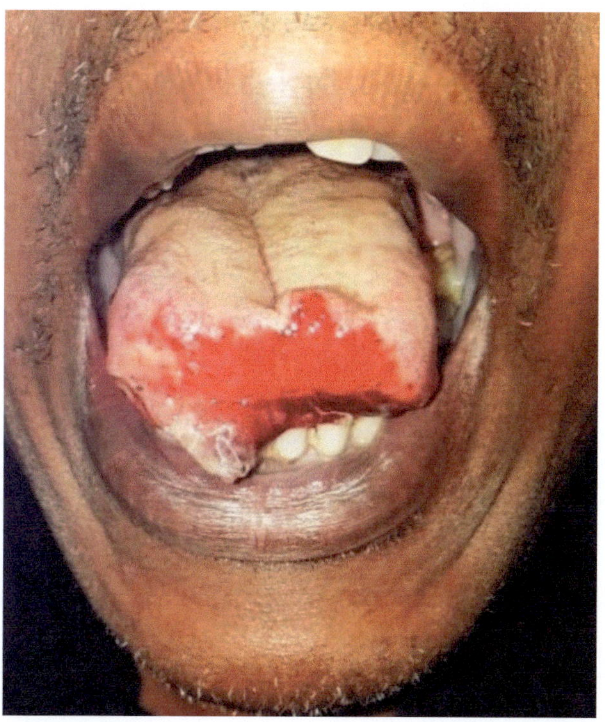

Fig. 18.1 Complete tongue amputation involving the anterior third in a 42-year-old gentleman

Tongue surgical repair in the setting of a total section requires integrity of arterial and venous flow, so anastomosis must be executed. There have been reports where venous repair cannot be attained due to the severity of the injury, with subsequent massive lingual edema; medical leeches have been used postoperatively and replantation has been reported successful [4]. The anastomosis of the lingual artery and vein is difficult; anastomosis of both increases the rate of success. When a primary anastomosis of the vein cannot be achieved, a vein graft can be applied.

In 1998, Buntic and Bunke reported the first successful tongue replant of an amputated segment measuring 5 × 4 cm with a 1.5-mm vessel diameter. Microsurgical reconnection of lingual artery and a venous autologous graft to the left facial vein was performed. Total ischemia time (TIT) was 8 h, and postoperative aspirin and dextran therapy was utilized [1].

Davis and Armstrong [8] reported a *failed* tongue replantation measuring 5 × 3.5 cm with a 0.5-mm vessel diameter. In this case, direct anastomoses of the left lingual artery and right lingual vein were performed. Ischemia time measured 10 h, and postoperative therapy with dextran and aspirin was utilized. Necrosis of the replant was noted on the fifth postoperative day resulting in failure of the replant [8].

In 2003, Toure et al. from Dakar, Senegal, reported successful emergency tongue replant for complete amputation of a portion of the tongue that occurred in a 12-year-old boy during a fight. The fragment of the tongue was brought to the emergency unit. It was placed in heparinized saline solution and replanted successfully 3 h after the trauma. The postoperative period was uneventful, and the tongue regained vitality and normal motion despite the occurrence of a slight retraction. They concluded that replantation of the tongue after complete section may not be successful, but should be attempted when possible [2].

Egozi et al. [6] reported the second successful replantation of an *incomplete* tongue amputation related to a motorcycle injury with massive facial trauma. Vessel diameter was less than 1 mm, and the left lingual artery and right lingual vein were used for microscopic revascularization. The total ischemia time (TIT) was rather long reaching 16 h, and postoperative dextran and aspirin therapy were utilized. One-centimeter necrosis of the tip of the tongue was noted [6].

This successful replantation demonstrated that the tongue can survive up to 16 h of ischemia and also suggests that arterial blood flow through a single lingual artery (unilateral revascularization) and a contralateral single vein may be adequate to perfuse the entire mobile tongue, despite the previously thought avascular median fibrous septum [6]. However, contralateral wound dehiscence may be more likely [3].

One year later, Kim et al. [3] replanted a small tongue segment measuring 2.5 × 1.7 cm, which had been amputated by the bite of another person. The vessels measured 0.7–0.8 mm in diameter. Only the left lingual artery was anastomosed using supermicrosurgical techniques, and no venous anastomosis was performed. Ischemia time was 9 h. Leech therapy, prostaglandin-E1 (PGE1), dipyridamole, and aspirin therapy were utilized in the postoperative period [3]. The result was that the state of the replanted tongue was relatively good both functionally and aesthetically, and the patient was very satisfied [3].

Later, in 2014, Hong and Eun replanted a tongue segment measuring 3.5 × 2 cm with vessel diameters of 0.8 and 0.9 mm in a patient with schizophrenia who attempted self-mutilation. Anastomosis of the right deep lingual artery and vein was performed under microscopy, with 14 h of ischemia time. To ensure that the patient did not make another mutilation attempt, he was kept under sedation in the intensive care unit, and a Denhardt mouth gag was placed for 5 days, and postoperative antipsychotic therapy was also initiated [4]. They reported that the pronunciation of the patient became close to normal, with recovery, to some degree, of somatic and gustatory sensation. In addition Hong and Eun emphasized that although it may be argued that the amputated tongue should be discarded, successful replantation can be achieved with high satisfaction for the patient and family, especially in a psychiatric patient [4].

Hernández-Méndez et al. [7] reported successful repair of a partial tongue amputation in a 25-year-old lady resulting from a motor vehicle accident that caused her to severely bite her tongue. There was a transverse partial-thickness laceration (7 × 3 cm) involving three quarters of the cross-sectional area of the tongue located at the junction of its middle and proximal thirds. The superior longitudinal muscle suffered complete section with only partial section of the inferior longitudinal and transverse muscles and median fibrous septum. Dissection of the muscle was made with mobilization of the distal and proximal parts, with debridement of the necrotic tissue [7].

The partial tongue amputation was approximated in layers using simple interrupted Polyglactin fine sutures resulting in good continuity of the tongue. Postoperatively, tongue swelling was present without respiratory compromise. Diet was initiated with rapid progression. She was discharged 72 h after surgery and recovered uneventfully with good functional result. The operative time was only 65 min. Hernández-Méndez et al. emphasized that in this patient "partial amputation" was the diagnosis since the tongue remained attached by the inferolateral border in which the arterial and venous vessels run. There were no signs of vascular compromise and the lingual nerve was intact. The surgical correction was applied under general anesthesia, and moderate tongue swelling was developed without respiratory compromise [7].

In 2017, Seitz et al. reported the first replantation of a *segmental amputation* of the tongue. Although segmental injuries can be a contraindication for replantation of digits or extremities, replantation of a segmental tongue amputation may be worthwhile. Patients with psychosis present an additional management challenge [5]. Seitz et al. reported that the victim was a 30-year-old male who suffered from a new-onset psychosis and amputated his tongue with scissors. Three separate pieces were brought on ice, including the tip (1.35 × 3.75 cm), a large central segment (2.7 × 5.9 cm), and a thin slice from the base of the tongue (0.5 × 5 cm). The large central segment was found suitable for replantation. The tip segment was reattached to the replanted segment as a *composite graft*, and the thin slice of amputated tongue was discarded. An interposition vein graft from the dorsum of the left hand was harvested. This was subsequently utilized for both the arterial and venous anastomoses performed to the left recipient lingual vessels located at the base of the remaining tongue. The arterial diameter in the amputated central segment was 0.7 mm, and the venous diameter was 0.5 mm. The operative sequence included anastomosis of the vein grafts to the amputated tongue vessel stumps with interrupted 11-0 nylon sutures using a supermicrosurgical parachute suture technique. The vein grafts were then anastomosed to the recipient left lingual artery and vein at the base of the tongue using interrupted 10-0 nylon sutures. Total ischemia time was 7 h. Postoperative management included a bite block, dextran drip, and leech therapy. The patient was sedated in the initial postoperative period, and antipsychotic medications were prescribed. The patient received in-patient speech therapy and had close psychiatric monitoring. He was discharged after 4 weeks [5].

The results of the reported tongue replantation in the literature from 1998 to 2017 are summarized in Table 18.1. These include six complete tongue amputations with success in five and failure in one, in addition to two successful repairs of partial tongue amputation.

Table 18.1 Summary of tongue replants in humans

Author (Year)	Injury	Segment size (L × W) (cm)	Vessel diameter (mm)	TIT (h)	Results/complications
Buntic and Bunke (1998) [1]	Complete amputation	5 × 4	1.5	8	Successful
Davis and Armstrong (2001) [8]	Complete amputation	5 × 3.5	0.5	10	Failed
					Graft necrosis on the fifth postoperative day
Toure et al. (2003) [2]	Complete amputation	–	–	3	Successful
					Slight retraction
Egozi et al. (2006) [6]	Partial amputation	–	1	16	Successful
					Necrosis of 1 cm at the tip
Kim et al. (2007) [3]	Complete amputation	2.5 × 1.7	0.7–0.8	9	Successful both functionally and esthetically
Hong and Eun (2014) [4]	Complete amputation	3.5 × 2	0.8 and 0.9	14	Successful
Hernández-Méndez et al. (2016) [7]	Partial amputation	–	–	–	Successful repair with no need for microvascular repair
Seitz et al. (2017) [5]	Complete amputation	Tip: 1.35 × 3.75	Lingual A: 0.7	7	Successful
		Central part: 2.7 × 5.9	Lingual vein: 0.5		At 6 months: excellent tongue mobility, regular diet, normal, intelligible speech
					At 4 years: patient regained near-complete sensation and taste

L length, *W* width, *A* artery, *V* vein, *TIT* total ischemia time

References

1. Buntic RF, Buncke HJ. Successful replantation of an amputated tongue. Plast Reconstr Surg. 1998;101(6):1604–7.
2. Toure S, Fall I, Diallo B-K, Diouf R, Sane J-C, Diouf M, et al. Emergency reimplantation of the tongue after complete traumatic amputation. Rev Stomatol Chir Maxillofac. 2003;104(1):52–4.
3. Kim JS, Choi TH, Kim NG, Lee KS, Han KH, Son DG, et al. The replantation of an amputated tongue by supermicrosurgery. J Plast Reconstr Aesthet Surg. 2007;60(10):1152–5.
4. Hong JM, Eun SC. Self-mutilation of the tongue in a patient with schizophrenia. J Craniofac Surg. 2014;25(02):e116–8.
5. Seitz IA, Pavone LA, Schechter LS. Successful tongue replantation following segmental autoamputation using supermicrosurgical technique. J Reconstr Microsurg Open. 2017;2:e132–5.
6. Egozi E, Faulkner B, Lin KY. Successful revascularization following near-complete amputation of the tongue. Ann Plast Surg. 2006;56(02):190–3.

7. Hernández-Méndez JR, Rodríguez-Luna MR, Guarneros-Zárate JE, Vélez-Palafox M. Traumatic partial amputation of the tongue. Case report and literature review. Ann Med Surg. 2016;5:110–3.
8. Davis C, Armstrong J. Replantation of an amputated tongue. Plast Reconstr Surg. 2001;108(05):1441–2.
9. Patel AK, Chaturvedi P, Panday RK, Sanyal B. Autoamputation of the tongue. Postgrad Med J. 2001;77(907):335.
10. Das UM, Gadicherla P. Lacerated tongue injury in children. Int J Clin Pediatr Dent. 2008;1:39–41.
11. Lo BM, Campbell BH. A traumatic swollen tongue. Resuscitation. 2010;81:267.
12. Lyos AT, Evans GR, Perez D, Schusterman MA. Tongue reconstruction: outcomes with the rectus abdominis flap. Plast Reconstr Surg. 1999;103:442–7.
13. Haughey BH. Tongue reconstruction: concepts and practice. Laryngoscope. 1993;103:1132–41.
14. Day TA, Tarr C, Zealear D, Burkey BB, Sullivan CA. Tongue replantation in an animal model. Microsurgery. 2000;20:105–8.
15. Bradley OC. Topographical anatomy of the dog. New York, NY: Macmillan; 1927. p. 176–7.
16. Finger ST, Duperon DF. The management of self-inflicted oral trauma secondary to encephalitis: a clinical report. ASDC J Dent Child. 1991;58:60–3.
17. Fenton SJ. Management of oral self-mutilation in neurologically impaired children. Spec Care Dent. 1982;2:70–3.
18. Romero MM, Ruiz DC, Vincent G. Management of oral lesions in Lesch-Nyham syndrome. J Clin Pediatr Dent. 2014;38:247–9.

Tongue Allotransplantation

19

19.1 Introduction

The tongue is a vital organ that is integral to many basic human functions, such as speech, eating, and swallowing. Many complex human social interactions require the proper form and function of this highly specialized and unique organ. However, the tongue is incapable of these intricate activities without the coordinated muscle activity of other key aerodigestive tract structures, namely the floor of mouth muscles, larynx, and pharynx [1].

Patients who undergo glossectomy experience postoperative difficulties with various oral functions when the excision defect is large. To improve the postoperative condition, flaps (local or free) or palatal augmentation prosthesis is typically used [2–7]. However, dysfunctional chewing and speaking often remain in many patients following such procedures, and swallowing difficulty recurs postoperatively due to atrophy of the flap. Suzuki et al. [8] reported that the average percent change in flap volume after free flap reconstructive surgery in patients with tongue cancer was 82.3% at 1 year postoperatively. In those patients, the quality of life became poor, and satisfaction with treatments was low, despite the controlled tumor growth.

When complete recovery of tongue function is required following glossectomy, reestablishment of the complex movements of the tongue is necessary. However, currently available methods for restoring those movements are inadequate, and there are no known techniques available for reconstruction of the ordinal structure of the tongue or augmentation of the function of other parts of the tongue [1]. Whole organ transplants with advancements in preventing transplant tissue rejection have revolutionized the ability to return function to organs such as the heart, lungs, kidneys, liver, and pancreas. Although the tongue is not a vital organ in sustaining life, it may be a vital organ in sustaining the will to live in many people.

© The Author(s), under exclusive license to Springer Nature Switzerland AG 2022
M. F. Sakr, *Tongue Lesions*, https://doi.org/10.1007/978-3-031-08198-9_19

19.2 Relevant Anatomy and Physiology

The tongue comprises muscle tissues and can change its shape or location freely by muscle movements. Furthermore, the movements of the tongue are delicate and enable precise control. The *intrinsic muscles* comprise bands of vertical, horizontal, and sagittal muscle fibers, which allow shape changes by cooperative movements. The *extrinsic muscles* play important roles in supporting and changing tongue position, such as thrusting forward and pulling back. The tongue also serves as a sensory organ that includes taste buds and anterior lingual salivary glands [9].

As mentioned before, the tongue plays an important role in many human functions including oral hygiene, mastication, deglutition, and speech. The tongue's mobility and acute sensory perception allow it to select food and debris for mastication, expulsion, or deglutition. Furthermore, the tongue's anterior-posterior mobility and obliteration of the oral cavity by contacting the hard and soft palate are critical to the oral phase of swallowing [10, 11]. Essential to the coordinated activity of the tongue's function is its sensory capabilities. Functional MRI has demonstrated a hierarchical overlap of the tongue, lips, and teeth in the primary somatosensory cortex [12]. Loss of this peripheral afferent input from the tongue has consequences in the central cortical control of mastication, deglutition, and speech [13]. In addition, the tongue provides the special visceral afferent sensation for taste. In today's reality, the tongue is an essential component of quality of life (QOL).

Although closely coordinated and structurally connected, for reconstructive purposes, the oral tongue and base of the tongue (BOT) are functionally distinct [14]. The oral tongue's function relies heavily upon its flexibility and mobility. It is critical to oral hygiene, speech, and the oral phase of swallowing. The oral tongue helps circulate saliva within the oral cavity and incorporates it into fragments of food. It positions food fragments between the teeth for mastication and creates the food bolus [15]. The base of tongue's function depends more on its volume and shape, although its mobility is also important. It plays a vital role in initiating pharyngeal swallowing by propelling the food bolus into the posterior pharyngeal wall. Its bulk promotes passage of the food bolus over and around the larynx for airway protection [14, 16, 17].

The tongue's multipurpose nature and almost whimsical mobility create difficult challenges for the head and neck reconstructive surgeon [1].

19.3 Current Modalities of Tongue Reconstruction

Generally, tongue reconstruction is defined by the volume and location of the tongue defect resulting from trauma (tongue amputation) or surgery (glossectomy or total glossectomy with resection of adjacent tissues). The location of the defect is generally described as oral tongue or base of the tongue (BOT).

Very small partial glossectomy defects require an epithelial reconstruction rather than the volumetric reconstruction that is needed for larger tongue defects. Healing by secondary intention, primary closure, split thickness skin grafts, or acellular dermis grafts may be utilized. Tongue reconstruction is performed in these cases, to prevent postoperative restriction of the tongue's mobility.

Other larger partial glossectomy defects are usually reconstructed with a split thickness skin graft, acellular dermis graft, or local tissue flaps, which have the limitation of the risk of compromised blood supply in the setting of a concurrent neck dissection. The buccinator muscle flap has been described for these types of tongue defects [18]. The limitation of this flap is the need for a secondary procedure to divide the pedicle and complete the flap inset. In addition, patients with good dentition are at risk for biting and injuring the flap pedicle, and there is also the possibility of postoperative trismus, especially in patients who may require postoperative radiation [18]. The submental island flap has also been used for tongue reconstruction [19]. Its primary limitation is the concern for oncological safety in patients with oral cancer, given the theoretical risk of nodal disease within the flap. Primary closure is traditionally *not* recommended for larger partial glossectomy defects; however, McConnel and colleagues [20] reported comparable speech and swallowing outcomes with both primary closure and complex flap reconstruction [20].

Larger hemiglossectomy, subtotal glossectomy, and total glossectomy defects require significant volumetric reconstruction. These defects have been addressed with distant pedicled flaps, such as the pectoralis major myocutaneous flap (PMMF) [21], but are now typically reconstructed with a free tissue transfer reconstruction. The radial forearm, anterolateral thigh, rectus abdominis, gracilis, and latissimus dorsi free flaps have all been used for tongue reconstruction [17, 21–23]. The radial forearm free flap (RFFF) provides a pliable skin paddle that is well suited for hemiglossectomy defects of the oral tongue, specifically the ventral tongue and floor of the mouth. This flap allows a static reconstruction of the multiform contour of the tongue but with limited utility for volumetric reconstruction. On the other hand, the anterolateral thigh and rectus abdominis free flaps provide significant soft tissue bulk that is well suited for near total and total glossectomy defects. These flaps allow a static volumetric reconstruction of the tongue's bulk but with limited ability to recreate the varied contour of the tongue and floor of the mouth. The radial forearm, anterolateral thigh, and rectus abdominis free flaps do not allow for the possibility of active intrinsic flap movement mediated by hypoglossal nerve reinnervation. The gracilis and latissimus dorsi free flaps provide soft tissue bulk with the potential for a dynamic reconstruction of the tongue defect. However, latissimus dorsi free flaps may suffer from loss of tissue bulk due to muscle atrophy over time [17].

Larger tongue defects co-existing with tissue loss in the floor of the mouth, mandible, buccal mucosa, lips, skin, pharynx, and larynx often require the utilization of free flaps with multiple skin paddles, vascularized bone, or the use of multiple free flaps. The scapular free flap with its multiple skin paddles, freedom of rotation, and vascularized bone stock is often an ideal single flap solution to complex oral cavity, oropharynx, and skin defects. The primary disadvantage lies in the need for patient positioning in the lateral decubitus position [24].

A special consideration involving large tongue resections is resultant "tissue ptosis" following reconstruction. Restoration of the structural integrity of the floor of the mouth and suspension of the reconstruction from the skull base are critical elements. Ptosis can be prevented by suspending the reconstructive tissue from the left to the right skull base by suturing to the pharyngeal constrictors or creating a supportive sling composed of polytetrafluoroethylene, fascia, or acellular dermis [17].

19.4 Challenges of Tongue Reconstruction

The primary challenges in tongue reconstruction lie in its unique form and function and the fact that complete functional rehabilitation is equally dependent on restoring sensory and motor functions. Haughey [17] described the ideal characteristics of the tissue used for subtotal and total glossectomy reconstruction [17]. He emphasized that it should not only have sufficient bulk to obliterate the oral cavity but also create a shelf superior to the laryngeal inlet to guide the food bolus into the hypopharynx during deglutition. The tissue should also be pliable enough to allow coordinated movement with residual tongue and muscles of deglutition. Ideally, this tissue should also be capable of intrinsic voluntary coordinated movement with an associated motor nerve that maybe anastomosed to the hypoglossal nerve. It should also have an associated donor sensory nerve that may be anastomosed to the recipient glossopharyngeal or lingual nerves to allow for sensory innervation of the neotongue.

19.4.1 Tongue Movement

While most skeletal muscles of the human body move in a single plane, or at most two dimensions, the tongue is able to move in three dimensions. Coupled with its ability to volumetrically change the dead space of the oral cavity, the tongue is able to manipulate sound waves, saliva, and food in a serpentine ballet of expansion and propulsion. With traditional methods of tongue reconstruction, some aspects of the tongue's form and function cannot be adequately restored [25].

19.4.2 Tongue Sensation

While neurovascular reconstruction can be performed, the tongue's refined sensation and taste cannot reliably be reconstructed at this time. Additionally, the tongue's complex movements cannot be replicated being only replaced by poorly coordinated gross muscle activity [25]. Function of the tongue relies mainly upon the cortical integration of sensory input from the oral cavity that is translated into coordinated muscle activity between the tongue, floor of the mouth muscles, larynx, and pharynx. Thus, complete functional rehabilitation is equally dependent on restoring sensory and motor functions [15].

19.4.3 Appropriately Sizing

Appropriately sizing the tongue reconstruction presents another challenge. The tongue's ability to obliterate the oral cavity is integral to its role in food bolus propulsion. More soft tissue bulk favors this ability in the reconstructed tongue. However, greater bulk also has the potential for oropharyngeal airway obstruction, tracheostomy dependence, or inability to achieve complete mouth closure.

19.4.4 Status of the Larynx

Critical to the reconstruction of the tongue is the status of the larynx in terms of not only presence but also function [26]. A nonfunctional larynx that is either prone to aspiration or tracheostomy dependence significantly alters the goals of the tongue reconstruction. A patient who is gastrostomy dependent due to aspiration has a little need for a large, dynamic tongue reconstruction to aid in deglutition. A patient who is tracheostomy dependent will better tolerate a larger, bulkier soft tissue reconstruction with the hope of restoring serviceable oral intake. In the tracheostomy- and gastrostomy-dependent patient, tongue reconstruction promotes oral hygiene by obliterating a potential reservoir for saliva pooling and maintains the native configuration of the mandible, which may undergo atrophy without the neotongue [1].

19.4.5 Reinnervation

If there is no graftable *hypoglossal nerve*, then there is no potential for intrinsic voluntary neotongue mobility. Additionally, if there is no viable hypoglossal nerve at all, then there is also no potential for extrinsic voluntary neotongue mobility based on the residual tongue's mobility. Neotongue mobility will rely upon extrinsic movement from the floor of mouth muscles and pharyngeal constrictors.

19.5 Tongue Allotransplantation

The complexity of tissue defects of the head and neck has fueled the development of composite tissue allotransplantations, a potential solution to these challenging problems [27–29]. While the development of allotransplantation remains a landmark event in head and neck reconstruction, the potential application is limited by the morbidity of immunosuppression. *The ideal recipient* of a composite tissue allotransplant is a young healthy patient with a tissue deficit following a traumatic injury, a benign tumor resection, or who is already on a posttransplant immunosuppression regimen [28]. *The indication* for tongue allotransplantation would be significant functional deficit following total or subtotal loss of tongue tissue with graftable hypoglossal and lingual nerves in the absence of other contraindication to oral intake.

19.5.1 Animal Models

In 1999, Haughey et al. first demonstrated that allotransplantation of the tongue was possible in a large mammal with long-term survival of tissue and recovery of sensory and motor function [25]. Haughey and colleagues successfully developed a canine model of hemi-tongue allotransplantation between same-sex, litter mates. Ten pairs of unmatched dogs underwent reciprocal exchange of the left hemi-tongue with micro-neurovascular replantation. The operated hemi-tongue acted as the control. Micro-vascular anastomosis was performed between the donor and recipient lingual artery and vein, hypoglossal nerve, and lingual nerve. The dogs were maintained under cyclosporine immunosuppression. Five dogs survived between 6 and 13 months with long-term evaluation (clinical observation, electromyography, force transduction studies, and histological examination). The remaining dogs succumbed to overwhelming infection or uncontrollable graft rejection that resulted from difficulty in delivery of cyclosporine.

Haughey et al. found that intrinsic transplanted tongue movement was achieved through ipsilateral reinnervation and not cross-neurotization from the native tongue. The contractile force of the transplanted hemi-tongue was approximately 68% of the native hemi-tongue (range, 47–97%). Preservation of muscle, mucosal, and stromal ultrastructure was seen with light microscopy of the transplanted tongue. However, it was not the finely coordinated movements of the native tongue [28]. In addition, Haughey et al. reported that histological study of the hypoglossal and lingual nerves showed anatomical evidence of reinnervation suggesting the potential for sensory recovery [25], a finding that is also seen in face transplant recipients who regained facial sensation [29]. From their animal model, Haughey et al. concluded that allotransplantation of the hemi-tongue and associated neurovascular apparatus is possible in a large mammalian model, with long-term survival of tissue being accompanied by partial recovery of contractile properties, and anatomical and clinical evidence of sensory recovery [25]. These data support the future possibility of employing a similar technique in glossectomy patients.

The rat model of composite face transplantation introduced by Kulahci and Sieminow in 2010 further demonstrated the feasibility and potential for tongue allotransplantation [30]. It also identified the potential immunosuppressive challenge of a higher antigenic load with tongue allotransplantation.

Recently, Isomura et al. [9] investigated the effects of hemi-tongue allotransplantations on the complete recovery of tongue function in eight pairs of unmatched beagle dogs. In each donor, the right side of the tongue, including lingual and hypoglossal nerves; extrinsic tongue muscles; mucous membrane of the oral floor;

lingual artery; and vein were exposed. In each recipient, the same tongue side was resected at the level of circumvallate papilla, and the recipient vessels (lingual artery and vein), nerves (lingual and hypoglossal), and extrinsic tongue muscles (genioglossus, hyoglossus, and styloglossus) were exposed [9].

A vascularized transplantation method was used with manual microsurgical anastomosis between the donor and recipient lingual artery and vein, hypoglossal nerve, and lingual nerve. Each of the intrinsic and extrinsic muscles and oral floor mucosa were sutured together. The dogs were maintained under tacrolimus immunosuppression [9].

Survival of the grafted tongue was only noted in one dog that died 5 days after transplantation. Isomura et al. believed that mortality resulted from nutritional deficiency or dehydration due to poor postoperative care, rather than hyperacute rejection of the transplant or technical failure of the microsurgical anastomosis. When the animal with the surviving graft died, Isomura et al. removed the grafted tongue and the opposite side of the tongue. This tissue was histologically examined. The grafted portion was partially connected to the recipient side of the tongue without a boundary line between the grafted and nongrafted sites. Infiltrating plasma cells and lymphocytes in the grafted site were observed indicating slight inflammation [9]. Isomura et al. concluded that even if tongue allograft including nerves and extrinsic muscles is performed, it seems to take a long time before the tongue recovers its functions and that expansive tongue allograft was too invasive a treatment for animals. They suggested that if this procedure is adopted in humans, the first trial in a human should be done without animal experiments, as was the case with face transplantations [9].

19.5.2 Human Tongue Allotransplantation

Compared with flap transplantation procedures, tongue allografts are regarded as the best method to restore normal tongue usage in patients. In addition to organ transplantation in humans, facial transplantations are commonly reported, and several facial allograft transplants have been performed worldwide [31–36]. However, no *successful* cases of tongue transplantation in humans have been reported. Tongue dysfunction is associated with a number of complications, and partial loss of tongue control can lead to near-fatal aspiration.

To date, Kermer et al. [37] published in 2008 the only case of allotransplantation of the human tongue alone without the face. A tongue was transplanted from an ABO-matched heart-beating donor into a 42-year-old man with T4N2bM0 squamous cell carcinoma (SCC) of the tongue with invasion of the floor of mouth and mandible. The tongue allotransplantation procedure was approved by the institution's ethics committee. The procedure was performed 6 weeks after chemoradiation therapy in conjunction with total glossectomy, right resection of floor of mouth, right hemimandibulectomy, and bilateral level I–III neck dissection. Donor allograft procurement was performed simultaneously with the ablative procedure. The donor hypoglossal nerves, lingual nerve, and lingual vessels were dissected. Anastomosis was performed to recipient bilateral hypoglossal nerves, left lingual nerve, and bilateral facial vessels. The recipient right lingual nerve was sacrificed at the time of tumor resection. The ischemic time for the allograft was 245 min, and it was flushed with a cold crystalloid organ preservative solution. The patient's immunosuppressive regimen included intraoperative methylprednisolone and postoperative antithymocyte globulin for 5 days, followed by daily doses of tacrolimus, mycophenolate mofetil, and prednisolone. The patient was started on speech therapy.

At 10 months postoperatively, the patient did not have clinically evident intrinsic tongue mobility, and electromyographic evaluation demonstrated only pathologic spontaneous activity. Videofluoroscopy demonstrated poor mobility, poor bolus preparation, and incomplete tongue-to-palate contact. His speech was intelligible, and he was able to swallow saliva and small quantities of pulp consistency foods without evidence of aspiration. Sensory evaluation revealed superficial discrimination to sharp and blunt contact on the left side of the tongue only. At 12 months postoperatively, a *recurrence* was found in the right neck, and the patient expired at home 1 month later. An autopsy was not performed. Since allograft transplantation in patients with cancer has the risk of recurrence of cancer due to immunosuppression, it is suggested that transplantation of a tongue is better to use for secondary and not immediate reconstruction by waiting for 5 years after an operation of cancer and checking that there is no recurrence before performing the allotransplantation [9].

In 2012, the most extensive facial allotransplantation to date was performed that included all facial skin, mimetic muscles, the tongue, the midface via Le Fort III osteotomy, and the mandible via sagittal split osteotomies [1]. The patient was a 37-year-old male who suffered a shotgun wound to his midface. Preoperatively, he was missing a portion of his tongue but tolerating an oral diet with intelligible speech. At 1-year postoperatively, the patient was noted to have intelligible speech and relearning to eat.

Recently, in 2016, the development of cancer has been reported in *face transplant* patients [38]. A recent report noted that 36 patients underwent face transplantation before 2016; of these, three developed cancer, of which two died because of cancer. However, this incidence is low in the context of immunosuppression. Other case reports described cancer in organ allografts; this was treated successfully in both cases [39, 40]. Furthermore, bone allograft reconstruction after malignant bone tumor resection (e.g., scapular, femur, or tibia) was performed in a few cases and showed good functional results [41–43]. These reports suggest the potential for successful transplantation of tongue allografts after tumor resection.

19.5.3 Challenges in Human Tongue Allotransplantation

19.5.3.1 Donor Tissue Procurement

Donor tissue procurement is one of the greatest challenges to human tissue allotransplantation. Similar to facial allotransplantation, consideration must be made for the donor's appearance after tissue procurement [44]. Given the tissue deficit is intraoral, replacing the donor tissue deficit is not a priority. However, masking the cutaneous incisions is important. The most aesthetically sensitive approach incorporates bilateral peri-auricular incisions with aura-clavicular incision at the midline. The tongue allograft is then released with intraoral mucosal incisions and delivered through the neck.

19.5.3.2 Timing of Allotransplantation

The timing of tongue reconstruction prior to the degeneration of the central and peripheral nervous pathways necessary for speech and deglutition is also a major consideration. Considering that the greatest need would be in head and neck cancer patients, full immunosuppression and tongue allotransplantation would have to wait several years, as mentioned before, for pending oncological outcome. Haughey suggested immediate tongue reconstruction with autogenous tissue with sensory and motor nerve anastomosis, followed by a waiting period—allowing for cancer surveillance and potential matched donor recruitment. If the patient remained free of cancer with persistent and severe functional deficits, then elective allotransplantation could be considered [25].

19.5.4 Immunosuppression for Composite Tissue Allotransplantation

The success of recent composite tissue allotransplantation is often attributed to improved microvascular techniques, but little consideration is given to the ongoing development of modern immunosuppressive techniques [31, 45]. Freedom from immunosuppression can only be achieved by inducing mixed chimerism and allograft tolerance. It is suggested that the inclusion of donor allograft containing lymphoid and vascularized bone marrow may be the key to developing and maintaining donor-specific chimerism [30, 46, 47]. The previously described full-face, double-jaw, and tongue transplant included vascularized bone marrow within the mandible and may offer additional insight into the development of donor tolerance [37]. As demonstrated in the first tongue allotransplantation, the concern for co-incident or recurrent cancer, while on immunosuppression is a serious consideration [37, 48]. Ironically, immunosuppression is known to lead to cancers of the lip and tongue [1].

19.6 Conclusion

Complex head and neck defects continue to remain a great challenge for reconstructive surgeons. Composite tissue allotransplantation may offer a solution to certain defects in certain patients, but consideration must be given to the morbidity of immunosuppression. It may be argued that composite tissue allotransplantation in the head and neck is for quality not the quantity of life [27]. It may also be suggested that although the tongue is not essential in sustaining life, it may be essential in sustaining the will to live [49]. Until new immunosuppressive methods are developed, conventional free tissue transfer reconstruction of glossectomy defects will remain the mainstay of treatment for head and neck cancer patients. Although the greatest need for tongue reconstruction exists in patients with head and neck cancer, the most recent cases of total face and tongue allotransplantation for trauma suggests a new application for tongue allotransplantation. The future of composite tissue allotransplantation—the tongue, larynx, face, or hands—may depend upon the development of organ-specific immunosuppression strategies and improved techniques for reinnervation [28]. However, the reconstructive goal remains the same: restore form and function with minimal morbidity to the patient. Considering the limitation of the flap reconstruction after the tongue resection, tongue allograft may be an expectant method for recovery of tongue function in long term [9].

References

1. Chi JJ, Haughey BH. Tongue transplantation. Curr Otorhinolaryngol Rep. 2014;2:178–83.
2. Lutz BS, Wei FC. Microsurgical workhorse flaps in head and neck reconstruction. Clin Plast Surg. 2005;32:421–30.
3. Wong CH, Wei FC. Microsurgical free flap in head and neck reconstruction. Head Neck. 2010;32:1236–45.
4. Hanasono MM, Matros E, Disa JJ. Important aspects of head and neck reconstruction. Plast Reconstr Surg. 2014;134:968e–80e.
5. Goll G. Design for maximal retention of obturator prosthesis for hemimaxillectomy patients. J Prosthet Dent. 1982;48:108–9.
6. Keyf F. Obturator prostheses for hemimaxillectomy patients. J Oral Rehabil. 2001;28:821–9.
7. Chen C, Ren W, Gao L, Cheng Z, Zhang L, Li S, et al. Function of obturator prosthesis after maxillectomy and prosthetic obturator rehabilitation. Braz J Otorhinolaryngol. 2016;82:177–83.
8. Suzuki T, Tanaka I, Osaka R, Baba A, Sato K, Yamauchi T, et al. Preliminary study of temporal change in free flap volume after tongue reconstruction. Bull Tokyo Dent Coll. 2017;58:269–75.
9. Isomura ET, Nakagawa K, Mitsui R, Shogen Y, Fujita T, Kogo M. Hemi-tongue allograft transplantation in dogs. Plast Reconstr Surg Glob Open. 2020;8(4):e2767.
10. Dodds WJ. Physiology of swallowing. Dysphagia. 1989;3:171–8.
11. Lazarus CL, Logemann JA, Pauloski BR, Rademaker AW, Larson CR, Mittal BB, et al. Swallowing and tongue function following treatment for oral and oropharyngeal cancer. J Speech Lang Hear Res. 2000;43:1011–23.
12. Miyamoto JJ, Honda M, Saito DN, Okada T, Ono T, Ohyama K, et al. The representation of the human oral area in the somatosensory cortex: a functional MRI study. Cereb Cortex. 2006;16:669–75.
13. Capra NF. Mechanisms of oral sensation. Dysphagia. 1995;10:235–47.
14. Lam L, Samman N. Speech and swallowing following tongue cancer surgery and free flap reconstruction—a systematic review. Oral Oncol. 2013;49:507–24.
15. Speksnijder CM, van der Bilt A, van der Glas HW, Koole R, Merkx MAW. Tongue function in patients treated for malignancies in tongue and/or floor of mouth; a one year prospective study. Int J Oral Maxillofac Surg. 2011;40:1388–94.
16. Urken ML, Moscoso JF, Lawson W, Biller HF. A systematic approach to functional reconstruction of the oral cavity following partial and total glossectomy. Arch Otolaryngol Head Neck Surg. 1994;120(6):589–601.
17. Haughey BH. Tongue reconstruction: concepts and practice. Laryngoscope. 1993;103:1132–41.

18. Woo SW, Jeong HS, Kim JP, Park JJ, Ryu J, Baek C-H. Buccinator myomucosal flap for reconstruction of glossectomy defects. Otolaryngol Head Neck Surg. 2013;149(2):226–31.
19. Sebastian P, Thomas S, Varghese BT, Iype EM, Balagopal PC, Mathew PC. The submental island flap for reconstruction of intraoral defects in oral cancer patients. Oral Oncol. 2008;44:1014–8.
20. McConnel FM, Pauloski BR, Logemann JA, Rademaker AW, Colangelo L, Shedd D, et al. Functional results of primary closure vs flaps in oropharyngeal reconstruction. Arch Otolaryngol Head Neck Surg. 1998;124:625–30.
21. Sultan MR, Coleman JJ. Oncologic and functional considerations of total glossectomy. Am J Surg. 1989;158:297–302.
22. Salibian AH, Allison G, Rappaport I. Total and subtotal glossectomy: function after microvascular reconstruction. Plast Reconstr Surg. 1989;85:513–24.
23. Kimata Y, Sakuraba M, Hishinuma S, Ebihara S, Hayashi R, Asakage T, et al. Analysis of the relations between the shape of the reconstructed tongue and postoperative functions after subtotal or total glossectomy. Laryngoscope. 2003;113:905–9.
24. Mitsimponas KT, Iliopoulos C, Stockmann P, Bumiller L, Nkeenke E, Neukam FW, et al. The free scapular/ parascapular flap as a reliable method of reconstruction in the head and neck region: a retrospective analysis of 130 reconstructions performed over a period of 5 years in a single department. J Craniomaxillofac Surg. 2014;42(5):536–43.
25. Haughey BG, Beggs JC, Bong J, Genden EM, Buckner A, et al. Microneurovascular allotransplantation of the canine tongue. Laryngoscope. 1999;109:1461–70.
26. Dziegielewski PT, Ho ML, Rieger J, Singh P, Langille M, Harris JR, et al. Total glossectomy with laryngeal preservation and free flap reconstruction: objective functional outcomes and systematic review of the literature. Laryngoscope. 2013;123:140–5.
27. Birchall M. Tongue transplantation. Lancet. 2004;363(9422):1663.
28. Birchall MA, Lorenz RR, Berke GS, Genden EM, Haughey BH, Siemionow M, et al. Laryngeal transplantation in 2005: a review. Am J Transplant. 2006;6:20–6.
29. Alam DS, Chi JJ. Facial transplantation for massive traumatic injuries. Otolaryngol Clin N Am. 2013;46(5):883–901.
30. Kulahci Y, Sieminow M. A new composite hemiface/mandible/tongue transplantation model in rats. Ann Plast Surg. 2010;64:114–21.
31. Devauchelle B, Badet L, Lengelé B, Morelon E, Teswtellin S, Michallet M, et al. First human face allograft: early report. Lancet. 2006;368:203–9.
32. Dubernard JM, Devauchelle B. Face transplantation. Lancet. 2008;372:603–4.
33. Guo S, Han Y, Zhang X, Lu B, Yi C, Zhang H, et al. Human facial allotransplantation: a 2-year follow-up study. Lancet. 2008;372:631–8.
34. Lantieri L, Meningaud JP, Grimbert P, Bellivier F, Lefaucheur J-P, Ortonne N, et al. Repair of the lower and middle parts of the face by composite tissue allotransplantation in a patient with massive plexiform neurofibroma: a 1-year follow-up study. Lancet. 2008;372:639–45.
35. Siemionow M, Papay F, Alam D, Bernard S, Djohan R, Gordon C, et al. Near-total human face transplantation for a severely disfigured patient in the USA. Lancet. 2009;374:203–9.
36. Kumamaru KK, Sisk GC, Mitsouras D, Schultz K, Steigner ML, George E, et al. Vascular communications between donor and recipient tissues after successful full face transplantation. Am J Transplant. 2014;14:711–9.
37. Kermer C, Watzinger F, Oeckher M. Tongue transplantation: 10 month follow-up. Transplantation. 2008;85(4):654–5.
38. Siemionow M. The miracle of face transplantation after 10 years. Br Med Bull. 2016;120:5–14.
39. Nagaraju S, Grethlein SJ, Vaishnav S, Sharfuddin AA, Pawelso JA, Fridell JA. Case report: primary de novo sarcoma in transplant pancreas allograft. Transplant Proc. 2017;49:2352–4.
40. Singh P, Visger Von J, Prosek J, Olencki T, Pandey D, Rovin B, et al. Preserved renal allograft function and successful treatment of metastatic Merkel cell cancer post nivolumab therapy. Transplantation. 2019;103:e52–3.
41. Capanna R, Totti F, Van der Geest IC, Muller DA. Scapular allograft reconstruction after total scapulectomy: surgical technique and functional results. J Shoulder Elb Surg. 2015;24:e203–11.

42. Pesenti S, Peltier E, Pomero V, Authier G, Roscigni L, Wiehweger E, et al. Knee function after limb salvage surgery for malignant bone tumor: comparison of megaprosthesis and distal femur allograft with epiphysis sparing. Int Orthop. 2018;42:427–36.
43. Campanacci DA. CORR insights: proximal tibia reconstruction after bone tumor resection: are survivorship and outcomes of endoprosthetic replacement and osteoarticular allograft similar? Clin Orthop Relat Res. 2017;475:683–5.
44. Quilichini L, Hivelin M, Benjoar MD, et al. Restoration of the donor after face graft procurement for allotransplantation: report on the technique and outcomes of seven cases. Plast Reconstr Surg. 2012;129(5):1105–11.
45. Petruzzo P, Lanzetta M, Dubernard JM, Landin L, Cavadas P, Margreiter R, et al. The international registry on hand and composite tissue transplantation. Transplantation. 2008;90(12):1590–4.
46. Sieminow M, Kulahci Y. Facial transplantation. Semin Plast Surg. 2007;21:259–68.
47. Ulusal BG, Ulusal AE, Ozmen S, Zins JE, Siemionow MZ, et al. A new composite facial and scalp transplantation model in rats. Plast Reconstr Surg. 2003;1112:1302–11.
48. Kermer C, Oeckher M. Wien Klin Wochenschr. 2004;116:643–4. German. English translation.
49. Day TA, Tarr C, Zealear D, Burkey BB, Sullivan CA. Tongue replantation in an animal model. Microsurgery. 2000;20:105–8.

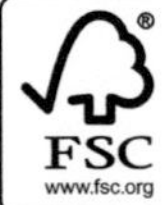

MIX
Papier aus verantwortungsvollen Quellen
Paper from responsible sources
FSC® C105338

If you have any concerns about our products, you can contact us on
ProductSafety@springernature.com

In case Publisher is established outside the EU, the EU authorized representative is:
Springer Nature Customer Service Center GmbH
Europaplatz 3, 69115 Heidelberg, Germany

Printed by Libri Plureos GmbH
in Hamburg, Germany